FOURTH EDITION

CARING for the VULNERABLE

Perspectives in Nursing Theory, Practice, and Research

The Pedagogy

Caring for the Vulnerable: Perspectives in Nursing Theory, Practice, and Research, Fourth Edition drives comprehension through various strategies that meet the learning needs of students, while also generating enthusiasm about the topic. This interactive approach addresses different learning styles, making this the ideal text to ensure mastery of key concepts. The pedagogical aids that appear in most chapters include the following:

CHAPTER OBJECTIVES

These objectives provide instructors and students with a snapshot of the key information they will encounter in each chapter. They serve as a checklist to help guide and focus study.

INTRODUCTIONS

Found at the beginning of each chapter, chapter introductory paragraphs provide an overview of the importance of the chapter's topic. They also help keep students focused as they read.

CASE STUDIES

Case studies encourage learning and promote critical thinking skills in learners. Students can ask questions, analyze the situation they are presented with, and solve problems.

CHAPTER CONCLUSIONS

Conclusions are included at the end of each chapter to provide a concise review of material covered in each chapter. These summaries highlight the most important points in the chapter.

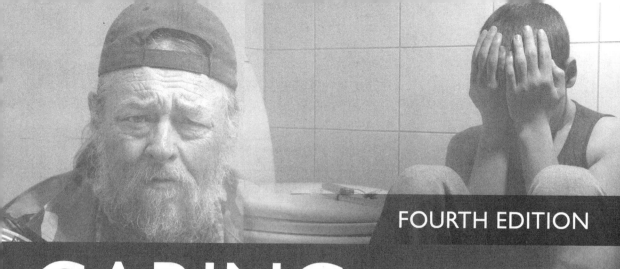

FOURTH EDITION

CARING for the VULNERABLE

Perspectives in Nursing Theory, Practice, and Research

Edited by

Mary de Chesnay, PhD, RN, PMHCNS-BC, FAAN
Professor, WellStar School of Nursing
Kennesaw State University
Kennesaw, Georgia

Barbara A. Anderson, DrPH, RN, CNM, FACNM, FAAN
Professor and Director, Doctor of Nursing Practice
Frontier Nursing University
Hyden, Kentucky

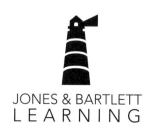

JONES & BARTLETT
L E A R N I N G

World Headquarters
Jones & Bartlett Learning
5 Wall Street
Burlington, MA 01803
978-443-5000
info@jblearning.com
www.jblearning.com

Jones & Bartlett Learning books and products are available through most bookstores and online booksellers. To contact Jones & Bartlett Learning directly, call 800-832-0034, fax 978-443-8000, or visit our website, www.jblearning.com.

08153-4

Production Credits

VP, Executive Publisher: David D. Cella
Executive Editor: Amanda Martin
Associate Acquisitions Editor: Rebecca Myrick
Editorial Assistant: Danielle Bessette
Production Manager: Carolyn Rogers Pershouse
Senior Marketing Manager: Jennifer Stiles
VP, Manufacturing and Inventory Control: Therese Connell
Composition: Cenveo® Publisher Services
Cover Design: Scott Moden
Rights and Media Manager: Joanna Lundeen
Rights and Media Research Coordinator: Ashley Dos Santos

Media Development Assistant: Shannon Sheehan
Cover Images: © Front Cover–top left © Brian Eichhorn/ShutterStock; top right © Di Studio/Shutterstock; middle © Lucian Coman/ShutterStock; bottom right © Edler von Rabenstein/Shutterstock; bottom left © absolut/ShutterStock. Spine: © Rasica/Shutterstock. Back Cover–top left © Olemac/Shutterstock; top right © John Gomez/Shutterstock; middle top © Diego Cervo/Shutterstock; middle bottom © bikeriderlondon/Shutterstock.
Printing and Binding: Edwards Brothers Malloy
Cover Printing: Edwards Brothers Malloy

Library of Congress Cataloging-in-Publication Data

Caring for the vulnerable : perspectives in nursing theory, practice, and research / edited by Mary de Chesnay, Barbara A. Anderson. -- Fourth edition.
    p. ; cm.
    Includes bibliographical references and index.
    ISBN 978-1-284-06627-2 (pbk.)
    I. De Chesnay, Mary, editor. II. Anderson, Barbara A. (Barbara Ann), 1944- , editor.
    [DNLM: 1. Community Health Nursing. 2. Vulnerable Populations. 3. Nursing Theory. 4. Transcultural Nursing. WY 106]
    RT86.5
    362.17'3--dc23
                  2015008690

6048

Printed in the United States of America
19 18 17 16 15   10 9 8 7 6 5 4 3 2 1

Dedication

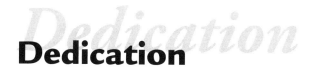

In memory of Dr. Michael Weber, retired provost and academic vice-president of Duquesne University, in appreciation for his guidance and leadership on behalf of a novice dean.

—*MdC*

In memory of my mother, who encouraged me in my childhood dream to care for the vulnerable, and for my daughters, Amanda, RN, and Suzanne, RN, who share the dream.

—*BA*

Contents

Preface   xiii

Foreword   xv

Contributors   xvii

Acknowledgments   xxi

About the Editors   xxiii

Unit I	Concepts and Theories	1

Chapter 1   Vulnerable Populations: Vulnerable People   3
             Mary de Chesnay

Chapter 2   Advocacy Role of Providers   19
             Mary de Chesnay and Vanessa Robinson-Dooley

Chapter 3   Cultural Competence and Resilience   33
             Mary de Chesnay, Patricia L. Hart, and Jane Brannan

Chapter 4   Social Justice in Nursing: A Review of the Literature   49
             Doris M. Boutain

Chapter 5   Low Literacy and Vulnerable Clients   67
             Toni Vezeau

Chapter 6   Nursing Theories and Models Applied to Vulnerable Populations:
             Examples from Turkey   91
             Behice Erci

Chapter 7 Applying Middle-Range Concepts and Theories to the Care of Vulnerable Populations 117
Nicole Mareno

Chapter 8 The Utility of Leininger's Culture Care Theory with Vulnerable Populations 141
Rick Zoucha

Chapter 9 Application of the Health Belief Model in Women with Gestational Diabetes 149
Janeen S. Amason and Shih-Yu (Sylvia) Lee

Chapter 10 Common Sense Model of Illness Behaviors: Older Adults Diagnosed with Acute Myocardial Infarction 165
Deonna S. Tanner

Unit II   Research 181

Chapter 11 Research with Vulnerable Populations: Implications for Developed and Developing Countries 183
Maria da Gloria M. Wright and Mary de Chesnay

Chapter 12 Sample Qualitative Research Proposal: A Study to Develop a Disclosure to Children Intervention for HIV/AIDS-Infected Women 197
Tommie Nelms

Chapter 13 Sample Quantitative Research Proposal: Effect of Video-Based Education on Knowledge and Perceptions of Risk for Breast Cancer Genes *BRCA1* and *BRCA2* in Urban Latinas 215
Janice B. Flynn and Janice M. Long

Chapter 14 Life History of Jim: "I Am Not Broken" 235
Mary de Chesnay and Anne Batson

Chapter 15 The Use of Community-Based Participatory Research to Understand and Work with Vulnerable Populations 243
Ellen F. Olshansky and Robynn Zender

Chapter 16 Decreasing Vulnerability in Birth: Waterbirth in Military Treatment Facilities 253
Elizabeth Nutter

Chapter 17 Women of Oman: A Systematic Review of Health Issues   263
Christie Emerson, Genie E. Dorman, Mary de Chesnay,
Diane Wilson, Bethany Francis, and Lisa McMasters

Unit III   **Practice and Programs**   285

Chapter 18 Transcultural Aspects of Perinatal Health Care of Somali Women   287
Danuta M. Wojnar and Robin A. Narruhn

Chapter 19 Navy Nurses: Vulnerable People Caring for Vulnerable Populations   303
Captain (Retired) Mary Anne White

Chapter 20 Pet Therapy in Nursing   311
Leslie Himot and Mary de Chesnay

Chapter 21 Undocumented Immigrants: Connecting with the Disconnected   321
Edwina Skiba-King

Chapter 22 Developing Population-Based Programs for the Vulnerable   329
Anne Watson Bongiorno and Mary de Chesnay

Chapter 23 Childhood Autism in a Rural Environment: Reaching
Vulnerable Children and Their Families   339
Ellyn E. Cavanaugh

Chapter 24 Developing a Nurse Practitioner–Run Center for Residents
in Rural Appalachia   357
Joyce M. Knestrick and Mona M. Counts

Chapter 25 Negotiating the World: Nursing Interventions for a Vulnerable Prison
Population Before and After Parole   365
Judi Daniels

Chapter 26 Role Transition for Immigrant Women: Vulnerabilities and Strengths   381
Lisa R. Roberts

Chapter 27 Youthful Resilience: Programs That Promote Health in Adolescence   391
Victoria L. Baker and Wendy Steinkraus

Chapter 28 Culture, Collaboration, and Community: Participatory Action
Anthropology in Development of Senior ConNEXTions   411
Rosemarie Santora Lamm

Chapter 29 Adolescents and Low Glycemic Control in Type 1 Diabetes Mellitus   419
Mary Katherine White

Unit IV   Teaching–Learning   427

Chapter 30 Teaching Nurses About Vulnerable Populations   429
Mary de Chesnay

Chapter 31 Caring for Vulnerable Populations: The Role of the DNP-Prepared Nurse   441
Barbara A. Anderson

Chapter 32 Community Action by Undergraduate Students on Behalf of Trafficked Children   449
Lady Collins, Kaitlin Chance, and Christine Meyers

Chapter 33 The College-Bound Adolescent with a Mental Health Disorder   461
Cara C. Young and Susan J. Calloway

Chapter 34 Homeless College Students   479
Jennifer A. Minick, Jennifer Emmons, Buffie Cole, Marcia A. Stidum, Joshua Gunn, and Mary de Chesnay

Chapter 35 Teaching Nurse Practitioners About Sex Trafficking: An Honors Capstone Project   493
Emily Peoples

Chapter 36 Family Nursing Clinical Immersion in Lac du Flambeau   509
Cheryl Ann Lapp

Chapter 37 Teaching Psychiatric and Community Health Simulations for Vulnerable Populations   523
Mary de Chesnay, Dori Cole, Johnathan Steppe, and Jennifer Bartlett

Unit V   Policy Implications   533

Chapter 38 Public Policy and Vulnerable Populations   535
Jeri A. Milstead

Chapter 39 The Samfie Man Revisited: Sex Tourism and Trafficking   549
Mary de Chesnay

Chapter 40 Impact of the Affordable Care Act on Health Policy and Advocacy
for Vulnerable Populations 561
Kathryn Osborne

Chapter 41 Health Systems and Human Resources for Health: New Dimensions
in Global Health Nursing 573
Patricia L. Riley and Maureen A. Kelly

Index 599

Preface

In the *Fourth Edition,* the editors retained material from previous editions that we consider basic, such as definitions, cultural competence, social justice, and health literacy. Additionally, we updated chapters on basic concepts and theories, programs, teaching–learning, and health policy. In the research section, we substituted a new lead chapter on the history of ethics in research and how research with human subjects differs in developed and developing countries. We also retained the sample research proposal for quantitative research, and we added a sample research proposal for qualitative research. New to this edition are chapters that represent the Patient Protection and Affordable Care Act, Doctor of Nursing Practice (DNP) capstone projects, and issues of immigrants. Based on the feedback from users of the previous editions, we asked new contributors to include more case examples and the *Fourth Edition* Instructor Guide will include more exercises, cases, and exam questions. Originally written for undergraduates, the book enjoys a wide audience and is used in courses at all levels. The new DNP degree was initiated under controversial conditions, but it has been shown to be effective and we are fortunate that Dr. Barbara Anderson, one of the editors, is a leader in this movement and can speak to the needs of DNP students. Although it is not possible to do justice to every diverse population in every edition, we give voice to a few in the hope that readers will be inspired to translate the ideas presented here to their own practices.

Foreword

W hen is the last time you cared for a patient who was poor, or old, or disabled? Did you ever care for an immigrant family or a fragile teen diabetic? What about caring for someone who does not speak English? Groups of patients like these may be vulnerable to the system, to society, and often to their own lack of knowledge and capacity. Who makes decisions for people with issues such as these? What is the role of the nurse? Are we their advocates, their guides, their partners in care? Where is the roadmap to follow? Who makes the rules? Who protects the patient and, also importantly, who protects the nurse?

Many of us in health care fumble through the day wondering if we are the only ones who ponder questions like these. As nurses, we need more than just a guidebook—more than a policy and procedure manual. We need to know the *how to's*, but we also need to know *how to think about* patients who fall into these categories.

Read this book. It will answer many of your questions and help you to think in a new way about groups of patients who are vulnerable. You will recognize your patient populations on the pages of this book.

As nurses, we usually employ an individualistic view for our patients, that is, we see our patients as individuals. We seldom see them in their social context because usually we care for immediate problems that require immediate action. Nurses really do not have time to be philosophical. We experience great urgency to take care of our patients and to resolve their immediate problems right away.

At the end of the day, and sometimes in the middle of the night, we do think more broadly about situations. We wonder what happened to certain patients and families, and sometimes we ask ourselves why things are the way they are. Who can help us ponder those questions? Where do we turn for help with those questions?

Reading this book will help you see the issues of vulnerable groups from another perspective—from a bird's eye view—using a wide-angle lens. Understanding vulnerable groups requires a broad context and fresh, unique approaches. Understanding why the problems of vulnerable groups are significant and why nurses should pay attention to them will give you a new energy and realization.

In the future, when you meet an immigrant family, a poor person, or a messed-up teenager you will have the knowledge this book provides to help you navigate your way with them. It will make you even more proud to be in nursing. Enjoy!

Karen Breda, PhD (Anthropology), MSN, BSN (Nursing)
Associate Professor, University of Hartford
West Hartford, Connecticut

Contributors

Janeen S. Amason, PhD, RN
Assistant Professor
Kennesaw State University

Victoria L. Baker, PhD, CNM, CPH
Associate Professor
Frontier Nursing University

Jennifer Bartlett, PhD, RN-BC, CNE
Assistant Professor/Simulation Coordinator
Kennesaw State University

Anne Batson, MSN, RN
Doctoral Student
Kennesaw State University

Anne Watson Bongiorno, PhD, APHN,
   BC, CNE
Adjunct Professor
Empire State College

Doris M. Boutain, PhD, RN
Associate Professor
University of Washington School of Nursing

Jane Brannan, EdD, RN
Professor
Kennesaw State University

Susan J. Calloway, PhD, RN, PMHNP-BC,
   FNP-BC, FAANP
Associate Professor
Frontier Nursing University

Ellyn E. Cavanagh, PhD, MN, ARNP
Pediatric Nurse Practitioner
The Everett Clinic in Washington State

Kaitlin Chance
Nursing Student
Mercer University

Buffie Cole
Nursing Student
Kennesaw State University

Dori Cole, MSN, RN
Nurse Educator

Lady Collins, RN, BSN
Children's Hospital of Atlanta

Mona M. Counts, PhD, CRNP, FNAP,
   FAANP, FAAN
Professor Emeritus
Penn State University

Judi Daniels, PhD, RN, APRN, PNP, FNP
Associate Professor
Frontier Nursing University

Genie E. Dorman, PhD, APRN, FNP-BC
Professor
Interim Associate Director, Graduate Nursing
 Programs
Kennesaw State University

Christie Emerson, MSN, RN, FNP
Senior Lecturer
Clinical Agency Liaison and BSN Part-Time
 Faculty Coordinator
Kennesaw State University

Jennifer Emmons
Nursing Student
Kennesaw State University

Behice Erci, PhD, RN
Professor
Inonu University, Turkey

Janice B. Flynn, PhD, RN
Associate Director WellStar School
 of Nursing
Undergraduate Program
Professor of Nursing
Kennesaw State University

Bethany Francis
Nursing Student
Kennesaw State University

Joshua Gunn, PhD
Director of Counseling and Psychological
 Services
Kennesaw State University

Patricia L. Hart, PhD, RN
Associate Professor of Nursing
Kennesaw State University

Leslie Himot, MSN
Clinical Lecturer
Kennesaw State University

Maureen A. Kelley, CNM, PhD, FACNM
Professor, Clinical Track
Nell Hodgson Woodruff School of Nursing
Emory University

Joyce M. Knestrick, PhD, CRNP, FAANP
Associate Professor and Online Program
 Director
Georgetown University

Rosemarie Santora Lamm, PhD, APRN
Director, Senior ConNEXTions
Lakeland, Florida

Cheryl Ann Lapp, PhD, MPH, RN
Professor of Nursing
University of Wisconsin-Eau Claire

Shih-Yu (Sylvia) Lee, PhD, RNC
Professor
Hungkuang University, Taiwan

Janice M. Long, RN, MSN, PhD
Associate Professor
Kennesaw State University

Nicole Mareno, PhD, RN
Assistant Professor
Kennesaw State University

Lisa McMasters
Nursing Student
Kennesaw State University

Christine Meyers
Nursing Student
Kennesaw State University

Jeri A. Milstead, PhD, RN
Milstead Innovations
Dublin, Ohio

Jennifer A. Minick, BSN, RN
WellStar Kennestone Hospital Oncology Unit

Robin A. Narruhn, MN, RN, PhD
Doctor of Nursing Science Student
University of Washington, School of Nursing

Tommie Nelms, PhD, RN
Professor and Director, WellStar School
    of Nursing
Kennesaw State University

Major Elizabeth Nutter, DNP, RN, CNM
Active Duty Army Officer
United States Army

Ellen F. Olshansky, PhD, RN, FAAN
Professor of Nursing
University of California, Irvine

Kathryn Osborne, PhD, RN, CNM, FACNM
Faculty
Rush University School of Nursing

Emily Peoples, BSN, RN
Nursing Student
Kennesaw State University

Patricia L. Riley, CNM, MPH, FACNM
Senior Technical Advisor in the Division of
    Global HIV/AIDS
U.S. Centers for Disease Control and
    Prevention
Atlanta, Georgia

Lisa R. Roberts, DPH, RN, FNP-BC
Associate Professor and Director of the FNP
    and AGNP Programs
Loma Linda University

Vanessa Robinson-Dooley, PhD, LCSW
Assistant Professor of Social Work
Kennesaw State University

Edwina Skiba-King, PhD, APN
Clinical Assistant Professor
Rutgers University

Wendy Steinkraus, DNP, FNP-BC
Family Nurse Practitioner
Lakeland Comprehensive Weight Loss Center
    and General Surgery Office
Niles, Michigan

Johnathan Steppe, RN, MSN, CCRN
Lecturer of Nursing
Kennesaw State University

Marcia A. Stidum, LCSW, MPA
Associate Director for Counseling
Psychological Services
CARE Center Coordinator
Kennesaw State University

Deonna S. Tanner, PhD, RN
Assistant Professor of Nursing
Clayton State University

Toni Vezeau, PhD, RNC, IBCLC
Associate Professor
Seattle University

Mary Anne White, PhD, RN
Captain (Retired) U.S. Navy Nurse Corps
Professor of Nursing
Kennesaw State University

Mary Katherine White, DNP, RN
Lecturer
Kennesaw State University

Diane Wilson
Nursing Student
Kennesaw State University

**Danuta M. Wojnar, PhD, RN, MEd,
    IBCLC, FAAN**
Associate Professor and Chair
Maternal/Child and Family Nursing
Seattle University, College of Nursing

Maria da Gloria M. Wright, PhD, RN
Former Coordinator Educational Development
  Program, Interamerican Drug Abuse Control
  Commission (CICAD)/Organization of
  American States (OAS)

Cara C. Young, PhD, RN, FNP-C
Assistant Professor
University of Texas

Robynn Zender, MS
Community Health Program Specialist
Institute of Clinical and Translational Research
University of California

Rick Zoucha, PhD, PMHCNS-BC, CTN-A
Professor and Chair of Advanced Role and PhD
  programs
Duquesne University School of Nursing

Acknowledgments

This book is a reflection of the talents of many people—first among them, both the new and returning contributing authors. That social justice and care for the vulnerable is a universal phenomenon among nurses is reinforced when we attend professional meetings and when we travel to our own fieldwork sites and see social justice in action in some of the poorest communities of the world. It is inspiring to hear these authors speak and an honor to provide a forum for all who read this book to hear about their work. We are deeply grateful to those scholars and practitioners around the world who contributed to this work.

There are always technical support people who labor quietly behind the scenes of any published venture. The editors and staff at Jones & Bartlett Learning made sure the work was published in a timely manner. We are grateful to Amanda Martin for her leadership as well as Rebecca Myrick, Danielle Bessette, and Renée Sekerak for their attention to detail.

The wonderful staff at Kennesaw State University, especially Cynthia Elery, enabled Mary de Chesnay to complete the book with the help of the invaluable student assistants, particularly Brad Garner. Two graduate students developed much of the material for the Instructor Guide, while maintaining a heavy course load in the doctoral program (Brenda Brown) and the master's degree program (Sheena Cole).

Finally, and perhaps most importantly, the editors would like to thank all of the vulnerable yet resilient people with whom they have worked during their many years of clinical practice and education. Working in every corner of the world, the editors time and time again encountered the strength of the human spirit and generosity of nature among people who have no reason to welcome strangers, yet who shared what they had and took the time to teach us about their cultures.

Mary de Chesnay
Barbara A. Anderson

About the Editors

Mary de Chesnay, PhD, RN, PMHCNS-BC, FAAN is professor of nursing at Kennesaw State University and secretary of the Council on Nursing and Anthropology (CONAA) of the Society for Applied Anthropology (SFAA). Her clinical practice and research program involve mostly women and children who have been abused or trafficked. She has conducted ethnographic fieldwork and participatory action research in Latin America and the Caribbean. She has taught a course in vulnerable populations and qualitative research at all levels in the United States and abroad in the roles of faculty, head of a department of research, dean, and endowed chair.

Barbara A. Anderson, DrPH, RN, CNM, FACNM, FAAN is professor of nursing and director of the post-master's DNP program at Frontier Nursing University. She serves on the Board of Directors of the American College of Nurse Midwives. She has worked with vulnerable populations in over 100 countries in public health program design and evaluation, nurse-midwifery, and the education of health professionals.

I

Concepts and Theories

Chapter 1

Vulnerable Populations: Vulnerable People

Mary de Chesnay

OBJECTIVES

At the end of this chapter, the reader will be able to

1. Distinguish between vulnerability as an individual concept and vulnerable population.
2. Identify at least five populations at risk for health disparities.
3. Discuss how poverty influences vulnerability.

In this chapter, key concepts are introduced to provide a frame of reference for examining healthcare issues related to vulnerability and vulnerable populations. The concepts presented in Unit I, as a whole, form a theoretical perspective on caring for the vulnerable within a cultural context in which nurses consider not only ethnicity as a cultural factor, but also the culture of vulnerability. The goal is to provide culturally competent care.

VULNERABILITY

Vulnerability incorporates two aspects, and it is important to distinguish between them. One is the individual focus, in which individuals are viewed within a system context; the other is an aggregate view of what would be termed *vulnerable populations*. Much of the literature on vulnerability is targeted toward the aggregate view, and nurses certainly need to address the needs of groups. Nevertheless, nurses also treat individuals, and this book is concerned with generating ideas about caring for both individuals and groups. It is critical for practitioners to keep in mind that groups are composed of individuals—we should not stereotype individuals in terms of their group characteristics. Yet, working with vulnerable populations is cost-effective because epidemiological patterns can be detected in groups and some standardized interventions can be developed that provide better quality health care to more people.

Vulnerability is a general concept meaning "susceptibility" and has a specific connotation in health care—"at risk for health problems." According to Aday (2001), vulnerable populations are those at risk for poor physical, psychological, or social health. Any person can be at risk statistically by way of having potential for certain illnesses based on genetic predisposition (Scanlon & Lee, 2007). Anyone can also be vulnerable at any given point in time as a result of life circumstances or response to illness or events. However, the notion of a vulnerable population is a public health concept that refers to vulnerability by virtue of status; that is, some groups are at risk at any given point in time relative to other individuals or groups.

To be a member of a vulnerable population does not necessarily mean a person is vulnerable. In fact, many individuals within vulnerable populations would resist the notion that they are vulnerable, because they prefer to focus on their strengths rather than their weaknesses. These people might argue that vulnerable population is just another label that healthcare professionals use to promote a system of health care that they, the consumers of care, consider patronizing. It is important to distinguish between a state of vulnerability at any given point in time and a labeling process in which groups of people at risk for certain health conditions are further marginalized.

Some members of society who are not members of the culturally defined vulnerable populations described in this book might be vulnerable in certain contexts. For example, nurses who work in emergency rooms are vulnerable to violence. Hospital employees and visitors are vulnerable to infections. Teachers in preschool and daycare providers are vulnerable to a host of communicable diseases because of their daily contact with young children. Individuals who work with heavy machinery are at risk for certain injuries. Patients are vulnerable to their nurses, who literally hold their lives in their hands.

Other examples of vulnerable groups might include people who pick up hitchhikers, drivers who drink alcohol, people who travel on airplanes during flu season, college students who are cramming for exams, and people who become caught in natural disasters. There is an unfortunate tendency in our culture to judge some vulnerable people as being at fault for their own vulnerability and to blame those who place others at risk. For example, rape victims have been blamed for enticing their attackers. People who pick up hitchhikers might be looked upon as foolish, even though their intentions might have been kindness and consideration for those stranded by car trouble. Airline passengers who continually sneeze might anger their seatmates, who feel at risk for catching a communicable disease. While it is logical to argue that we should be more cautious about personal protection in societies in which dangers exist in so many contexts, that concept is quite different from blaming the victim. In the final analysis, criminals and predators need to be held accountable for criminal behavior. Victims can be taught self-defense tactics, but they need to be reassured that the crime was not their fault simply because they were in the wrong place at the wrong time.

VULNERABLE POPULATIONS

Who are the vulnerable in terms of health care? Vulnerable populations are those with a greater-than-average risk of developing health problems (Aday, 2001; Sebastian, 1996) by virtue of their marginalized sociocultural status, their limited access to economic resources, or their personal characteristics such as age and gender. For example, members of ethnic minority groups have traditionally been marginalized even when they are highly educated and earning good salaries. Immigrants and the poor (including the working poor) have limited access to health care because of the way health insurance is obtained in the United States. Children, women, and the elderly are vulnerable to a host of healthcare problems—notably violence, but also specific health problems associated with development or aging. Developmental examples might include susceptibility to poor influenza outcomes for children and the elderly, psychological issues of puberty and menopause, osteoporosis and fractures among older women, and Alzheimer's disease.

Bezruchka (2000, 2001), in his provocative work, not only addressed the correlation between poverty and illness but also asserted that inequalities in wealth distribution are responsible for the state of health of the U.S. population. Bezruchka argued that the economic structure of a country is the single most powerful determinant of the health of its people. He noted that Japan, with its small gap between rich and poor, has a high percentage of smokers but a low percentage of mortality from smoking. Bezruchka advocated redistribution of wealth as a solution to health disparities.

The prescription drug benefit for Medicare recipients highlights Bezruchka's observations about disparities in the United States. Senior citizens are among the most vulnerable in any society, including in the United States, where Medicare is an attempt to address some of their healthcare costs. However, while a philosophy of social justice might be valued by practitioners (Larkin, 2004), the implementation of social justice is usually balanced with cost. In the case of the Medicare prescription drug benefit, the cost is projected to exceed $700 billion over the period from 2006 to 2015 (Gellad, Huskamp, Phillips, & Haas, 2006). The difficulties created by attempting to balance social justice with cost illustrate how difficult it is to implement Bezruchka's ideas in the United States.

CONCEPTS AND THEORIES

Aday (2001) published a framework for studying vulnerable populations that incorporated the World Health Organization's (1948) dimensions of health (physical, psychological, and social) into a model of relationships between individual and community on a variety of policy levels. In Aday's framework, which is still applicable, the variables of access, cost, and quality are critical for understanding the nature of health care for vulnerable populations. Access refers to the ability of people to find, obtain, and pay for health care. Costs can be either direct or indirect: Direct costs are the dollars spent by healthcare facilities to provide care, whereas indirect costs are losses resulting from decreased patient productivity (e.g., absenteeism from work). Quality refers to the relative inadequacy, adequacy, or superiority of services.

Other authors who have addressed the conceptual basis of vulnerable populations include Sebastian (1996; Sebastian et al., 2002), who focused on marginalization as a factor in resource allocation, and Flaskerud and Winslow (1998), who emphasized resource availability in the broad sense of socioeconomic and environmental resources. Karpati, Galea, Awerbuch, and Levins (2002) argued for an ecological approach to understanding how social context influences health outcomes. Lessick, Woodring, Naber, and Halstead (1992) described the concept of vulnerability in relationship to a person within a system context. Although the study applied the model to maternal–child nursing, the authors argued that the model is appropriate in any clinical setting.

Spiers (2000) argued that epidemiological views of vulnerability are insufficient to explain human experience and offered a new conceptualization based on perceptions that are both etic (externally defined by others) and emic (defined from the point of view of the person). Etic approaches are helpful in understanding the nature of risk in a quantifiable way. Emic approaches enable one to understand the whole of human experience and, in so doing, help people capitalize on their capacity for action.

HEALTH DISPARITIES

In 1998, President Bill Clinton made a commitment to reduce health disparities that disproportionately affect racial and ethnic minorities in the United States by the year 2010. The Department of Health and Human Services selected six areas to target: infant mortality, cancer screening and management, cardiovascular disease, diabetes, human immunodeficiency virus (HIV) infection and acquired immune deficiency syndrome (AIDS), and immunization (National Institutes of Health [NIH], n.d.). Subsequently, the NIH announced a strategic plan for 2002–2006 that committed funding for three major goals related to research, research infrastructure, and public information/community outreach (NIH, 2002). It is clear from the recent healthcare reform actions taken by President

Barack Obama that he intends to carry out the mission of improving health care for all. The *Healthy People* objectives are even more important today than when first envisioned.

When Flaskerud et al. (2002) reviewed 79 research reports published in *Nursing Research*, they concluded that although nurse researchers have systematically addressed health disparities, they have tended to ignore certain groups (e.g., indigenous peoples). They also inappropriately lump together as Hispanic, members of disparate groups with their own cultural identity (e.g., Puerto Ricans, Mexicans, Cubans, Dominicans).

Aday (2001) emphasized certain groups as vulnerable populations, and the 2010 priorities showcase obvious needs within these groups:

- *High-risk mothers and infants-of-concern.* This population reflects the currently high rates of teenage pregnancy and poor prenatal care, leading to birth-weight problems and infant mortality. Affected groups include very young women, African American women, and poorly educated women, all of whom are less likely than middle-class white women to receive adequate prenatal care due to limited access to services.
- *Chronically ill and disabled persons.* Individuals in this category not only experience higher death rates than comparable middle-class white women as a result of heart disease, cancer, and stroke, but are also subject to prevalent chronic conditions such as hypertension, arthritis, and asthma. The debilitating effects of such chronic diseases lead to lost income resulting from limitations in activities of daily living. African Americans, for example, are more likely to experience ill effects and to die from chronic diseases.
- *Persons living with HIV/AIDS.* In the past decade or so, advances in tracing and treating AIDS have resulted in declines in deaths and increases in the number of people living with HIV/AIDS. This increase is also due, in part, to changes in transmission patterns from largely male homosexual or bisexual contact to transmission through heterosexual contact and sharing needles among intravenous (IV) drug users.
- *Mentally ill and disabled persons.* The population with mental illness is usually defined broadly to include individuals with mild anxiety and depression. Prevalence rates are high with age-specific disorders, and severe emotional disorders seriously interfere with activities of daily living and interpersonal relationships.
- *Alcohol and other substance abusers.* The wide array of substances that are abused includes drugs, alcohol, cigarettes, and inhalants (such as glue). Intoxication results in chronic disease, accidents, and, in some cases, criminal activity. Young male adults in their late teens and early twenties are more likely to smoke, drink, and take drugs.
- *Persons exhibiting suicide- or homicide-prone behavior.* Rates of suicide and homicide differ by age, sex, and race, with elderly white and young Native American men being most likely to kill themselves and young African American, Native American, and Hispanic men being most likely to be killed by others.

- *Abusive families.* Children, the elderly, and spouses (overwhelmingly women) are likely targets of violence within the family. Although older children are more likely to be injured, young female children older than 3 years of age are consistently at risk for sexual abuse.
- *Homeless persons.* Because of ongoing problems in identifying this population, it is reasonably certain that the estimated prevalence rates at any given time are low and vary across the country. Generally, more young men are homeless, but all homeless individuals are likely to suffer from chronic diseases and are vulnerable to violence.
- *Immigrants/refugees.* Health care for immigrants, refugees, and temporary residents is complicated by the diversity of languages, health practices, food choices, culturally based definitions of health, and previous experiences with American bureaucracies.

Aday (2001) provided much statistical information for these vulnerable groups, but prevalence rates for specific conditions change periodically. Readers are referred to the website of the National Center for Health Statistics (www.cdc.gov/nchs) for updated information.

Trends in families over the last 5 decades (the lifetime of the baby boomers) show marked changes in the demographics of families, and these changes, in turn, affect health disparities. At present, more men and women are delaying marriage, with greater numbers of people choosing to live together first. Divorce rates are higher, with a concurrent increase in single-parent families. Out-of-wedlock births have increased, partially due to decreases in marital fertility. There is a sharp and sustained increase in maternal employment (Hofferth, 2003).

The most recent *Healthy People* report documents health disparities as a major issue both in the health of individuals and that of the healthcare system, in the sense that our structures are not addressing the needs of all citizens. While there is an emphasis on culturally competent care for all, our health professions fall far short of the goals we have set for the nation. Racial and ethnic disparities still exist and increase the cost of health care. When prevention programs are differentially applied, health status decreases and acuity levels rise—with a corresponding cost increase not only in monetary but also in human terms.

Complicating discussions about health disparities is the tendency of the literature to treat race and socioeconomic status (SES) separately. Because a disproportionate number of minorities are poor, it is hard to tell if race or income is more important. Dubay and LeBrun (2012) studied the two together and found that within each racial/ethnic group, a greater proportion of low- versus high-SES individuals was in poor health, and a lower proportion had healthy behaviors and access to care. Unsurprisingly, for either socioeconomic level, minorities had poorer health outcomes than whites.

The populations discussed in this chapter represent a small proportion of those who are vulnerable. Anyone can be considered vulnerable at a specific point in time, but when we discuss vulnerable populations we usually think of people who are members of at-risk groups for certain health disparities, whether short-term or long-term. Efforts have been made in each edition of this book to include authors who have expertise with a variety of vulnerable populations.

INSTITUTE OF MEDICINE STUDY

The U.S. Congress directed the Institute of Medicine (IOM) to study the extent of racial and ethnic differences in health care and to recommend interventions to eliminate health disparities (IOM, 2003). The IOM found consistent evidence of disparities across a wide range of health services and illnesses. Although these racial and ethnic disparities may occur within a wider historical context, they are unacceptable, as the IOM pointed out. It urged a general public acknowledgment of the problem and advocated specific cross-cultural training for health professionals. Other recommendations included specific legal, regulatory, and policy interventions that speak to fairness in access; increases in the number of minority health professionals; and better enforcement of civil rights laws. IOM recommendations with regard to data collection should serve to monitor progress toward the goal of eliminating health disparities based on different treatment for minorities.

Vulnerability to Specific Conditions or Diseases

A large portion of the research that has been done on specific conditions and diseases was generated from psychological data and predates much of the medical and nursing literature on disparities. Researchers on vulnerability to these specific conditions tend to take an individual approach, in that conditions or diseases are treated from the point of view of how a particular individual responds to life stressors and how that response can cause the condition to develop or continue.

Researchers have focused on conditions too numerous to report here, but a search quickly turned up references to alcohol consumption in women and vulnerability to sexual aggression (Testa, Livingston, & Collins, 2000); rape myths and vulnerability to sexual assault (Bohner, Danner, Siebler, & Stamson, 2002); self-esteem and unplanned pregnancy (Smith, Gerrard, & Gibbons, 1997); lung transplantation (Kurz, 2002); coronary angioplasty (Edell-Gustafsson & Hetta, 2001); adjustment to lower limb amputation (Behel, Rybarczyk, Elliott, Nicholas, & Nyenhuis, 2002); reaction to natural disasters (Phifer, 1990); reaction to combat stress (Aldwin, Levensen, & Spiro, 1994; Ruef, Litz, & Schlenger, 2000); homelessness (Morrell-Bellai, Goering, & Boydell, 2000; Shinn, Knickman, & Weitzman, 1991); mental retardation (Nettlebeck, Wison, Potter,

& Perry, 2000); anxiety (Calvo & Cano-Vindel, 1997; Strauman, 1992); and suicide (Schotte, Cools, & Payvar, 1990).

Depression

Many authors have focused on cognitive variables in an attempt to explain vulnerability to depression (Alloy & Clements, 1992; Alloy, Whitehouse, & Abramson, 2000; Hayes, Castonguay, & Goldfried, 1996; Ingram & Ritter, 2000). Others have explored gender differences (Bromberger & Mathews, 1996; Soares & Zitek, 2008; Whiffen, 1988). In a major analysis of the existing literature on depression, Hankin and Abramson (2001) explored the development of gender differences in depression. They noted that although both male and female rates of depression rise during middle adolescence, incidence in girls rises more sharply after age 13 or puberty. This model of general depression might account for gender differences based on developmentally specific stressors and implies possible treatment options.

Variables related to attitudes present a third area of focus in the literature (Brown, Hammen, Craske, & Wickens, 1995; Joiner, 1995; Zuroff, Blatt, Bondi, & Pilkonis, 1999). In a study of 75 college students, researchers found that a high level of "perfectionistic achievement attitudes," as indicated on the Dysfunctional Attitude Scale, correlated with a specific stressor (e.g., poorer than expected performance on a college exam) to predict an increase in symptoms of depression (Brown et al., 1995).

Situational factors also produce vulnerability to depression. For example, the stress of providing care to patients with Alzheimer's disease can produce or exacerbate symptoms of depression. In a study of family caregivers of Alzheimer's patients, Neundorfer and colleagues (2006) found that caregivers with prior depressive symptoms were not necessarily more prone to depression than others, but rather that all subjects were more likely to experience depression when the dependency of the patient was high.

Despite the current trend to regulate depression via chemical means, promising evidence suggests that vulnerability to depression can be modified by emotion regulation instruction. Ehring and colleagues (2010) conducted an experiment in which they showed short films with sad content to people with depression as well as to a control group. According to the researchers, if subjects were vulnerable to depression, they would spontaneously use dysfunctional emotional regulation strategies, however they were able to use more functional techniques if instructed to do so.

Schizophrenia

Smoking has been observed to be a problem in individuals with schizophrenia, and there is some evidence that smokers have a more serious course of mental illness than nonsmokers. The theory proposed to explain this relationship is that schizophrenic patients smoke as a way to self-medicate (Lohr & Flynn, 1992). In a twin study investigating lifetime prevalence of smoking and nicotine withdrawal, Lyons et al. (2002) found that the association between smoking and schizophrenia may be related to familial vulnerability to schizophrenia.

Other authors have examined the relationship between schizophrenia and personality. This relationship remains largely unexplored, but might provide a new direction in which to search for knowledge about vulnerability to schizophrenia. In their meta-analysis, Berenbaum and Fujita (1994) found a significant relationship between introversion and schizophrenia; they suggested that studies on this link might provide new knowledge about the covariation of schizophrenia with mood disorders, particularly depression. In a thoughtful analysis of the literature on the role of the family in schizophrenia, Wuerker (2000) presented evidence for the biological view, concluding that there is a unique vulnerability to stress in schizophrenic patients and that communication difficulties within families with schizophrenic members may be due to a shared genetic heritage.

Eating Disorders

Acknowledgment of food as a common focus for anxiety has become a way of life. Canadian researchers refer to "food insecurity" to describe the phenomenon of nutritional vulnerability resulting from food scarcity and insufficient access to food by welfare recipients and low-income people who do not qualify for welfare (McIntyre et al., 2003; Tarasuk, 2003). In the United States, eating disorders are often a result of body image problems, which are particularly prevalent in gay men and heterosexual women (Siever, 1994). In a prospective study of gender and behavioral vulnerabilities related to eating disorders, Leon, Fulkerson, Perry, and Early-Zaid (1995) found significant differences among girls in the variables of weight loss, dieting patterns, vomiting, and use of diet pills. They reported a method for predicting the occurrence of eating disorders based on performance scores on risk-factor status tests in early childhood.

HIV/AIDS

In a meta-analysis of 32 HIV/AIDS studies involving 15,440 participants, Gerrard, Gibbons, and Bushman (1996) found empirical evidence to support the commonly known motivational hypothesis. This hypothesis is derived from the Health Belief Model (Becker & Rosenstock, 1987). The authors found that perceived vulnerability was the major force behind prevention behavior in high-risk populations but cautioned that studies were not available for low-risk populations. They also discovered that risk behavior shapes perceptions of vulnerability—that is, people who engage in high-risk behavior tend to see themselves as more likely to contract HIV than those who engage in low-risk behavior.

Evidence that high-risk men tend to relapse into unsafe sex behaviors is provided in a longitudinal study of results of an intervention in which researchers were able to successfully predict relapse behavior (Kelly, St. Lawrence, & Brasfield, 1991). In a gender study on emotional distress predictors, Van Servellen, Aguirre, Sarna, and Brecht (2002) found that although all subjects had scores indicating clinical anxiety levels, HIV-infected women had more symptoms and poorer functioning than HIV-infected men.

In a study that used a vulnerable populations framework, Flaskerud and Lee (2001) considered the role that resource availability plays in the health status of informal female caregivers of people with HIV/AIDS ($n = 36$) and age-related dementias ($n = 40$). Not surprisingly, the caregivers experienced high levels of both physical and mental health problems. However, the use of the vulnerable populations framework explained the finding that the resource variables of income and minority ethnicity made the greatest contribution to understanding health status. In terms of the risk variables, anger was more common in caregivers for HIV-infected patients and was significantly related to depressive mood, which was also common among these caregivers.

Gender differences among HIV-infected people can exacerbate their response to the disease. Murray et al. (2009) interviewed Zambian women infected with HIV about their reasons for taking or not taking antiretroviral drugs. The key informants revealed fears of abandonment by their husbands, a decision to stop the medications when they felt better, choosing instead to die, and fear of having to take medications for the rest of their lives. These women are vulnerable not only to the disease but also to their family's reaction; the barriers to taking medication that could save their lives may be overshadowed by these risks, making them even more vulnerable.

Substance Abuse

In a study of 288 undergraduates, Wild, Hinson, Cunningham, and Bacchiochi (2001) examined the inconsistencies between a person's perceived risk of alcohol-related harm and motivation to reduce that risk. These researchers found a general tendency for people to view themselves as less vulnerable than their peers regardless of their risk status; notably, however, the at-risk group rated themselves more likely to experience harm than the not-at-risk group. The authors concluded that motivational approaches to reducing risk should emphasize not only why people drink but also why they should reduce alcohol consumption. Additional support for the motivational hypothesis—that perceived vulnerability influences prevention behavior—extends to marijuana use (Simons & Carey, 2002) and to early onset of substance abuse among African American children (Wills, Gibbons, Gerrard, & Brody, 2000).

Finally, in a study of family history of psychopathology in families of the offspring of alcoholics, researchers demonstrated that male college student offspring of these families are a heterogeneous group and that the patterns of heterogeneity are related to familial types in relation to vulnerability to alcoholism. Three different family types were identified:

- Low levels of family pathology with moderate levels of alcoholism
- High levels of family antisocial personality and violence with moderate levels of family drug abuse and depression
- High levels of familial depression, mania, anxiety disorder, and alcoholism with moderate levels of familial drug abuse (Finn et al., 1997)

Students and Faculty as Vulnerable Populations

The April 2007 shootings at Virginia Tech highlighted the fact that college students in the United States face a relatively new kind of threat, much as the Columbine tragedy did for high school students. Alienated young people who stalk and kill their classmates, for whatever reasons, seem logical to them, and represent a new type of terrorist. Yet, the literature has not documented either the experience of these alienated students, nor have we found effective ways of treating and preventing violent behavior among them.

Some attempts have been made to document types of violence toward students. The American College Health Association (ACHA) has published a white paper on the topic (Carr, 2007). This paper largely focuses on the most frequent types of student-directed violence, such as sexual assault, hazing, suicide, celebratory violence, and racial/gender/ sexual orientation–based violence. While spree killings are mentioned, not much attention can be given until more is known about these killers.

Some attention has been given to the relationship between alcohol use and violence. Marcus and Swett (2003) studied precursors to violence among 451 college students at two sites and used the Violence Risk Assessment tool to establish the relationship of patterns related to gender, peer pressure, and alcohol use. Nicholson and colleagues (1998) examined the influence of alcohol use in both sexual and nonsexual violence.

A British study on responding to students' mental health needs illustrates how the previously discussed categories of mental illnesses can be exacerbated in the vulnerable population of college students with mental illnesses. Using surveys and focus groups, Stanley and Manthorpe (2001) assessed college students with mental illnesses and identified many issues related to the problems of providing care to students. The authors noted that high rates of suicide and need for antidepressant medication strained the National Health Service's resources and that colleges varied widely in their ability to provide effective interventions.

In an Australian study, the researchers found a significantly high level of food insecurity among college students. Food insecurity was measured by a "yes" response to a survey question about running out of food and not being able to buy more (Hughes,

Serebryanikova, Donaldson, & Leveritt, 2011). Implications are not only related to student retention, progression, and success but also to long-term health effects.

DalPezzo and Jett (2010) identified nursing faculty as a vulnerable population. They noted student incivility, horizontal violence, and abuse of power by administrators as examples of the pressures faced by faculty.

While these studies document some issues related to campus violence, they do not go far enough to explain and prevent the types of spree killings students have experienced during the last decade. The threat of copycat attacks has engendered continuing fears among students, parents, and teachers alike. More research is needed on personal characteristics of these young killers, potential interventions, and prevention strategies.

CONCLUSION

A growing body of literature has focused on the concept of vulnerability as a key factor of concern to practitioners who work with clients with many different kinds of presenting problems. Vulnerability may be explored on two levels, in that vulnerability is both an individual concept and a group concept. In public health, the group concept is dominant, and intervention is directed toward aggregates. Other practitioners and researchers focus on individual vulnerabilities to specific conditions or diseases. When working with clients from vulnerable populations, it is critical to understand that they might not view themselves as vulnerable and may actually resent labels that imply they are not autonomous.

REFERENCES

Aday, L. (2001). *At risk in America*. San Francisco, CA: Jossey-Bass.

Aldwin, C., Levensen, M., & Spiro, A. (1994). Vulnerability and resilience to combat exposure: Can stress have lifelong effects? *Psychology and Aging, 9*, 34–44.

Alloy, L., & Clements, C. (1992). Illusion of control invulnerability to negative affect and depressive symptoms after laboratory and natural stressors. *Journal of Abnormal Psychology, 101*, 234–245.

Alloy, L., Whitehouse, W., & Abramson, J. (2000). The Temple-Wisconsin cognitive vulnerability to depression project: Lifetime history of axis I psychopathology in individuals at high and low cognitive risk for depression. *Journal of Abnormal Psychology, 109*, 403–418.

Becker, M., & Rosenstock, I. (1987). Comparing social learning theory and the health belief model. In W. B. Ward (Ed.), *Advances in health education and promotion* (Vol. 2, pp. 245–249). Greenwich, CT: JAI Press.

Behel, J., Rybarczyk, B., Elliott, T., Nicholas, J., & Nyenhuis, D. (2002). The role of perceived vulnerability in adjustment to lower extremity amputation: A preliminary investigation. *Rehabilitation Psychology, 47*(1), 92–105.

Berenbaum, H., & Fujita, F. (1994). Schizophrenia and personality: Exploring the boundaries and connections between vulnerability and outcome. *Journal of Abnormal Psychology, 103*, 148–158.

Bezruchka, S. (2000). Culture and medicine: Is globalization dangerous to our health? *Western Journal of Medicine, 172,* 332–334.

Bezruchka, S. (2001). Societal hierarchy and the health olympics. *Canadian Medical Association Journal, 164,* 1701–1703.

Bohner, G., Danner, U., Siebler, F., & Stamson, G. (2002). Rape myth acceptance and judgments of vulnerability to sexual assault: An Internet experiment. *Experimental Psychology, 49,* 257–269.

Bromberger, J., & Mathews, K. (1996). A "feminine" model of vulnerability to depressive symptoms: A longitudinal investigation of middle-aged women. *Journal of Personality and Social Psychology, 70,* 591–598.

Brown, G., Hammen, C., Craske, M., & Wickens, T. (1995). Dimensions of dysfunctional attitudes as vulnerabilities to depressive symptoms. *Journal of Abnormal Psychology, 104,* 431–435.

Calvo, M., & Cano-Vindel, A. (1997). The nature of trait anxiety: Cognitive and biological vulnerability. *European Psychologist, 2,* 301–312.

Carr, J. (2007). Campus violence white paper. *Journal of American College Health, 55*(5), 304–319.

DalPezzo, N., & Jett, K. (2010). Nursing faculty: A vulnerable population. *Journal of Nursing Education, 49*(3), 132–136.

Dubay, L., & LeBrun, L. (2012). Health, behavior, and health care disparities: Disentangling the effects of income and race in the United States. *International Journal of Health Services, 42*(4), 607–625.

Edell-Gustafsson, U., & Hetta, J. (2001). Fragmented sleep and tiredness in males and females one year after percutaneous transluminal coronary angioplasty (PTCA). *Journal of Advanced Nursing, 34*(2), 203–211.

Ehring, J., Tuschen-Caffier, B., Schulke, J., Fischer, S., & Gross, J. (2010). Emotion regulation and vulnerability to depression: Spontaneous versus instructed suppression and reappraisal. *Emotion, 10*(4), 563–572.

Finn, P., Sharkansky, E., Viken, R., West, T., Sandy, J., & Bufferd, G. (1997). Heterogeneity in the families of sons of alcoholics: The impact of familial vulnerability type on offspring characteristics. *Journal of Abnormal Psychology, 106,* 26–36.

Flaskerud, J., & Lee, P. (2001). Vulnerability to health problems in female informal caregivers of persons with HIV/AIDS and age-related dementias. *Journal of Advanced Nursing, 33*(1), 60–68.

Flaskerud, J., Lesser, J., Dixon, E., Anderson, N., Conde, F., Kim, S., ... Koniak-Griffin, D. (2002). Health disparities among vulnerable populations: Evolution of knowledge over five decades in *Nursing Research* publications. *Nursing Research, 51*(2), 74–85.

Flaskerud, J., & Winslow, B. (1998). Conceptualizing vulnerable populations in health-related research. *Nursing Research, 47*(2), 69–78.

Gellad, W., Huskamp, H., Phillips, K., & Haas, J. (2006). How the new Medicare drug benefit could affect vulnerable populations. *Health Affairs, 25*(1), 248–255.

Gerrard, M., Gibbons, F., & Bushman, B. (1996). Relation between perceived vulnerability to HIV and precautionary sexual behavior. *Psychological Bulletin, 119,* 390–409.

Hankin, B., & Abramson, L. (2001). Development of gender differences in depression: An elaborated cognitive vulnerability-transactional stress theory. *Psychological Bulletin, 127,* 773–796.

Hayes, A., Castonguay, L., & Goldfried, M. (1996). Effectiveness of targeting the vulnerability factors of depression in cognitive therapy. *Journal of Consulting and Clinical Psychology, 64,* 623–627.

Hofferth, S. (2003). The American family: Changes and challenges for the 21st century. In H. Wallace, G. Green, & K. Jaros (Eds.), *Health and welfare for families in the 21st century* (pp. 71–79). Sudbury, MA: Jones and Bartlett.

Hughes, R., Serebryanikova, I., Donaldson, K., & Leveritt, M. (2011). Student food insecurity: The skeleton in the university closet. *Nutrition and Dietetics, 68,* 27–32.

Ingram, R., & Ritter, J. (2000). Vulnerability to depression: Cognitive reactivity and parental bonding in high-risk individuals. *Journal of Abnormal Psychology, 109,* 588–596.

Institute of Medicine (IOM), National Academy of Sciences. (2003). Unequal treatment: Confronting racial and ethnic disparities in health care. Retrieved from www.nap.edu

Joiner, T. (1995). The price of soliciting and receiving negative feedback: Self-verification theory as a vulnerability to depression. *Journal of Abnormal Psychology, 104,* 364–372.

Karpati, A., Galea, S., Awerbuch, T., & Levins, R. (2002). Variability and vulnerability at the ecological level: Implications for understanding the social determinants of health. *American Journal of Public Health, 92,* 1768–1773.

Kelly, J., St. Lawrence, J., & Brasfield, T. (1991). Predictors of vulnerability to AIDS risk behavior relapse. *Journal of Consulting and Clinical Psychology, 59*(1), 163–166.

Kurz, J. M. (2002). Vulnerability of well spouses involved in lung transplantation. *Journal of Family Nursing, 8,* 353–370.

Larkin, H. (2004). Justice implications of a proposed Medicare prescription drug benefit. *Social Work, 49*(3), 406–414.

Leon, G., Fulkerson, J., Perry, C., & Early-Zaid, M. (1995). Prospective analysis of personality and behavioral vulnerabilities and gender influences in the later development of disordered eating. *Journal of Abnormal Psychology, 104*(1), 140–149.

Lessick, M., Woodring, B., Naber, S., & Halstead, L. (1992). Vulnerability: A conceptual model. *Perinatal and Neonatal Nursing, 6,* 1–14.

Lohr, J., & Flynn, K. (1992). Smoking and schizophrenia. *Schizophrenia Research, 8,* 93–102.

Lyons, M., Bar, J., Kremen, W., Toomey, R., Eisen, S., Goldberg, J., & Tsuang, M. (2002). Nicotine and familial vulnerability to schizophrenia: A discordant twin study. *Journal of Abnormal Psychology, 111,* 687–693.

Marcus, R., & Swett, B. (2003). Multiple precursor scenarios: Predicting and reducing campus violence. *Journal of Interpersonal Violence, 18*(5), 553–571.

McIntyre, L., Glanville, N., Raine, K., Dayle, J., Anderson, B., & Battaglia, N. (2003). Do low-income lone mothers compromise their nutrition to feed their children? *Canadian Medical Association Journal, 168*(6), 686–691.

Morrell-Bellai, T., Goering, P., & Boydell, K. (2000). Becoming and remaining homeless: Qualitative investigation. *Issues in Mental Health Nursing, 21,* 581–604.

Murray, L., Semrau, K., McCurley, E., Thea, D., Scott, N., Mwiya, M., … Bolton, P. (2009). Barriers to acceptance and adherence of antiretroviral therapy in urban Zambian women: A qualitative study. *AIDS Care, 21*(1), 78–86.

National Institutes of Health. (n.d.). Addressing health disparities: The NIH program of action. Retrieved December 4, 2003, from http://healthdisparities.nih.gov/whatare.html

National Institutes of Health. (2002). *Strategic research plan and budget to reduce and ultimately eliminate health disparities*. Washington, DC: US Department of Health and Human Services.

Nettlebeck, T., Wison, C., Potter, R., & Perry, C. (2000). The influence of interpersonal competence on personal vulnerability of persons with mental retardation. *Journal of Interpersonal Violence*, *15*(1), 46–62.

Neundorfer, M., McLendon, M., Smyth, K., Strauss, M., & McCallum, T. (2006). Does depression prior to caregiving increase vulnerability to depressive symptoms among caregivers of persons with Alzheimer's disease? *Aging and Mental Health*, *10*(6), 606–615.

Nicholson, M., Maney, D., Blair, K., Wamboldt, P., Mahoney, B., & Yuan, J. (1998). Trends in alcohol-related campus violence: Implications for prevention. *Journal of Alcohol and Drug Education*, *43*(3), 34–52.

Phifer, J. (1990). Psychological distress and somatic symptoms after natural disaster: Differential vulnerability among older adults. *Psychology and Aging*, *5*, 412–420.

Ruef, A., Litz, B., & Schlenger, W. (2000). Hispanic ethnicity and risk for combat-related posttraumatic stress disorder. *Cultural Diversity and Ethnic Minority Psychology*, *6*(3), 235–251.

Scanlon, A., & Lee, G. (2007). The use of the term vulnerability in acute care: Why does it differ and what does it mean? *Australian Journal of Advanced Nursing*, *24*(3), 54–59.

Schotte, D., Cools, J., & Payvar, S. (1990). Problem-solving deficits in suicidal patients: Trait vulnerability or state phenomenon? *Journal of Consulting and Clinical Psychology*, *58*, 562–564.

Sebastian, J. (1996). Vulnerability and vulnerable populations. In M. Stanhope & J. Lancaster (Eds.), *Community health nursing: Promoting health of individuals, aggregates and communities* (4th ed., pp. 403–417). St. Louis, MO: Mosby.

Sebastian, J., Bolla, C. D., Aretakis, D., Jones, K. J., Schenk, C., & Napolitano, M. (2002). Vulnerability and selected vulnerable populations. In M. Stanhope & J. Lancaster (Eds.), *Foundations of community health nursing* (pp. 349–364). St. Louis, MO: Mosby.

Shinn, M., Knickman, J., & Weitzman, B. (1991). Social relationships and vulnerability to becoming homeless among poor families. *American Psychologist*, *46*, 1180–1187.

Siever, M. (1994). Sexual orientation and gender as factors in socioculturally acquired vulnerability to body dissatisfaction and eating disorders. *Journal of Consulting and Clinical Psychology*, *62*(2), 252–260.

Simons, J., & Carey, K. (2002). Risk and vulnerability for marijuana use: Problems and the role of affect dysregulation. *Psychology of Addictive Behaviors*, *16*(1), 72–75.

Smith, G., Gerrard, M., & Gibbons, F. (1997). Self-esteem and the relation between risk behavior and perceptions of vulnerability to unplanned pregnancy in college women. *Health Psychology*, *16*(2), 137–146.

Soares, C. N., & Zitek, B. (2008). Reproductive hormone sensitivity and risk for depression across the female life cycle: A continuum for vulnerability? *Journal of Psychiatry and Neuroscience*, *33*(4), 331–343.

Spiers, J. (2000). New perspectives on vulnerability using etic and emic approaches. *Journal of Advanced Nursing*, *31*(3), 715–721.

Stanley, N., & Manthorpe, J. (2001). Responding to students' mental health needs: Impermeable systems and diverse users. *Journal of Mental Health, 10*, 41–52.

Strauman, T. (1992). Self-guides, autobiographical memory, and anxiety and dysphoria: Toward a cognitive model of vulnerability to emotional distress. *Journal of Abnormal Psychology, 101*, 87–95.

Tarasuk, V. (2003). Low income, welfare and nutritional vulnerability. *Canadian Medical Association Journal, 168*, 709–710.

Testa, M., Livingston, J., & Collins, R. (2000). The role of women's alcohol consumption in evaluation of vulnerability to sexual aggression. *Experimental and Clinical Psychopharmacology, 8*(2), 185–191.

Van Servellen, G., Aguirre, M., Sarna, L., & Brecht, M. (2002). Differential predictors of emotional distress in HIV-infected men and women. *Western Journal of Nursing Research, 24*(1), 49–72.

Whiffen, V. (1988). Vulnerability to post-partum depression: A prospective multivariate study. *Journal of Abnormal Psychology, 97*, 467–474.

Wild, T. C., Hinson, R., Cunningham, J., & Bacchiochi, J. (2001). Perceived vulnerability to alcohol-related harm in young adults: Independent effects of risky alcohol use and drinking motives. *Experimental and Clinical Psychopharmacology, 9*(1), 1064–1297.

Wills, T. A., Gibbons, F., Gerrard, M., & Brody, G. (2000). Protection and vulnerability processes relevant for early onset of substance use: A test among African American children. *Health Psychology, 19*(3), 253–263.

World Health Organization. (1948). Constitution. Geneva, Switzerland.

Wuerker, A. (2000). The family and schizophrenia. *Issues in Mental Health Nursing, 21*, 127–141.

Zuroff, D., Blatt, S., Bondi, C., & Pilkonis, P. (1999). Vulnerability to depression: Reexamining state dependence and relative stability. *Journal of Abnormal Psychology, 108*, 76–89.

Chapter 2

Advocacy Role of Providers

Mary de Chesnay and Vanessa Robinson-Dooley

OBJECTIVES

At the end of this chapter, the reader will be able to

1. Compare and contrast the concept of advocacy from the points of view of nursing and social work.
2. Identify key features of the role of patient advocate.
3. Provide an analysis of one's own patient cases from the point of view of the social worker or nurse.

INTRODUCTION

People are vulnerable to illness, injury, and psychological trauma in many contexts of their lives and it would seem they should be safe in the arms of their healthcare providers. Nothing could be further from the truth. As healthcare practitioners, we sometimes believe that we know best and, although we often do know best technically, we do not always frame our interventions in consultation with our clients, nor do we consult with one another for the good of the client. The political nature of health care means that we often make decisions for the good of the organization rather than for the good of the patient. An example of this kind of decision making is limiting visiting hours in intensive care units. In the old days, visits by family members were limited to 5 minutes every hour, justified on the basis that staff members were too busy caring for patients to deal with visitors. Now, hours are more liberal even though patient acuity levels are higher.

Written by a nurse and a social worker, this chapter describes advocacy as a team effort and demonstrates through case studies how the practitioner can function as an advocate and how a team of healthcare professionals can work together for the good of their clients. The literatures in nursing and social work are reviewed separately because the roles of each professional are distinct in most ways. The case studies bring the two disciplines together to show how the roles can complement each other. We hope that readers will be inspired to look for ways in which they can to collaborate—to bring the skills and talents of many disciplines together for the sake of the patients, all of whom are vulnerable when they need our services.

REVIEW OF THE NURSING LITERATURE

The Concept of Patient Advocacy

The nursing literature on patient advocacy seems to be divided into conceptualization of advocacy (Hyland, 2002) and role functions of an advocate. Bu and Jewesky (2006) conducted a concept analysis of patient advocacy by using Walker and Avant's (1995) procedure. The concept analysis generated a mid-range theory with three attributes of patient advocacy: safeguarding autonomy, acting on the patient's behalf, and championing social justice. These attributes give recognition to the vulnerability of patients, the need for some protection within the healthcare system while respecting autonomy, and the international recognition of the role of patient advocate.

The attributes described here are consistent with the role of advocate that institutional review boards (IRBs) play in research involving human and animal subjects. The federal regulations for composition of IRBs mandate inclusion of lay members specifically for the purpose of keeping researchers honest by ensuring that investigators consider the needs of the study population and effects of the study on the people who participate. Mmatli (2009) goes even further in his paper on including people with disabilities in evidence-based research, by arguing that such individuals need to be involved not only in designing studies but also in making decisions about application of the research.

In a critical review of the nursing literature on advocacy, Mallik (1997) argued that the literature lacks clarity in the operationalization of the concept of advocacy, suggesting that authors tend to focus more on defending the role of advocate than on explaining it. Historical reasons for justifying the need for the role are explained by cultural shifts in the roles of physicians and patients' rights. Over time, distrust of experts and technology created a climate of fear, resulting in a higher level of participation by patients in decision making about their own care. The result was creation of a Patient's Bill of Rights and the role of patient advocate (Annas, 1988).

Annas also believed that the nurse is in an ideal position to serve as an advocate (Annas & Healey, 1974). Nurses have certainly filled this role quite ably, and there are many examples of nurses taking on healthcare organizations as whistleblowers. Nevertheless, members of other disciplines may also serve as effective advocates. For example, social workers might be even more effective than nurses in this role because they do not act directly in the medical care of patients and do not participate in historical doctor–nurse games. Even so, to claim the role for any one discipline is not only disrespectful to our colleagues in health care, but self-serving and inconsistent with the spirit of advocacy. What seems clear is the need to understand the context of the advocacy role both for the profession mindful of the rules and regulations and for the professional and the practice setting (Jugessur & Iles, 2009).

In a provocative paper discussing advocacy, Zomorodi and Foley (2009) clarified the thin line between advocacy and paternalism. As healthcare providers who are experts in the treatment of disease, we can easily cross the line between speaking for a patient's right to self-determination and deciding we know what is best for the patient. In fact, this is an occupational hazard for nurses and physicians. Consider the case of a 45-year-old small business owner hospitalized for myocardial infarction. His heart attack comes the day his most trusted employee resigns and the night before a major sales presentation. If he does not get the contract, his business could go under. Because he is the breadwinner, his wife and five children are also at risk if he cannot work. The patient recovers nicely from the acute episode and is in the ICU asking for a phone to make some calls to explain his absence at the meeting. The staff knows that rest and medications are the best treatment and that he should be prevented from becoming upset by anything. They assume that allowing him to talk about business would place him at risk for another heart attack. Unfortunately, denying him the use of the phone causes his anxiety to escalate, which creates a paradoxical effect: His heart rate increases and his blood pressure skyrockets as he sees his life's work destroyed for lack of 10 minutes' access to a phone.

The paternalistic approach is particularly prevalent in settings in which multidisciplinary teams are used to deliver patient care. While nurses tend to use the language of advocacy, physicians often use the language of medical decision making (McGrath, Holewa, & McGrath, 2006). As one physician put it, "of course, we are a team and I am the captain." Fortunately, the nursing profession has evolved from an individual perspective to a systemic perspective in which nurses collectively act to change institutional culture (Mahlin, 2010).

The Role of Patient Advocate

Pullen (1995) makes the case that the role of nurse as advocate is essential to modern health care as a result of paternalism in health care. Paternalism reduces the patient to a passive recipient of care and forces the patient to depend on the integrity and self-regulation of the providers. Yet, patients are often unable to make decisions for themselves without help, either because of ignorance of their own complex health issues or because of temporary incapacitation. The nurse as advocate can play a major role in helping patients regain autonomy. In the example described earlier, the nurse as advocate might have offered to stay near the monitoring equipment in the nurses' station while the patient made the call to make sure he would be safe. However, there are also cultural factors that can interfere with the professional's view of treatment. An example that is seen with greater frequency as immigration increases from developing countries, is the practice of female genital cutting (McCrae & Mayer, 2014). How do nurses balance respect for different cultural traditions with ideas about sanitation, rights of female children, and acculturation to a society that does not approve of female genital cutting?

Community-based participatory action research enables communities to generate relevant knowledge to benefit their own people. Similarly, patient advocacy groups can benefit healthcare consumers. Lara and Salberg (2009) describe how advocacy groups may play a role in health policy by linking patients and consumers of healthcare services with policy makers. Patients, for their part, have realized that they can serve as their own advocates. As a consequence, they are increasingly educating themselves by searching the Internet for information on their diseases or symptoms and coming to appointments armed with more sophisticated questions for which they demand answers.

Further support for the value of partnerships between patients or consumers and providers comes from a study of 405 patients and 118 nurses in 12 hospital units in Finland. Vaartio, Leino-Kilpi, Suominen, and Puukka (2009) found that patients varied in their acts of advocacy and nurses applied principles of advocacy in a haphazard way when caring for patients with postsurgical pain. They concluded that patients perceived care as being good most of the time but not all of the time, while nurses were quite content with their level of advocacy. The explanation for the patients' perception was, either they were not asked about their preferences, or they did not know to ask. At any rate, this lack of participation can be construed as a failure of nurses to provide sufficient information about options for patients and to invite patients to participate more fully in decision making.

In a survey of 5000 medical–surgical nurses registered in the state of Texas, Hanks (2010) found that the nurses, when describing their role as advocates, most often cited certain role behaviors. Education of patients and families emerged as the key response, closely followed by communicating with others on the team and ensuring adequate care. Issues of safety and ensuring that patients' rights were protected were also considered important responsibilities for advocates.

While it is clear that communicating effectively is a key component of effective patient advocacy, little has been done to determine what effective communication in advocacy looks like. In a grounded theory study of 12 nurses at 8 Midwestern hospitals, Martin and Tipton (2007) used the constant comparative method to develop a typology of communication roles that included liaison, feedback remediation, counseling and support, system monitor, troubleshooter, investigator, and group facilitator. An example of the liaison role is communicating with the physician on behalf of patient and family. Feedback remediation includes informing nurses when their behavior toward a patient indicates a less than therapeutic approach. Counseling and support include behaviors such as providing refreshments as well as the traditional counseling activities of listening and problem solving. System monitoring is an important action in terms of environmental issues such as poor room temperature. The troubleshooter makes sure that problems are resolved immediately, sometimes through informal connections such as calling the pharmacy to hurry a prescription. When serious problems occur, the investigator takes action to discover the causes and fix them. Finally, the group facilitator holds meetings with family members, staff, and physicians to make difficult decisions such as those involving end-of-life care.

The literature seems clear about role functions and behaviors of nurses who are successful advocates, but how did they get to be so effective? Advocacy is learned behavior, implying the importance of teaching role behaviors to students. In a synthesis of qualitative studies from 1993–2005, MacDonald (2006) found that, while advocacy is a complex concept, it can be studied within the context of relational ethics and, therefore, can be learned. The starting place is recognizing the vulnerability of patients or clients, not just the developmentally disabled (Jenkins, 2012), but all clients who are temporarily unable to advocate for themselves. Case studies can help students identify the "authentic" wishes of the patient by helping students to clarify their own values as they learn to help patients clarify theirs.

REVIEW OF THE SOCIAL WORK LITERATURE

Definitions

Advocacy has been defined in numerous ways within the social work literature. It has been called one of the "cornerstone" activities of the profession (Clark, 2007, p. 3). Even though advocacy is often viewed as one of the major roles for the generalist social worker, Dorfman (1996) states that advocacy is also the role of the clinical social worker. The *Encyclopedia of Social Work* defines advocacy as the "act of directly representing, defending, intervening, supporting, or recommending a course of action on behalf of one or more individuals, groups, or communities, with the goal of securing or retaining social justice" (Hoefer, 2006, p. 8; Mickelson, 1995, p. 95). *The Social Work Dictionary* defines advocacy as the "act of directly representing or defending others" (Barker, 1995, p. 11; Hoefer, 2006, p. 8). Both definitions speak to what social workers do in their roles as advocates.

Lens (2004) noted that advocacy could be viewed from the perspective of the activity that the individual is performing. Activities such as brokering, case advocacy, and cause advocacy are all part of social work practice (Lens, 2004). Pierce (1984) defined "class advocacy" as a form of advocacy in which social workers use their training and skills to influence social policies and programs that are created to assist a particular group or potential client. Class advocacy is an activity that is addressed in social workers' professional code of ethics (Brawley, 1997). This form of advocacy focuses on ensuring that clients receive the services to which they are entitled in the human service arena (Sheafor & Horejsi, 2003). Sosin and Caulum (1983) defined advocacy through "activities" when they sought to conceptualize advocacy by involving the actions of three social actors: the advocate, the client, and the decision maker. This conceptualization resulted in advocacy being defined as the following:

> *An attempt, having a greater than zero probability of success, by an individual or group to influence another individual or group to make a decision that would not have been made otherwise and that concerns the welfare or interests of a third party who is in a less powerful status than the decision maker.* (p. 13)
>
> Sosin, M., & Caulum, S. (1983, January–February). Advocacy: A conceptualization for social work practice. Social Work, 12–17.

Advocacy has also been defined in the literature as an action that is defined by the setting in which it is performed. Schneider and Lester (2000) note that advocacy involves the relationship between the client and a particular system and the social worker working to influence the decision-making process on behalf of the client. Hospitals are a familiar setting for social workers and their advocacy efforts. Advocacy in this setting involves the social worker intervening on behalf of the patient to access needed resources when the organization is not meeting his or her needs (Faust, 2008).

In spite of the varying definitions of advocacy found in the literature, it is clear that the meanings are similar and that advocacy is an important role for the social worker (Gilbert & Specht, 1976; Lynch & Mitchell, 1995; Sosin & Caulum, 1983), both today and historically.

A Brief History of Advocacy and Social Work

Advocacy has been an integral part of the social work profession since its inception. Such advocacy efforts have usually occurred in response to the social needs of the time.

During the Civil War era and World War I, for example, social work focused on responding to the major changes of these time periods brought about by industrialization. Issues such as working hours, work conditions, and safety became the focus of the advocacy efforts of social workers (Kirst-Ashman & Hull, 2009). The increased migration from rural areas all over the United States to larger cities was fueled by the hopes of prosperity through employment. Individuals came from rural areas with dreams of finding work in cities, but instead were often met with overcrowded neighborhoods and living conditions that promoted health concerns for many (Kirst-Ashman & Hull, 2009). The settlement house movement of the 1880s represented a response to these poor inner-city living conditions. Settlement houses were places where religious leaders and others moved into neighborhoods to interact with the poor and "advocate for child labor laws, women's suffrage, public housing, and public health" (Smith, 1995, p. 2130).

In contrast to the settlement movement, the Charity Organization Societies (COS) of the early 1900s focused on "curing individuals rather than on empowering communities"

(Kirst-Ashman & Hull, 2009, p. 35). Faust (2008) observed that during the early period of the CSO, at the turn of the 20th century, these "friendly visitors" were concerned with the current social conditions. Although their work sought to address what were perceived as "moral deficiencies" at that time, the ensuing activities, discussions, and work focused on eradicating the wretched conditions that plagued urban cities (Faust, 2008; Miley, O'Melia, & DuBois, 2009). As Gilbert and Specht (1976) point out, this attention to therapeutic and clinical interventions prevailed as the major theme of social work from 1935 to 1960.

Although advocacy was a part of the profession long before this time, it became an especially prominent activity of social workers in the 1960s (Gilbert & Specht, 1976). The turbulent 1960s were the period of the civil rights movement, and the pressures for social justice exerted as part of that movement reaffirmed social workers' need to focus on advocacy as a profession (Gilbert & Specht, 1976). "The 1960s produced a new focus on social change versus individual pathology" (Kirst-Ashman & Hull, 2009, p. 36), which required the social work profession to revisit its earlier days of working to empower clients and moving beyond therapeutic interventions. In 1969, an Ad Hoc Committee on Advocacy publication included four major papers addressing the need for advocacy-related work in social work (Gilbert & Specht, 1976). The significance of this committee was that it was established by the national organization for the social work profession, the National Association of Social Workers (NASW) Task Force on Urban Crisis and Public Welfare Problems. "The Ad Hoc Committee of NASW reminded social workers of their social obligation [to advocacy]" (Faust, 2008, p. 293). NASW has, throughout the years, continued to affirm the importance of advocacy for the social work profession. The NASW Code of Ethics (NASW, 1994) details the responsibilities of social workers, including the responsibility to work to "promote general welfare and social justice" (Lynch & Mitchell, 1995, p. 9).

Thus advocacy on behalf of clients has been an important role of social workers for more than 130 years. Advocating on behalf of clients has historically been the responsibility of social workers whether they are working as case workers, general practitioners, researchers, or clinical social workers. Advocacy has come to be something that all social workers are expected to incorporate into their professional role and identity (Gilbert & Specht, 1976, p. 288).

INTERDISCIPLINARY BENEFITS AND APPROACH

In a world where social service organizations have seen their budgets shrink, staff diminish, and ability to provide services cut due to difficult economic times, the interdisciplinary approach to providing services has become even more essential. Working to provide services in an era characterized by limited resources has resulted in clients working with multiple agencies and multiple professions. In this challenging environment, an interdisciplinary team approach to service provision is the best approach.

Social work and the nursing profession are well suited to be in the forefront of the interdisciplinary service provision movement. Compartmentalized problem focus by clients is often a result of having to seek services from multiple organizations. The interdisciplinary team approach to service lessens compartmentalization of problems by clients and can be found in many mental health and medical settings (Johnson, 1995). "Medical settings also make use of the interdisciplinary team approach in providing for both the psychosocial and the physical needs of the patients; diagnostic centers also make considerable use of this type of team approach" (p. 119). When agencies work together and take an interdisciplinary team approach to helping, the client recognizes, respects, and benefits from this practice. Most importantly, the professions and social service community ensure the most effective and efficient use of public resources.

CASE STUDIES

Case 1: Mrs. Smith

Laura Smith is a 24-year-old mother of three who lives in a one-room motel unit and works at a low-paying waitress job at a local café. Although the restaurant chain where she works offers health insurance, she cannot qualify because she is scheduled to work 29 hours per week.

Recently, one of Mrs. Smith's children developed a cough and fever. Mrs. Smith was able to have her child seen at the local emergency room, but the treatment was limited, covering only medication for 3 days of treatment. Mrs. Smith was told she should follow up with the child's primary care physician and have some testing done to confirm that the cough was not something more serious. The emergency room doctor also recommended that the child receive a vaccine that might prevent future problems. Mrs. Smith explained to the doctor that she did not have a regular physician or insurance, and she could not afford to pay out of pocket for a vaccine or any future doctor visits. The emergency room doctor made a referral to the social work department in the hospital and asked if someone could assist Mrs. Smith with accessing resources to meet her medical needs. The emergency room nurse, who had been working with Mrs. Smith and her son, completed the referral to the social work department and asked the social worker to come and meet with Mrs. Smith as soon as possible given Mrs. Smith's limited flexibility with her employer.

The social worker came to the emergency room and met with Mrs. Smith and her child. The emergency room nurse remained in the room because Mrs. Smith was becoming agitated and nervous about the numerous individuals asking her for personal and medical information during this hospital visit. The nurse thought her presence might provide Mrs. Smith with a sense of consistency and assist with calming her fears about the presence of the social worker.

The social worker met with Mrs. Smith and collected background information about her current home environment, employment, and potential social support network. After determining that Mrs. Smith would need community resources beyond what the hospital could provide, the social worker and the nurse met to discuss community agencies that might be able to assist Mrs. Smith and her family. The nurse recalled the opening of a community health clinic about 1 mile from the motel where Mrs. Smith resided. Given the proximity to Mrs. Smith's current home, this was an ideal option for follow-up for her child's medical needs. The social worker agreed to make a call to the clinic to determine if Mrs. Smith might qualify for services.

The social worker was told by the clinic staff that the clinic provided services to families who were underinsured or uninsured. The clinic also had a sliding-scale policy that it used if families could afford to pay a small amount. Mrs. Smith was referred to the clinic and received the following services:

1. Mrs. Smith was scheduled to come to the clinic and complete her intake and income assessment paperwork. A social work intern was assigned to assist her with completing her paperwork.
2. Mrs. Smith's son was seen by the nurse practitioner to evaluate his cough and other symptoms.
3. It was recommended to Mrs. Smith that she be given a brief physical examination, because she had not been seen by a doctor for several years. Her primary focus had been work and her children, and it was suggested that a physical might provide Mrs. Smith with some knowledge about her own health status. Her physical examination was completed by the nurse practitioner.
4. The social worker at the clinic asked Mrs. Smith if there were any other areas in which she might need assistance. Mrs. Smith stated that she could use some assistance with housing, employment, and food. The social worker and the social work intern provided Mrs. Smith with a contact name and direct number for the local housing authority to determine if she would qualify for assistance with Section 8 housing (housing assistance provided to families meeting federal guidelines). Mrs. Smith was also provided with a referral for a food bank (in the same building as the clinic) so that she would be able to get food after her time at the clinic. Finally, she was referred to an employment support program (provided with an actual contact name and direct number) to assist her with locating full-time employment.
5. The nurse practitioner at the clinic provided Mrs. Smith with a prescription for the medications she needed for her child. The social worker assisted Mrs. Smith with completing prescription assistance paperwork to qualify for prescription assistance from the pharmaceutical company.

Case 2: Mr. Jackson

Marty Jackson is a 35-year-old homeless man who has had repeated incarcerations for alcohol abuse, public drunkenness, and simple assaults when drunk. Mr. Jackson's most recent arrest occurred while he was loitering in a local park in a downtown urban area. Individuals at the park called the police and reported that a man was "harassing" individuals in the park. The police arrived at the park to find Mr. Jackson incoherent and disoriented. The police officer observed that Mr. Jackson had an alcoholic odor and had difficulty walking. The officer also observed that Mr. Jackson had an open wound on his hand that had been hastily wrapped in a soiled bandage.

The police officer transported Mr. Jackson to the local hospital for observation. During the ride in the police car, Mr. Jackson complained that "Marvin" was taking up too much of the backseat and was threatening him with a knife. The only occupants in the vehicle were the police officer and Mr. Jackson. Upon arrival at the hospital, the police officer noted to the intake nurse that Mr. Jackson might be hallucinating and recounted his comments on the ride to the hospital. The intake nurse placed Mr. Jackson in an area of the hospital where he could be observed and asked the police officer if he could remain with Mr. Jackson until a psychiatric evaluation could be completed.

The nurse then requested a psychiatric consult from the Mental Health Unit in the hospital. The Mental Health Unit used an interdisciplinary approach to service provision, in which patients were seen by a team consisting of a psychiatrist, a psychiatric nurse specialist, a clinical social worker, and a psychologist. A clinical social worker (LCSW) was sent to the emergency room and interviewed Mr. Jackson.

The clinical social worker conducted a bio-psycho-social assessment of Mr. Jackson that included an evaluation of whether he posed any harm to himself (suicide) or to others (homicide). The clinical social worker's assessment found that Mr. Jackson was not homicidal or suicidal, but noted that there was a possibility of some mental instability. Mr. Jackson did meet all of the risk markers for alcoholism. He adamantly stated he wanted to stop drinking but claimed the alcohol subdued his "moments of confusion and voices."

The clinical social worker called for a consult from another member of the mental health team, the psychiatric nurse. The psychiatric nurse reviewed the initial assessment and assessed Mr. Jackson for mental health risk. The nurse and clinical social worker met and conferred about their assessment findings and determined that Mr. Jackson had bipolar disorder and needed medication to be able to function without continued intervention by law enforcement. The psychiatric nurse and social worker worked together to create the following treatment plan for Mr. Jackson:

1. Mr. Jackson was given a 3-day regimen of medication for bipolar disorder and scheduled for a follow-up consultation with the psychiatric team at the county services board. The clinical social worker contacted the mental health worker on the crisis intervention team at the county services board and scheduled an appointment for Mr. Jackson. Initially, the scheduler indicated he could not be seen for at least 3 weeks. The social worker emphasized that Mr. Jackson was an alcoholic and had expressed a desire to stop drinking if he could get some help. The social worker reminded the scheduler that withdrawal from alcohol could have serious medical complications and Mr. Jackson would need to be seen within 3 days to prevent serious medical harm. His appointment was scheduled for 3 days from the current day.
2. The psychiatric nurse followed up with the intake nurse to be sure Mr. Jackson had received the needed treatment for his hand wound and to ascertain if he would need additional medications.
3. The social worker called the local shelter for men dealing with the issue of homelessness to inquire if they had a bed for Mr. Jackson. The shelter intake worker indicated that he would be able to stay at the shelter but would need to remain sober and would be drug tested. The shelter staff indicated that their program included Alcoholics Anonymous (AA) meetings and residents were required to attend.

4. The psychiatric nurse contacted a colleague (and fellow psychiatric nurse) at a local health clinic to determine if Mr. Jackson would qualify for follow-up services for his wound (physical health) and monitoring until his appointment with the county services board. The community clinic had a partnership with the local men's shelter and agreed to schedule an appointment to follow up with Mr. Jackson the next morning.
5. Mr. Jackson was allowed to regain his sobriety in the hospital that evening. Once he was able to travel, he was provided with bus fare to travel to the shelter. The social worker called the shelter to notify the staff there of his impending arrival. The nurse called a few hours later to confirm Mr. Jackson had arrived at the shelter and reviewed his medical and mental health needs with his shelter case worker (with a signed release from the patient).

IMPLICATIONS FOR PRACTICE

These cases suggest how social work and nursing professionals can work effectively as an interdisciplinary team. The role of the social worker and nurse, in each of the cases, was that of advocate—in each instance, the social worker and nurse sought out resources that would be useful to the client and enhance the client's ability to function in his or her everyday life. The role of advocate played by the professionals in each case scenario was critical to the client's health. The interdisciplinary team worked together to avoid compartmentalizing each client's issues, which ensured the delivery of more effective and efficient services for the client.

REFERENCES

Annas, G. (1988). The hospital: A human rights wasteland. In G. Annas (Ed.), *Judging medicine*. (pp. 9–29). Clifton, NJ: Human Press.

Annas, G., & Healey, J. (1974). The patients' rights advocate. *Journal of Nursing Administration*, 4, 25–31.

Barker, R. (1995). *The social work dictionary* (3rd ed.). Washington, DC: NASW Press.

Brawley, E. A. (1997). Teaching social work students to use advocacy skills though mass media. *Journal of Social Work Education*, 33(3), 445–460.

Bu, X., & Jewesky, M. A. (2006). Developing an id-range theory of patient advocacy through concept analysis. *Journal of Advanced Nursing*, 57(1), 101–110.

Clark, E. J. (2007). Advocacy: Profession's cornerstone. *NASW News*, 52(7), 3.

Dorfman, R. A. (1996). *Clinical social work: Definition, practice, and vision*. New York: Brunner/Mazel.

Faust, J. R. (2008). Clinical social worker as patient advocate in a community mental health center. *Clinical Social Work Journal*, 36, 293–300.

Gilbert, N., & Specht, H. (1976). Advocacy and professional ethics. *Social Work*, 21(4), 288–293.

Hanks, R. (2010). The medical–surgical nurse perspective of advocate role. *Nursing Forum*, 45(2), 97–107.

Hoefer, R. (2006). *Advocacy practice*. Chicago, IL: Lyceum Books.

Hyland, D. (2002). An exploration of the relationship between patient autonomy and patient advocacy: Implications for nursing practice. *Nursing Ethics, 9*(5), 472–482.

Jenkins, R. (2012). Using advocacy to safeguard older people with learning disabilities. *Nursing Older People, 24*(6), 31–36.

Jugessur, T., & Iles, I. (2009). Advocacy in mental health nursing: An integrative review of the literature. *Journal of Psychiatric and Mental Health Nursing, 16*(2), 187–195.

Johnson, L. (1995). *Social work practice: A generalist approach* (5th ed.). Boston, MA: Allyn & Bacon.

Kirst-Ashman, K. K., & Hull, Jr., G. (2009). *Generalist practice with organizations and communities* (4th ed.). Belmont, CA: Brooks/Cole.

Lara, A., & Salberg, L. (2009). Patient advocacy: What is its role? *Pacing and Clinical Electrophysiology, 32*(suppl. 2), S83–S85.

Lens, V. (2004). Principled negotiation: A new tool for case advocacy. *Social Work, 49*(3), 506–513.

Lynch, R., & Mitchell, J. (1995) Justice system advocacy: A must for NASW and the social work community. *Social Work, 40*(1), 9–12.

MacDonald, H. (2006). Relational ethics and advocacy in nursing: Literature review. *Journal of Advanced Nursing, 57*(2), 119–126.

Mahlin, M. (2010). Individual patient advocacy, collective responsibility, and activism within the professional nursing associations. *Nursing Ethics, 17*(2), 247–254.

Mallik, M. (1997). Advocacy in nursing: A review of the literature. *Journal of Advanced Nursing, 25,* 130–138.

Martin, D., & Tipton, B. (2007). Patient advocacy in the USA: Key communication role functions. *Nursing and Health Sciences, 9,* 185–191.

McGrath, P., Holewa, H., & McGrath, Z. (2006). Nursing advocacy in an Australian multidisciplinary context: Findings on medico-centrism. *Scandinavian Journal of Caring Science, 20,* 394–402.

McCrae, N., & Mayer, F. (2014). The role of nurses in tackling female genital mutilation. *International Journal of Nursing Studies, 51*(6), 829–832.

Mickelson, J. S. (1995). Advocacy. In R. L. Edwards (Ed.), *Encyclopedia of social work* (19th ed., Vol. 1, pp. 95–100). Washington, DC: NASW Press.

Miley, K. K., O'Melia, M., & DuBois, B. (2009). *Generalist social work practice: An empowering approach* (6th ed.). Boston, MA: Pearson.

Mmatli, T. (2009). Translating disability-related research into evidence-based advocacy: The role of people with disabilities. *Disability and Rehabilitation, 31*(1), 14–22.

National Association of Social Workers. (1994). *NASW code of ethics.* Washington, DC: Author.

Pierce, D. (1984). *Policy for the social work practitioner.* New York: Longman.

Pullen, F. (1995). Advocacy: A specialist practitioner role. *British Journal of Nursing, 4*(5), 275–278.

Schneider, R., & Lester, L. (2000). *Social work advocacy: A new framework for action.* Belmont, CA: Brooks/Cole.

Sheafor, B., & Horejsi, C. R. (2003). *Techniques and guidelines for social work practice* (6th ed.). Boston, MA: Allyn and Bacon.

Smith, R. F. (1995). Settlements and neighborhood center. In R. L. Edwards (Ed.), *Encyclopedia of social work* (19th ed., Vol. 3, pp. 2129–2135). Washington, DC: NASW Press.

Sosin, M., & Caulum, S. (1983). Advocacy: A conceptualization for social work practice. *Social Work, 28*(1), 12–17.

Vaartio, H., Leino-Kilpi, H., Suominen, T., & Puukka, P. (2009). Nursing advocacy in procedural pain care. *Nursing Ethics, 16*(3), 340–362.

Walker, L., & Avant, P. (1995). *Strategies for theory construction in nursing* (3rd ed.). Norwalk, CT: Appleton & Lange.

Zomorodi, M., & Foley, B. J. (2009). The nature of advocacy vs paternalism in nursing: Clarifying the "thin line." *Journal of Advanced Nursing, 65*(8), 1746–1752.

Chapter 3

Cultural Competence and Resilience

Mary de Chesnay, Patricia L. Hart, and Jane Brannan

OBJECTIVES

At the end of this chapter, the reader will be able to

1. Define the term cultural competence, as differentiated from cultural sensitivity.
2. Compare and contrast the models of cultural competence.
3. Analyze the concept of resilience from the points of view of the patient who is resilient and the nurse who is attempting to promote resilience.

INTRODUCTION

This chapter examines two key concepts that are particularly useful in caring for people who are vulnerable. *Cultural competence* is a way of providing care that takes into account cultural differences between the nurse and the patient while meeting the health needs of the patient. *Resilience* is both a characteristic and a desired outcome; it is the capacity for transcending obstacles, which is present to some degree in all human beings. A goal of nursing is to enhance resilience. The central idea of the chapter is that the concepts of cultural competence and resilience relate in specific ways that enable nurses to frame care within a cultural context, not just for vulnerable populations but for all clients.

CULTURAL COMPETENCE

Cultural competence is a way of practicing one's profession by being sensitive to the differences in cultures of one's constituents and acting in a way that is respectful of the client's values and traditions while performing those activities or procedures necessary for the client's well-being. In nursing, the outcomes are positive changes in health status or lifestyle changes expected to prevent disease.

A social justice view of cultural competence should take into account what Hall (Hall, 1999; Hall, Stevens, & Meleis, 1994) described as marginalization. Marginalized people experience discrimination, poor access to health care, and resultant illnesses and traumas from environmental dangers or violence that make them vulnerable to a wide range of health problems. In a life history study of successful African American adults, for example, the effect of racism was pronounced; success at overcoming racism emphasizes the importance of culture in reducing health disparities (de Chesnay, 2005). Culturally competent practitioners, then, not only would seem to concern themselves with superficial skills of learning about other cultures, but also would view marginalized patients within a wider system context and intervene within that context.

Historically, nursing has moved from a view of cultural sensitivity (focus on awareness) to one of cultural competence (focus on behavior). In other words, nurses aspire to cultural competence not because the concept is trendy or politically correct as described by Poole (1998), but because nurses are pragmatists who understand that recognizing cultural differences enables them to interact with patients and their families in ways that enable them to heal.

Zoucha (2001) urged that we put aside deep-seated feelings of ethnocentrism and accept the value that every health worldview is equally valid. Locsin (2000) proposed that cultural blurring might be a technique that bridges the gaps in cultural differences by enabling the practitioner to merge the best of both worlds. Cultural competence then becomes a practice with broad appeal in all of the service professions. Teachers, social workers, and physicians all understand the usefulness of this concept as not just politically correct, but good practice (Bonder, Martin, & Miracle, 2001; Dana & Matheson, 1992; Gutierrez & Alvarez, 1996; Leavitt, 2003; Sutton, 2000).

MODELS OF CULTURAL COMPETENCE

As an exciting theoretical development in nursing, several models have been introduced to explore the dimensions of cultural competence. In reference to community health nursing, Kim-Godwin, Clarke, and Barton (2001) constructed a model derived from concept analysis that focuses on the relationship between cultural competence and health outcomes for diverse populations. They suggested that the four dimensions of cultural competence are caring, cultural sensitivity, cultural knowledge, and cultural skills. These authors developed a cultural competence scale that measures all dimensions except caring; items cover both the affective and cognitive domains. When they tested the scale in a sample of 192 senior undergraduate and graduate nursing students, the authors found factors that loaded on two dimensions, sensitivity and skill, explaining 72% of the variance and providing evidence of construct validity.

A second model portrayed cultural competence as a process in which the healthcare provider integrates cultural awareness, cultural knowledge, cultural skill, cultural encounters, and cultural desire (Campinha-Bacote, 2002). This model assumes variations exist both within groups and between groups—an important distinction for those who would treat members of ethnic groups as if they are exactly like everyone else within their group, thereby constructing new stereotypes instead of developing cultural knowledge. Campinha-Bacote (2003, 2005) updated her model to elaborate on several of the key concepts and to suggest the relevance of cultural competence to Christianity and moral reasoning.

Taking a different direction, Purnell (2000, 2002, 2012, 2014) and Purnell and Paulanka (2003) integrated the concepts of biocultural ecology and workforce issues into his model for cultural competence. Purnell asserted that healthcare providers and recipients of care have a mutual obligation to share information to obtain beneficial outcomes. In this sense, the patient is both a teacher of culture and a client of the provider; the provider, in turn, becomes a teacher of the culture of health care. Derived from many disciplines and including many domains, the Purnell model might be seen as a diagram encompassing the patient within a series of concentric circles that include family, community, and global society.

A third view of cultural competence states that existing models are insufficient and the term itself is limiting. Wells (2000) argued for extending the concept of cultural competence into cultural proficiency. According to this author, cultural competence is not adequate; rather, proficiency is a higher-order concept for institutions in that proficiency indicates mastery of a complex set of skills. The process of moving toward proficiency requires overcoming barriers that are both affective and cognitive. The most serious barrier is the unwillingness to examine one's own assumptions about people who are different from oneself. Wells would say that the most effective way to develop cultural proficiency is to maintain an open attitude and to interact with people who are different, allowing them to become your teachers or coaches.

Except for Leininger's (1970, 1995) extensive work, most nursing theories do not include cultural competence because they were published long before its emergence as a major concept for nursing. The application of several of the nursing theories to caring for vulnerable populations is discussed elsewhere in Unit II of this book. However, Watson's theory of caring deserves special note. In a theoretical review of Watson's theory, Mendycka (2000) explored the relationship of culture and care, providing a clinical example of how the nurse and the patient become more human through their interaction. In his description of a case of an American Indian who is HIV positive, Mendycka showed how a nurse practitioner trying to treat the patient with a traditional Western medical approach comes into conflict with the patient's cultural belief system. On the one hand, the nurse wants to see the patient more often and suggests pharmacotherapy to prevent progression of the HIV infection to full-blown AIDS. On the other hand, the patient wants to use the healing practices of his tribe: sweat baths, herbs, and prayer. Unless the nurse practitioner can find a way to work with the tribe's medicine man, she is doomed to failure because the patient will place his own cultural belief system above the uncertainties of Western medical practice.

Other authors have recognized the need for institutional change to develop culturally competent models of intervention for the populations served by diverse providers. For example, home care nurses must manage cultural issues with their patients (DiCicco-Bloom & Cohen, 2003). Andrews (1998) applied the process of developing cultural competence to administration in an assessment process leading to organizational change in cultural competence. Holistic nursing, which views patients within a series of contexts, has cultural competence as a core value. In a review of the concept in the holistic nursing literature, however, Barnes, Craig, and Chambers (2000) found that only 9.6% of the abstracts made reference to concepts of culture or ethnicity; these authors raised the question of whether the sample sizes were large enough to address cultural differences or whether the researchers lacked awareness of these issues. Finally, authors in psychiatric nursing (Craig, 1999; Kennedy, 1999) and oncology (Kagawa-Singer, 2000) have addressed the need for practitioners to develop cultural competence at both individual and institutional levels.

LEARNING CULTURAL COMPETENCE

Although many methods and ideas for developing cultural competence are described in the literature, there is general agreement on certain precepts—namely, that cultural competence happens on affective, cognitive, and behavioral levels and that self-awareness is a critical indicator of success. Campinha-Bacote (2006) suggests that standardization of nursing curricula might be effective in ensuring that nurses address issues related to cultural competence.

Simulation activities provide a setting in which participants can practice communication and problem solving as well as develop self-awareness (Meltzoff & Lenssen, 2000). Cross-cultural communication exercises for physicians can help them develop the skills needed to overcome barriers in this regard (Shapiro, Hollingshead, & Morrison, 2002).

Immersion programs are powerful learning experiences at all levels because they enable participants to experience different cultures out of their usual safe context.

Immersion programs are probably the best way to induce cultural competence, although they are costly and time consuming. There are several examples in this book, which explore in detail how undergraduate students and graduate nursing students can conduct fieldwork that leads to cultural competence. One example of an immersion program used in nutrition studies is a food travel course in which participants learn diverse dietetic preferences and practices (Kuczmarski & Cole, 1999). Another example is a population-based program with the Hutterites of the United States and Canada (Fahrenwald, Boysen, Fischer, & Maurer, 2001).

Didactic materials can be prepared for developing knowledge about groups and are a useful point of reference for practitioners who are under enormous pressure to function with diverse patients in high-acuity settings. An innovative program at the University of Washington used action research as the basis for developing culture clues—a series of documents that enable practitioners to see at a glance the dominant preferences of the diverse cultural groups served by the hospital. These documents cover perception of illness, patterns of kinship and decision making, and comfort with touch. They were written for a variety of cultures, including Korean, Russian, Latino, Albanian, Vietnamese, and African American (Abbot et al., 2002).

The didactic approach was also used in Sweden, which is becoming more diverse as immigration into the country increases, largely from Eastern Europe and Iraq. The researchers used Leininger's theory to guide development of a curriculum for undergraduate nursing students with specific content areas at all levels (Gebru & Willman, 2003).

Didactic programs are easier and less costly to operate than immersion programs, perhaps because cognitive outcomes are easier to measure than affective outcomes. In one multicultural training course for counseling students, outcomes included development of multicultural knowledge and skill and increased comfort with discussing differing worldviews; the program was less successful at getting participants to examine themselves as racial–cultural beings, however (Tomlinson-Clark, 2000).

RESILIENCE

Resilience is the ability of individuals to bounce back or to cope successfully despite adverse circumstances (Rutter, 1985). The *Merriam-Webster Online Dictionary* (2014) defines resilience as "an ability to recover from or adjust easily to change or misfortune" and the *American Heritage Online Dictionary* (2011) defines it as "the ability to recover quickly from illness, depression, change, or misfortune; buoyancy." Resilience has been referred to as both a personality trait and a dynamic process (Luthar, Cicchetti, & Becker, 2000). Dyer and McGuinness (1996) define resilience as "a global term describing a process whereby people bounce back from adversity and go on with their lives. It is a dynamic process highly influenced by protective factors" (p. 277).

Two concept analyses have been conducted for resilience (Earvolino-Ramirez, 2007; Gillespie, Chaboyer, & Wallis, 2007). Both studies used Walker and Avant's (2005) method of inquiry to guide the approach for the concept analysis. In this analytical technique, antecedents are the events or incidents that occur before the occurrence of the concept, whereas consequences are circumstances that result from the concept (Walker & Avant, 2005). Earvolino-Ramirez (2007) found that the main antecedent to resilience is adversity. Gillespie et al. (2007) found that, in addition to adversity, three other antecedents to resilience exist—interpretation of the event as either physically and/ or psychologically traumatic, the cognitive ability to interpret adversity, and a realistic worldview rather than a false optimism or depressive attitude. Integration, control, adjustment, growth (Gillespie et al., 2007), effective coping, mastery, and positive adaptation (Earvolino-Ramirez, 2007) were found to be consequences of resilience. Walker and Avant (2005) describe defining attributes as the cluster of characteristics that are most frequently associated with the concept and that are consistently present when the concept occurs. Earvolino-Ramirez (2007) found the defining attributes of resilience to be rebounding/reintegration, high expectancy/self-determination, positive relationships/ social support, flexibility, sense of humor, and self-esteem/self-efficacy, while Gillespie et al. (2007) found them to be self-efficacy, hope, and coping. The importance of conducting concept analyses is to acquire an understanding of the concept so that theoretical models can subsequently be developed to test the concept; the investigation then progresses to research studies that examine the effectiveness of strategies and interventions to help build resilience in vulnerable populations.

Resilience has been studied in numerous vulnerable populations, such as children, older adults, women, and survivors of disasters. Resilience research has also been explored in the nursing profession.

Children

Resilience in children has been studied in many different populations and situations. Research has been conducted on children in poverty (Anthony, 2008; Fotso, Holding, & Ezeh, 2009; Sanders, Lim, & Sohn, 2008), children with a parent who suffers from mental illness (Foster, O'Brien, & Korhonen, 2012; Fraser & Pakenham, 2008; Rounding, Hart, Hibbard, & Carroll, 2011), children of divorced parents (Regev & Ehrenberg, 2012), children with chronic and terminal illness (Betancourt et al., 2011; Im & Kim, 2012: Tonks et al., 2011), children suffering from child abuse and neglect (Jaffee, Caspi, Moffitt, Polo-Tomas, & Taylor, 2007), and homeless children (Rew, Taylor-Seehafer, Thomas, & Yockey, 2001), to identify but a few populations. Children who are resilient are able to respond to adversity by adapting to their circumstances, coping with and managing major life problems and events, and succeeding despite immeasurable disadvantages in life (Dent & Cameron, 2003).

Family resiliency has been found to comprise a series of complex interactions between risk and protective factors operating at individual (locus of control; emotional regulation; belief systems; self-efficacy; effective coping skills; education, skills, and training; health; temperament; and gender), family (family structure, intimate-partner relationship stability, family cohesion, supportive parent–child interaction, stimulating environment, social support, family of origin influences, stable and adequate income, and adequate housing), and community (involvement in the community, peer acceptance, supportive mentors, safe neighborhoods, access to quality schools and child care, and access to quality health care) levels (Benzies & Mychasiuk, 2009). Risk factors for families may change over time, so different protective factors may be more beneficial at different times resulting in a variety of outcomes. Several intervention programs have been conducted to build resilience in children, such as the Keeping Families Strong program (Riley et al., 2008), Coping and Promoting Strength Program (CAPS) (Ginsburg, 2009), and the Bridge Project (Anthony, Alter, & Jenson, 2009) to name a few.

Women

Resilience has been studied in various situations with women. McGrath, Wiggin, and Caron (2010), for example, found a relationship between body image dissatisfaction and resilience. In the study, college women who had a positive relationship with their parents were more resilient and, therefore, demonstrated less body image dissatisfaction. In a phenomenological study conducted by Singh, Hays, Chung, and Watson (2010), the researchers found resilience strategies used by Asian immigrant women in the United States who survived child sexual abuse. The resilience strategies used by these women included use of silence, sense of hope, South Asian social support, social advocacy, and intentional self-care. These strategies allowed the women to heal and move on with their lives.

Kinsel (2005) identified factors that were salient to resilience in older women. Having a social connectedness with family, friends, and the community provided support mechanisms as well as allowed these women to extend themselves to help others. Spiritual grounding was important to the women in providing a higher power to lean on, which gave meaning and purpose to their lives. Resilient older women took a "head-on" approach to adversity to move forward through life challenges (Kinsel, 2005).

Older Adults

Many adults face adversity in their older years, as evidenced by decreasing functional status, declining health, increasing stress, poorer living conditions, and experiencing negative life events (Hildon, Montgomery, Blane, Wiggins, & Netuveli, 2010). Protective attributes of more resilient older adults include good quality relationships, integration in the community, and use of developmental and adaptive coping styles. Older adults who receive support from family, have a broad network of friends (Wells, 2009), and have confiding relationships with others are found to be more resilient than those without these types of relationships (Hildon et al., 2010; Hildon, Smith, Netuveli, & Blane, 2008). Terminally ill older adults facing death demonstrate resilient behaviors by redefining their self, embracing religion and spirituality in times of uncertainty, maintaining social relationships, and defending their independence as the end of their life approaches (Nelson-Becker, 2006).

Cultural values also play an important part in how older individuals exhibit resilience. Becker and Newsom (2005) found that older African Americans responded to their disabling illnesses by demonstrating determination, perseverance, and tenacity as resilient behaviors leading to a culturally specific philosophy of resilience.

Survivors of Disasters

Several studies have been conducted to explore resilience in survivors of disasters. Bonanno, Galea, Bucciarelli, and Vlahov (2007) examined the role of demographics, resources, and life stress on psychological resilience of individuals in New York City after the September 11, 2001, terrorist attacks. The researchers found that the "prevalence of resilience was uniquely predicted by participant gender, age, race/ethnicity, and education level; by the absence of depression and substance use; by less income loss, social support, and fewer chronic diseases; and by less direct impact of September 11 and fewer recent life stressors, fewer past prior traumatic events, and not having experienced an additional traumatic event since September 11" (p. 676).

Greene (2007) reviewed three case study transcripts of older adult survivors of Hurricane Katrina to identify themes of survivorship that promoted resilience in these older adults. These themes were resolving to live, obtaining food and shelter, choosing survival strategies, keeping family ties, connecting with community, and giving testimony. Kanji, Drummond, and Cameron (2007), in a review of resilience in Afghan children and their families, postulated that protective factors that influenced their survival and abilities to rebuild their lives while still facing a magnitude of challenges included faith in Allah (God), family support, and community support.

Nurses

Factors contributing to the need for resilient behaviors in nurses include challenging workplaces, psychological emptiness, diminishing inner balance, and a sense of dissonance in the workplace (Glass, 2009; Hart, Brannan, & de Chesnay, 2014; Hodges, Keeley, & Troyan, 2008). To date, however, very little research has been conducted on resilience in nurses (Ablett & Jones, 2007; Gillespie, Chaboyer, & Wallis, 2009; Gillespie, Chaboyer, Wallis, & Grimbeck, 2007; Glass, 2009; Hart et al., 2012; Hodges et al., 2008; Simoni,

Larrabee, Birkhimer, Mott, & Gladden, 2004). Characteristics found in resilient nurses include hope, self-efficacy, coping, control, competence, flexibility, adaptability, hardiness, sense of coherence, skill recognition, and nondeficiency focusing. Nurses employed cognitive reframing, grounding connections and work–life balance, critical reflection, and reconciliation as strategies to build resilience (Ablett & Jones, 2007; Glass, 2009; Hart et al., 2012; Hodges et al., 2008).

Additional nursing research needs to be conducted on resilience and resilient attributes to enhance the resilience process in vulnerable, diverse populations and situations. Better understanding of how some individuals remain resilient despite facing adversity may lead to successful implementation of strategies and interventions for others. Nurses are in key positions to perform resiliency assessments and intervene to promote well-being and positive outcomes in vulnerable populations (Ahren, 2006).

CASE STUDY

Case Study: Donna

The following example illustrates the relationship of cultural competence and resilience. Although fictional and representing only a small type of population, this case study shows that helping patients to become more resilient is a cross-cultural strategy.

Donna swung her new vehicle into a parking space, grabbed her lunch sack, and trotted upstairs to the cardiovascular rehabilitation unit at Morris Center. Her assignment was already posted, and she noted that she was still working with Mr. Hernandez, a 60-year-old man who had suffered a cerebrovascular accident (CVA or stroke) and who continued to have hemiparesis on his left side. Donna sighed and prepared for care.

Mr. Hernandez had immigrated to the United States from Cuba 5 years ago. He worked for a local food distribution company. His family had been literally swarming around him each day in his room. His wife and grown daughter were there every day. In addition, his two sons, his brother, his elderly mother, and her sister arrived periodically to tend to him. It wasn't so much that they were present frequently (although it did pose a challenge to provide care when weaving among the people); rather, Donna's larger concern was the effect that the family's hovering had on Mr. Hernandez's physical rehabilitation and recovery. Lately, he did not seem to be coping well with his limitations. He seemed depressed, anxious, and fatigued—more so now than when he arrived at the unit 2 weeks ago.

Donna entered the room and found Mrs. Hernandez shaving her husband. She stated, "Oh my—Mrs. Hernandez, he should do that for himself. Your husband is quite capable of shaving himself. Don't you remember us saying it several days ago, that he must become more independent?" Mrs. Hernandez scurried aside, head bowed, eyes downcast, and mumbling an apology. Donna continued her morning assessment, and provided information to the patient and family about his physical state and the physical therapy he was doing today. But she was annoyed. Didn't they listen? Don't they understand that they were hindering care? Every day Mrs. Hernandez continued to do things for her husband that he could do for himself.

The situation was frustrating. Mr. Hernandez's progress was slower than Donna expected, and she didn't seem to be able to help him deal with his depression. The illness had really hit him hard emotionally. It seemed as if the family was undermining Donna's care—doing everything for the patient and not allowing him to regain his strength.

Later that afternoon, Donna expressed her concerns at a multidisciplinary team meeting. Margarite, the new nurse educator (who was originally from Puerto Rico) spoke up: "I think what you are seeing is very much what is considered a display of love and concern in this family. Independence and self-care during an illness is not particularly a value for them. The pampering and indulgence by his family are expected by Mr. Hernandez. Maybe we can talk about ways Mrs. Hernandez can still provide care that does not alter his treatment. We also should discuss how we can help Mr. Hernandez deal with the overwhelming concern about how his life has changed with this illness and help him develop some strategies to address his concerns." Donna realized that she had misinterpreted the actions of the Hernandez family by not having a clear understanding of their cultural mores.

Working together, the team made a plan for working with Mr. Hernandez to enhance his coping and resilience. His family priest and counselors at the center began meeting with him and his family. His family also was consulted regarding activities they could do to assist Mr. Hernandez to move forward in his physical development, while still allowing them to care for him. Mrs. Hernandez was asked to help minimally by providing morning care and bringing favorite meals from home for him to eat. Other family members accompanied Mr. Hernandez to physical therapy activities during the day to learn how they might help him continue these exercises at home.

Based on Donna's experience working with the Hernandez family, she orchestrated a cultural competency program for the staff working in the rehabilitation hospital. The program focused on caring for patients from various ethnicities and backgrounds to ensure that the staff understood and were sensitive to cultural traditions and relationships within families.

CONCLUSION

Cultural competence is a set of behaviors that transcend mere good intentions. Accepting that cultural differences exist reflects an open mind, which in turn leads to exploring the client's own strengths and adaptive capabilities. Using cultural resources at the client's disposal concurrently with "best practices" in nursing and medicine is not only culturally appropriate, it is also likely to develop resilience. Both cultural competence and resilience have much relevance to nursing practice.

REFERENCES

Abbot, P., Short, E., Dodson, S., Garcia, C., Perkins, J., & Wyant, S. (2002). Improving your cultural awareness with culture clues. *Nurse Practitioner*, 27(2), 44–49.

Ablett, J. R., & Jones, R. S. P. (2007). Resilience and well-being in palliative care staff: A qualitative study of hospice nurses' experience of work. *Psycho-Oncology*, 16(8), 733–740.

Ahren, N. R. (2006). Adolescent resilience: An evolutionary concept analysis. *Journal of Pediatric Nursing*, 21(3), 175–185.

Andrews, M. (1998). A model for cultural change. *Nursing Management, 29*(10), 62–66.

Anthony, E. K. (2008). Cluster profiles of youths living in urban poverty: Factors affecting risk and resilience. *Social Work Research, 32*(1), 6–17.

Anthony, E. K., Alter, C. F., & Jenson, J. M. (2009). Development of a risk and resilience-based out-of-school time program for children and youths. *Social Work, 54*(1), 45–55.

Barnes, D., Craig, K., & Chambers, K. (2000). A review of the concept of culture in holistic nursing literature. *Journal of Holistic Nursing, 18*(3), 207–221.

Becker, G., & Newsom, E. (2005). Resilience in the face of serious illness among chronically ill African Americans in later life. *Journal of Gerontology Series B: Psychological Sciences and Social Sciences, 60B*(4), S214–S223.

Benzies, K., & Mychasiuk, R. (2009). Fostering family resiliency: A review of the key protective factors. *Child and Family Social Work, 14*, 103–114.

Betancourt, T. S., Meyers-Ohki, S., Stulac, S. N., Barrera, A. E., Mushashi, C., & Beardslee, W. R. (2011). Nothing can defeat combined hands (Abashize hamwe ntakibananira): Protective processes and resilience in Rwandan children and families affected by HIV/AIDS. *Social Science & Medicine, 73*(5), 693–701.

Bonanno, G. A., Galea, S., Bucciarelli, A., & Vlahov, D. (2007). What predicts psychological resilience after disaster? The role of demographics, resources, and life stress. *Journal of Consulting and Clinical Psychology, 75*(5), 671–682.

Bonder, B., Martin, L., & Miracle, A. (2001). Achieving cultural competence: The challenge for clients and healthcare workers in a multicultural society. *Generations, 25*(1), 35–43.

Campinha-Bacote, J. (2002). The process of cultural competence in the delivery of health care services: A model of care. *Journal of Transcultural Nursing, 13*(3), 180–184.

Campinha-Bacote, J. (2003). *The process of cultural competence in the delivery of healthcare services: A culturally competent model of care* (4th ed.). Cincinnati, OH: Transcultural CARE Associates.

Campinha-Bacote, J. (2005). A biblically based model of cultural competence in healthcare delivery. *Journal of Multicultural Nursing and Health, 11*(2), 16–22.

Campinha-Bacote, J. (2006). Cultural competence in nursing curricula: How are we doing 20 years later? *Journal of Nursing Education, 45*(7), 243–244.

Craig, A. B. (1999). Mental health nursing and cultural diversity. *Australian and New Zealand Journal of Mental Health Nursing, 8*, 93–99.

Dana, R., & Matheson, L. (1992). An application of the agency cultural competence checklist to a program serving small and diverse ethnic communities. *Psychosocial Rehabilitation Journal, 15*(4), 101–106.

de Chesnay, M. (2005). "Can't keep me down": Life histories of successful African Americans. In M. de Chesnay (Ed.), *Caring for the vulnerable: Perspectives in nursing theory, practice and research* (pp. 221–234). Sudbury, MA: Jones and Bartlett.

Dent, R. J., & Cameron, R. J. (2003). Developing resilience in children who are in public care: The educational psychological perspective. *Educational Psychology in Practice, 19*(1), 3–20.

DiCicco-Bloom, B., & Cohen, D. (2003). Home care nurses: A study of the occurrence of culturally competent care. *Journal of Transcultural Nursing, 14*(1), 25–31.

Dyer, J. G., & McGuinness, T. M. (1996). Resilience: Analysis of the concept. *Archives of Psychiatric Nursing, 10*(5), 276–282.

Earvolino-Ramirez, M. (2007). Resilience: A concept analysis. *Nursing Forum, 42*(2), 73–82.

Fahrenwald, N., Boysen, R., Fischer, C., & Maurer, R. (2001). Developing cultural competence in the baccalaureate nursing student: A populations-based project with the Hutterites. *Journal of Transcultural Nursing, 12*(1), 48–55.

Foster, K., O'Brien, L., & Korhonen, T. (2012). Developing resilient children and families when parents have mental illness: A family-focused approach. *International Journal of Mental Health Nursing, 21*(1), 3–11.

Fotso, J. C., Holding, P. A., & Ezeh, A. C. (2009). Factors conveying resilience in the context of urban poverty: The case of orphans and vulnerable children in the informal settlements of Nairobi, Kenya. *Child & Adolescent Mental Health, 14*(4), 175–182.

Fraser, E., & Pakenham, K. I. (2008). Evaluation of a resilience-based intervention for children of parents with mental illness. *Australian & New Zealand Journal of Psychiatry, 42*(12), 1041–1050.

Gebru, K., & Willman, A. (2003). A research-based didactic model for education to promote culturally competent nursing care in Sweden. *Journal of Transcultural Nursing, 14*(1), 55–61.

Gillespie, B. M., Chaboyer, W., & Wallis, M. (2007). Development of a theoretically derived model of resilience through concept analysis. *Contemporary Nurse, 25*(1), 124–135.

Gillespie, B. M., Chaboyer, W., & Wallis, M. (2009). The influence of personal characteristics on the resilience of operating room nurses: A predictor study. *International Journal of Nursing Studies, 46*(7), 968–976.

Gillespie, B. M., Chaboyer, W., Wallis, M., & Grimbeck, P. (2007). Resilience in the operating room: Developing and testing of a resilience model. *Journal of Advanced Nursing, 59*(4), 427–438.

Ginsburg, G. S. (2009). The child anxiety prevention study: Intervention model and primary outcomes. *Journal of Consulting and Clinical Psychology, 77*(3), 580–587.

Glass, N. (2009). An investigation of nurses' and midwives' academic/clinical workplaces. *Holistic Nursing Practice, 23*(3), 158–170.

Greene, R. R. (2007). Reflections of Hurricane Katrina by older adults: Three case studies in resiliency survivorship. *Journal of Human Behavior in the Social Environment, 16*(4), 57–74.

Gutierrez, L., & Alvarez, A. (1996). Multicultural community organizing: A strategy for change. *Social Work, 41*(5), 501–509.

Hall, J. M. (1999). Marginalization revisited: Critical, postmodern and liberation perspectives. *Advances in Nursing Science, 22*(1), 88–102.

Hall, J. M., Stevens, P., & Meleis, A. (1994). Marginalization: A guiding concept for valuing diversity in nursing knowledge development. *Advances in Nursing Science, 16*(4), 23–41.

Hart, P. L., Brannan, J. D., & de Chesnay, M. (2014). Resilience in nurses: An integrative review. *Journal of Nursing Management, 22*, 720–734.

Hildon, Z., Montgomery, S. M., Blane, D., Wiggins, R. D., & Netuveli, G. (2010). Examining resilience of quality of life in the face of health-related and psychosocial adversity at older ages: What is "right" about the way we age? *Gerontologist, 50*(1), 36–47.

Hildon, Z., Smith, G., Netuveli, G., & Blane, D. (2008). Understanding adversity and resilience at older ages. *Sociology of Health & Illness, 30*(5), 1–15.

Hodges, H. F., Keeley, A. C., & Troyan, P. J. (2008). Professional resilience in baccalaureate-prepared acute care nurses: First steps. *Nursing Education Perspectives, 29*(2), 80–89.

Im, Y. J., & Kim, D. H. (2012). Factors associated with the resilience of school-aged children with atopic dermatitis. *Journal of Clinical Nursing, 21*(1/2), 80–88.

Jaffee, S. R., Caspi, A., Moffitt, T. E., Polo-Tomas, M., & Taylor, A. (2007). Individual, family, and neighborhood factors distinguish resilient from non-resilient maltreated children: A cumulative stressors model. *Child Abuse & Neglect, 31*(3), 231–253.

Kagawa-Singer, M. (2000). Addressing issues for early detection and screening in ethnic populations. *Oncology Nursing Forum, 27*(9), 55–61.

Kanji, Z., Drummond, J., & Cameron, B. (2007). Resilience in Afghan children and their families: A review. *Paediatric Nursing, 19*(2), 30–33.

Kennedy, M. (1999). Cultural competence and psychiatric nursing. *Journal of Transcultural Nursing, 10*(1), 11–18.

Kim-Godwin, Y. S., Clarke, P., & Barton, L. (2001). A model for the delivery of culturally competent care. *Journal of Advanced Nursing, 35*(6), 918–926.

Kinsel, B. (2005). Resilience as adaptation in older women. *Journal of Women & Aging, 17*(3), 23–39.

Kuczmarski, M., & Cole, R. (1999). Transcultural food habits travel courses: An interdisciplinary approach to teaching cultural diversity. *Topics in Clinical Nutrition, 15*(1), 59–71.

Leavitt, R. L. (2003). Developing cultural competence in a multicultural world: Part II. *Magazine of Physical Therapy, 11*(1), 56–70.

Leininger, M. (1970). *Nursing and anthropology: Two worlds to blend.* New York: John Wiley & Sons.

Leininger, M. (1995). *Transcultural nursing: Concepts, theories, research and practice.* New York: McGraw-Hill.

Locsin, R. (2000). Building bridges: Affirming culture in health and nursing. *Holistic Nursing Practice, 15*(1), 1–4.

Luthar, S., Cicchetti, D., & Becker, B. (2000). The construct of resilience: A critical evaluation and guidelines for future work. *Child Development, 71*(3), 543–562.

McGrath, R. J., Wiggin, J., & Caron, R. M. (2010). The relationship between resilience and body image in college women. *International Journal of Health, 10*(2). Retrieved from http://www.ispub.com/journal/the_internet_journal_of_health/volume_10_number_2_12/article_printable/the-relationship-between-resilience-and-body-image-in-college-women.html

Meltzoff, N., & Lenssen, J. (2000). Enhancing cultural competence through simulation activities. *Multicultural Perspectives, 2*(1), 29–35.

Mendycka, B. (2000). Exploring culture in nursing: A theory-driven practice. *Holistic Nursing Practice, 15*(1), 32–41.

Nelson-Becker, H. B. (2006). Voices of resilience: Older adults in hospice care. *Journal of Social Work in End-of-Life & Palliative Care, 2*(3), 87–106.

Poole, D. (1998). Politically correct or culturally competent? *Health and Social Work*, 23(3), 163–167.

Purnell, L. (2000). A description of the Purnell model for cultural competence. *Journal of Transcultural Nursing*, 11(1), 40–46.

Purnell, L. (2002). The Purnell model for cultural competence. *Journal of Transcultural Nursing*, 13(3), 193–196.

Purnell, L. (2012). *Transcultural health care: A culturally competent approach* (4th ed.). Philadelphia: F.A. Davis.

Purnell, L. (2014). *Guide to culturally competent healthcare* (3rd ed.). Philadelphia: F.A. Davis.

Purnell, L., & Paulanka, B. (2003). *Transcultural health care: A culturally competent approach* (2nd ed.). Philadelphia: F.A. Davis.

Regev, V. R., & Ehrenberg, M. F. (2012). A pilot study of a support group for children in divorcing families: Aiding community program development and marking pathways to resilience. *Journal of Divorce & Remarriage*, 53(3), 220–230.

Resilience. (2011). *The American heritage online dictionary*. Retrieved from http://dictionary.reference.com/browse/resilience

Resilience. (2014). *Merriam-Webster online dictionary*. Retrieved from http://www.merriam-webster.com/dictionary/resilience

Rew, L., Taylor-Seehafer, M., Thomas, N. Y., & Yockey, R. D. (2001). Correlates of resilience in homeless adolescents. *Journal of Nursing Scholarship*, 33(1), 33–43.

Riley, A. W., Valdez, C. R., Barrueco, S., Mills, C., Beardslee, W., Sandler, I., & Rawal, P. (2008). Development of a family-based program to reduce risk and promote resilience among families affected by maternal depression: Theoretical basis and program description. *Clinical Child and Family Psychology Review*, 11(1/2), 12–29.

Rounding, K., Hart, K. E., Hibbard, S., & Carroll, M. (2011). Emotional resilience in young adults who were reared by depressed parents: The moderating effects of offspring religiosity/spirituality. *Journal of Spirituality in Mental Health*, 13(4), 236–246.

Rutter, M. (1985). Resilience in the face of adversity: Protective factors and resistance to psychiatric disorder. *British Journal of Psychiatry*, 147, 598–611.

Sanders, A. E., Lim, S., & Sohn, W. (2008). Resilience to urban poverty: Theoretical and empirical considerations for population health. *American Journal of Public Health*, 98(6), 1101–1106.

Shapiro, J., Hollingshead, J., & Morrison, E. (2002). Primary care resident, faculty and patient views of barriers to cultural competence and the skills needed to overcome them. *Medical Education*, 36, 749–759.

Simoni, P. S., Larrabee, J. H., Birkhimer, T. L., Mott, C. L., & Gladden, S. D. (2004). Influence of interpretive styles of stress resiliency on registered nurse empowerment. *Nursing Administration Quarterly*, 28(3), 221–224.

Singh, A. A., Hays, D. G., Chung, Y. B., & Watson, L. (2010). South Asian immigrant women who have survived child sexual abuse: Resilience and healing. *Violence Against Women*, 16(4), 444–458.

Sutton, M. (2000). Cultural competence. *Family Practice Management*, 7(9), 58–61.

Tomlinson-Clark, S. (2000). Assessing outcomes in a multicultural training course: A qualitative study. *Counseling Psychology Quarterly*, *13*(2), 221–232.

Tonks, J., Yates, P., Frampton, I., Williams, W. H., Harris, D., & Slater, A. (2011). Resilience and the mediating effects of executive dysfunction after childhood brain injury: A comparison between children aged 9–15 years with brain injury and non-injured controls. *Brain Injury*, *25*(9), 870–881.

Walker, L., & Avant, K. (2005). *Strategies for theory construction in nursing* (4th ed.). Upper Saddle River, NJ: Pearson Prentice Hall.

Wells, M. (2000). Beyond cultural competence: A model for individual and institutional cultural development. *Journal of Community Health Nursing*, *17*(4), 189–200.

Wells, M. (2009). Resilience in rural community-dwelling older adults. *Journal of Rural Health*, *25*(4), 415–419.

Zoucha, R. (2001). President's message. *Journal of Transcultural Nursing*, *12*(2).

Chapter 4

Social Justice in Nursing: A Review of the Literature

Doris M. Boutain

OBJECTIVES

At the end of this chapter, the reader will be able to

1. Define social justice for nursing.
2. Compare and contrast the definitions of social justice used in the nursing literature.
3. Present a concise statement summarizing the state of the art for social justice as a concept for further development in nursing scholarship.

INTRODUCTION

This chapter explores how social justice was conceptualized in the nursing literature between the years 2000 and 2014. Analysis of this literature reveals that various authors ascribed to social, distributive, and market views of justice. Most authors, however, do not explicitly attend to the differences among these concepts. The three predominant models of justice are reviewed first in this chapter, and then a framework for how nurses can focus on injustice awareness, amelioration, and transformation as forms of social justice is presented. The multiple methods of promoting a social justice agenda, from consciousness raising to the re-creation of social policies, are also delineated. Recognizing the many ways to promote social justice can have a transformational impact on how nurses teach, research, and practice.

Although social justice is not a new concept, the nursing literature lacks a coherent and complex understanding of its implications for studying societal health (Buettner-Schmidt

& Lobo, 2012; Drevdahl, Kneipp, Canales, & Dorcy, 2001; Grace & Willis, 2012; Lipscomb, 2011). Social justice is often mentioned only briefly, as an afterthought to elaborate discussions about ethics. When ethics is defined in the forefront, the concept of social justice often recedes to the background, appearing fleetingly in the conclusion section of articles. Inattention to the subtle variations in how social justice is conceived can inadvertently result in nursing practice, research, and education that are antithetical to a social justice agenda.

LITERATURE SEARCH METHODOLOGY

A search of the Cumulative Index to Nursing and Allied Health Literature (CINAHL) database using the terms "social justice and nursing" from the years 2000 to 2014 identified a total of 184 publications which used the terms "social justice" as a major subject heading. A major subject heading is ascribed by the manuscript authors to classify the main focus of their work. The publications using social justice as a major subject heading included academic journal publications ($n = 156$), magazine publications ($n = 24$), dissertations ($n = 4$), continuing education units ($n = 4$), and a book ($n = 1$).

Only resources written in English were reviewed for this chapter. Two articles were not written in English. Thus, the total number of publications reviewed was 182. Although all English written resources were reviewed, only publications emphasizing uncommon points are included in the reference list to limit the chapter's length. The literature reviewed in the sections about views of justice in nursing education, research, and practice is limited to resources written within the stated time frame. Publications from nursing, sociology, social work, philosophy, public health, and religious studies supplement the literature analysis in the sections about the literature review critique and implications. Many of these resources were written prior to the literature review timeframe.

This chapter will first define how the concept of justice is used in nursing. Then, different ways of viewing justice are explored. Examples are provided about how social justice is articulated in articles focused on nursing education, research, and practice. Lastly, an alternative view of social justice is provided before the chapter summary.

Defining Justice in Nursing

The ethical principle of justice was referenced frequently in the nursing literature surveyed. More than half of the publications retrieved equated justice with what is fair. Authors primarily described ethics as a framework for understanding how values, duties, principles, and obligations informed one's sense of societal fairness. The notion that two orientations to ethics exist was also highlighted in the literature (Mathes, 2004, 2005; Woods, 2012). Specifically, ethics can be defined by a care orientation or by a justice orientation. For example, ethics can be defined by universal truths (justice orientation) or in relationship to caring for others in context (care orientation) (Mathes, 2004, 2005).

Although many authors mentioned justice, few articles actually defined justice beyond notions of ethical fairness (Drevdahl et al., 2001; Harris, 2005; Kneipp & Snider, 2001) or ethical relationship formation (Myhrvold, 2003). Most articles focused on caring for persons after injustice had already occurred, not changing policies or environments to promote justice. Two articles focused on the contradictions of working for justice in the context of unjust nursing environments (Galon & Wineman, 2010; Giddings, 2005a). Only one article examined the theoretical connection between social justice and spirituality (Pesut, Fowler, Reimer-Kirkham, Taylor, & Sawatzky, 2009).

Exploring the philosophical underpinnings of justice, Drevdahl et al. (2001) compared the concepts of social justice, distributive justice, and market justice. They posited that most nurses neither consider the distinction among concepts related to justice (Drevdahl et al., 2001) nor distinguish between social justice and social analysis (Stys, 2008). A few authors broaden the discussion of ethics to globalization (Falk-Rafael, 2006) or structural inequality (Sistrom & Hale, 2006) as having implications for social justice.

Without an intricate understanding of the different views of justice, nurses may limit their problem-solving abilities when attempting to understand how unjust social conditions influence health status, access, and delivery. Although concepts such as care (Boersma, 2006) and culture (Jackson, 2003) are not mutually exclusive to a justice ideology, inattention to the distinctions between care and justice may result in limited theoretical analysis and thus action. A review of the American Nurses Association's *Code of Ethics for Nurses with Interpretive Statements*, *Nursing's Social Policy Statement,* and *Nursing Scope and Standards of Practice*, for example, revealed inconsistent and superficial conceptualizations of social justice (Bekemeier & Butterfield, 2005). These points were also a cause for debate in review of the Canadian Nurses Association's (CNA) 2002 revised *Code of Ethics for Registered Nurses* (Hubert, 2004; Kikuchi, 2004). The disjunctions between practice, policy, and politics of justice; however, have a long history in nursing (Murphy, Canales, Norton, & DeFilippis, 2005). For this reason, it is important to explore the most prominent forms of justice in nursing literature today.

Social, Distributive, and Market Justice: Within and Beyond the Nursing Literature

Social, distributive, and market justice are the most common forms of justice referenced in the nursing literature. Social justice is often defined as a concern for the equitable measuring of benefits and burdens in society (Redman & Clark, 2002). Social justice is also—albeit less often—defined as changing social relationships and institutions to promote equitable relationships (Drevdahl et al., 2001). Distributive justice is discussed in reference to the equal distribution of goods and services in society (Silva & Ruth, 2003).

Market justice posits that people are entitled only to those goods and services that they acquire according to guidelines of entitlement (Young, 1990).

Although these forms of justice may appear similar at first glance, there are distinct differences between them when using multidisciplinary sources (Beauchamp, 1986; Whitehead, 1992). Social justice is concerned with making equitable the balance between societal benefits and burdens. It posits that social rights exist, but that collateral responsibilities come with those rights (Lebacqz, 1986). Social beings both give and receive in equitable measure, using equity as a framework for relating to one another. Equity, derived from the Greek word *epiky,* means that persons must conduct themselves with reasonableness and moderation when exercising their rights (Whitehead, 1992). Distributive justice involves equality more than equity; this concept is used most often to discuss the allocation or distribution of goods and services in society (Young, 1990). Equality focuses on giving the same access and resources to different socially vulnerable groups, without consideration for what factors created those differences.

Social justice advocates explore social relationships, including how those relationships form the basis for the allocation of goods and services (Young, 1990). Social justice focuses on equity, not equality or sameness. Thus the concepts of social and distributive justice are somewhat parallel, yet have different primary foci of study (Drevdahl et al., 2001).

Market justice is also viewed as a form of justice in nursing (Drevdahl, 2002). It is based on honoring the rights of those who have earned entitlement to those privileges. Market justice permits inequality as long as those inequalities result from a fair market system. That is, only those who earn rights can receive their entitled privileges in a market system. Those who earn no rights do not have secured privileges.

Critics of the market justice agenda note that using the word *market* as an adjective for *justice* is itself an oxymoron (Beauchamp, 1986). Justice is a word most often used to discuss fairness, equity, or the process of deliberation. The term *market* is most often concerned with the balance between monetary value and goods allocation. Thus, according to these critics, the two terms do not work together when discussing equity. Simply "applying the word 'justice' to 'market' does not bring the concept into the realm of justice" (Drevdahl et al., 2001, p. 24). Social justice is not a parallel model to market justice; rather, it is antithetical to a market model (Beauchamp, 1986). These two ways of viewing the world, therefore, diametrically oppose each other and simultaneously coexist.

An example may clarify the difference between social, distributive, and market justice. Using a social justice framework, everyone in the United States would be entitled to health care as needed if health care were deemed a right of citizenship. Health care, using a social justice view, is a moral obligation and a right of citizenship. A distributive justice framework would give a certain level of health care to everyone as a result of citizenship. The leveling of health care is needed to make sure that enough health care services are available for all citizens to receive at least minimal benefit. Within a distributive justice model, health is a right of citizens but not necessarily a moral responsibility. In a market system, people can receive health care as a result of how much they can pay for those services. The focus of a market system is not on moral or citizenship rights, but rather on making sure that those citizens who want the good of health care, for example, can pay for those services.

All forms of justice, although somewhat distinct, may coexist to varying degrees. For example, some healthcare services in the United States are given as needed, such as the care given to children who are orphaned. In other cases, minimal health care is given, such as the medical and dental benefits associated with Medicaid. Persons who can afford more treatment or faster treatment may get those services if they can pay a particular price; an example is healthcare clinics that are designed to give expanded services if clients pay certain access fees. Although these three forms of justice are noted in the nursing literature to varying degrees, seldom is it discussed how these views of justice guide nursing education, research, or practice.

Views of Justice in Nursing Education Articles

Most resources about nursing education and justice focus on the clinical preparation of undergraduate students to meet the needs of a culturally diverse population (Ezeonwu, 2013; Herman & Sassatelli, 2002; Leuning, 2001; Mohammed, 2014; Redman & Clark, 2002; Scanlan, Care, & Gessler, 2001). Simulations are currently viewed as novel ways to educate future nurses using a social justice framework (Menzel, Willson, & Doolen, 2014). Other publications proclaim the need for a global consciousness (Leuning, 2001; Messias, 2001), critical thinking (Pereira, 2006), culturally sensitive evidence-based practice (McMurray, 2004), and human rights education (Fitzpatrick, 2003) among nurses as the starting point for justice awareness. Also present in the nursing literature are curricular considerations (Fahrenwald et al., 2005; MacIntosh & Wexler, 2005; Myrick, 2005; Vickers, 2008), teaching models (Bond, Mandleco, & Warnick, 2004; Boutain, 2005; Fahrenwald, 2003; Lapum et al., 2012; Leuning, 2001), clinical evaluation frameworks (Boutain, 2008), case examples, and service-learning experiences (Herman & Sassatelli, 2002; Redman & Clark, 2002) that use justice as a framework to educate undergraduate students. A limited number of articles focus on teaching justice content in general (Abrams, 2009) or in graduate education (Browne & Tarlier, 2008; Shattell, Hogan, & Hernandez, 2006). Only one article was found exploring how teaching social justice affects faculty directly (Fahrenwald, Taylor, Kneipp, & Canales, 2007). Few articles use social justice as a theoretical framework for educational scholarship (Kirkham, Hofwegen, & Harwood, 2005; Moule, 2003) or as a means to understand how to conduct educational research in nursing (Comer, 2009).

Although some nurse educators discuss the practical application of justice principles, few distinguish between the use of social justice and distributive justice concepts. For instance, authors may define social justice using distributive justice principles of equality or as working with vulnerable populations (Redman & Clark, 2002). One manuscript introduces justice in terms of contractual justice, meaning the fair and honest contract between equals (Oddi & Oddi, 2000). In one instance, the term "social justice" was used but never defined (Herman & Sassatelli, 2002). Rarely is social justice used as a framework to critique nursing education models, student–faculty relationships (Oddi & Oddi, 2000; Scanlan et al., 2001), or develop a comprehensive curriculum (Snyder, 2014).

Even fewer articles focused on advancing theoretical insights about social justice. Giddings (2005b) described a model for how nurses may develop a social consciousness. A three position, flexible model was proposed. It focused on understanding (1) acquired, (2) awakened, and (3) expanded social consciousness among nurses. The contextualized model offers a way to work with nurses in light of the different ways to acquire social justice knowledge.

Views of Justice in Nursing Research Articles

Most articles about justice and nursing research focus on the care of vulnerable populations or working with those who are marginalized in society (Alderson, 2001; Barnes & Brannelly, 2008; Dresden, McElmurry, & McCreary, 2003; Guenter et al., 2005; Lind, Prinsloo, Wardie, & Pyrch, 2010; McKane, 2000; Mill & Ogilvie, 2002; Rew, Taylor-Seehafer, & Thomas, 2000; Thomas, 2004). Nurses (Alexis & Vydelingum, 2004; Giddings, 2005a, 2005b; Mantler, Armstrong-Stassen, Horsburgh, & Cameron, 2006; Spence Laschinger, 2004) and nursing students (Grant, Giddings, & Beale, 2005; Thuma-McDermond, 2011) were the most common study participants in research studies exploring issues of justice.

Few scholars researched how social justice was defined or used by patients or clients, from their point of view. One such study was by Carifio and Nasser (2012). Carifio and Nasser (2012) researched how elders' beliefs in a just world informed their ability to cope with anxiety, fear and life transitions. Those who scored high on belief in a just world scored low on depression, and vice versa.

Nevertheless, few articles explicitly stated and defined how social justice was used as a theoretical research framework (Blondeau et al., 2000; Clark, Barton, & Brown, 2002; Giddings, 2005a, 2005b; Grant et al., 2005), as a measurement parameter for understanding concepts related to nursing (Altun, 2002), or as an outcome of a particular methodological approach (Sullivan-Bolyai, Bova, & Harper, 2005). Messias, McDowell, and Estrada (2009), for example, highlight how social justice is useful to consider while practicing language interpreting.

However, more researchers identify how the concept of social justice was used in the research process (Guo & Phillips, 2006; Mohammed, 2006; Racine, 2002; Tee & Lathlean, 2004) in the United States and globally (Bathum, 2007). Overall, social justice is infrequently defined as a framework for guide nursing research, as a theory to develop research instruments to assess values (Weis & Schank, 2009), or as a way to measure justice concepts in practice (Rodwell, Noblet, Demir, & Steane, 2009). A growing number of research articles do state the social justice implications for the research area studied (Andrews & Heath, 2003; Lynam et al., 2003).

Views of Justice in Nursing Practice Articles

Articles about how justice relates to nursing practice focus on how ethics is useful in making moral judgments about care of individuals or populations (Baisch, 2009; Bell, 2003; Hildebrandt & Ford, 2009; Lawson, 2005; MacKinnon, 2009; McMurray, 2006; Peter & Morgan, 2001; Phillips & Phillips, 2006; Pieper & Dacher, 2004; Purdy & Wadhwani, 2006; Stinson, Godkin, & Robinson, 2004; Turkoski, 2005; Williams, 2004). In the last decade, a growing number of articles focused on using justice as a concept to guide nursing administration and leadership (Curtin & Arnold, 2005a, 2005b; Waite & Brooks, 2014; Williams, 2006), nursing practice (Bell & Hulbert, 2008; Falk-Rafael, 2005; MacKinnon, 2009; Sutton, 2003), and healthcare management (Williams, 2005). Crock (2009) is one of few authors to focus on how nursing practice is increasingly connected to and lured by organized power in other disciplines.

When used in clinical nursing practice, justice is often defined as treating people fairly. Justice is also viewed as a social obligation for nurses to understand how practice is influenced by assumptions and social inequalities that guide the design of health care and society (Benner, 2005; Drevdahl, 2002; Ervin & Bell, 2004; Leung, 2002; Ludwick & Silva, 2000; Russell, 2002). Most authors agree that discussions of justice are needed to assess how the work of individual nurses and the profession at large contribute to the formation of a just healthcare system and society (Haddad, 2002).

Despite the recognition that exploring justice is needed, most articles on this topic do not define justice beyond notions about fairness. Alternatively, if justice is defined more elaborately in relationship to nursing practice, authors often use a distributive justice framework (Silva & Ruth, 2003). Authors using a distributive justice viewpoint assert that all persons have equal political and social access to opportunities. The belief that persons are equal forms the basis for the even allocation of goods and services. A main limitation of the distributive view of justice is the lack of acknowledgment that social groups are often regarded unequally on the basis of gender, class, and race; thus the allocation of goods and services is also unequal in U.S. society (Young, 1990). Even fewer authors use social justice as a lens through which to view how nurses practice in unjust healthcare settings (Anderson et al., 2009). Few authors acknowledge the limits of the distributive paradigm or focus on educating nurses to change laws, public institutions, and communities in order to promote social justice.

SOCIAL JUSTICE: DEFINITIONAL LIMITATIONS IN THE NURSING LITERATURE

There are two main concerns with definitions of social justice in nursing. First, social injustice is viewed as a result of a personal act, and thus justice is seen as an individual response to that act. This assumes that justice can be achieved by multiple individual acts, versus by institutional changes and reform processes. The individualization of social justice is historically related to how nurses conceive the person as the primary site of, and remedy to, unjust conditions. Rarely is it highlighted how injustice nationally or globally (Austin, 2001) is created by power imbalances in the distribution of wealth, resources, and access. Moreover, seldom is it acknowledged that the unequal distribution of resources and access influences healthcare delivery, health status, and health actualization or achievement of optimal health.

The second main concern with publications about social justice in nursing is the way social justice is presented. Lipscomb (2011) noted that social justice claims are inadequately detailed in the nursing literature. Social justice is asserted by authors as a result without adequate evidence that their theories or practices promoted social justice. Social justice is a popularly used phrase in most publications without substantiation.

Often the articles about social justice in nursing limit the focus to underrepresented, vulnerable, or populations of people of color (Herman & Sassatelli, 2002; Redman & Clark, 2002). In the last decade, however, more focus has been directed toward the practices of nurses in terms of enabling or limiting justice. Nevertheless, nursing literature rarely addresses how inequitable conditions contribute to diminished health actualization in majority groups as well. Deaton and Lubotsky (2003), for example, determined that death rates in U.S. states with more income inequality were higher for all groups than the corresponding rates in states with more equal income distributions. After considering the racial and ethnic composition of those states, it remained unclear why the mortality of the majority group of white Americans was related to racial composition and income inequality (Deaton & Lubotsky, 2003).

There is also a tendency to compare health indicators of people of color to white Americans, even though white Americans as a population may not experience the best health outcomes nationally or globally for certain conditions. Thus, the standard reference to white Americans, without considering the best population health indicators more globally or broadly, may promote reference comparison bias. In part, this bias exists because of a lack of research into how inequality contributes to poor health outcomes for both minority *and* majority members of society. Despite this consideration, some litera-ture suggests that injustice lessens the presence of optimal health for all (Subramanian, Blakely, & Kawachi, 2003). Even on a global level, poor environments foster poor health locally and nationally (Subramanian, Blakely, & Kawachi, 2003).

Considerations such as this remain under-documented in the nursing literature for several reasons. Most nurses have a limited view of social justice (Drevdahl, 2002) and inadequate social policies to guide their depth of thinking about social justice (Bekemeier & Butterfield, 2005; Kikuchi, 2004). When justice is defined in relationship to individual equality and fairness, the social dimensions of justice and injustice are also minimized. Fairness and equality are not the same concepts. Given the historic disadvantages encoun-tered by underrepresented groups in the United States, for instance, to give equal treat-ment would not remedy current or past ills.

Social justice asserts that vulnerable persons should be protected from harm and pro-moted to achieve full status in society. The dynamics of being perceived as privileged or vulnerable require further exploration. Particularly relevant would be an investigation of how nurses themselves are influenced by privilege as they espouse their role as social jus-tice advocates. One question becomes critical in this kind of research: Can nurses really promote a social justice agenda when that promotion will result in the critique and dis-mantlement of their own advantage?

Social justice critique means, for example, that one must recognize the social fac-tors that construe persons as privileged or vulnerable at different points in time. A social justice agenda necessitates transforming systems that promote subordination or disad-vantage in the long term and the immediate conditions that limit self-actualization in the short term (Kirkham & Anderson, 2002). It requires a consistent focus on understanding how concepts are developed to limit or promote justice (Lutz & Bowers, 2003). A focus on multiple simultaneous sites of social justice action is needed to address the short- and long-term oppressive situations that create social injustice and limit access to health and health care. A multifocal approach to social justice is needed but as yet has not been fully articulated in the nursing literature.

ALTERNATIVE VIEWS OF SOCIAL JUSTICE

Definitions of social justice vary across disciplines and over time. Theories about social justice are espoused in philosophy (Young, 1990), public health science (Beauchamp, 1986), and religious studies (Lebacquz, 1986). The use of social justice by nurses as a research framework gained momentum in the early 1990s with the application of wom-anist, feminist, and social critical theories (Boutain, 1999), in the late 1990s with the use of postcolonial perspectives (Kirkham & Anderson, 2002), and in the early 2000s with a focus on indigenous knowledge creation. Authors who use critical theories to critique nursing education, research, and practice help guide the nursing profession toward a social justice agenda. Unfortunately, many of these works were not developed to give explicit attention to the multiple ways to understand social justice as a concept.

One useful framework for nurses to consider is based on the work of Holland (1983). He argues that to be effective in promoting justice, scholars must think of addressing injustice on many fronts. Specifically, scholars must deal with the antecedents of injustice, the processes of injustice, and the results of injustice in society. These stages of injustice creation and re-creation will help focus nursing on points of intervention. Nurses can then address social justice in terms of social justice awareness, amelioration, or transformation.

SOCIAL JUSTICE AWARENESS, AMELIORATION, AND TRANSFORMATION

Social justice awareness entails exploring how one perceives others as either vulnerable or privileged. Awareness involves asking critical questions about how systems of domination and oppression foster categorizations such as vulnerability and privilege. An example may be helpful in understanding social justice awareness.

Homelessness is a major health and social concern. A focus on social justice awareness may involve conducting a self-interview and client interview on how housing influences health. For example, think about how health is related to housing. Write your thoughts prior to interviewing clients with and without a home. Talk with clients who have homes and those who do not. Ask them about how having or not having a home influences their health and record their point of view.

Conduct a literature review on housing, home ownership, and health. Questions to consider include these: How does having a home relate to health? What is the health status of those who have homes? What is the health status of those who do not have homes? Compare your initial thoughts to the knowledge gained in the interview and review of relevant literature. You may discover that your awareness of the relationship between housing and health increases.

Social justice awareness is an ongoing process. To alter the analogy described by Lebacquz (1986), injustice is like the proverbial elephant standing right next to you. You cannot appreciate the entire view, and you may not fully recognize how you are affected by or are affecting the elephant. You must continue to move, sensing each part of the elephant at different angles and with different senses. Social justice awareness is temporal and dependent on your frame of reference. Being aware is a start, but it is not enough.

Social justice amelioration involves addressing the immediate results or antecedents to unjust conditions. To continue with the example of health and homelessness, amelioration entails a direct attempt to address the situation of the clients who are homeless. How that situation is addressed, however, is often to treat the most immediately seen concerns of a person experiencing homelessness. Obtaining grants to provide temporary shelter, food, clothing, or health care to the homeless, for example, is an illustration of social justice amelioration. In the short term, amelioration remedies urgent or semi-urgent concerns, but it does not really change the conditions that will cause others to become homeless over and over again.

Social justice transformation also involves critically deliberating about the conditions of home dwelling and homelessness in relationship to health in order to proactively change those conditions. Who are the people most likely to have homes? Which conditions were present that allowed them to have homes? Who are the people most likely to be homeless? Which conditions led them to become known as homeless? How does housing relate to health services allocation, current health status, or future health attainment? Social justice transformation advocates seek to answer these questions as part of their attempts to change or develop just housing and health policies. Their aim is to eliminate or limit the conditions that result in homelessness. Social justice transformation is devoted to redressing unjust conditions by changing the structures that foster those unjust situations. Transformation focuses individual actions toward long-range systematic solutions to unjust situations.

The work of Iris Young (1990) is helpful in further understanding social justice transformation. She argues that distributive justice (similar to social justice amelioration) is based on a false system of distributing services and rights to those who are already marginalized (as a result of social injustice). Thus, the rendering of service re-creates the system of privilege by allowing those who give the services (the privileged) to remain in a position of power over those who receive those services (the needy). In the short term, this strategy addresses the immediate needs of those who had already become vulnerable; in the long term however, the system does not change because those privileged few in power maintain their positions. Young believes it is most helpful to restructure systems so that certain services, such as homeless shelters, are needed only infrequently or are no longer needed. System restructuring is accomplished by recognizing, confronting, and diminishing entrenched inequalities associated with gender, class, and racial inequalities in society (Young, 1990).

CONCLUSION

A social justice agenda recognizes both the privileged and inequitable organization of social groups based on the systems that support the distribution of power and resources among those social groups. Social justice gives moral privilege to the needs of the most vulnerable groups in an effort to promote justice within the society at large. As vulnerability among persons is eliminated or minimized, the moral agency of those privileged can be simultaneously elevated. This view of social justice is not clearly articulated in the literature on nursing education, research, and practice, however.

Discussions about social justice remain conceptually limited in the majority of published works in nursing. Without a more complex and nuanced view of social justice, nurses are less able to fully utilize this concept as a framework to redress unjust conditions in healthcare delivery and health attainment. Social justice is regarded as central to the nursing profession, despite the need to critically revisit discussions about this concept. Nurses can contribute much to understanding how the interdisciplinary concept of social justice is useful in promoting just health and social relationships in society.

ACKNOWLEDGMENTS

Support for the first edition of this chapter was provided by grants from the National Institute of Child Health and Human Development (HD-41682); the National Institute of Nursing Research (F31 NR07249-01); and the Centers for Disease Control and Prevention (U48/CCU009654-06). Support for the second edition of the chapter was provided by National Institute of Child Health and Human Development (HD-41682), an Intramural Award from the University of Washington School of Nursing, and Community Award from the the March of Dimes. The University of Washington School of Nursing supported the funding of the third and fourth chapter editions. The author wishes to thank Joseph Fletcher III.

REFERENCES

Abrams, S. (2009). Education at the margins and beyond borders. *Public Health Nursing*, 26(6), 487–488.

Alderson, P. (2001). Prenatal screening, ethics, and Down's syndrome: A literature review. *Nursing Ethics*, 8, 360–374.

Alexis, O., & Vydelingum, V. (2004). The lived experience of overseas black and minority ethnic nurses in the NHS in the south of England. *Diversity in Health and Social Care*, 1(1), 13–20.

Altun, I. (2002). Burnout and nurses' personal and professional values. *Nursing Ethics*, 9, 269–278.

Anderson, J., Rodney, P., Reimer-Kirkham, S., Browne, A., Khan, K., & Lynam, M. (2009). Inequalities in health and healthcare viewed through the ethical lens. *Advances in Nursing Science*, 32(4), 282–294.

Andrews, J., & Heath, J. (2003). Women and the global tobacco epidemic: Nurses call to action. *International Council of Nurses*, 50, 215–228.

Austin, W. (2001). Nursing ethics in an era of globalization. *Advances in Nursing Science*, 24, 1–18.

Baisch, M. (2009). Community health: An evolutionary concept analysis. *Journal of Advanced Nursing*, 65(10), 2464–2476.

Barnes, M., & Brannelly, T. (2008). Achieving care and social justice for people with dementia. *Nursing Ethics*, 15 (3), 384–395.

Bathum, M. (2007). Global health research to promote social justice: A critical perspective. *Advances in Nursing Science*, 30(4), 303–314.

Beauchamp, D. (1986). Public health as social justice. In T. Mappes & J. Zembaty (Eds.), *Biomedical ethics* (pp. 585–593). New York: McGraw-Hill.

Bekemeier, B., & Butterfield, P. (2005). Unreconciled inconsistencies: A critical review of the concept of social justice in three national nursing documents. *Advances in Nursing Science, 28*(2), 152–162.

Bell, S. (2003). Community health nursing, wound care, and … ethics? *Journal of Wound, Ostomy and Continence Nurses Society, 30*(5), 259–265.

Bell, S. E., & Hulbert, J. (2008). Translating social justice into clinical nurse specialist practice. *Journal for Advanced Nursing Practice, 22*(6), 293–301.

Benner, P. (2005). Honoring the good behind the rights and justice in healthcare when more than justice is needed. *American Journal of Critical Care, 14*(2), 152–156.

Blondeau, D., Lavoie, M., Valois, P., Keyserlingk, E., Hebert, M., & Martineau, I. (2000). The attitude of Canadian nurses towards advance directives. *Nursing Ethics, 7,* 399–411.

Boersma, R. (2006). Integrating the ethics of care and justice—or are they mutually exclusive? *International Journal for Human Caring, 10*(2), 21.

Bond, A., Mandleco, B., & Warnick, M. (2004). At the heart of nursing: Stories reflect the professional values in AACN's *Essentials* document. *Nurse Educator, 29*(2), 84–88.

Boutain, D. (1999). Critical nursing scholarship: Exploring critical social theory with African-American studies. *Advances in Nursing Science, 21,* 37–47.

Boutain, D. (2005). Social justice as a framework for professional nursing. *Journal of Nursing Education, 44*(9), 404–408.

Boutain, D. (2008). Social justice as a framework for undergraduate community health clinical experiences in the United States. *International Journal of Nursing Education Scholarship, 5*(1), 13.

Browne, A., & Tarlier, D. (2008). Examining the potential of nurse practitioners from a critical social justice perspective. *Nursing Inquiry, 15*(2), 83–93.

Buettner-Schmidt, K., & Lobo, M. (2012). Social justice: A concept analysis. *Journal of Advanced Nursing, 68*(4), 948–958.

Carifio, J., & Nasser, R. (2012). Belief in a just world and depression in elderly nursing home residents. *Work, 43*(3), 303–312.

Clark, L., Barton, J., & Brown, N. (2002). Assessment of community contamination: A critical approach. *Public Health Nursing, 19,* 354–365.

Comer, S. (2009). The ethics of conducting educational research on your own students. *Journal of Nursing, 13*(4), 100–105.

Crock, E. (2009). Ethics of pharmaceutical company relationships with the nursing profession: No free lunch or no more pens? *Contemporary Nurse: A Journal for the Australian Nursing Profession, 33*(2), 202–209.

Curtin, L., & Arnold, L. (2005a). A framework for analysis: Part I. *Nursing Administration Quarterly, 29*(2), 183–187.

Curtin, L., & Arnold, L. (2005b). A framework for analysis: Part II. *Nursing Administration Quarterly, 29*(3), 288–291.

Deaton, A., & Lubotsky, D. (2003). Mortality, inequality and race in American cities and states. *Social Science and Medicine, 56,* 1139–1153.

Dresden, E., McElmurry, B., & McCreary, L. (2003). Approaching ethical reasoning in nursing research through a communitarian perspective. *Journal of Professional Nursing, 19*(5), 295–304.

Drevdahl, D. (2002). Social justice or market justice? The paradoxes of public health partnerships with managed care. *Public Health Nursing, 19*(3), 161–169.

Drevdahl, D., Kneipp, S., Canales, M., & Dorcy, K. (2001). Reinvesting in social justice: A capital idea for public health nursing. *Advances in Nursing Science, 24*, 19–31.

Ervin, N., & Bell, S. (2004). Social justice issues related to uneven distribution of resources. *Journal of the New York State Nurses Association, 35*, 8–13.

Ezeonwu, M. (2013). A nurse-managed health fair to promote social justice in community health pedagogy. *Communicating Nursing Research, 46*, 217.

Fahrenwald, N. (2003). Teaching social justice. *Nurse Educator, 28*(5), 222–226.

Fahrenwald, N., Bassett, S., Tschetter, L., Carson, P., White, L., & Winterboer, V. (2005). Teaching core nursing values. *Journal of Professional Nursing, 21*(1), 46–51.

Fahrenwald, N., Taylor, J., Kneipp, S., & Canales, M. (2007). Academic freedom and academic duty to teach social justice: A perspective and pedagogy for public health nursing faculty. *Public Health Nursing, 24*(2), 190–197.

Falk-Rafael, A. (2005). Advancing nursing theory through theory-guided practice: The emergence of a critical caring perspective. *Advances in Nursing Science, 28*(1), 38–49.

Falk-Rafael, A. (2006). Globalization and global health: Toward nursing praxis in the global community. *Advances in Nursing Science, 29*(1), 2–14.

Fitzpatrick, J. (2003). From the editor: Social justice, human rights, and nursing education. *Nurse Educator, 28*(5), 222–226.

Galon, P., & Wineman, N. (2010). Coercion and procedural justice in psychiatric care: State of the science and implications for nursing. *Archives of Psychiatric Nursing, 24*(5), 307–316.

Giddings, L. (2005a). Health disparities, social injustice, and the culture of nursing. *Nursing Research, 54*(5), 304–312.

Giddings, L. (2005b). A theoretical model of social consciousness. *Advances in Nursing Science, 28*(3), 224–239.

Grace, P., & Willis, D. (2012). Nursing responsibilities and social justice: An analysis in support of disciplinary goals. *Nursing Outlook, 60*(4), 198–207.

Grant, B. M., Giddings, L., & Beale, J. (2005). Vulnerable bodies: Competing discourses of intimate bodily care. *Journal of Nursing Education, 44*(11), 498–503.

Guenter, D., Majumdar, B., Willms, D., Travers, R., Browne, G., & Robinson, G. (2005). Community-based HIV education and prevention workers respond to a changing environment. *Journal of the Association of Nurses in AIDS Care, 16*(1), 29–36.

Guo, G., & Phillips, L. (2006). Key informants' perceptions of health for elders at the U.S.–Mexico border. *Public Health Nursing, 23*(3), 224–233.

Haddad, A. (2002). Fairness, respect, and foreign nurses. *RN, 65*(7), 25–28.

Harris, G. (2005). Ethical issues in community care. *Journal of Community Nursing, 19*(11), 12–16.

Herman, C., & Sassatelli, J. (2002). DARING to reach the heartland: A collaborative faith-based partnership in nursing education. *Journal of Nursing Education, 41*(10), 443–445.

Hildebrandt, E., & Forde, S. (2009). Justice and impoverished women: The ethical implications of work-based welfare. *Policy, Politics, & Nursing Practice, 10*(4), 295–302.

Holland, J. (1983). *Social analysis: Linking faith and justice.* Maryknoll, NY: Orbis Books.

Hubert, J. (2004). Continuing the dialogue: A response to Kikuchi's critique of the 2002 CNA Code of Ethics. *Canadian Journal of Nursing Leadership, 17*(4), 10–13.

Jackson, D. (2003). Epilogue: Culture, health and social justice. *Contemporary Nurse, 15*(3), 347–348.

Kikuchi, J. (2004). 2002 CNA Code of Ethics: Some recommendations. *Canadian Journal of Nursing Leadership, 17*(3), 28–33.

Kirkham, S., & Anderson, J. (2002). Postcolonial nursing scholarship: From epistemology to method. *Advances in Nursing Science, 25*(1), 1–17.

Kirkham, S., Hofwegen, L., & Harwood, C. (2005). Narratives of social justice: Learning in innovative clinical settings. *International Journal of Nursing Education Scholarship, 2*(1), Article 28.

Kneipp, S., & Snider, M. (2001). Social justice in a market model world. *Journal of Professional Nursing, 17*(3), 113.

Lapum, J., Hamzavi, N., Veljkovic, K., Mohamed, Z., Pettinato, A., Silver, S., & Taylor, E. (2012). A performance and poetical narrative of critical social theory in nursing education: An ending and threshold of social justice. *Nursing Philosophy, 13*(1), 27–45.

Lawson, L. (2005). Furthering the search for truth and justice. *Journal of Forensic Nursing, 1*(4), 149–150.

Lebacqz, K. (1986). *Six theories of justice.* Minneapolis, MN: Augsburg.

Leung, W. (2002). Why the professional–client ethic is inadequate in mental health care. *Nursing Ethics, 9*(1), 51–60.

Leuning, C. (2001). Advancing a global perspective: The world as classroom. *Nursing Science Quarterly, 14*(4), 298–303.

Lind, C., Prinsloo, I., Wardie, M., & Pyrch, T. (2010). Social justice: Hearing voices of marginalized girls expressed in theatre performance. *Advances in Nursing Science, 33*(3), E12–E23.

Lipscomb, M. (2011). Challenging the coherence of social justice as a shared nursing value. *Nursing Philosophy, 12*(1), 4–11.

Ludwick, R., & Silva, M. (2000, August 14). Nursing around the world: Cultural values and ethical conflicts. *Online Journal of Issues in Nursing 5*(3). Retrieved from http://www.nursingworld.org/MainMenuCategories/ANAMarketplace/ANAPeriodicals/OJIN/Columns/Ethics/Cultural-ValuesandEthicalConflicts.html

Lutz, B., & Bowers, B. (2003). Understanding how disability is defined and conceptualized in the literature. *Rehabilitation Nursing, 28*(3), 74–78.

Lynam, M., Henderson, A., Browne, A., Smye, V., Semeniuk, P., Blue, C., & Singh, S. (2003). Healthcare restructuring with a view and efficiency: Reflections on unintended consequences. *Canadian Journal of Nursing Leadership, 16*(1), 112–140.

MacIntosh, J., & Wexler, E. (2005). Interprovincial Partnership in Nursing Education. *Canadian Nurse*, *101*(4), 17–20.

MacKinnon, C. (2009). Applying feminist, multicultural, and social justice theory to diverse women who function as caregivers in end-of-life and palliative home care. *Palliative & Supportive Care*, *7*(4), 501–512.

Mantler, J., Armstrong-Stassen, M., Horsburgh, M., & Cameron, S. (2006). Reactions of hospital staff nurses to recruitment incentives. *Western Journal of Nursing Research*, *28*(1), 70–84.

Mathes, M. (2004). Ethical decision making and nursing. *Medsurg Nursing*, *13*(6), 429–431.

Mathes, M. (2005). Ethical decision making and nursing. *Dermatology Nursing*, *17*(6), 444–458.

McKane, M. (2000). Research, ethics and the data protection legislation. *Nursing Standard*, *2*(14), 36–41.

McMurray, A. (2004). Culturally sensitive evidence-based practice. *Collegian*, *11*(4), 14–18.

McMurray, A. (2006). Peace, love and equality: Nurses, interpersonal violence and social justice. *Contemporary Nurse*, *21*(2), vii–x.

Menzel, N., Willson, L, & Doolen, J. (2014). Effectiveness of a poverty simulation in Second Life: Changing nursing student attitudes toward poor people. *International Journal of Nursing Education Scholarship*, *11*(1), 1–7.

Messias, D. (2001). Globalization, nursing, and health for all. *Journal of Nursing Scholarship*, *33*(1), 9–11.

Messias, D., McDowell, L., & Estrada, R. (2009). Language interpreting as social justice work: Perspectives of formal and informal healthcare interpreters. *Advances in Nursing Science*, *32*(2), 128–143.

Mill, J., & Ogilvie, L. (2002). Ethical decision making in international nursing research. *Qualitative Health Research*, *12*(6), 807–815.

Mohammed, S. (2006). Moving beyond the "exotic": Applying postcolonial theory in health research. *Advances in Nursing Science*, *29*(2), 98–109.

Mohammed, S. (2014). Exploring root issues of American Indian health: Social justice in nursing pedagogy. *Communicating Nursing Research*, *46*, 215.

Moule, P. (2003). ICT: A social justice approach to exploring user issues? *Nurse Education Today*, *23*, 530–536.

Murphy, N., Canales, M., Norton, S., & DeFilippis, J. (2005). Striving for congruence: The interconnection between values, practice, and political action. *Policy, Politics, & Nursing*, *6*(1), 20–29.

Myhrvold, T. (2003). The exclusion of the other: Challenges to the ethics of closeness. *Nursing Philosophy*, *4*, 33–43.

Myrick, F. (2005). Educating nurses for the knowledge economy. *International Journal of Nursing Education Scholarship*, *2*(1), Article 20.

Oddi, L., & Oddi, S. (2000). Student–faculty joint authorship: Ethical and legal concerns. *Journal of Professional Nursing*, *16*(4), 219–227.

Pereira, A. (2006). Critical thinking, *Dynamics*, *17*(3), 4–5.

Pesut, B., Fowler, M., Reimer-Kirkham, S., Taylor, E., & Sawatzky, R. (2009). Particularizing spirituality in points of tension: Enriching the discourse. *Nursing Inquiry*, *16*(4), 337–346.

Peter, E., & Morgan, K. (2001). Explorations of a trust approach to nursing ethics. *Nursing Inquiry*, *8*, 3–10.

Phillips, L., & Phillips, W. (2006). Better reproductive healthcare for women with disabilities: A role for nursing leadership. *Advances in Nursing Science*, *29*(2), 134–151.

Pieper, B., & Dacher, J. (2004). Looking backward toward our future: Creating the nexus between community health nursing and palliative care. *Journal of the New York State Nurses Association*, *35*(1), 20–24.

Purdy, I., & Wadhwani, R. (2006). Embracing bioethics in neonatal intensive care. Part II: Case histories in neonatal ethics. *Neonatal Network*, *25*(1), 43–53.

Racine, L. (2002). Implementing a postcolonial feminist perspective in nursing research related to non-Western populations. *Nursing Inquiry*, *10*(2), 91–102.

Redman, R., & Clark, L. (2002). Service-learning as a model for integrating social justice in the nursing curriculum. *Journal of Nursing Education*, *41*, 446–449.

Rew, L., Taylor-Seehafer, M., & Thomas, N. (2000). Without parental consent: Conducting research with homeless adolescents. *Journal of the Society of Pediatric Nurses*, *5*, 131–138.

Rodwell, J., Noblet, A., Demir, D., & Steane, P. (2009). Supervisors are central to work characteristics affecting nurse outcomes. *Journal of Nursing Scholarship*, *41*(93), 310–319.

Russell, K. (2002) Silent voices. *Public Health Nursing*, *19*(4), 233–234.

Scanlan, J., Care, W., & Gessler, S. (2001). Dealing with unsafe students in clinical practice. *Nurse Educator*, *26*(1), 23–27.

Shattell, M., Hogan, B., & Hernandez, A. (2006). The interpretive research group as an alternative to the interpersonal process recording. *Nurse Educator*, *31*(4), 178–182.

Silva, M., & Ruth, L. (2003). Ethics and terrorism: September 11, 2001 and its aftermath. *Online Journal of Issues in Nursing*, *8*(1), 21–24.

Sistrom, M., & Hale, P. (2006). Integrative review of population health, income, social capital and structural inequality. *Journal of Multicultural Nursing & Health*, *12*(2), 21–27.

Snyder, M. (2014). Emancipatory knowing: Empowering nursing students toward reflection and action. *Journal of Nursing Education*, *53*(2), 65–69.

Spence Laschinger, H. (2004). Hospital nurses' perceptions of respect and organizational justice. *Journal of Nursing Administration*, *34*(7/8), 354–364.

Stinson, C., Godkin, J., & Robinson, R. (2004). *Dimensions of Critical Care Nursing*, *23*(1), 38–43.

Stys, J. (2008). Social analysis formation for nurse educators. *Nursing Education Perspectives*, *29*(6), 366–369.

Subramanian, S., Blakely, T., & Kawachi, I. (2003). Income inequality as a public health concern: Where do we stand? *Health Services Research*, *38*, 153–167.

Sullivan-Bolyai, S., Bova, C., & Harper, D. (2005). Developing and refining interventions in persons with health disparities: The use of the qualitative description. *Nursing Outlook*, *53*, 127–133.

Sutton, J. (2003). The ethics of theatre nurse practice under the microscope. *British Journal of Perioperative Nursing*, *13*(10), 405–408.

Tee, S., & Lathlean, J. (2004). The ethics of conducting a co-operative inquiry with vulnerable people. *Journal of Advanced Nursing*, *47*(5), 536–543.

Thomas, S. (2004). School connectedness, anger behaviors, and relationship of violent and nonviolent American youth. *Perspectives in Psychiatric Care*, 40(40), 135–148.

Thuma-McDermond, W. (2011). *A focused ethnography: Nursing students' perceptions of cultural competences and social justice*. Chester, PA: Widener University School of Nursing.

Turkoski, B. (2005). Culturally sensitive healthcare. *Home Healthcare Nurse*, 23(6), 355–358.

Vickers, D. (2008). Social justice: A concept for undergraduate nursing curricula? *Southern Online Journal of Nursing Research*, 8(1), 18.

Waite, R., & Brooks, S. (2014). Cultivating social justice learning and leadership skills: A timely endeavor for undergraduate student nurses. *Nurse Education Today*, 34(6), 890–893.

Weis, D., & Schank, M. (2009). Development and psychometric evaluation of the Nurses Professional Values Scale—Revised. *Journal of Nursing Measurement*, 17(3), 221–231.

Whitehead, M. (1992). The concepts and principles of equity and health. *International Journal of Health Services*, 22(3), 429–445.

Williams, A. (2004). Nursing, health and human rights: A framework for international collaboration. *Association of Nurses in AIDS Care*, 15(3), 75–77.

Williams, A. (2005). Thinking about equity in health care. *Journal of Nursing Management*, 13, 397–402.

Williams, L. (2006). The fair factor in matters of trust. *Nursing Administration Quarterly*, 30(1), 30–37.

Woods, M. (2012). Exploring the relevance of social justice within a relational nursing ethic. *Nursing Philosophy*, 13(1), 56–65.

Young, I. (1990). *Justice and the politics of difference*. Princeton, NJ: Princeton University Press.

Chapter 5

Low Literacy and Vulnerable Clients

Toni Vezeau

OBJECTIVES

At the end of this chapter, the reader will be able to

1. Describe the current status of health literacy in the United States.
2. Explain how health literacy affects vulnerability.
3. Provide solutions that healthcare providers might implement to reverse the negative effects of health illiteracy.

INTRODUCTION

Effective health care requires skills on the part of both providers and clients. Providers must have a strong knowledge base and successful communication skills that match the needs of their clients. Clients must be able to take in information, make sense of it, apply it to their own situations, and retain the information for future use. These skills are the hallmarks of literacy. Without literacy as a base client skill, there is little chance that healthcare interactions will meet their intended goals. This chapter presents literacy as a primary driver of vulnerability in health care. The discussion explores the current status of literacy skills in the United States, client and provider aspects of the problem, and recommendations for current practice.

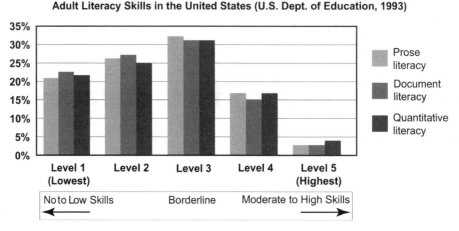

Figure 5-1 Adult literacy skills in the United States.

Data from US Department of Education, Office of Educational Research and Improvement, National Center for Educational Statistics, 1993.

WHAT IS THE STATUS OF LITERACY IN THE UNITED STATES?

The National Adult Literacy Survey (NALS), first conducted in 1992, defined literacy as the use of printed information to maneuver in society, meet one's goals, and develop one's knowledge and abilities (Kirsch, Jungeblut, Jenkins, & Kolstad, 1993). Doak, Doak, and Root (2001) modified this definition to include comprehension and retention of verbal and gestural information. The 2003, the last National Assessment of Adult Literacy (NAAL) assessment included life skills (ability to read everyday documents) and basic quantitative skills in their assessment. While there has been some equalization of outcomes between genders noted in 2003, basic literacy skills have not meaningfully changed since the initial national assessment (National Center for Education Statistics [NCES], 2014).

The 2003 NAAL remains the largest study on adult literacy carried out in the United States (*n* = 26,000). This study went far beyond establishing the reading grade level of participants and tested their performance in three areas (**Figure 5-1**):

1. *Prose literacy*: printed word in connected sentences and passages; implies skill in finding information and integrating information from several sections of the text
2. *Document literacy*: structured prose in arrays of columns and rows, lists, and maps; implies skill in locating information, repeating the search as often as needed, and integrating information

3. *Quantitative literacy*: information displayed in graphs, charts, and in numerical form; in addition to locating information, implies that one can infer and apply the needed arithmetic

Participants were tested on a wide variety of tasks encountered at work, home, and in community activities, such as signing a mock Social Security card and filling out personal information on a simple job application.

Current NAAL data suggested that one-third of American adults are functionally illiterate and an approximately equal number have marginal literacy skills that disallow full functioning in society (NCES, 2014). Essentially, half of the adult population in the United States has poor to nonexistent skills in reading, listening, and computation. Minor proportions of the NAAL were learning disabled (5%) and spoke English as a second language, if at all (15%). Current smaller surveys suggest that the proportion of the total U.S. population who are primary speakers of a language other than English and who cannot speak or read English well is 8.7% and increasing (U.S. Census, 2013). However, most were white and born in America. Although education correlated with literacy, generally those adults who had a tenth-grade education read at the seventh- to eighth-grade level. Participants receiving Medicaid had an average of a fifth-grade reading level. One-third of the NAAL sample demonstrated basic functionality in understanding and using written information. Only 20% of the sample demonstrated a level of proficiency in handling information to perform complex reading and computation tasks. When these data were recomputed using 2003 data and released in 2006 (NCES, 2006), the results showed a slightly worsening trend.

The NAAL data suggested that certain groups fared much worse in their literacy skills than the general population. Of those adults who tested at the lowest reading level:

- 41–44% were poor
- 33% were older than 65 years of age
- 25% were immigrants
- 62% did not finish high school (disproportionately represented by Hispanic, African American, and Asian Pacific participants)
- 12% had physical, mental, or health conditions that disallowed participation in work or school settings
- 75% of the subfunctional group had a mental health problem
- 63% of prisoners tested below functional levels; those with GED or high school diploma fared slightly better (NCES, 2007)

Participants in the lowest literacy level had difficulty performing usual tasks of daily living based on printed information and in performing complex tasks that required following directions and computation. Interestingly, members of the group who were considered to have no or minimal functional literacy did not acknowledge themselves as vulnerable, related to their illiteracy. This group noted that they could read "adequately to very well," and fewer than 25% of these participants stated that they received help with information from family and friends.

A meta-analysis of U.S. studies on literacy in 2005 (Paasche-Orlow, Parker, Gazmararian, Neilsen-Bohlman, & Rudd, 2005) reviewed literature from January 1963 through January 2004 and, based on a pool of 85 articles, essentially validated the same prevalence rates mentioned earlier. The authors concluded that limited literacy is highly prevalent, negatively affects health, and is consistently associated with education, ethnicity, and age.

WHAT IS THE RELATIONSHIP BETWEEN LITERACY AND HEALTH VULNERABILITY?

Kirsch et al. (1993) discussed literacy as currency in the United States, because those with less literacy are much less likely to meet the needs of daily living and to pursue life goals. From this perspective, illiteracy has the potential to create health risks and exacerbate existing health conditions.

Literacy as a Predictor of Vulnerability

Aday's (2001) model of vulnerability and health posits that although all humans are vulnerable to illness, certain segments of the community are much more vulnerable to ill health in terms of initial susceptibility and in their response. Illiteracy is related to each of Aday's (2001) predictors of vulnerability. Persons with poor reading skills who are unable to perform basic literacy functions, such as reading a bus schedule or following directions in completing a task, generally have low social status outside of their immediate social ties. For example, low social status is often associated with low-paying jobs that offer no or minimal health insurance. Low status also can affect a provider's perception of client abilities, resulting in care that is "edited" based, at times, on misperceptions (Aday, 2001).

Social Status

Social status has been correlated with poor health (Duncan, Daly, McDonough, & Williams, 2002), in that persons with low status are more likely to use disproportionately more healthcare services, receive substandard care and less information about their illness, and be presented with fewer options. Kirsch et al. (1993) identified that persons with low literacy have much greater difficulty in accessing what Aday (2001) calls human capital (e.g., jobs, schools, income, and housing) than people with functional literacy skills. Similarly, NAAL data are congruent with Aday's third driver of vulnerability, lack of social capital, in that persons who are illiterate are more likely to be single or divorced, live in single-parent homes, and be loosely connected to their own communities.

Access to Care

Additionally, Aday (2001) addresses relationships of vulnerability to access to health care, cost of care, and quality of care. Accessing care in the United States most often requires complex language skills that are applied to the following tasks:

- Identifying and evaluating possible providers of care
- Negotiating appropriate entry points into the system
- Contacting and communicating needs to obtain an appointment
- Successfully traveling to and finding the actual site of care
- Interpreting written materials and relating to clock and calendar skills

Access to care is seriously challenged when clients have low literacy skills.

Consequences of Vulnerability

Quality of Care

The literature published during the last decade documents how illiteracy has affected the cost of care and the quality of care (Agency for Healthcare Research and Quality, 2004; Baker et al., 2002; Institute of Medicine [IOM], 2003). Illiteracy is a significant component of client adherence to care regimens and hospitalizations in the following health contexts: pregnancy, diabetes, AIDS, asthma, sexually transmitted diseases, women's health, rural residents, immigrants, mental health, advanced age, cardiac surgery, rheumatoid arthritis, prostate cancer, psychiatric clients, older adults, cardiac surgical clients, and payer status.

Without exception, the populations just cited have high prevalence of illiteracy, in proportions that mirror the findings from the NAAL data. Studies have shown that persons with literacy problems do not understand instructions and demonstrate less comprehension of their illness or condition.

Costs

Healthy People 2020 (Department of Health and Human Services [HHS], 2013) notes that the consequences of illiteracy include both poorer health outcomes and increased healthcare costs; in fact, costs of health care may be as much as four times greater for clients who read at or below the second-grade level than for the general populace.

Baker et al. (2002) reported that clients with documented low literacy had a 52% higher risk of hospital admission compared with clients with functional literacy, even after controlling for age, social and economic factors, and self-reported health. In another study, client illiteracy was the highest predictor of poor asthma knowledge and ineffective use of metered-dose inhalers (Williams, Baker, Honig, Lee, & Nowlan, 1998).

Acknowledging the pervasive influence of illiteracy on the quality of care in the United States, the IOM has identified literacy as one of the top three areas that cut across all other priorities for improvement in the nation's health. As noted by the IOM, literacy is also required for self-management and collaborative care, the other two priority cross-cutting areas.

REDEFINING THE FOCUS

Since the mid-1990s, the medical literature began to use a new term—*health literacy*—to address the literacy problem. The Ad Hoc Committee on Health Literacy for the Council on Scientific Affairs of the American Medical Association (1999) defined an individual's functional health literacy as "the ability to read and comprehend prescription bottles, appointment slips, and other essential health-related materials required to successfully function as a patient." To this definition, the National Health Education Standards added, the importance of understanding of basic health information and effectively communicating consent forms (Williams, 2000). Most recently, navigating Medicare and Affordable Care Act (ACA) information has been folded into the health literacy conversation (Center for Health Care Strategies, 2010). *Health literacy* has now become the preferred term when referring to this intersection of health concerns and literacy skills. Williams is articulate in describing the complexity of this nexus, which requires listening, analytical, decision-making, computational, and application skills.

International healthcare work has addressed health literacy in these terms for a much longer time; related literature exists from the 1960s onward. Interestingly, the issues discussed in international literature correspond well to current Western health literature. Watters (2003) comprehensively summarized the healthcare implications of no or low literacy in international work: increased use of health systems and costs, late entry into care, secondary to poor interpretation of symptoms, poor participation in preventive care, shame over literacy status eliminating self-identification of needs to care providers, self-administration medication errors related to literacy errors, and inconsistent shows at appointments. Each of these health concerns related to literacy has been documented in the United States as well (Baker, 1999; Kripalani et al., 2006; Wolf et al., 2007).

After remaining long silent on this issue, The Joint Commission's National Patient Safety Goals now include systematic approaches to address low-literacy clients by focusing on organizational strategies and policy development (Joint Commission, 2007; Murphy-Knoll, 2007).

In summary, research has supported Aday's (2001) theoretical work on health vulnerability. It is clear that—as yet without exception—literacy strongly influences the health of individuals and populations. The problems with literacy, however, are jointly owned and created by clients and providers. It is important to understand specific literacy problems of clients and to consider how providers have contributed to these problems.

HOW DOES ILLITERACY SPECIFICALLY INCREASE HEALTH RISKS OF CLIENTS?

Clients with no or low literacy cannot read or interpret pamphlets, directions on prescribed or over-the-counter medications, or diet instructions. A mismatch of vocabulary and skill is just one of the problems. Comprehension of graphics and pictures pose additional and, for many clients, insurmountable challenges (Doak et al., 2001; NCES, 2006).

Literacy is a complex skill requiring much more than the simple reading of words. It has many components, such as decoding, comprehension, and retention of information. In addition, the development of literacy involves a series of stages. Finally, literacy is not a "free-standing" skill, but rather involves integration of related life skills to navigate the healthcare system, effectively perform self-care, and make healthcare decisions.

Health and health care add unique aspects to the concern for client literacy. The effects of health and health care on literacy skills can be either temporary or sustained. Such situations as anesthesia due to surgery, blood loss, or acute pain may temporarily impair one's decoding, comprehension, and recall skills. Moreover, sustained medical conditions can interfere with mentation, cognition, and attention on a longer-term basis. Delayed mental development; neurological conditions, such as Alzheimer's disease; cerebral vascular accidents; and psychological disorders, such as depression or anxiety, may affect literacy skills and the ability of the client to interact effectively with providers. Understandably, clients who have sensory impairments are likely to have literacy difficulty. Visual and hearing difficulties were noted in 20% of the NAAL sample that tested in the lowest level of literacy (HHS, 2014a).

Medications may also negatively affect clients' abilities to effectively use their literacy skills, there by increasing risk for the client. Drug categories such as opiates, anticonvulsants, antidepressants, glucocorticosteroids, some antihypertensives, and thyroid and ovarian hormones are but a few medications that are known to affect information processing.

Providers need to appreciate how certain therapies and health conditions affect the client's ability to use his or her literacy skills. For those clients with low literacy skills, the health situations noted provide serious challenges to a client's ability to use healthcare information.

HOW DO HEALTHCARE PROVIDERS INFLUENCE THE LITERACY PROBLEM?

Clients come to providers with unique characteristics and abilities related to health literacy. In the past, providers, in their listening, speaking, and written interactions with clients, generally have ignored the literacy variable in care and, in most cases, continue to do so and increase the literacy challenge for their clients (Doak et al., 2001; Hohn, 1998; Karsenty, Landau, & Ferguson, 2013). A review of the literature reveals several threads addressing how providers have influenced health literacy: readability of client health education text, measurement of clients' reading levels in specific healthcare settings, and client–provider communications.

Readability of Written Healthcare Education Materials

Since 1988, the literature has documented that the readability of written healthcare instructions, booklets, and informed consent forms has not matched the skills of clients in the general care population (Cutilli, 2007; Doak et al., 2001; Forbis & Aligne, 2002; Ryan et al., 2014). Health education materials have been tested but often only a few at a time. When Doak et al. (2001) evaluated 1,234 health education materials, they found that more than 50% were written at or above the 10th-grade level. It is important to remember that education levels of clients do not generally match their reading skill levels. Specifically, reading skill levels average four to five grades lower when tested compared with level of educational attainment (Cutilli, 2007). Thus, the news is even more dire: If a client population has a mean of 10th-grade education, most educational materials in current use would outstrip the client skill level (Doak et al., 2001) (**Figure 5-2**). Studies have documented discharge instructions and client educational materials to be written well above a ninth-grade level of difficulty (Gannon & Hildebrandt, 2002; Ryan et al., 2014). Recent studies have confirmed that the readability level of commercially produced materials that are targeted to lower-literacy populations is far above the skill level of most clients (Cutilli, 2007; Sanders, Federico, Klass, Abrams, & Dreyer, 2009).

Consent forms, contracts, and commonly used self-report diagnostic tools are consistently documented as having a readability score higher than a ninth-grade level. For example, clients who read at a sixth-grade level or lower did not demonstrate comprehension of 54% of the items on the Beck Depression Scale; good readers experienced difficulty with one-third of the items (Sentell & Ratcliff-Baird, 2003). Similarly, in a study of 1,014 adults completing the Baltimore STD and Behavior Survey, 28% of the adults read at or lower than the eighth-grade level; this group showed a high error rate in comprehending survey items. The error rate in item comprehension decreased significantly

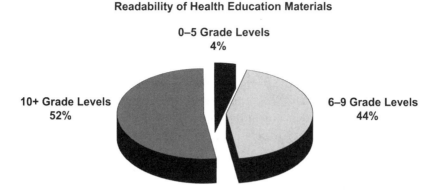

Figure 5-2 Readbility of health education materials.
Data from Doak, Doak, and Root, 2001. Readability levels of 1,234 healthcare materials.

as the literacy level increased ($p < 0.0001$) (Al-Tayyib, Rogers, Gribble, Villarroel, & Turner, 2002).

Studies investigating the literacy challenge of informed consent have consistently rated forms above the 12th-grade level and noted that institutional review boards typically do not take reading difficulty of consent forms into account (Raich, Plomer, & Coyne, 2001). When institutional review boards do act on this matter, the effect is generally to lower the reading level merely by one grade level (Raich et al., 2001). Readable consents, congruent with the lower literacy levels found in the local population, are now viewed as ethical imperatives, not just in the United States, but internationally (*Journal of Empirical Research on Human Research Ethics*, 2013).

Clients with no or low literacy who are given materials that directly affect their understanding of their health condition, who sign written forms that direct care, or who are tested using self-report tools are vulnerable to a host of negative consequences, including inadequate understanding of healthcare instructions, agreeing to procedures they do not fully understand, and faulty diagnosis.

Provider–Client Interactions and Communication

Interactions with low-literacy clients are just beginning to be studied. Provider–client interactions are influenced by perceptions of both client and provider. Both U.S. Census Bureau literacy data and NAAL data indicate that people with low literacy state to others that they read well enough to meet their needs. For healthcare providers, it is important to understand that such clients generally do not self-identify or discuss their literacy status because of the stigma associated with illiteracy (Doak et al., 2001; Easton, Entwistle, & Williams, 2013; Safeer & Keenan, 2005). Not only do low-literacy clients not admit to difficulties with literacy to their care providers, but they may also hide their need for help from their spouses and families (Easton et al., 2013).

Stigma and Shame

Stigma is both self-imposed, in the form of shame, and evident in how providers interact with clients. When Baker et al. (1996) interviewed clients who tested as having no to low literacy, they found that participants in the study held a deep sense of shame, which was exacerbated when healthcare providers became distressed or irritated when clients had difficulty filling out forms or reading instructions. Study participants stated that accessing care is daunting because of problems with registration and forms. In many cases, these clients avoided seeking care because of poor interactions with their care providers. Low literacy has been found to inhibit client questions, and it may be a major factor in over-all participation in a healthcare encounter (Arthur, Geiser, Arriola, & Kripalani, 2009; Easton et al., 2013; Katz, Jacobson, & Kripalani, 2007; Wolf et al., 2007).

Myths and Misidentification

Providers are generally not knowledgeable about illiteracy and interact differentially with clients who admit to literacy problems (Easton et al., 2013; Schillinger et al., 2003). Few providers have had any formal training in identification of and approaches to low-literacy clients (Easton, Entwistle, & Williams, 2012 Jukkala, Deupree, & Graham, 2009; Schlicting et al., 2007). As a consequence, there are a number of common myths held by providers (Doak et al., 2001, p. 6):

- "Illiterates are dumb and learn slowly if at all."
- "Most illiterates are poor, immigrants, or minorities."
- "Years of schooling are a good measure of literacy level."

Research refutes each of these myths (Easton et al., 2013). A person's measurement of intelligence does not correlate strongly with literacy skills; the correlation with income level is better. In terms of raw numbers, most persons with illiteracy in the United States are white native-born Americans in all areas of society; minorities and foreign-born groups in the United States have disproportionately high percentages of persons with no to minimal literacy. Years of schooling show the amount of education the person was exposed to, not the skill level achieved.

Incorrectly, providers may believe they can identify which clients need extra support related to their literacy needs. Bass, Wilson, Griffith, and Barnett (2002) conducted a study to see whether medical residents could correctly identify persons with low literacy from of a pool of 182 clients. The residents identified 90% of the clients as having no literacy problem. Of this client group, 36% tested as functionally illiterate. Only 3 of 182 clients were thought to have literacy problems when they did not test as such. Schlichting et al. (2007) found that the typical provider in their survey of 803 primary care providers could identify 41% and 43% of low-literacy, English-speaking and Spanish-speaking clients, respectively.

Only recently have nurses been studied, with similar results. In one study, bachelor's degree–prepared nurses could identify the risks and consequences of low literacy, but could not identify elderly clients as an important low-literacy population and could not identify interventions for working with low-literacy clients (Cormier & Kotrlik, 2009). A 2013 study compared nurses' estimates to the actual patient literacy level using the Newest Vital Sign tool. The nurses incorrectly identified clients with low literacy with overestimations outstripping underestimations 6:1 (Dickens, Lambert, Cromwell, & Piano (2013). Both studies suggest that providers seriously underestimate the literacy problem in their client group.

Inattention to Literacy Needs

Another study observed senior physicians interacting during several outpatient visits with 74 diabetic clients who spoke only English and tested as having no or low literacy (Schillinger et al., 2003). Even when made aware of the literacy needs of their clients, provider use of language was assessed as being well above the literacy level of their clients. The physicians in 80% of encounters did not test their clients' comprehension and recall. Those clients whose physicians did test for understanding and short-term recall had significantly greater glycemic control.

Rootman and Ronson (2005) stated the following:

> [W]e are mired in a state of denial over literacy. The immensity of the issue has paralyzed our public institutions, which seem to spend as much energy holding strategy sessions or denying responsibility as they do actually supporting programs of proven success. . . . It's hardly a promising time for a major national crusade against anything—especially poor literacy, which has no quick fix. (p. 62)
>
>> *Rootman, I., & Ronson, B. (2005). Literacy and health research in Canada: Where have we been and where have we gone? Canadian Journal of Public Health, 96(suppl 2), S62–S77.*

HOW CAN PROVIDERS DECREASE THE HEALTH RISK DUE TO ILLITERACY?

The literature reports a variety of approaches to decrease vulnerability of clients related to literacy problems. Currently, many websites, developed by private and public agencies, exist as clearinghouses to guide clinicians on preferred approaches to working with low-literacy clients (**Table 5–1**).

Identification

Many studies have emphasized a personal approach in discreetly asking about literacy status (Feifer, 2003; Nutbeam, 2008). Nevertheless, given the breadth of the literacy

Table 5-1 Helpful Websites on Health Literacy

- National Assessment of Adult Literacy
  http://nces.ed.gov/NAAL/
- National Center for Education Statistics
  http://nces.ed.gov/pubsearch/pubsinfo.asp?pubid=2006483
- National Institute for Literacy
  https://www.federalregister.gov/agencies/national-institute-for-literacy
- National Cancer Institute, Clear and Simple: Developing Effective Print Materials for Low-Literate
  Readers
  http://www.cancer.gov/cancertopics/cancerlibrary/clear-and-simple
- U.S. Census Bureau: Education Statistics
  http://www.census.gov/hhes/socdemo/education/
- Center for Health Care Strategies: Fact Sheets on Literacy
  http://www.chcs.org/publications3960/publications_show.htm?doc_id=291711#.UzW1uE1OWvE
- National Institutes of Health: Clear Communication
  http://www.nih.gov/clearcommunication/healthliteracy.htm
- Pfizer Clear Health Communication: The Newest Vital Sign Toolkit
  http://www.pfizer.com/health/literacy/public_policy_researchers/nvs_toolkit/
- Center for Medicare Education: Communicating With Clients in Person and Over the Phone
  http://www.healthliteracy.com/uploads/CME_IssueBrief.pdf
- *Healthy People 2020*: Health Communication and Health Information Technology
  http://www.healthypeople.gov/2020/topicsobjectives2020/overview.aspx?topicid=18

problem and the reading demand placed on clients in the United States, a systematic approach to address literacy in a client population is indicated. It is now recommended that as part of routine primary care, literacy should be a measured baseline, comparable with many baselines obtained in the course of quality health care.

A first step in intervention for low literacy is to identify clients with literacy deficits. One study compared physicians who screened for literacy issues among their clients and physicians who did not. It was found that physicians overestimated 62% of the time and voiced more dissatisfaction with the client visit (Seligman et al., 2005). In contrast, other researchers have found that residents have increased comfort and skill in working with low-literacy clients after completing a training program (Rosenthal, Werner, & Dubin, 2004). Sadly, health literacy may not be a consistent part of the core curriculum of residency programs (Ali, 2013).

Several researchers have identified tools to efficiently screen clients:

- The Rapid Estimate of Adult Literacy in Medicine (REALM) is a 2-minute test that measures a client's recognition and ability to pronounce common healthcare words (Davis et al., 1993).
- The Test of Functional Health Literacy in Adults (TOFHLA) uses hospital-written materials to test both reading comprehension and basic computational skills. This test takes much longer to administer, approximately 20 to 25 minutes. A shortened version of this test (S-TOFHLA) takes 10 to 15 minutes to administer. These tests may be useful to assess individual clients with specific needs. Recent testing suggests that using just 3 of the 16 S-TOFHLA questions was effective in identifying low-literacy clients ("How often do you have someone help you read hospital materials?" "How confident are you filling out medical forms by yourself?" "How often do you have problems learning about your medical condition because of difficulty understanding written information?") (Chew, Bradley, & Boyko, 2004).
- The Newest Vital Sign is a nutrition label that is accompanied by six questions; it takes 3 minutes to give to a client and broadly screens for low literacy (Johnson & Weiss, 2008; Mackert, Champlin, Pasch, & Weiss, 2013; Weiss et al., 2005). A 2013 study paired this easily used tool with measurement of eye-tracking to identify the effects of distraction and understanding of written information.
- The most recently introduced test, the Single Item Literacy Screener (SILS; Morris, MacLean, Chew, & Littenberg, 2006), was used to evaluate 999 adults with diabetes, 169 of whom had low literacy. SILS asks, "How often do you need to have someone help you when you read instructions, pamphlets, or other written material from your doctor or pharmacy?" The sensitivity of this test was reported to be 54%, and specificity was 83%. Similarly, a one-question screen ("How confident are you filling out forms by yourself?") was found to be the best predictor of low literacy and as good as more time-consuming formal evaluations of literacy (Chew et al., 2008). In a similar vein, a study compared the use of the SILS with a two-item literacy screener ("What was the last grade you completed?" and "Can you estimate your reading ability with one of the following: I frequently read complete books, I read the newspaper, I occasionally need help with the newspaper, or I frequently need help with the newspaper."). The study concluded that use of the single-item tool had similar outcomes and was easier to use (Brice et al., 2014).

Although it takes time and other resources to obtain literacy measures, recent research suggests that this effort may be as simple as asking a single question. Proper identification of client literacy levels can give clear guidance in effective client education.

Within those systems that do not routinely screen clients, asking blunt questions regarding reading abilities may not yield accurate responses. As discussed earlier, clients with low literacy generally do not disclose their difficulties related to reading. They may deliberately conceal their literacy problems or, in some cases, may be unaware of their level of difficulty. Schultz (2002) and Doak et al. (2001) have identified several potential indicators of literacy problems: reading text upside down, difficulty orienting to a brochure, excuses for not reading in front of others (e.g., forgot glasses), mispronouncing words (for English speakers), reluctance to ask questions, missed appointments, difficulty following verbal instructions, relying on family members to fill out forms, and tiring quickly when reading text. When such client behaviors are noticed, it is important for the provider to explore the underlying issues.

Education Strategies

Low-literacy clients may learn better when multiple modes are used to deliver information, such as audiovisual materials, pictographs, and small-group classes, if they are thoughtfully constructed and pretested (HHS, 2014b; Hahn & Cella, 2003; Houts, Wismer, Egeth, Loscalzo, & Zabora, 2001; Oermann, Webb, & Ashare, 2003). At the same time, it is important to understand that changing the mode of communication by itself does not decrease the literacy demand of the message—the decoding, comprehension, and recall components remain the same. However, if there is careful use of language, appropriate use of pictographs and vignettes, client control over the pacing of the information, and provider follow-up to assess comprehension and to individualize the message, then these strategies can prove successful (HHS, 2014a; Hahn & Cella, 2003; Houts et al., 2001).

Such a combination of strategies is now being tested. DeWalt et al. (2006) included picture-based educational materials, training sessions, a digital scale, and frequent telephone follow-up in a heart-failure management program and found that it reduced hospitalization and death.

Readability of Written Materials

Readability of written materials for health care can be vastly improved. Indeed, both the IOM (2003) and original Healthy People list evidence-based health communication as a high-priority item for the improvement of health care. Multiple tools exist that can be used to assess the reading level of materials (Doak et al., 2001); SMOG, FOG, Flesch, and Fry are among the most frequently used readability tools. The formulae employed in these measures are simple, and calculations can often be done by hand or by using widely available software programs, taking only a few minutes (National Cancer Institute, 2003).

The means used to assess the reading demand of text have encountered much criticism in recent years. The tools noted previously evaluate aspects of reading demand, such as word familiarity, length of sentences, punctuation, and number of prepositional words. More recently, new formulae have been introduced that address other variables that affect readability. The Singh Readability Assessment Instrument, for example, includes handwriting or typography that is legible, interest level of the text, and style of writing when evaluating the reading demand of written materials (Singh, 2003).

Given the expense and importance of written materials in today's healthcare environment for vulnerable clients, written materials need to be tested in a systematic fashion (National Cancer Institute, 2003) before their use with actual patient populations. Given the alarming findings based on the NAAL data, all systems of health care need to systematize how written materials are evaluated before their dissemination (IOM, 2003).

English as a Second Language Clients

Addressing the needs of English as a second language (ESL) clients is very complex. Providers generally have taken shortcuts in providing simple English or translated pamphlets that are far above the skill level of such clients—an especially critical shortcoming given that these individuals tend to have significantly longer hospital stays than English-speaking patients (Schillinger & Chen, 2004). Clients with limited English proficiency, even if skilled in their primary language, may be more likely to have children with a fair to poor health status (Flores, Abreu, & Tomany-Korman, 2005). Tools to measure literacy in languages other than English have just begun to be introduced (Lee, Bender, Ruiz, & Cho, 2006). Such development is particularly important because research suggests that a significant number of clients who report proficiency in English in healthcare settings actually have very limited English literacy (Zun, Sadoun, & Downey, 2006).

Use of Computers and the Internet

A number of studies have suggested that technology can be used to address the learning needs of low-literacy clients. One primary drawback, however, is that the reading level of most health-related information (83%) in both English and Spanish on the Internet has been found to require a 12th-grade reading level or higher to ensure adequate comprehension (Berland et al., 2001). Friedman, Hoffman-Goetz, and Arocha (2004) found that cancer-related information was often written at a college level. This finding was validated in a 2006 study of websites providing colorectal cancer information: Not only did the material have a high reading level, but access and skills in the use of such technology represented barriers for those with low literacy.

One study reported a high level of client satisfaction with using the Internet to obtain healthcare information, but also found that low-literacy users greatly overestimated their reading skill in relation to access and comprehension of such information (Birru et al., 2004). Three-fourths of the low-literacy subjects in this investigation did not look past the first page on Google search retrievals, stating that the first page always gives them what they need. Seligman et al. (2005) found similar results in a study of diabetic patients with limited literacy. Specifically, the Internet education strategy alone did not result in significant changes in weight, hypertension, knowledge, and self-efficacy. Programs that had an adaptive component so that each user used a tailored educational approach yielded more positive results (Nebel et al., 2004). Current research questions whether the use of the Internet to solve literacy challenges does pose an unnecessary and unhelpful barrier to clients with low literacy (Jones & DeWalt, 2013). What is now referred to as "e-health literacy" is required to access, decode, comprehend, and use health information found online. Additionally, the consumer would also need regular access to digital resources for this to be a viable option of patient education. Focus groups with an underserved population in Hawaii identified significant obstacles, mirroring the digital divide in our society (Connolly & Crosby, 2014).

IMPROVING LITERACY THROUGH HEALTH CARE

Potential strategies to address illiteracy in health care focus on ways to identify and work with individual clients so that providers' styles of oral and written communication fit with their clients' skill levels. However, these approaches may essentially be skirting the core issue related to client vulnerability.

As reviewed in this chapter, literacy problems themselves create health risks. By using methods that ignore or accommodate the literacy deficit, providers essentially perpetuate the illiteracy problem. This approach, in which providers address the consequences of such core problems as illiteracy, perpetuates the predominant tertiary care focus in the current system of health care. Literacy affects the lives of our clients in foundational ways: the creation of social stigma and prejudicial attitudes; the ability to navigate within complex systems throughout society, including and beyond health care; housing; and money management. Literacy is a core driver of vulnerability in the United States and needs to be addressed as a foundational aspect of health care.

Healthy People 2020 and the IOM state that providers need to improve their communication skills related to literacy needs to improve the quality of health care. In addition, healthcare providers can and should improve their clients' health by increasing their literacy. As David Baker, a researcher in health literacy, has stated (Marwick, 1997) how critical the need is to find better ways of communicating with people to change their learning capabilities in order to achieve health literacy

The literature review for this chapter found few clinical intervention recommendations that spoke to the need to directly improve client literacy skills. Miles and Davis

(1995) recommended that healthcare providers partner with community-wide agencies, such as the school and neighborhood settings where the opportunity to become literate initially foundered. In 2005, Parker evaluated more community approaches to improve literacy by working with libraries to address the long-term nature of low literacy and interventions. Uniquely, she asserted that proper design of all healthcare information—whether written, verbal, or electronic—aligned with the Plain Language Initiative of the National Institutes of Health is a necessary first step. University of Wisconsin-Madison School of Medicine and Public Health has partnered with the Literacy Network, in an "English for Health" program. These classes for the public teach learners how to access the healthcare system, talk more effectively with care providers, take medications safely, and develop healthier lifestyles. In this program, medical students are assigned to classes for 8 weeks and serve as teaching assistants, enabling them to gain experience in working directly with low-literacy clients (Robbins, 2014).

Improvements in provider sensitivity and skills in working with low-literacy clients are required. Providers must be aware of their tendency to overestimate literacy levels, especially in individuals with altered health states. Alternative approaches, such as use of pictures, can be useful. Slowing down, bringing other family members into the discussion, and consistent evaluation of learning for all clients are needed. Use of therapeutic relationships and meaningful interactions can change outcomes dramatically. Paasche-Orlow et al. (2005), for example, studied a "teach to goal" strategy that used a multiple-method and multiple-encounter approach that emphasized effective evaluation of learning. Even with well-planned, focused, and simplified instruction, one-third of the clients were unable to demonstrate comprehension of instructions on first evaluation. The authors note that this approach is very time intensive, but the outcomes were significantly different than the more typical single-encounter, single-method approach in health care.

Similarly, a "teach back" approach to education of clients with low literacy was developed to improve retention and understanding for low-literacy clients. After viewing a multimedia diabetes education program, participants were asked questions about their comprehension and memory of program information. When missed or poorly understood information was immediately "taught back" to the participant, there were no improved outcomes for the program after 2 weeks for the participants (Kandula, Malli, Zei, Larsen, & Baker, 2011). Although this method shows promise, there remains the inherent issue of provider identification. Current research suggests that providers are selectively choosing which patients require a teach-back strategy (Jager & Wynia, 2012).

International literature has already reported programs in which the development of literacy occurs in tandem with healthcare interventions. Watters (2003) presented a fascinating model that integrates linguistics, literacy, nursing, community partnership, and anthropology, which shows potential for use in the United States. Watters reviewed the international programs, citing one in Nepal that noted initially greater costs of a combined maternal nutrition and literacy program, when compared with simply administering vitamin A. The combined approach, however, decreased infant and child mortality by 50%. Such programs can help the community first gain the needed tools in literacy, then subsequently provide for long-term health benefits and decreased vulnerability in the community.

As Baker (1999) stated, in the United States, this kind of approach would require a paradigm shift. Rather than compartmentalizing the skills needed to decrease health vulnerability, healthcare providers could actively work to address core issues that lead to clients' need to access care.

CONCLUSION

Functional illiteracy directly creates health vulnerability in clients. Illiteracy is pervasive in client populations, and clinicians cannot rely on education level or self-disclosure to identify all clients with these needs. Those clients who have the greatest health needs are the same clients who do not have the tools to navigate the complex U.S. healthcare system. Currently, there is a major mismatch between provider communication styles and materials and client literacy skills. Solutions addressing this intersection of healthcare needs and illiteracy have typically been client focused and administered on a micro level. We propose that providers partner with communities to develop literacy skills in their members and, thereby, decrease their health risk. International models may provide models for trial in the United States.

REFERENCES

Aday, L. A. (2001). *At risk in America: The health and health care needs of vulnerable populations in the United States* (2nd ed.). San Francisco: Jossey-Bass.

Ad Hoc Committee on Health Literacy for the Council on Scientific Affairs of the American Medical Association. (1999). Retrieved from http://www.ncbi.nlm.nih.gov/pubmed/10022112

Agency for Healthcare Research and Quality. (2004). Literacy and health outcomes (Evidence Report/Technology Assessment No. 87). Retrieved from www.ahrq.gov

Ali, N. D. (2013). Are we training residents to communicate with low health literacy patients? *Journal of Health Communication*, 7. Retrieved from http://www.jchimp.net/index.php/jchimp/article/view/19238/html

Al-Tayyib, A. A., Rogers, S. M., Gribble, J. N., Villarroel, M., & Turner, C. F. (2002). Effect of low medical literacy on health survey measurements. *American Journal of Public Health*, 92(9), 1478–1480.

Arthur, S. A., Geiser, H. R., Arriola, K. R., & Kripalani, S. (2009). Health literacy and control in the medical encounter: A mixed-method analysis. *Journal of the National Medical Association*, 101(7), 677–683.

Baker, D. (1999). Reading between the lines: Deciphering the connections between literacy and health. *Journal of General Internal Medicine, 14*, 315–317.

Baker, D. W., Gazmararian, J. A., Williams, M. V., Scott, T., Parker, R. M., Green, D., . . . Peel, J. (2002). Functional health literacy and the risk of hospital admission among Medicare managed care enrollees. *American Journal of Public Health, 92*(8), 1278–1283.

Baker, D. W., Parker, R. M., Williams, M. V., Pitkin, K., Parikh, N. S., Coates, W., & Imara, M. (1996). The health care experience of patients with low literacy. *Archives of Family Medicine, 5*(6), 329–334.

Bass III, P. F., Wilson, J. F., Griffith, C. H., & Barnett, D. R. (2002). Residents' ability to identify patients with low literacy skills. *Academic Medicine, 77*(10), 1039–1041.

Berland, G. K., Elliott, M. N., Morales, L. S., Algazy, J. I., Kravitz, R. L., Broder, M. S., . . . McGlynn, E. A. (2001). Health information on the Internet: Accessibility, quality, and readability in English and Spanish. *Journal of the American Medical Association, 285*(20), 2612–2621.

Birru, B. A., Monaco, V. M., Drew, L., Njie, V., Bierria, B. A., Detlefsen, E., & Steinman, R. A. (2004). Internet usage by low-literacy adults seeking health information: An observational analysis. *Journal of Medical Internet Research, 6*(3), e25.

Brice, J. H., Foster, M. B., Principe, S., Moss, C., Shofer, F. S., Falk, R. J., Ferris, M. E., & DeWalt, D. A. (2014). Single-item or two-item literacy screener to predict the S-TOFHLA among adult hemodialysis patients. *Patient Education and Counseling, 94*.

Center for Health Care Strategies. (2010). Health literacy implications of the Affordable Care Act. Retrieved from http://www.unboundmedicine.com/medline/citation/24169024/Single_item_or_two_item_literacy_screener_to_predict_the_S_TOFHLA_among_adult_hemodialysis_patients_

Chew, L. D., Bradley, K. A., & Boyko, E. J. (2004). Brief questions to identify patients with inadequate health literacy. *Family Medicine, 36*(8), 588–594.

Chew, L. D., Griffin, J. M., Partin, M., Noorbaloochi, S., Grill, J., Snyder, A., . . . Vanryn, M. (2008). Validation of screening questions for limited health literacy in a large VA outpatient population. *Journal of General Internal Medicine, 23*(5), 561–566.

Connolly, K. K., & Crosby, M. E. (2014). Examining e-Health literacy and the digital divide in an underserved population in Hawaii. *Hawaii Journal of Medicine & Public Health, 73*(2), 44–48.

Cormier, C., & Kotrlik, J. (2009). Health literacy knowledge and experience of senior baccalaureate nursing students. *Journal of Nursing Education, 48*(5), 237–248.

Cutilli, C. (2007). Health literacy in geriatric patients: An integrative review of the literature. *Orthopaedic Nursing, 26*(1), 43–48.

Davis, T. C., Long, S. W., Jackson, R. H., Mayeaux, E. J., George, R. B., Murphy, P. W., . . . Crouch, M. A. (1993). Rapid estimate of adult literacy in medicine: A shortened screening instrument. *Family Medicine, 1993*(25), 391–395.

Department of Health and Human Services (HHS). (2013). Health communications and health information technology. Retrieved from http://www.healthypeople.gov/2020/topics objectives2020/overview.aspx?topicid=18

Department of Health and Human Services (HHS). (2014a). Health literacy and older adults. Retrieved from http://www.health.gov/communication/literacy/olderadults/visual.htm

Department of Health and Human Services (HHS). (2014b). Strategies: Improve the usability of health information. Retrieved from http://www.health.gov/communication/literacy/quickguide/healthinfo.htm

DeWalt, D. A., Malone, R. M., Bryant, M. E., Kosnar, M. C., Corr, K. E., Rothman, R. L., . . . Pignone, M. P. (2006). A heart failure self-management program for patients of all literacy levels: A randomized, controlled trial. *BMC Health Services Research, 6*, 6–30.

Dickens, C., Lambert, B. L., Cromwell, T., & Piano, M. R. (2013). Nurse estimation of patients' health literacy. *Journal of Health Communication, 18*, 62–69.

Doak, C. C., Doak, L. G., & Root, J. H. (2001). *Teaching patients with low literacy skills* (2nd ed.). Philadelphia: Lippincott.

Duncan, G. J., Daly, M. C., McDonough, P., & Williams, D. (2002). Optimal indicators of socioeconomic status for health research. *American Journal of Public Health, 92*(7), 1151–1158.

Easton, P., Entwistle, V. A., & Williams, B. (2012). Health in the 'hidden' population of people with low literacy: A systematic review of the literature. *BMC Health Services Research,10*, 459–469.

Easton, P., Entwistle, V. A., & Williams, B. (2013). How the stigma of low literacy can impair patient–professional spoken interactions and affect health: Insights from a qualitative investigation. *BMC Health Services Research, 13. Retrieved from http://www.biomedcentral.com/1472-6963/13/319*

Feifer, R. (2003). How a few simple words improve patients' health. *Managed Care Quarterly, 11*(2), 29–31.

Flores, G., Abreu, M., & Tomany-Korman, S. C. (2005). Limited English proficiency, primary language at home, and disparities in children's health care: How language barriers are measured matters. *Public Health Reports, 120*(4), 418–430.

Forbis, S., & Aligne, C. (2002). Poor readability of asthma management plans found in national guidelines, *Pediatrics, 109*, e52.

Freidman, D. B., Hoffman-Goetz, L., & Arocha, J. F. (2004). Readability of cancer information on the Internet. *Journal of Cancer Education, 19*(2), 117–122.

Gannon, W., & Hildebrandt, E. (2002). A winning combination: Women, literacy, and participation in health care. *Health Care of Women International, 23*(6–7), 754–760.

Hahn, E. A., & Cella, D. (2003). Health outcomes assessment in vulnerable populations: Measurement challenges and recommendations. *Archives of Physical Medicine and Rehabilitation, 84*(4 suppl 2), S35–S42.

Healthy People 2010. (2000). Retrieved from http://www.healthypeople.gov/2010/document/pdf/uih/2010uih.pdf?visit=1

Hohn, M. D. (1998). Empowerment health education in adult literature: A guide for public health and adult literacy practitioners, policy makers, and funders. Retrieved from http://www.nifl.gov/nifl/fellowship/reports/hohn/HOHN.HTM

Houts, P. S., Wismer, J. T., Egeth, H. E., Loscalzo, M. J., & Zabora, J. R. (2001). Using pictographs to enhance recall of spoken medical instruction. *Patient Education and Counseling, 43*(3), 231–242.

Institute of Medicine (IOM). (2003). *Priority areas for national action: Transforming health care quality*. Washington, DC: National Academies Press.

Jager, A. J., & Wynia, M. K. (2012). Who gets a teach-back? Patient-reported incidence of experiencing a teach back. *Journal of Health Communication, 17*, 294–302.

Johnson, K., & Weiss, B. (2008). How long does it take to assess literacy skills in clinical practice? *Journal of the American Board of Family Medicine, 21*(3), 211–214.

Jones, C. D., & DeWalt, D. A. (2013). Lost in translation: Are we reaching the target audience with Internet-based education materials? *Journal of Vascular & Interventional Radiology, 24* (4), 474–475.

Joint Commission (2007). "What did the Doctor say?:" Improving health literacy to protect patient safety." Retrieved from http://www.jointcommission.org/assets/1/18/improving_health_literacy.pdf

Jukkala, A., Deupree, J., & Graham. (2009). Knowledge of limited health literacy at an academic health center. *Journal of Continuing Education in Nursing, 40*(7), 298–302.

Kandula, N., Malli, T., Zei, C. P., Larsen, E., & Baker, D. W. (2011). Literacy and retention of information after a multimedia diabetes educations program and teach-back. *Journal of Health Communication, 16*, 89–102.

Karsenty, C., Landau, M., & Ferguson, R. (2013). Assessment of medical resident's attention to the health literacy level of newly admitted patients. *Journal of Community Hospital Internal Medicine Perspectives, 17*(3), 3–4.

Katz, M., Jacobson, E., & Kripalani, S. (2007). Patient literacy and question-asking behavior during the medical encounter: A mixed-methods analysis. *Journal of General Internal Medicine, 22*(6), 782–786.

Kirsch, I. S., Jungeblut, A., Jenkins, L., & Kolstad, A. (1993). Executive summary of adult literacy in America: A first look at the results of the National Adult Literacy Survey. Retrieved from http://nces.ed.gov/pubs93/93275.pdf

Kripalani, S., Henderson, L., Chiu, E., Robertson, R., Kohm, P., & Jacobson, T. (2006). Predictors of medication self-management skill in a low-literacy population. *Journal of General Internal Medicine, 21*(8), 852–856.

Lee, S. Y., Bender, D. E., Ruiz, R. E., & Cho, Y. I. (2006). Development of an easy-to-use Spanish health literacy test. *Health Services Research, 41*(4 Pt 1), 1392–1412.

Mackert, M., Champlin, S. E., Pasch, K. E., & Weiss, B. D. (2013). Understanding health literacy measurement through eye tracking. *Journal of Health Communication, 18*, 185–196.

Marwick, D. (1997). Patients' lack of literacy may contribute to billions of dollars in higher hospital costs. *Journal of the American Medical Association, 278*(12), 971–972.

Miles, S., & Davis, T. (1995). Patients who can't read: Implications for the health care system. *Journal of the American Medical Association, 274*(21), 1677–1682.

Morris, N. S., MacLean, C. D., Chew, L. D., & Littenberg, B. (2006). The Single-Item Literacy Screener: Evaluation of a brief instrument to identify limited reading ability. *BMC Family Practice, 7*(21), 107.

Murphy-Knoll, L. (2007). Low health literacy puts patients at risk. *Journal of Nursing Care Quality, 22*(3), 205–209.

National Cancer Institute. (2003). Clear and simple: Developing effective print materials for low-literate clients. Retrieved from http://www.nci.nih.gov/cancerinformation/clearandsimple

National Center for Education Statistics. (2006). The health literacy of adults: Results from the 2003 National Assessment of Adult Literacy. Retrieved from http://nces.ed.gov/pubs2006/2006483.pdf

National Center for Education Statistics. (2007). Literacy behind bars: Results from the 2003 National Assessment of Literacy. Retrieved from http://nces.ed.gov/pubs2007/2007473_2.pdf

National Center for Education Statistics. (NCES). (2014). National assessment of adult literacy—Gender & Literacy. Retrieved from https://nces.ed.gov/naal/health_results.asp#GenderHealth Literacyasp&PageID=158

Nebel, I. T., Klemm, T., Fasshauer, M., Muller, J., Verlohren, H. J., Klaiberg, A., & Paschke, R. (2004). Comparative analysis of conventional and an adaptive computer-based hypoglycaemia education programs. *Patient Education and Counseling, 53*(3), 315–318.

Nutbeam, D. (2008). The evolving concept of health literacy. *Social Science & Medicine, 6*(8), 2072–2078.

Oermann, M. H., Webb, S. A., & Ashare, J. A. (2003). Outcomes of videotape instruction in clinic waiting area. *Orthopedic Nursing, 22*(2), 102–105.

Paasche-Orlow, M., Parker, R., Gazmararian, J., Neilsen-Bohlman, L., & Rudd, R. R. (2005). The prevalence of limited health literacy. *Journal of General Internal Medicine, 20*, 175–184.

Paasche-Orlow, M., Reikert, K. A., Bilderback, A., Chanmugam, A., Hill, P., Rand, C., . . . Krishnan, J. A. (2005). Tailored education may reduce health literacy disparities in asthma self-management. *American Journal of Respiratory and Critical Care Medicine, 172*(8), 980–986.

Parker, R. (2005). Library outreach: Overcoming health literacy challenges. *Journal of the Medical Library Association, 93*(3), S81–S85.

Powell, C., & Kripalani, S. (2005). Resident recognition of low literacy as a risk factor in hospital readmission. *Journal of General Internal Medicine, 20*(11), 1042–1044.

Raich, P. C., Plomer, K. D., & Coyne, C. A. (2001). Literacy, comprehension, and informed consent in clinical research. *Cancer Investigation, 19*(4), 437–445.

Robbins, K. (2014). UW-Madison University/Community Partnership Award. Retrieved from http://ahec.wisc.edu/community-partnership-award

Rootman, I., & Ronson, B. (2005). Literacy and health research in Canada: Where have we been and where have we gone? *Canadian Journal of Public Health, 96*(suppl 2), S62–S77.

Rosenthal, M. S., Werner, M. J., & Dubin, N. H. (2004). The effect of a literacy training program on family medicine residents. *Family Medicine, 36*(8), 582–587.

Ryan, L., Logsdon, M. C., McGill, S., Stikes, R., Senior, B., Helinger, B., . . . Davis, D. W. (2014). Evaluation of printed health education materials for use by low-education families. *Journal of Nursing Scholarship.*

Safeer, R. S., & Keenan, J. (2005). Health literacy: The gap between physicians and patients. *American Family Physician, 72*(3), 463–468.

Sanders, L. M., Federico, S., Klass, P., Abrams, M. A., & Dreyer, B. (2009). Literacy and child health. *Archives of Pediatric and Adolescent Medicine, 163*(2), 131–140.

Schillinger, D., & Chen, A. (2004). Literacy and language: Disentangling measures of access. *Journal of General Internal Medicine, 19*, 288–290.

Schillinger, D., Piette, J., Grumbach, K., Wang, F., Willson, C., Daher, C., . . . Bindman, A. B. (2003). Physician communication with diabetic patients who have low literacy. *Archives of Internal Medicine, 163*(1), 83–90.

Schlichting, J., Quinn, M., Heuer, L., Schaefer, C., Drum, M., & Chin, M. (2007). Provider perceptions of limited health literacy in community health centers. *Patient Education and Counseling, 69*(1), 114–120.

Schultz, M. (2002). Low literacy skills needn't hinder care. *RN, 65*(4), 45–48.

Seligman, H. K., Wang, F. F., Palacios, J. L., Wilson, C. L., Haher, C., Piette, J. D., & Schillinger, D. (2005). Physician notification of their diabetes patients' limited health literacy: A randomized controlled study. *Journal of General Internal Medicine, 20*, 1001–1007.

Sentell, T., & Ratcliff-Baird, B. (2003). Literacy and comprehension of Beck Depression Inventory response alternatives. *Community Mental Health Journal, 39*(4), 323–331.

Singh, J. (2003). Research briefs reading grade level and readability of printed cancer education materials. *Oncology Nursing Forum, 30*(5), 867–870.

U.S. Census, American Community Survey Reports. (2013). *Language use in the U.S. 2011.* Retrieved from http://www.census.gov/prod/2013pubs/acs-22.pdf

Watters, E. K. (2003). Literacy for health: An interdisciplinary model. *Journal of Transcultural Nursing, 14*(1), 48–54.

Weiss, B. D., Mays, M. Z., Martz, W., Castro, K. M., DeWalt, D., Pignone, M., . . . Hale, F. A. (2005). Quick assessment of literacy in primary health care: The newest vital sign. *Annals of Family Medicine, 31*(6), 514–522.

Williams, M. V. (2000). Definition of "health literacy." Message posted to National Institute for Literacy list server. Retrieved from http://www.nifl.gov/nifl-health/2000/0439.html

Williams, M. V., Baker, D., Honig, E. G., Lee, T. M., & Nowlan, A. (1998). Inadequate literacy as a barrier to asthma knowledge and self-care. *Chest, 114*, 1008–1015.

Wolf, M. S., Williams, M. V., Parker, R. M., Pariskh, N. S., Nowlan, A. W., & Baker, D. W. (2007). Patients' shame and attitudes toward discussing the results of literacy screening. *Journal of Health Communication, 12*(8), 721–732.

Zun, L. S., Sadoun, T. A., & Downey, L. (2006). English-language competency of self-declared English-speaking Hispanic patients using written tests of health literacy. *Journal of the National Medical Association, 98*(6), 912–919.

Chapter 6

Nursing Theories and Models Applied to Vulnerable Populations: Examples from Turkey

Behice Erci

OBJECTIVES

At the end of this chapter, the reader will be able to

1. Identify the key concepts of the theories and models discussed in this chapter.
2. Compare and contrast the application of theories and models with the same patient for each example given.
3. Explain how the application of the theories and models might differ with patients from cultures other than Turkey.

INTRODUCTION

Nursing must continue to develop distinctive, if not unique, knowledge if it is to take its place as a legitimate professional discipline. Within the last 30 years, nurse theorists and modelers have made extensive contributions in defining the essence of nursing practice and in delineating the role nurses play in supporting the health and well-being of clients (Villarruel, Bishop, Simpson, Jemmott, & Fawcett, 2001).

This chapter describes the areas in which nursing models and theories guide nursing practice related to vulnerable populations. Three nursing theories and seven nursing models are presented, with detailed clinical examples offered for several of the theories believed to be most applicable. Readers are referred to the primary sources for complete description and explanation of the theoretical concepts. In addition, this chapter briefly reviews prior discussion concerning the theory–practice split, including the major concerns regarding the contribution of theory to practice in the design of instruction (or lack thereof) as well as proposals and progress made by scholars to address those concerns. We suggest, however, that the gap between theory and practice has yet to be satisfactorily resolved and that an alternative way of thinking about this long-standing problem, and about theory per se, can improve attempts to generate usable theoretical understanding. As we explicate this alternative perspective, we suggest several of its implications for future theorizing and inquiry in the field (Yanchar & South, 2009).

The Importance of Theories and Models in Advanced Nursing Practice

The dilemma for nurse educators is how best to prepare nurses for advanced practice roles. Are nursing theories and models important? Do they contribute to clinical practice? Which theories and models form sound foundations for advanced practice? Theories and models exist to challenge existing practice, create new approaches to practice, and remodel the structure of rules and principles. Furthermore, theories and models should ultimately improve nursing practice. Usually, this goal is achieved by using theories or portions of theories and models to guide practice.

Defining the scope of advanced practice requires that the role of nurses be perceived as unique. For nursing practice to be viewed as professional, it is essential that practice is based on theory and model. Theory and theoretical frameworks are intended to provide guidance and rationale for professional practice, but as advanced practice roles evolve in nursing, the incorporation of nursing theory becomes problematic. Some critics have suggested that the wide variety of definitions and concepts discussed in most nursing theories do not explain or predict anything and, therefore, cannot practically be applied to clinical situations and are of little use to nurses in advanced practice.

Future of Nursing Theory and Model

Theoretical systems are active and give direction to future research studies and administrative, educational, and practice applications. Theoretical works developed in a discipline affect the nature of the questions asked, the methods used to answer the questions, and the scope of knowledge addressed. Nursing models and theories exhibit characteristics of Kuhn's criteria for normal science; that is, a scientific community uses research based on scientific achievements as the foundation of practice. Expansion of the philosophy of nursing science has increased the use of qualitative theory development in addition to use of quantitative methods and has greatly increased the development and use of middle range theory. Global communities of nurse scholars have emerged as a result of the expanded communication opportunities on the Internet (Alligood, 2006).

LEININGER'S THEORY OF CULTURE CARE

Leininger's interest in the cultural dimensions of human care and caring led to the development of her theory (Leininger, 2002). This author subscribed to the central tenet that "care is the essence of nursing and the central, dominant, and unifying focus of nursing" (McFarland, 2006, p. 472). The unique focus of Leininger's theory is care, which she believes to be inextricably linked with culture. She defines culture as "the learned, shared, and transmitted values, beliefs, norms, and life ways of a particular group that guides their thinking, decisions, and actions in patterned ways" (Leininger, 1991, p. 47). The ultimate purpose of care is to provide culturally congruent care to people of different or similar cultures to "maintain or regain their well-being and health or face death in a culturally appropriate way" (Leininger, 1991, p. 39).

Example

A group of Iraqi refugees fled to a city in southeastern Turkey to seek refuge from political unrest, persecution, and extreme poverty. Providing culturally congruent nursing care to this group of people is difficult because of differences in language, which in turn leads to difficulty in understanding the lifeways of this group. The children have diarrhea, and it is difficult for the nurse to observe, interview, and collect data related to cultural practices that might explain the diarrhea. The nurse helps the group to preserve favorable health and caring lifestyles related to their poverty and diarrhea. The nurse assists group members in accomplishing cultural adaptation, negotiation, or adjustment to the refugees' health and lifestyles. To do so, the nurse can reconstruct or alter designs to help clients change their health or life patterns in ways that are meaningful to them.

WATSON'S THEORY OF HUMAN CARING

The caring model or theory can also be considered a philosophical and moral–ethical foundation for professional nursing and part of the central focus for nursing at the disciplinary level. Watson's model of caring is both art and science; it offers a framework that embraces and intersects with art, science, humanities, spirituality, and new dimensions of mind–body–spirit. Key concepts in this theory include nursing, person, health, human care, and environment. Watson's theory has particular relevance to nursing ethics (Watson, 2005).

Application to Vulnerable Populations

Watson emphasizes that it is possible to read, study, learn about, and even teach and research the caring theory; however, to truly "get it," one has to personally experience it. Thus, the model is both an invitation and an opportunity to interact with the ideas, to experiment with them, and to grow through their application. If one chooses to use the caring perspective as theory, model, philosophy, ethic, or ethos for transforming self and practice or self and system, then asking a variety of questions related to one's view of caring and what it means to be human might help in clarifying the theory's application (McCance, McKenna, & Boore, 1999; Watson, 1996; Watson & Smith, 2002).

Example

Nesim is 60 years old, married, and lives with his family. His primary diagnosis is hypertension. Under older models of care, this patient might be convinced that he would simply overcome his hypertension—that it would "go away." In the Watson model, however, the nurse should aim to sustain a helping–trusting, authentic, caring relationship to develop the capacity of the patient to problem solve and to teach him and his family proper care of his condition. The nurse educates the patient about hypertension and about improving self-health, thereby enabling and authenticating the deep belief system of the patient. The nurse is supportive of the expression of both positive and negative feelings by the patient. Nesim improves as the nurse creates a healing environment at all levels (physical as well as nonphysical).

The patient should be assisted in the creative use of self and all ways of knowing as part of the caring process. The nurse must engage Nesim in the artistry of caring-healing practices that are "human care essentials," and that facilitate alignment of mind–body–spirit, wholeness, and unity of being in all aspects of care (Watson, 1996, p. 157). The patient should be followed to evaluate the medical and dietary treatment of hypertension.

KOLCABA'S COMFORT THEORY

The Theory of Comfort has already made significant contributions to nursing and is poised for greatly expanded use in the discipline. Kolcaba's energy for disseminating her theory through presentations, publications, and websites is as great as her energy for developing and applying her theory. This committed theoretician is a model of excellence for the nursing community in her drive to further the discipline's domain of knowledge and to promote patient-focused care.

Application to Vulnerable Populations

Comfort is defined as the state that is experienced by recipients of comfort measures. It is the immediate and holistic experience of being strengthened through having needs met for the three types of comfort (relief, ease, and transcendence) in four contexts of experience (physical, psycho-spiritual, social, and environmental) (Kolcaba, 1994; 2003.)

Nursing is the intentional assessment of comfort needs, design of comfort measures to address those needs, and reassessment of comfort levels after implementation compared with the baseline. Assessment and reassessment can be intuitive or subjective or both, such as when a nurse asks if the patient is comfortable, or objective, such as in observations of wound healing, changes in laboratory values, or changes in behavior. Assessment can be achieved through the administration of visual analog scales or traditional questionnaires, both of which Kolcaba (2003) has developed. The first part of the theory, predicting that effective nursing interventions offered over time will demonstrate enhanced comfort, has been tested and supported with women with breast cancer.

Example

Meryem, a 16-year-old female patient diagnosed with leukemia, was admitted in a semiprivate ward in the oncology unit. She was about to receive her combination chemotherapy when the nurse noticed her alone and crying silently while lying on her bed.

Taxonomic Structure of Meryem's Comfort Needs

- *Relief*
  - o Physical: mouth sores, nausea and vomiting, neuropathy, diarrhea/constipation
  - o Psycho-spiritual: anxiety, alopecia, radiation recall
  - o Environmental: cold room, patients cohorted in a single room
  - o Sociocultural: absence of family
- *Ease*
  - o Physical: comfortable resting position to facilitate sleep and relaxation to deter fatigue
  - o Psycho-spiritual: anticipation of social stigma toward baldness and skin problems
  - o Environmental: deviation from aseptic technique and standard precautions, lack of privacy
  - o Sociocultural: failure of effective communication due to language barrier
- *Transcendence*
  - o Physical: patient resumes most of her leukemia treatment with all the side effects controlled
  - o Psycho-spiritual: actual need for reassurance and support from the healthcare team and significant others
  - o Environmental: need for calm and positive atmosphere that strictly adheres to infection control guidelines; need for privacy for personal hygiene routine care
  - o Sociocultural: need for family support and reinforcement

When nurses are committed to provide satisfyingly holistic comfort care, the needs for relief, ease, and/or transcendence are routinely identified throughout the practice. Assessment could go back and forth to relief, ease, and transcendence until the main focus of health care is identified and be addressed. However as the patient's condition varies, it is essential that the nurse identify correctly which context the patient and his family's concerns entails for priority of comfort measures. When comfort needs are addressed in one context, total comfort is enhanced in the remaining contexts.

Nurses are the mighty front lines in the healthcare institution. As active participants in strengthening and enhancing comfort for every patient, they engage themselves in activities to achieve and maintain a certain level of their optimal health. They tend to be the advocates of patients, leading them to be the patients' first link to normalcy once they face a frightening or painful experience.

Comfort Interventions

Standard comfort. Assessment for development and complaints of the side effects of the chemotherapy (may use comfort daisies, comfort behavior, checklist, etc.); Frequently check vitals and watch out for fever or signs of nosocomial infections; Administer medications or treatments to relieve the side effects of chemotherapy; Agent: nurse/consultation with family and doctors.

Coaching. Avoiding the word "pain" upon assessment, obtaining data, and rendering health teaching for a paediatric patient; Initiate patient and family education as needed; Agent: doctors/nurses consultation with family.

Comfort food for the soul. Practice guided imagery to eliminate factors that could increase physical discomfort; Provide privacy as Marie is entering pubescent stage when she will be concerned about her body image and privacy; Agent: nurse/family.

Comfort interventions have three categories: (a) standard comfort interventions to maintain homeostasis and control pain; (b) coaching, to relieve anxiety, provide reassurance and information, instill hope, listen, and help plan for recovery; and (c) comfort food for the soul, those extra nice things that nurses do to make children and families feel cared for and strengthened, such as massage or guided imagery (Kolcaba, 2003).

OREM'S SELF-CARE MODEL

Orem's self-care theory (Berbiglia & Saenz, 2000; Orem, 2001) links patient assessments with nursing diagnosis, expected patient outcomes, discharge planning, quality assurance, clinical research, and external agency reports. This theory includes three subtheories:

- The *theory of self-care deficit* details how individuals can benefit from nursing because they are subject to health-related or self-derived limitations.

- The *theory of self-care* states that care is a learned behavior that purposely regulates human structural integrity, functioning, and development.
- The *theory of nursing systems* describes how nurses use their abilities to prescribe, design, and provide nursing care.

Application to Vulnerable Populations

To provide nursing care, Orem identifies operations that are specifically professional–technological, including diagnostic, prescriptive, treatment, or regulatory and case management. The application of Orem's theory to nursing practice is relevant as a framework in a variety of settings, including acute care units, ambulatory clinics, community health programs, high-rise senior centers, nursing homes, hospices, and rehabilitation centers. The theory is applied to patients with specific diseases or conditions, including adolescents with chronic disease, alcoholics, the chronically ill, patients who have undergone head and neck surgery, patients with rheumatoid arthritis, and patients with cardiac conditions (Conway, McMillan, & Solman, 2006; Taylor, Geden, Issaramalai, & Wongvatunyu, 2000). The theory is also applied to selected age groups, including the aged, children, coronary care, prenatal and postnatal care, and mothers with newborns.

Example

Yeliz is 29 years old, married, and 5 months pregnant. She has anemia, is underweight, and is under the care of a primary healthcare center. Complete data have been compiled from this client's records and a home visit. The nurses are concerned that Yeliz's self-care requisites (or requirements) are not being met—specifically, food, healthy activity, and rest. Yeliz requires assistance in food preparation but can eat on her own. Her priority diagnoses are inadequate food intake, low activity level, and fatigue due to inadequate rest.

Diagnostic and Prescriptive Operations

All three of these priority diagnoses are related to preventing health deterioration. In this client's case, the self-care deficit theory of nursing proposes a supportive educational nursing system that is designed to individualize her care. The individualization of the nursing system is accomplished through the overlay of basic conditioning factors and developmental self-care requisites (or requirements for life and health) on the therapeutic self-care demands (those processes necessary to maintain life or health). The expected outcome is health status maintenance, health promotion, and prevention of further health deterioration through the strengthening of the self-care agency. Unless expected outcomes are provided, the nursing system design will change.

Regulatory Operations

The self-care deficit theory of nursing is especially useful with this client. It shifts the focus away from disease and toward the strengths and weaknesses of the self-care agent. It is evident that this client does seek to prevent or manage the conditions threatening her health, yet she requires assistance in this area. The most significant self-care deficit is in the area of nutrition. Guided by the theory, the nurse analyzed the self-care agency from the perspective of the basic conditioning factors. Cultural variety should be considered in reaching for the expected outcome.

Data collection for Yeliz in terms of her self-care requisites led to the following proposed outcomes: maintenance of the healthy environment, ability of the client to feed herself, and discussion of her condition and medical regimen with the home health nurse and aide and the client's family. The nursing diagnosis showed a potential for anemic complications such as falls and decreased mobility. Methods of help and intervention included teaching, guiding, and providing and maintaining direction in an environment that supported personal development. Self-care agency is inadequate and implies the necessity to gain better understanding of the cause and subsequent prevention of problems. The nursing diagnosis is "potential for exacerbation and increased disability related to knowledge deficits concerning problems." Teaching, guiding, and directing are methods of helping. For the nursing diagnosis, "inability to maintain ideal body weight related to cultural attitudes toward eating and weight gain and meal preparation by aide," the methods of helping are to provide and maintain an environment that supports personal development.

ROY'S ADAPTATION MODEL

Roy drew upon expanded insights in relating spirituality and science to present a new definition of adaptation and related scientific and philosophical assumptions (Connerley, Ristau, Lindberg, & McFarland, 1999; Lopes, Pagliuca, & Araujo, 2006). Roy believes that adaptation involves human response to stimuli within the system. According to Roy, a person's response may be either adaptive or ineffective during interaction with the environment (Ducharme, Ricard, Duquette, Levesque, & Lachance, 1998; Roy, 1997). Her philosophical stance articulates that nurses see persons as coextensive with their physical and social environments. Furthermore, nurse scholars take a value-based stance rooted in beliefs and hopes about the human person, and they develop a discipline that participates in enhancing the well-being of persons and of the earth. Roy views persons and groups as adaptive systems, for which cognator and regulator subsystems act to maintain adaptation in the four modes: physiological–physical, self-concept–group identity, role function, and interdependence.

Application to Vulnerable Populations

Roy used a problem-solving approach for gathering data, identifying the capacities and needs of the human adaptive system, selecting and implementing approaches for nursing care, and evaluating the outcome of the care provided. This approach includes assessment of behavior and stimuli and is consistent with the nursing process of assessment, diagnosis, planning, implementation, and evaluation.

Example

Hasan is a 35-year-old man who was recently admitted to the oncology nursing unit for evaluation after undergoing surgery for class IV prostate cancer. He has smoked approximately two packs of cigarettes per day for the past 9 years. Hasan is married and lives with his wife. He has done well after surgery except for being unable to completely empty his urinary bladder. Hasan is having continued postoperative pain. When he goes home, it will be necessary for him to perform intermittent self-catheterization. His home medications are an antibiotic and an analgesic as needed. In addition, he will be receiving radiation therapy on an outpatient basis.

Hasan is extremely tearful. He expresses great concern over his future. He believes that this illness is a punishment for his past life.

Physiological Adaptive Mode

This client's health problems are complex. It is impossible to develop interventions for all of his health problems within this chapter. Therefore, only representative examples are given. The physiological adaptive mode refers to the basic and complex biological processes necessary to maintain life.

Assessment of Behavior

Postoperatively, the patient is unable to completely empty his urinary bladder. He states that he is "numb" and unable to tell when he needs to void. Catheterization for residual urine reveals that he is retaining 300 mL of urine after voiding. As a consequence, this patient needs to perform intermittent self-catheterization at home. Unsanitary conditions at Hasan's home place him at high risk for developing a urinary tract infection. He states that he is scared about performing self-catheterization.

Assessment of Stimuli

In this phase of the nursing process, the nurse searches for the stimuli responsible for certain observed behaviors. After the stimuli are identified, they are classified as focal, contextual, or residual. The focal stimulus for Hasan's urinary retention is his disease process. Contextual stimuli include tissue trauma resulting from surgery and radiation therapy. Anxiety is a residual stimulus. Infection is a potential problem.

The focal stimulus is the need for intermittent self-catheterization. Contextual stimuli include altered skin integrity related to surgical incision, poor understanding of aseptic principles, and unsanitary conditions at Hasan's home.

Nursing Diagnosis

From the assessment of behaviors and the assessment of stimuli, the following nursing diagnoses are made:

- *Altered elimination*: urinary retention related to surgical trauma, radiation therapy, and anxiety
- *Potential for infection*: related to intermittent self-catheterization, altered skin integrity resulting from surgical incision, poor understanding of aseptic principles, and unsanitary conditions at the client's home

Goal Setting

Goals are mutually set between the nurse and the client for each of the nursing diagnoses. The goals are: (1) complete urinary elimination every 4 hours as evidenced by correct demonstration of the procedure for intermittent self-catheterization, and (2) continued absence of signs of infection of the surgical incision and urinary tract.

Implementation

To help the client attain these goals, the following nursing interventions were implemented:

- To address the issue of incomplete elimination, the client is taught the importance of performing intermittent self-catheterization every 4 hours to prevent damage to the urinary bladder. He is taught to assess his abdomen for bladder distension and the proper procedure for intermittent self-catheterization. He is instructed to keep a record of the exact time and amount of voiding and catheterizations. In addition, the client is taught relaxation techniques to facilitate voiding so it will not be necessary for him to catheterize himself as often.
- To address the potential for infection, the client is taught the importance of washing hands before touching the surgical incision or doing incision care. After the nursing staff demonstrates the procedure for incision care, the client is asked to perform a return demonstration. After the intermittent self-catheterization procedure is explained and demonstrated, the client is asked to perform a return demonstration.

Evaluation

An evaluation of the client's adaptive level is performed during each shift.

Self-Concept Adaptive Mode

Assessment of Behavior

The client is extremely tearful and expresses great concern over his future. Exploration of the client's tearfulness revealed that the client is afraid of dying. Also, the client has not asked the nurse any questions about sexuality. His hesitancy to introduce the subject may be related to his cultural background. In this case, the nurse introduces the topic. Salient findings are as follows: (1) the client recently learned of his diagnosis of prostate cancer, (2) he has undergone a recent operation, (3) he is receiving radiation therapy in the hospital and this therapy will continue when he leaves the hospital, and (4) the client has a lack of information about the impact of prostate cancer and chemotherapy on sexuality.

Assessment of Stimuli

The client is an adult, married, and has a fifth-grade education. He is in an emotionally distant and sometimes abusive relationship. Being diagnosed with prostate cancer at an early age has resulted in a maturational crisis for the client, which is further complicated by the fact that several of his relatives have died of cancer. It is important for the nurse to assess coping strategies. One coping strategy that is mentioned is that the client is frequently tearful.

Nursing Diagnosis

The following nursing diagnoses are made:

- Fear and anxiety of dying related to medical diagnosis and witnessing other family members' deaths as a result of cancer
- Spiritual distress related to severe life-threatening illness and perception of the moral–ethical–spiritual self
- Sexual dysfunction related to the disease process, need for radiation therapy at home, weakness, fatigue, pain, anxiety, and a lack of information about the impact of prostate cancer and chemotherapy on sexuality
- Grieving related to body image disturbance, lack of self-ideal, and potential for premature death

Goal Setting

To help the client achieve adaptation in the self-concept adaptive mode, the following goals are set:

- Decrease fear and anxiety of dying, as evidenced by less tearfulness, relaxed facial expression, relaxed body movements, verbalization of new coping strategies, and fewer verbalizations of fear and anxiety
- Decrease spiritual distress, as evidenced by verbalization of positive feelings about the value and meaning of his life, and less tearfulness
- Resume sexual relationship that is satisfying to both partners, as evidenced by verbalization of self as sexually capable and acceptable, and verbalization of alternative methods of sexual expression during the first 10 weeks after surgery
- Progression through the grieving process as evidenced by verbalization of feelings regarding body image, self-ideal, and potential for premature death

Implementation

The following nursing interventions are implemented to help achieve these goals in the self-concept adaptive mode:

Fear and anxiety of dying related to the medical diagnosis and witnessing other family members' deaths as a result of cancer. Although the client's prognosis appeared to be good, he remained fearful of dying. Time is taken to sit with the client, make eye contact, and actively listen. The client is asked to share an extremely difficult experience he encountered in the past. He is asked how he coped with that experience. Once his present coping strategies are assessed, new coping strategies are suggested.

In addition, the client is encouraged to express his feelings openly. After allowing the client adequate time to express his feelings, truthful and realistic hope based on the client's medical history is offered. A cancer support group meets each week in the hospital where the client is a patient. The client is given a schedule of the meeting times and topics. He and his partner are encouraged to attend the cancer support group meetings.

Spiritual distress related to severe life-threatening illness and perception of the moral–ethical–spiritual self. The client is encouraged to express his feelings openly about his illness. It is suggested that times of illness are good times to renew spiritual ties. The client is supported in positive aspects of his life.

Sexual dysfunction related to the disease process, need for radiation therapy at home, weakness, fatigue, pain, anxiety, and a lack of information about the impact of prostate cancer and chemotherapy on sexuality. A complete sexual assessment is conducted to evaluate the perceived adequacy of the client's sexual relationship and to elicit concerns or issues about sexuality before his diagnosis with prostate cancer. A private conversation is initiated with the client to gain an understanding of his sexual concerns resulting from his therapy and his beliefs about the effects of prostate cancer in regard to sexual functioning. The client is instructed regarding possible changes in sexual functioning, such as a temporary inability to achieve or sustain an erection, which may last for several months.

Grieving related to body image disturbance, loss of self-ideal, and potential for premature death. The client's perceptions regarding the impact of the diagnosis of prostate cancer on his body image, self-ideal, roles, and his future are explored. Hasan is encouraged to verbally acknowledge the losses he is experiencing. He is observed to determine which stage of the grief process he currently experiences. The grieving process is explained to the client and to his family, and they are assured that grieving is a normal process. The nursing staff should offer realistic reassurance about the client prognosis. The client is encouraged to attend the cancer support group so he can talk to others who better understand his grief.

Evaluation

Behavior change is expected.

KING'S INTERACTING SYSTEMS MODEL

The focus of King's (1997) theory is on individuals whose interactions in groups within social systems influence behavior within the systems (Sieloff, 2006). In other words, the perceptions that people experience as a result of their surroundings influence their own behavior. King's theory is system based. Concepts of self-growth and development and body image are important (Frey & Norris, 1997; Sieloff, 2006). King's conceptual system provides a comprehensive view of three dynamic interacting systems—personal, interpersonal, and social. Her theory of goal attainment has been used as the basis for practice, education, research, and administration, examples of which are presented here (King, 1997). According to this theory, the goal of nursing is to help individuals maintain their health so they can function in their roles.

Application to Vulnerable Populations

It is within the nurse–client interpersonal system that the traditional steps of the nursing process are carried out. Nurse and client meet in some situation, perceive each other, make judgments about the other, take some mental action, and react to each one's perceptions of the other. Because these behaviors cannot be directly observed, one can only draw inferences from them. The next step in the process is interaction that can be directly observed. When interactions lead to transactions, goal attainment behaviors are exhibited. An assumption underlying the interaction process is that of reciprocally contingent behavior in which the behavior of one person influences the behavior of the other, and vice versa (Sieloff, 2006).

Example

Elif is 50 years old and has heart failure. She is married and lives with her husband. She describes him as emotionally distant and abusive at times. Elif is having continued cardiac pain and palpitation. She will be receiving cardiac therapy on an outpatient basis. Elif is extremely tearful and anxious, and she expresses great concern over her future.

Within King's framework, Elif is conceptualized as a personal system in interaction with other systems. Many of these interactions influence her health. In addition, her recent diagnosis of heart failure influences her health. Together Elif and the nurse communicate, engage in mutual goal setting, and make decisions about the means to achieve goals.

Nursing care for Elif begins with assessment, which includes collection, interpretation, and verification of data. Sources of data primarily include Elif herself: her perceptions, behavior, and past experiences. In addition, the nurse uses knowledge of concepts in the systems framework, critical thinking skills, the ability to use the nursing process, and medical knowledge about the treatment and prognosis of heart failure. Care should cover the full range of nursing practice: maintenance and restoration of health, care of the sick, and promotion of health.

The nurse forms an interpersonal system with Elif. The transaction process includes perception, judgments, mental actions, and reactions of both individuals. The nurse assesses and applies her knowledge of concepts and processes. Critical concepts are perception, self-coping, interaction, role, stress, power, and decision making. The nurse's perception serves as a basis for gathering and interpreting information. Elif's perceptions influence her thoughts and actions and are assessed through verbal and nonverbal behaviors. Because perceptual accuracy is important to the interaction process, the nurse analyzes her own perceptions and her interpretation of Elif's perceptions collaboratively with Elif. It is expected that perceptions might be influenced by her emotional state, stress, or pain.

According to King, self is the conception of who and what one is; it includes one's subjective totality of attitudes, values, experiences, commitments, and awareness of individual existence. Elif reveals important information about herself. She is tearful and expresses fear and concern. Her past behavior provides some basis for her present feelings, in that Elif has not taken actions to promote and maintain her own health. Clearly, her feelings about herself and the situation are psychological stressors.

Elif has physical and interpersonal stressors as well. The physical stressors are a result of her illness. Cardiac function, pain, and palpitation are identified as immediate problems. In the interpersonal system, Elif identifies a distant and abusive relationship with her husband. She is experiencing a major lack of emotional support during this very difficult time. Her husband's inability to provide basic emotional support is likely to change Elif's physical status.

An additional stressor is Elif's living situation. It is also possible that the lack of personal and perhaps family space contributes to stress. Coping with personal and interpersonal stressors is likely to influence both health and illness outcomes. Elif may need additional resources to help her cope with the immediate situation and the future.

Communication is the key to establishing mutuality and trust between Elif and the nurse, which are key components needed to establish patient priorities and move the interaction process toward goal setting. Elif is expected to participate in identifying goals. However, direction from the nurse will likely be necessary because of Elif's overwhelming needs and lack of resources.

Nurses can find direction for assisting patients in identifying goals based on the assumptions that underlie King's systems framework. They assist patients to adjust to changes in their health status. Decisions about goals must be based on the capabilities, limitations, and priorities of the patient, as well as the unique situation. In this case, the immediate goals seem to be control of cardiac pain and palpitation, although this needs validation by Elif.

The first nursing action is to perform a psychological assessment and provide crisis intervention. Other important goals and actions will be directed toward mobilizing resources, especially support from Elif's husband. However, it is possible that nursing goals and client goals may be incongruent. Continuous analysis, synthesis, and validation are critical to keep this process on track.

In addition to decisions about goals, Elif is expected to be involved in decisions about actions to meet goals. Involving Elif in decision making may be a challenge because of her sense of powerlessness over the illness, treatment, and ability to contribute to family functioning. Yet empowering Elif is likely to increase her sense of self, which in turn can reduce her level of stress, improve her coping ability, change her perceptions, and lead to positive changes in her physical state.

Goal attainment needs ongoing evaluation. For Elif, follow-up on pain, palpitation, and cardiac function after discharge is necessary. An option might be to arrange for in-home nursing services. Having a professional in the home would also contribute to further assessment of the family, validation of progress toward goals, and modifications in plans to achieve goals. According to King, if transactions are agreed upon and carried out, goals will be attained. Goal attainment can improve or maintain health, control illness, or lead to a peaceful death. If goals are not attained, the nurse needs to reexamine the nursing process, critical thinking process, and transaction process.

ROGERS'S UNITARY HUMAN BEINGS MODEL

Rogers formulated a theory to describe humans and the life process in humans (Daily et al., 1994; Rogers, 1992, 1994). Over the ensuing years, four critical elements emerged that are basic to the proposed system: energy fields, open systems, pattern, and pandimensionality (Rogers, 1992). The final concept, *pandimensionality*, was previously known as multidimensionality and four-dimensionality. Although Rogers never updated her work, the theory still provides much that is useful (Malinski, 2006).

Application to Vulnerable Populations

Within Rogers' model, the critical-thinking process can be divided into three components: pattern appraisal, mutual patterning, and evaluation. The critical-thinking process begins with a comprehensive pattern appraisal. The life process possesses its own unity and is inseparable from the environment; thus a holistic appraisal requires the identification of patterns that reflect the whole. Pattern appraisal is a comprehensive assessment.

Knowledge gained in the appraisal process occurs via cognitive input, sensory input, intuition, and language. The nurse gains a great deal of appraisal knowledge during the interview with the client by using the feeling or sensing level of knowing. Often described as instinctual, such intuitive knowledge is best realized through reflection. Reflection, in turn, assists in appraising patterns. Manifestations of patterns are not static, but rather partial perceptions of the synthesis of the past, present, and future. These perceptions provide the basis for intuitive knowing. Manifestation, patterns, and rhythms are an indication of evolutionary emergence of the human field. Pattern appraisal and rhythm identification, along with reflection, provide the content for appraisal validation with the patient.

Once the client and the nurse have reached a consensus with respect to the appraisal, then nursing action centers on mutual patterning of the client's human–environmental field. The goal of the nursing action is to bring about and promote "symphonic interaction" between human and environment. This interaction is intended to strengthen the coherence and integrity of the human field and to "direct and redirect patterning of the human and environmental fields" (Rogers, 1992, p. 122). Patterning activities can be devised with respect to the initial pattern appraisal.

The evaluation process is ongoing and fluid as the nurse reflects on his or her intuitive knowing. During the evaluation phase, the nurse repeats the pattern appraisal process to determine the level of dissonance perceived. These perceptions are then shared with the client and his or her family and friends. Further mutual patterning is directed by the perceptions found during the evaluation process. This process continues as long as the nurse–client relationship continues (Bultmeier, 1997).

Example

Ayse is a 32-year-old woman who was recently admitted to the infection nursing unit for evaluation after experiencing urinary infection and late-stage AIDS. Her weight is 58 kilograms, down from her usual weight of 80 kilograms. She has smoked approximately one pack of cigarettes per day for the past 16 years. Ayse has two children; she is married and lives with her husband in conditions that she describes as less than sanitary. She describes her husband as emotionally distant and abusive at times. She is having continued pain and nausea. It will be necessary for her to perform intermittent self-catheterization at home. Her home medications are an antibiotic, an analgesic, and an antiemetic. She will soon be receiving radiation therapy on an outpatient basis.

Ayse is extremely tearful. She expresses great concern over her future and the future of her two children. She believes that this illness is a punishment for her past life.

Within the Rogerian model, the process of caring for Ayse begins with pattern appraisal, which is seen as the most important component of the nursing process. The nurse must engage in caring–healing practices that are human care essentials. The purpose is to potentiate alignment, followed by engagement in mutual patterning and evaluation.

Pattern Appraisal

The history provides a major portion of the pattern appraisal. Ayse has a pattern of smoking, which has been associated with poor health. This visible rhythmical pattern is a manifestation of evolution toward dissonance. In addition, Ayse has a pattern manifestation that has been labelled AIDS. This emergent pattern manifests as dissonant. Ayse has a low educational level, which is relevant as patterning activities are introduced. The nurse has reported that Ayse has a manifestation of fear; she reports the fear of dealing with her life after this illness, and the nurse senses this manifestation of fear. Ayse's self-knowledge links the illness to her personal belief of being punished for past mistakes. History and focusing on the "relative present" to explore the pattern of punishment is imperative. It is important that the nurse appraise the environment of the hospital and of the others who share her existence.

The pain and fear are dissonant manifestations. Dissonance can be perceived in many aspects of Ayse's appraisal: her unsanitary living conditions, her relationship with her husband, the manifestations of AIDS, weight loss, pain, nausea, and tobacco use. Likewise, dissonance is conceptualized as fear and is manifested in the emotional distance that Ayse feels.

On completion of the pattern appraisal, the nurse presents the analysis to the patient. Emphasis can be placed on areas in which dissonance and harmony are noted in the personal and environmental field manifestations. Consensus needs to be reached with Ayse before patterning activities can be suggested and implemented.

Mutual Patterning

Patterning can be approached from many directions, but must always be mutual between nurse and patient. Medications are patterning modalities, for example, and Ayse is receiving medications. Decisions are made in conjunction with Ayse regarding the use of the medications and the patterning that emerges with the introduction of these modalities. Personal knowledge regarding the medications empowers Ayse to be a vital agent in the selection of modalities. She possesses freedom and involvement in these decisions. Options include therapeutic touch, humor, meditation, visualization, and imagery.

Therapeutic touch can be introduced to Ayse, particularly to reduce her pain. Touch in combination with medications provides patterning that Ayse can direct. The nurse can introduce the process of touch to Ayse's husband and teach him how to incorporate touch into her care. Another option would be to teach Ayse how to center her energy and channel it to the area that is experiencing pain.

Patterning directed at the manifestation of Ayse's fear is critical. Options to alter her current pattern include imagery, music, light, and meditation. Fear is manifested as her apprehension about self-catheterization, for example. Emphasis needs to be placed on having Ayse direct how, where, when, and with whom the self-catheterization is taught. Establishing a rhythm to the catheterization schedule that is harmonious with Ayse's life would reduce dissonance. Patterning of nutrition and catheterization based on the pattern appraisal can assist in empowering Ayse to learn self-catheterization. A rhythm will evolve that is harmonious with Ayse and her energy field rhythm and that empower Ayse to direct this phase of her treatment.

Human–environment patterning needs to involve the other individuals who share Ayse's environment, including her husband and children. Options relate to increased communication and sanitation patterns. The nurse talks with the family and Ayse to determine what Ayse would prefer to change in her environment to improve sanitation. Options are introduced that allow pattern evolution to be integral with her environment in way that is not perceived as dissonant.

Evaluation

The evaluation process centers on the perceptions of dissonance that exist after the mutual patterning activities are implemented, to determine whether they were successful. Specific emphasis is placed on emergent patterns of dissonance that are still evident.

Manifestations of pain, fear, and tension with family members are appraised. The nurse continually evaluates the amount of dissonance that is apparent with respect to Ayse as he or she cares for her. A summary of the dissonance or harmony that the nurse perceives is then shared with Ayse, and mutual patterning is modified or instituted as indicated based on the evaluation.

ROPER, LOGAN, AND TIERNEY'S ACTIVITIES OF LIVING MODEL

In the United Kingdom, the model of nursing used most predominantly is that developed by Roper, Logan, and Tierney (2002), which bases its principles on a model of living. This model consists of five components: activities of daily living, life span, dependence–independence continuum, factors influencing activities of daily living, and individuality in living. Roper et al. suggest that these five components are as applicable to a model of living as they are to a model of nursing. Their work has applicability to a variety of clinical situations (Mooney & O'Brien, 2006; Timmins, 2006).

Example

Hatice is 55 years old. She has difficult respiration and constipation. She cannot do her own cleaning.

First, considering 12 activities of daily living and affecting factors, the nurse collects data about the client and sets nursing diagnoses, goals, and activities.

Diagnosis: Difficult breathing

Goal setting: Effective breathing

Activity: The nurse monitors Hatice's breathing patterns and respirations and ensures that her room is clean and at a normal temperature.

Diagnosis: Constipation

Goal setting: Normal defecation

Activity: The nurse provides warm water for the client every morning and encourages appropriate exercise. After these activities, the nurse should evaluate the results.

PEPLAU'S INTERPERSONAL RELATIONS MODEL

Pearson, Vaughan, and Fitzgerald (2005, p. 179) describe Hildegard Peplau as "one of the earliest American theorists to recognize and respond to the need for changes in nursing practice," Peplau's primary area of interest was psychiatric nursing, but her work can be applied to other fields as well (Pearson et al., 2005).

Peplau's interpersonal relations model relates to the meta-paradigm of the discipline of nursing (Forchuk, 1993) and includes four concepts: the view of the person, health, nursing, and environment. This model describes the individual as a system with physiological, psychological, and social component. The individual is viewed an unstable system for which equilibrium is a desirable state but occurs only through death. This perspective is supported by Peplau's statement that "man is an organism that lives in an unstable equilibrium (i.e., physiological, psychological, and social fluidity) and life is the process of striving in the direction of stable equilibrium (i.e., a fixed pattern that is never reached except in death)" (Peplau, 1992, p. 82). Despite the fact that her model was developed some years ago, Peplau's work continues to have high applicability (McCamant, 2006; Moraes, Lopes, & Brage, 2006; Stockmann, 2005; Vandemark, 2006).

Application to Vulnerable Populations

The interpersonal relationship between the nurse and the client as described by Peplau (1992) has four clearly discernible phases: orientation, identification, exploitation, and resolution. These phases are interlocking and require overlapping roles and functions as the nurse and the client learn to work together to resolve difficulties in relation to health problems.

During the *orientation* phase of the relationship, the client and the nurse come together as strangers meeting for the first time. At this stage, the development of trust and empowerment of the client are primary considerations. This is best achieved by encouraging the client to participate in identifying the problem and allowing the client to be an active participant. By asking for and receiving help, the client will feel more at ease expressing needs, knowing that the nurse will take care of those needs. Once orientation has been accomplished, the relationship is ready to enter the next phase.

During the *identification* phase of the relationship, the client, in partnership with the nurse, identifies problems. Once the client has identified the nurse as a person willing and able to provide the necessary help, the main problem and other related problems can then be worked on, in the context of the nurse–client relationship. Throughout the identification phase, both the nurse and the client must clarify each other's perceptions and expectations, as these considerations affect the ability of both to identify problems and the necessary solutions. When clarity of perceptions and expectations is achieved, the client will learn how to make use of the nurse–client relationship. In turn, the nurse will establish a trusting relationship. Once identification has occurred, the relationship enters the next phase.

During the *exploitation* phase, the client takes full advantage of all available services. The degree to which these services are used reflects the needs and interests of the client. During this time, the client begins to feel like an integral part of the helping environment and starts to take control of the situation by using the help available from the services offered. In other words, the client begins to develop responsibility and become more independent. From this sense of self-determination, the client develops an inner strength that allows him or her to face new challenges. This point is best described by Peplau: "Exploiting what a situation offers gives rise to new differentiations of the problem and to the development and improvement of skill in interpersonal relations" (Peplau, 1992, pp. 41–42).

As the relationship passes through all the aforementioned phases and the needs of the client have been met, the relationship passes to closure that is, the *resolution* phase.

The strength of Peplau's model derives from its focus on the nurse–client relationship. This emphasis allows for the nurse and the client to work together as partners in problem solving. Peplau's model encourages and supports empowerment of the client by encouraging the client to accept responsibility for well-being. The focus on the partnership of the nurse and the client and the emphasis on meeting the identified needs of the client make this model ideal for short-term crisis intervention. Although it is often applied to getting sick people well, the model is also appropriate for health promotion. Indeed, its clear focus on the nurse–client relationship provides a foundation for many types of interactions between the nurse and the client that can enhance health.

Example

Tarkan is a 46-year-old married man who is scheduled to undergo a heart operation next week. He has had a few hospitalizations and is anxious about the operation.

The first phase of Peplau's model is orientation. Because this client has previously been cared for at the hospital, he is familiar with the layout of the facility as well as the general rules and regulations of the facility. Thus orientation is quickly established.

In the next phase of the relationship (identification), the nurse and Tarkan identify problems that require attention, including his feelings about the operation and potential for death as a result. The nurse determines that the client is experiencing mixed emotions about the operation because he understands it is necessary. The nurse then identifies that this client requires additional support because he has been relatively stable for a time, yet now requires an operation.

In the third phase (exploitation), Tarkan quickly begins making use of the available resources and services at his disposal and talks with the nurse about his fears and hopes. He expresses feelings of mixed emotions, and the nurse comforts him by reminding him that his feelings are normal. In turn, he expresses relief.

Because the client had been hospitalized twice within a 1-year period, the client is provided with information on services that can be accessed to assist him further should the need arise. With the client making full use of the available services, the nurse–client relationship then enters the final phase, resolution. During resolution, the client becomes less dependent on the nurse for one-on-one interactions and no longer seeks further assistance.

NEUMAN'S HEALTHCARE SYSTEMS MODEL

The Neuman healthcare systems model (Neuman, 2002) is related here to the meta-paradigm of the discipline of nursing. As in other models of nursing, the major concepts are the person, health, nursing, and the environment. Neuman, however, uses a systems approach to explain how these elements interact in ways that provide nurses with guidance to intervene with patients, families, or communities. Her view of health seems to be that of a continuum rather than a dichotomy of health versus illness (Freese, 2006). Not much is found in the current nursing literature on Neuman's model, as newer models have developed. Nevertheless, her legacy should be honored. For example, this model has been successfully used in the examination of anxiety (August-Brady, 2000).

Example

Dilek is a 25-year-old woman experiencing violence from her husband and auditory and visual hallucinations. An intrapersonal stressor for Dilek is the limited effectiveness of her current medication regimen in relieving her acute symptoms, including difficulty sleeping. Other interpersonal and extrapersonal stressors are also exacerbating her distress. The interpersonal stressors include a strained relationship with her husband related to the charges brought against him for sexual and physical abuse. The extrapersonal stressor comprises inadequate community resources that could help her stay in her home. Once the stressors have been identified, a determination of the level of prevention required to strengthen the flexible line of defense is made.

In Dilek's situation, the identified stressors have penetrated the line of defense, so the goal is to prevent further regression. This is a tertiary level of intervention in this case, focused on maintaining and supporting the existing strengths of the client. Such an intervention is best achieved through intensive conversations of the nurse with the client to emphasize her existing strengths. Dilek is encouraged to express her mixed feelings of relief and sadness about her relationship with her husband, and her feelings are validated as normal. The alleviation of her psychiatric symptoms is achieved without alteration to her established medication regimen.

The primary level of intervention is aimed at health promotion. One of the identified stressors is inadequate community resources. The client attends the local mental health center on a regular basis, but these appointments take place only once per month. The client should be provided with information about crisis centers, emergency support, and grief counselling. The nurse follows up to ensure that the client makes contact with these resources to strengthen the flexible line of defence.

CONCLUSION

This chapter reviewed some of the major nursing theories and models. Although the examples presented here are from Turkey, the elements of these models are global and timeless.

REFERENCES

Alligood, M. R. & Tomey, A. M. (Eds.). (2010). Nursing theorists and their work (7th ed.). Maryland Heights, (MO): Mosby-Elsevier.

August-Brady, M. (2000). Prevention as intervention. *Journal of Advanced Nursing*, *31*(6), 1304–1308.

Berbiglia, V. A., & Saenz, J. (2000). Design, implementation, and evaluation of a self-care undergraduate elective. *The International Orem Society Newsletter*, *8*(1), 2–5.

Bultmeier, K. (1997). Rogers' science of unitary human being in nursing practice. In M. Alligood & A. Marriner-Tomey (Eds.), *Nursing theory utilization and application* (pp. 283–306). St. Louis, MO: Mosby-Year Book.

Connerley, K., Ristau, S., Lindberg, C., & McFarland, M. (1999). The Roy model in nursing practice. In Roy, C. (Ed.), *The Roy adaptation model* (2nd ed., pp. 515–534). Stamford, CT: Appleton & Lange.

Conway, J., McMillan, M., & Solman, A. (2006). Enhancing cardiac rehabilitation nursing through aligning practice to theory: Implications for nursing education. *Journal of Continuing Education in Nursing 37*(5), 233–238.

Daily, L. S., Maupin, J. S., Murray, C. A., Satterly, M. C., Schnell, D. L., & Wallace, T. L. (1994). Martha E. Roger: Unitary human beings. In A. Marriner-Tomey (Ed.), *Nursing theorists and their work* (3rd ed., pp. 211–230). St. Louis, MO: C. V. Mosby.

Ducharme, F., Ricard, N., Duquette, A., Levesque, L., & Lachance, L. (1998). Empirical testing of a longitudinal model derived from the Roy adaptation model. *Nursing Science Quarterly*, *11*(4), 149–159.

Forchuk, C. (1993). *Hildegarde E. Peplau: Interpersonal nursing theory*. Newbury Park, CA: Sage.

Freese, B. T. (2006). Betty Neuman: Systems model. In A. M. Tomey & M. R. Alligood (Eds.), *Nursing theorists and their work* (pp. 318–334). St. Louis, MO: Mosby.

Frey, M. A., & Norris, D. (1997). King's system framework and theory in nursing practice. In M. Alligood & A. Marriner-Tomey (Eds.), *Nursing theory utilization and application* (pp. 181–206). St. Louis, MO: Mosby-Year Book.

King, I. M. (1997). King's theory of goal attainment in practice. *Nursing Science Quarterly*, *10*(4), 180–185.

Kolcaba, K. (1994). A theory of holistic comfort for nursing. *Journal of Advanced Nursmg 19*, 1178–1184.

Kolcaba, K. (2003). *Comfort theory and practice: A vision for holistic health care and research.* New York: Springer Publishing Company.

Leininger, M. M. (1991). *Culture care diversity and universality: A theory of nursing.* New York: National League of Nursing Press.

Leininger, M. (2002). Essential transcultural nursing concepts, principles, example, and policy statements. In M. Leininger & M. R. McFarland (Eds.), Transcultural nursing: Concepts, theories, research, and practice (3rd ed., pp. 45–69). New York: McGraw-Hill Medical Publishing Division.

Lopes, M. V. O., Pagliuca, L. M. F., & Araujo, T. L. (2006). Historical evolution of the concept environment proposed in the Roy adaptation model. *Revista Latino-Americana de Enfermagem, 14*(2), 259–265.

Malinski, V. (2006). Rogerian science-based nursing theories. *Nursing Science Quarterly, 19*(1), 7–12.

McCamant, K. (2006). Humanistic nursing, interpersonal relations theory and the empathy-altruism hypothesis. *Nursing Science Quarterly, 19*(4), 334–338.

McCance, T., McKenna, H., & Boore, J. (1999). Caring: Theoretical perspectives of relevance to nursing. *Journal of Advanced Nursing, 30*, 1388–1395.

McFarland, M. (2006). Madeleine Leininger: Culture care theory of diversity and universality. In A. M. Tomey & M. R. Alligood (Eds.), *Nursing theorists and their work* (pp. 472–496). St. Louis, MO: Mosby.

Mooney, M., & O'Brien, F. (2006). Developing a plan of care using the Roper, Logan and Tierney model. *British Journal of Nursing, 15*(16), 887–892.

Moraes, L., Lopes, M., & Brage, V. (2006). Analysis of the functional components of Peplau's theory and its confluence with the group reference. *Acta Paulista de Enfermagem, 19*(2), 228–233.

Neuman, B. (2002). *The Neuman systems model definition.* In B. Neuman & J. Fawcett (Eds.), *The Neuman systems model* (4th ed., pp. 322–324). Upper Saddle River, NJ: Prentice-Hall.

Orem, D. E. (2001). *Nursing concepts of practice* (6th ed.). St. Louis, MO: Mosby.

Pearson, A., Vaughan, B., & Fitzgerald, M. (2005). The self-care models for nursing. In Orem, D. (Ed.), *Nursing models for practice* (3rd ed., pp. 103–122). Philadelphia: Butterworth-Heinemann, Elsevier.

Peplau, H. E. (1992). *Interpersonal relations in nursing.* New York: Springer.

Rogers, M. E. (1992). Window on science of unitary human beings. In M. O'Toole (Ed.), *Miller-Keane encyclopedia and dictionary of medicine, nursing and allied health* (p. 1339). Philadelphia: W. B. Saunders.

Rogers, M. E. (1994). The science of unitary human beings: Current perspectives. *Nursing Science Quarterly, 7*(1), 33–35.

Roper, N., Logan, W., & Tierney, A. (2002). *The elements of nursing* (4th ed.). Edinburgh: Churchill Livingstone.

Roy, C. (1997). Future of the Roy model: Challenge to redefine adaptation. *Nursing Science Quarterly, 10*(1), 42–48.

Sieloff, C. L. (2006). Imogene King: Interacting systems of goal attainment. In A. M. Tomey & M. R. Alligood (Eds.), *Nursing theorists and their work* (pp. 297–318). St. Louis, MO: Mosby.

Stockmann, C. (2005). A literature review of the progress of the psychiatric nurse–patient relationship as described by Peplau. *Issues in Mental Health Nursing, 26,* 911–919.

Taylor, S. G., Geden, E., Issaramalai, S., & Wongvatunyu, S. (2000). Orem's self-care deficit nursing theory: Its philosophic foundation and the state of the science. *Nursing Science Quarterly, 13*(2), 104–108.

Timmins, F. (2006). Conceptual models used by nurses working in coronary care units: A discussion paper. *European Journal of Cardiovascular Nursing, 5*(4), 253–257.

Vandemark, L. (2006). Awareness of self and expanding consciousness: Using nursing theories to prepare nurse therapists. *Issues in Mental Health Nursing, 27*(6), 605–615.

Villarruel, A. M., Bishop, T. L., Simpson, E. M., Jemmott, L. S., & Fawcett, J. (2001). Borrowed theories, shared theories, and the advancement of nursing knowledge. *Nursing Science Quarterly, 14*(2), 158–163.

Watson, J. (1996). Watson's theory of transpersonal caring. In P. H. Walker & B. Neuman (Eds.), *Blueprint for use of nursing models: Education, research, practice, and administration* (pp. 141–184). New York: NLN Press.

Watson, J. (2005). Caring science: Belonging before being as ethical cosmology. *Nursing Science Quarterly, 18*(4), 304–305.

Watson, J., & Smith, M. (2002). Caring science and the science of unitary human beings: A transtheoretical discourse for nursing knowledge development. *Journal of Advanced Nursing, 37,* 452.

Yanchar, S. C., & South J. B. (2009). Beyond the theory–practice split in instructional design: The current situation and future directions. In M. Orey et al. (Eds.), *Educational media and technology yearbook.* New York: Springer Science-Business Media.

Chapter 7

Applying Middle-Range Concepts and Theories to the Care of Vulnerable Populations

Nicole Mareno

OBJECTIVES

At the end of this chapter, the reader will be able to

1. Describe how middle-range theories in nursing apply to vulnerable populations.
2. Apply at least one theory to a specific population of interest to the reader.
3. Provide at least one research example that uses a middle-range theory.

INTRODUCTION

The disciplinary focus of the nursing profession is to improve the quality of life and health of individuals, families, communities, and society (McCurry, Hunter Revell, & Roy, 2010). Contemporary nursing care is heavily influenced by knowledge development that is happening within a dynamic, evolving social and environmental healthcare context (McCurry et al., 2010). Risjord (2010) argued that nursing knowledge development, which he termed the *nursing standpoint* starts from "nurses lives" (p. 74), or that the problems and solutions in nursing are identified within nurses' daily practice. Problem identification leads to the development, refinement, and dissemination of knowledge, with theory providing the foundation (Risjord, 2010). Risjord posits that appropriate theories for the nursing profession address nursing problems, whether they are proposed by nurses, or borrowed from other disciplines.

Middle-range theories are useful in addressing the problems of nursing, especially among vulnerable populations. Although middle-range theories address specific phenomena within nursing practice, the theories are broad enough to be applied to a variety of patient populations, and across many practice settings. Middle-range concepts and theories selected for this chapter were adapted from content in a graduate-level family nurse practitioner course on healthcare theory. In the course, family nurse practitioner students applied middle-range concepts and theories to practice. Either the concept or an associated theory are discussed and applied to the care of the vulnerable. Concepts from this chapter could be used in doctoral courses for concept analysis and explored in the context of vulnerability.

In this chapter, eight middle-range concepts or theories will be discussed. Individual-level middle-range theories, social middle-range theories, and middle-range theories that integrate multiple perspectives will be presented. Definitions of the concepts comprising each middle-range theory will be provided. The middle-range concept or theory will be applied to the care of vulnerable populations using a specific example from the literature. Practical application of each middle-range concept or theory in the care of vulnerable populations will be given.

INDIVIDUAL-LEVEL MIDDLE-RANGE THEORIES

In proposing solutions to problems of vulnerability, it is essential to begin by understanding individual-level factors. Once the concepts are understood from an individual level, the influence of families, communities, and populations can be examined. The individual-level middle-range concepts or theories of self-efficacy, adherence, and change will be discussed.

Self-Efficacy

Self-efficacy has been defined as a system of self-monitoring where an individual judges his or her capability to carry out a behavior or course of action (Bandura & Perloff, 1967; Bandura, 1977). Cognitive processing, in the form of reflective thought, helps individuals to set standards for their behavior and then generate skills necessary to accomplish behavioral goals. Bandura and Perloff (1967) noted that individuals generate self-prescribed rewarding or punishing consequences that they apply depending on how their behavior compares to a self-selected external evaluation criterion. An assumption of self-efficacy theory is that individuals have the cognitive ability to exercise behavioral control and create evaluation criteria to judge their abilities.

In social cognitive theory, Bandura (1986) asserted that self-efficacy was an important mediator within the triad of reciprocity among behavior, cognition, and other personal/environmental influences. Bandura (1977) proposed two components of self-efficacy: self-efficacy expectations and outcome expectations. Bandura defined self-efficacy expectations as an individual's belief that he or she can successfully carry out a behavior to produce an anticipated outcome. Bandura defined outcome expectations as a person's estimation that a particular behavior will lead to a particular outcome. An individual may believe that a particular behavior leads to a certain outcome (outcome expectations), but may or may not possess the belief that they can successfully carry out the behavior (self-efficacy expectations).

Bandura and colleagues' early work with individuals who suffered from snake phobias provided the foundation for self-efficacy theory (Bandura, Blanchard, & Ritter, 1969). Bandura (1977) asserted that individuals who are motivated by fear avoid threatening situations that they believe exceed their coping abilities, whereas individuals who believe themselves capable will unquestionably handle situations or problems. Self-efficacy expectations influence the amount of effort an individual expends in making a behavioral change, and how likely an individual is to persist with accomplishing the behavioral change in spite of obstacles (Bandura, 1977). Bandura was careful to note that expectations alone do not produce behavioral changes, and individuals may be capable of change but do not possess the incentive to engage in the process.

Self-Efficacy Sources

Bandura (1986) proposed that individuals use four informational self-efficacy sources that work in a reciprocal manner: (1) enactive attainment, (2) vicarious experience, (3) verbal persuasion, and (4) physiological feedback.

Enactive Attainment

Enactive attainment is defined as personal mastery experiences or the actual performance of the behavior (Bandura, 1977, 1986). Bandura (1995) acknowledged that an individual's perception of the difficulty of the behavioral change, amount of effort required, context/environment of the behavioral change, and past pattern of successes and failures had an impact on self-efficacy. Bandura (1977, 1986) theorized that mastery of one behavioral change can have a carry-over effect in the execution of other behavioral changes.

Vicarious Experience

Bandura (1977) defined *vicarious experience* as expectations that are derived from seeing others perform a behavioral change (or threatening activity) without experiencing negative consequences. The observer subsequently self-models the behavior and uses social comparison to persuade him or herself that he or she is capable of making the change with effort and perseverance. Bandura argued that an individual needs to have clear performance outcomes, otherwise improvements in self-efficacy may be based on the observed individual's successful performance of the behavioral change.

Verbal Persuasion

Verbal persuasion is defined as leading individuals, through verbal suggestion, into believing that they can successfully make behavioral changes (Bandura, 1977). Bandura stated that verbal persuasion is less effective than enactive attainment because an individual is not authentically experiencing success with the change and can easily be derailed by a disconfirming experience.

Physiological Feedback

Bandura (1977) asserted an individual's judgment of their ability to successfully make changes depends, in part, by their acknowledgement and response to physiological indicators (e.g., anxiety). Bandura originally termed this *emotional arousal* (p. 198). If the individual experiences negative physiological symptoms, he or she may be less inclined to engage in the behavioral change process.

Application to Vulnerable Populations

Vulnerability may increase the likelihood of threatening situations or obstacles to success. In order to support individuals who embark on the behavioral change process, nurses can use self-efficacy theory in order to understand barriers and facilitators to self-efficacy. Nursing interventions can be used to increase the opportunity for personal mastery experiences (enactive attainment), include family or support systems as role models in the behavioral change process (vicarious experience), use professional communication skills to help patients and families identify facilitators to change (verbal persuasion), and provide nursing care that helps to mitigate anxiety (physiological feedback). Assisting patients to improve self-efficacy in the behavioral change process can occur in any setting (e.g., long-term care), and among any population or subpopulation (e.g., pregnant adolescents).

Enhancing self-efficacy among vulnerable populations requires attention to the patient's (and family's) socioeconomic status, strength of the support system relationships, primary language spoken, literacy level, educational level, and the context/environment in which the patient and family lives. Opportunities for personal mastery experiences may be limited, for example, by lack of financial means or community safety issues. Nurses are well positioned to assess for barriers to self-efficacy, including demoralization from past efforts to change. Professional, empathetic communication is critical when helping to enhance self-efficacy among vulnerable populations.

Research Example

Sharoni and Wu (2012) examined self-efficacy with managing type 2 diabetes among a sample of 388 adults in Malaysia. Self-efficacy of diabetes management was measured using the Diabetes Management Self-Efficacy Scale (DMSES) (van der Bijl, van Poelgeest-Eeltink, & Shortridge-Baggett, 1999). The DMSES is a Likert-type scale that addresses an individual's confidence in managing blood glucose, diet, and exercise (van der Bijl et al., 1999). Sharoni and Wu (2012) assessed self-efficacy and correlated self-efficacy score with self-care behavior. Self-care behavior was measured by a patient's level of glycosylated hemoglobin, which is indicative of glycemic control. The participants reported a moderately high level of self-efficacy in managing their type 2 diabetes. Sharoni and Wu (2012) found that participants who reported higher levels of self-efficacy had better glycemic control. Lower levels of education impacted self-efficacy and glycemic control in a negative manner; this finding has implications for vulnerable patients who do not possess high levels of formal education.

Practical Application

Brenda is a 19-year-old woman, recently divorced from a physically abusive husband, and has just given birth to her first child. The vaginal delivery was without incident; both mother and child are recovering on the postpartum unit. Brenda has had three unsuccessful attempts to breastfeed her daughter. Brenda's primary nurse is concerned that it is an issue of low self-efficacy with breastfeeding. The primary nurse outlined several interventions to promote Brenda's breastfeeding self-efficacy including: (1) two sessions with a lactation consultant to increase opportunities for personal mastery (enactive attainment), (2) encouraging Brenda to observe her roommate who has been successful with breastfeeding attempts (vicarious experience), and (3) use of encouraging words (verbal persuasion) and empathetic listening to reduce anxiety (physiological feedback). After two sessions with the lactation consultant to practice breastfeeding techniques, and self-modeling after watching her roommate breastfeed, Brenda was successfully able to breastfeed her daughter.

ADHERENCE

In order to provide patient and family-centered nursing care to vulnerable populations, understanding the attributes of the concept of adherence, and factors impacting adherence is critical. Through concept analysis Cohen (2009) defined adherence as an agreement (or goal concordance) between or among a patient, family, and healthcare provider in determining necessary persistence in the practice and maintenance of desired, recommended health behaviors. McBride, Bryan, Bray, Swan, and Green (2012) argued that adherence differs from other health change outcomes because the focus is on persistence in practicing and maintaining treatment recommendations from a healthcare provider.

Cohen (2009) identified four attributes of adherence including: (1) patient (and family) behaviors align with provider treatment recommendations, (2) patient (and family) increase health knowledge and master the new behavior, (3) patient/family and healthcare provider have concordant goals with plans to overcome barriers, and (4) ongoing support for maintaining treatment recommendations.

Conceptually, adherence involves a group of characteristics that leads to an outcome of improved health outcomes. Characteristics of adherence include communication, goal setting, practice of health behaviors/skills, and self-management. Since adherence can apply to a variety of treatment recommendations (e.g., taking a medication, engaging in physical activity) the way the concept is operationalized can vary. In general, adherence has been operationalized as percentage of time that an individual correctly or properly fulfills a treatment recommendation. For example, Walsh, Mandalia, and Gazzard (2002) measured 30-day medication adherence using a self-report diary, while Colbert, Sereika, and Erlen (2012) used electronic event monitoring (a medication cap containing a microchip that records the date and time the bottle is opened) to assess the percentage of prescribed medication administrations taken.

Application to Vulnerable Populations

There is a constellation of personal, family, social, economic, religious, environmental, and societal factors that impact an individual's ability to adhere to a healthcare provider's treatment recommendations. In addition to sociodemographic factors including age and educational level, researchers have explored an individual's functional health literacy (Colbert et al., 2012) and self-efficacy (Nokes et al., 2012) as factors impacting adherence to treatment recommendations. While Colbert and colleagues did not find a strong association between functional health literacy and adherence to treatment, Nokes and colleagues found that self-efficacy was a significant predictor of treatment adherence. The treatment itself, especially if the treatment creates untoward side effects, can be a barrier to adherence.

When caring for vulnerable populations, sensitivity to an individual's or family's life circumstances including family income, employment status, ability to afford health insurance, environmental living conditions, transportation issues, and personal beliefs/value systems is necessary. While a desire to adhere to treatment recommendations may be present, social or financial issues may impact adherence. As Cohen (2009) noted, two critical attributes of adherence are ongoing support and plans to overcome barriers to treatment adherence.

Research Example

Fair, Monahan, Russell, Zhao, and Champion (2012) examined perceived benefits and risks of adherence to yearly mammograms among a group of 299 African American women in Indiana. Fair and colleagues defined mammography adherence as a woman's fulfillment of a yearly screening mammogram via self-report. Fair et al. interviewed women to understand their perception of benefits (e.g., decreased death from cancer) and risks (e.g., fear of finding cancer) to engaging in yearly screenings, as well as their readiness to fulfill the annual screening. Fair et al. reported low rates of mammography adherence among women with high perceived risk and low perceived benefit toward mammography. Conversely, Fair et al. found that women who perceived mammography to be low risk had higher mammography adherence. Understanding factors related to mammography adherence can help to build interventions tailored to the needs of at-risk populations who historically do not participate in recommended health screenings.

Practice Application

George is a 57-year-old attorney who was recently diagnosed with hypertension. The nurse practitioner caring for George has recommended dietary modifications and physical activity, in addition to a low dose of an antihypertensive medication. George comes to his follow-up visit and tells the nurse practitioner that he stopped taking the antihypertensive medication after 2 days because he "felt funny." George shares that he does not have time to exercise, and has to eat at restaurants frequently with clients. The nurse practitioner begins to explore George's beliefs, values, and perceptions of the situation. George expresses fear about having to make lifestyle changes and take a medication for his blood pressure. George and the nurse practitioner come up with three manageable goals for George, discuss potential side effects of the medications and how to manage them, and give George a diary to keep track of his progress. On his next visit, George has been able to incorporate two walks per week into his schedule, has been taking his daily medications more than 85% of the time, and has been making an effort to have fruit or vegetables for a snack instead of potato chips or cookies.

CHANGE

In order for nurses to assist patients in successfully making behavioral changes, it is important to understand an individual's decision-making process as it pertains to behavioral change. In this section, the Transtheoretical Model of Change (Prochaska, 1979; Prochaska & DiClemente, 1982; Prochaska & DiClemente, 1983) will be discussed. The Transtheoretical Model of Change (TTM) is an individual-level theory that is useful for understanding medical decisions that start a behavioral change process in patients that nurses may historically label *nonadherent* or *resistant to change*.

The TTM was developed to assess readiness for change among a population of individuals who smoked (Prochaska & DiClemente, 1983). A guiding principle of the TTM is that healthcare providers may be more successful in helping patients change behaviors if their interventions are tailored to a patient's place in the change process. Philosophically, a nurse using the TTM respects the patient's self-determinism and autonomy in the decision-making process. Individual-level change theories involve numerous assumptions including, but not limited to: (1) individuals value good health; (2) individuals will make necessary changes to reduce unhealthy behaviors; (3) behavior is under volitional control; and (4) an individual's beliefs, values, attitudes, and perception drive health behaviors (Crosby, Kegler, & DiClemente, 2009).

Central Constructs of the TTM

The TTM has four central constructs: stages of change, processes of change, self-efficacy, and decision-making ability.

Stages of Change

The TTM has six stages of change including precontemplation, contemplation, preparation, action, maintenance, and termination (Prochaska, 1979; Prochaska & DiClemente, 1982). The stages of change are temporal, or have a time orientation. Individuals progress through the following stages of change: (1) precontemplation, the individual has no intention of making a behavioral change in the next 6 months; (2) contemplation, the individual intends to make a behavioral change in the next 6 months; (3) preparation, the individual intends to make a behavioral change in the next 30 days; (4) action, the individual is actively making behavioral changes for fewer than 6 months; (5) maintenance, the individual has maintained the behavioral change for greater than 6 months; and (6) termination, the individual has incorporated the behavioral change into their daily life and they have no temptation to relapse, or revert, to old behaviors (Prochaska, Redding, & Evers, 1997). At any stage an individual may relapse into old behaviors and is at risk for restarting the process.

Processes of Change

In order for behavioral change to take place, 10 processes, both overt and covert, are used to progress through each stage (Prochaska & DiClemente, 1983; Prochaska, Velicer, DiClemente, & Fava, 1988). The first five processes are cognitive, and are primarily used by individuals in the precontemplation, contemplation, and preparation stages. The last five processes are behavioral and are used by individuals who are in the action and maintenance stages. The 10 processes include: (1) consciousness raising, or increasing awareness about a problem behavior; (2) dramatic relief, emotional release about the problem behavior; (3) environmental reevaluation, a social reappraisal of how the problem behavior affects the environment; (4) social liberation, an individual's appraisal of how there are opportunities within their environment to make the change easier; (5) self-reevaluation, an individual's appraisal of themselves with or without the problem behavior; (6) stimulus control, an individual reengineers his or her environment to remove things that remind him or her of the problem behavior; (7) helping relationships, identification of support persons to help with the change process; (8) counter conditioning, an individual learns to substitute healthy behaviors for problem behaviors; (9) reinforcement management, an individual rewards him or herself for avoiding the problem behavior; and (10) self-liberation, an individual makes a commitment to maintain the new healthy behavior (Prochaska & DiClemente, 1983; Prochaska, Velicer, DiClemente, & Fava, 1988).

Self-Efficacy

Self-efficacy (Bandura, 1977) was discussed earlier in the chapter. In terms of the change process, high levels of self-efficacy are especially important in high-risk situations when individuals are confronted with the opportunity to relapse into old behaviors.

Decision-Making Ability

A final construct of the TTM is decision-making ability; the weighting of pros and cons, or consideration of risks and benefits. Janis and Mann (1977) theorized that individuals experience decisional conflicts and proposed responses that an individual might use to resolve decisional conflicts. Janis and Mann (1977) proposed that individuals weigh the benefits of the decision to self and others, approval of self and others to make the decision, costs of the decision to self and others, and disapproval of self and others in making the decision.

Application to Vulnerable Populations

Labeling individuals as nonadherent to treatment recommendations or nursing plans of care has the potential of threatening the therapeutic relationship, especially among individuals who may be vulnerable based on age, gender, race, ethnicity, sexual orientation, or socioeconomic status. Using active listening, nurses can assess a patient's readiness for change using the TTM as a guide. Careful consideration of a patient's sociocultural needs is warranted. A patient might be amenable and ready to change; however, family issues, finances, cultural or environmental factors could have an impact on an individual's ability to move through the change process. Designing nursing interventions based on a patient's stage of change is important, especially if barriers to the change process are identified and managed in the treatment plan.

Research Example

Fahrenwald and Shangreaux (2006) examined the relationship between the TTM stages and physical activity behavior among a group of 30 American Indian mothers attending a Women, Infants, and Children (WIC) program on a South Dakota Indian reservation. Fahrenwald and Shangreaux noted that low-income American Indian mothers in South Dakota are at an increased risk of leading sedentary lifestyles. A descriptive correlational research design was used. The participants completed five instruments including: a 7-day activity recall (Blair et al., 1985), stage of exercise adoption tool (Marcus, Rakowski, & Rossi, 1992), Pros and Cons of Exercise tool (Marcus, Rakowski et al., 1992), Self-Efficacy for Exercise scale (Marcus, Selby, Niaura, & Rossi, 1992), and Processes for Exercise Adoption tool (Marcus, Selby et al., 1992).

Fahrenwald and Shangreaux (2006) found that increased physical activity and increased self-efficacy correlated significantly with advancing stage of change. For example, a woman who was categorized within the action phase was meeting the minimum weekly standard for moderate physical activity and reported a high level of self-efficacy. The processes of change followed the pathway proposed by the TTM, and women who were categorized in earlier stages reported significantly lower pros and decisional balance (Fahrenwald & Shangreaux, 2006). The results of the study have implications in the design of interventions specific to a population of low-income mothers residing on an Indian reservation in South Dakota.

Practice Application

Jeremiah is a student at a state university. He makes an appointment at the student health center on campus because he has gained 30 pounds since starting at the university, and is scared about developing health problems associated with being overweight. The nurse working at the student health center assesses Jeremiah; his body mass index is 32, putting him in the category of obese. Jeremiah expresses his desire to begin a reduced calorie diet and exercise program within the next 2 weeks. The nurse assesses that Jeremiah is in the preparation stage of the TTM. Using two processes of change, social liberation and self-reevaluation, the nurse and Jeremiah discuss opportunities on the college campus to make his change easier, and how Jeremiah sees himself currently being overweight and after he loses weight. Jeremiah identifies that the school track is in walking distance from his dorm, and the dining hall offers a salad bar where he can make a side salad instead of eating French fries with his meals. Jeremiah tells the nurse that he sees himself becoming more confident without his weight problem. The nurse plans to see Jeremiah in 2 weeks at the health center to assess where he is with the change process.

SOCIAL MIDDLE-RANGE THEORIES

Social middle-range concepts and theories address the structure and interactions of social support systems within relationships. Social support systems can include family members, significant others, friends, and community groups. A middle-range theory of social support is discussed in this section.

Social Support

An individual's social network can impact their health status and health outcomes. The term social support was coined by Cassel (1974), who theorized that supportive persons might play a role in improving an individual's health status and helping an individual cope with stressors. Bowlby's (1971) attachment theory, which addressed an individual's ability to form and maintain socially supportive relationships, served as a basis for contemporary theories of social support. Bowlby maintained that if an individual experienced secure attachments in childhood this would translate into an ability to engage in well-adjusted adult social relationships.

Finfgeld-Connett's (2005) conceptual model of social support was selected for this section. Finfgeld-Connett's conceptual model is based on a concept analysis of social support which included four key aspects: (1) emotional support, or comforting behaviors that one person provides to another person in order to alleviate anxiety, uncertainty, or hopelessness; (2) instrumental support, when one person provides tangible goods or services to assist another person; (3) structural support, the involvement of a network of support persons including relatives, friends, coworkers, and community support groups; and (4) functional support, the provision of assistive information.

Application to Vulnerable Populations

When caring for vulnerable populations, it is important for nurses to identify social networks and support systems that are, or may be, influential in improving an individual's health status and health outcomes. Assessment of supportive individuals or groups includes the strength of the relationships and resources available. Of equal importance is identification of individuals or groups who may serve to threaten an individual's health status or health outcomes; minimizing or avoiding the inclusion of unsupportive individuals or groups in the nursing plan of care may help to overcome barriers that threaten the health of vulnerable populations.

Research Example

Sjolander and Ahlstrom (2012) explored the meaning of social support by interviewing 17 family members of persons newly diagnosed with advanced-stage lung or gastrointestinal cancer in Sweden. Using content analysis, the researchers sought to validate Finfgeld-Connett's (2005) conceptual model of social support. Sjolander and Ahlstrom found that the primary attribute of social support was the theme of confirmation through togetherness, which incorporated two of Finfgeld-Connett's aspects of social support: emotional support (e.g., encouragement) and functional support (e.g., information from the spiritual community). Sjolander and Ahlstrom noted three additional subthemes as antecedents to social support including the need for support, the desire to establish deeper relationships with relatives/family, and identification of a social network to turn to. The findings of this study can be useful for nurses to help families identify critical support persons within their social networks that can provide emotional support and information.

Practice Application

Chad has been experiencing intimate partner violence for the last 2 years. His boyfriend, Phillip, has been verbally and physically abusive towards Chad. Chad has sought assistance from a local shelter in order to remove himself from the abusive situation. The nurse at the local shelter helps Chad to identify sources of social support. Chad tells the nurse that he has a tenuous relationship with his parents. He identifies two friends that can provide comforting words to him (emotional support). One of his friends has offered to drive Chad to and from his job as a store manager at a local coffeehouse (instrumental support). Chad identifies additional coworkers that will be supportive and protective of Chad's safety at work as he transitions away from his relationship with Phillip (structural support). Finally, Chad identifies functional support systems, including a local community support group for persons who have experienced intimate partner violence.

INTEGRATIVE MIDDLE-RANGE CONCEPTS AND THEORIES

Integrative middle-range concepts and theories incorporate multiple perspectives. Integration may include individual-level, social, community, or societal factors. The concepts or middle-range theories of health-related quality of life, health promotion, resilience, and chronic care will be discussed in this section.

Health-Related Quality of Life

Historically, scholars have had difficulty defining the concept of quality of life because multiple definitions of the concept exist (Sandau, Bredow, & Peterson, 2013). Despite multiple definitions of the concept, quality of life has been broadly defined as satisfaction with life, and has three primary aspects: assessment of well-being, broad domains (e.g., physical, psychological, economic, spiritual, social), and the definition includes components of each domain (Spiker, 1996). Health-related quality of life (HRQOL) shares the central aspects of quality of life, and has been characterized as multidimensional, temporal, and subjective (Sandau et al., 2013).

Wilson and Cleary's (1995) conceptual model of HRQOL will be discussed. Wilson and Cleary proposed that HRQOL comprises five dimensions that exist across a biologically, socially, and psychologically complex continuum. The five dimensions include:

(1) biological factors, (2) symptoms experienced, (3) functional status, (4) general perceptions of health status, and (5) overall quality of life. Wilson and Cleary proposed that individual characteristics, psychological support, social support, economic support, individual value/preferences, personality/motivation, and environmental factors have an impact on the five dimensions, and on quality of life overall.

Application to Vulnerable Populations

Vulnerable populations have unique sociocultural needs that impact HRQOL. Biological factors, including racial or ethnic disparities in disease prevalence, and lack of access to health services put individuals at risk for poorer health outcomes and lower levels of HRQOL (Institute of Medicine , 2003). As Wilson and Cleary (2005) proposed, the dimensions of HRQOL exist across a continuum; environmental, social, and economic issues experienced by the vulnerable have an impact on HRQOL. HRQOL is subjective, thus individual perception of health status can have an impact on the experience of disease symptoms and life satisfaction.

Research Example

Ozanne, Strang, and Persson (2011) examined HRQOL among patients diagnosed with amyotrophic lateral sclerosis (ALS) and their primary caregivers. Ozanne and colleagues noted that HRQOL for the individual diagnosed with ALS, and for the caregiver can be impacted during the long-term trajectory of the disease. Thirty five pairs (patients and caregivers) were recruited for the study. Ozanne et al. used a descriptive design. The dyads completed two instruments: the SF-36 (measures dimensions of HRQOL) and the Hospital Anxiety and Depression Scale (a self-assessment scale for anxiety and depression). The patients and their caregivers reported higher levels of depression and anxiety than the general population in Sweden. Ozanne and colleagues found that there was a positive correlation between the patients' and caregivers' levels of anxiety. Ozanne et al. concluded that an important nursing role is to address mental health needs of both patients with ALS and their caregivers.

Practice Application

Amelia, an 18-year-old woman, has recently been diagnosed with anorexia nervosa. Her current weight is 89 pounds and she is 5'4" tall. Amelia has entered an inpatient eating-disorder treatment facility. She has begun counseling with a psychiatric-mental health clinical nurse specialist. Amelia shares that the eating disorder has impacted her quality life in the areas of overall life satisfaction, body satisfaction, and has impaired her physical functioning. She perceives her health status to be poor and fears that the eating disorder "will kill her soon." The clinical nurse specialist incorporates several dimensions of HRQOL into

Amelia's treatment plan including symptom management, assessment of personality and motivation, identification of psychological and social support systems, and economic support for Amelia's continued recovery after she leaves the inpatient program.

HEALTH PROMOTION

Health promotion integrates several concepts and constructs including self-efficacy, social support, and change. Health has come to be defined as more than the absence of disease; Pender, Murdaugh, and Parsons (2010) define health as an individual's drive toward achieving their fullest potential, which includes times of wellness and illness. Pender and colleagues' definition of health encompasses an individual's lifestyle, social relationships, and environmental factors.

The Health Promotion Model (HPM) (Pender, 1996; Pender et al., 2010) is a framework for delivering nursing care to support health promotion behaviors. The HPM was originally developed to target individuals; however the framework can be used to target families, groups, or communities. The HPM comprises three primary areas that nurses can use to assess health promotion behaviors: (1) personal characteristics and experiences, (2) behaviors-specific cognition and affect, and (3) behavioral outcome (Pender, 1996; Pender et al., 2010).

Personal characteristics and experiences include prior behavior and personal factors (e.g., biological, sociocultural) (Pender, 1996; Pender et al., 2010). Behavior-specific cognitions include perception of benefits/barriers to action, perception of self-efficacy, and movement (affect) toward actively engaging in health promotion behaviors (Pender, 1996; Pender et al., 2010). Interpersonal influences (e.g., social support) and situational/environmental influences are proposed to have an effect on cognition and activity-related movement. Finally, the HPM incorporates elements of the change process including commitment to a plan of action and acknowledgement of competing demands (Pender, 1996; Pender et al., 2010). The final outcome is engagement in health promotion behaviors.

Application to Vulnerable Populations

Health promotion, especially preventive care, is essential for ethnic minority groups and the economically disadvantaged—groups who often lack access to safe, effective, timely, equitable, and patient-centered care (Agency for Healthcare Research and Quality, 2008; Richardson & Norris, 2010). Understanding personal factors (e.g., lack of finances to afford health insurance), and an individual's perception of the benefits and barriers of engaging in health promotion behaviors is an important component of a nursing assessment. When working with vulnerable populations, screening recommendations and health promotion practices can be tailored to the patient's and family's cultural values and beliefs, finances, and access to support within the community.

Research Example

Attentional barriers to health promotion among community dwelling elders were examined by Stark, Chase, and DeYoung (2010). Attentional barriers were defined as: (1) physical/environmental (e.g., stairs), (2) informational (e.g. hearing changes), (3) behavioral (e.g., vulnerability related to mobility changes), and (4) affective (worries). Stark and colleagues recruited 141 community dwelling elders from senior centers and churches. The participants completed two questionnaires; one questionnaire on health promotion behaviors (e.g., nutrition, physical activity, stress relief, spiritual resources) and one questionnaire on attentional demands. Stark et al. found that elders who reported increased attentional demands participated in fewer health-promoting behaviors. Nurses can include attentional demands in an assessment and tailor interventions to promote access to health promotion activities for elderly populations.

Practice Application

A community health nurse, who is a faculty member at a school of nursing, partners with an activities director at an apartment complex for economically disadvantaged families. The apartment activities director is concerned with the number of renters (adults and children) who are overweight or obese. The activities director wants to work with the nursing faculty member to establish a weekly family-oriented physical activity session at the apartment complex. The nurse understands that engagement in health promotion activities starts with understanding the families' past experience with physical activity, cultural values related to physical activity, perceived benefits and barriers to participating in the sessions, and commitment to a plan of action. The apartment complex is a tight-knit community of Hispanic families who interact socially on regular basis. Prior to planning the sessions, the nurse hosts two family dinner meetings to discuss the aforementioned issues so that the physical activity sessions can be tailored to the families, thereby increasing the likelihood that families will participate.

RESILIENCE

Vulnerable populations face varying types of adversity including, but not limited to, chronic health conditions. Positive adjustment to adverse life experiences is termed resilience (Haase & Peterson, 2013). Haase and Peterson state that understanding resilience helps nurses to improve health outcomes, especially among at-risk populations.

Resilience has been defined as a dynamic concept occurring as a personal quality enabling success, a process, and/or an intrinsic force that exists within individuals or groups (Richardson, 2002). Ahern's (2006) concept analysis of resilience will be used to describe key attributes of the concept. Ahern studied a population of adolescents;

however, the attributes of resilience Ahern proposed can be used to guide nursing interventions for populations across the lifespan.

Ahern (2006) defined the concept of resilience as a process that an individual undertakes to adapt to adversity or risk by using personal characteristics, family and social support, and community resources. In this context, Ahern defined risks as being either internal or external to the individual. Ahern identified several attributes including individual protective factors (e.g., competence, coping ability, sense of humor, connectedness, and health risk knowledge) and sociocultural protective factors (e.g., family connectedness and availability of community resources). Several of the attributes, including competence, are subjective perceptions of abilities in dealing with adversity; the degree of adversity is also subjective and unique to the individual.

Application to Vulnerable Populations

Internal (e.g., chronic disease) and external (e.g., physical abuse) risks experienced by vulnerable populations vary in degree and severity. Although adversity can be defined broadly, it is important for nurses to thoroughly assess an individual or family's knowledge of the health risk, perception of personal/family competency, coping mechanisms, sense of humor, social support networks, and resources available in the individual or family's community. Interventions can be designed to incorporate an individual or family's key strengths and to access resources in the community that best enable the individual or family to overcome adversity.

Research Example

Kornhaber (2011) explored Australian burn nurses' abilities to build resilience as a strategy for dealing with the exhaustion and distress of caring for patients who have experienced traumatic and disfiguring burns. Seven burn nurses were recruited for the study. Kornhaber conducted a qualitative phenomenological study using semistructured interviews to explore nurses' lived experiences in caring for severely burned patients. Kornhaber noted several themes about building resilience including: toughening up, emotional toughness, coping with challenges, regrouping, and emotional detachment. The findings of Kornhaber's study have implications for nurse managers in the areas of staff orientation and continuing staff education.

Practice Application

A nurse working in a public high school is planning interventions to address a recent act of violence on the high school campus. The nurse wants to engage the adolescents and their families in an intervention to promote personal and family competence in coping with the traumatic event. The nurse plans a series of support groups/debriefing sessions for the adolescents alone, parents alone, and for families to encourage verbalization of fears and concerns within a supportive environment. The debriefing sessions will also be used for the adolescents and their parents to make plans for how to continue to ensure safety on the campus using resources within the community.

CHRONIC CARE

The chronic care model (CCM) is a population-based model that outlines a planned approach to chronic disease care delivery. The goal of the CCM is to provide high quality, comprehensive care that helps to improve chronic disease management, mitigate complications of chronic diseases, and improve health outcomes at the population level (Coleman, Austin, Brach, & Wagner, 2009). In the CCM, chronic conditions are defined as any condition that requires ongoing adjustments by the affected individual or family and continuing interaction with the healthcare system (Coleman et al., 2009).

The CCM has two major dimensions: community and health systems (Coleman et al., 2009). Within the two major dimensions there are subdimensions including self-management support, delivery system design, decision support, and clinical information systems. Self-management support, a subdimension of community, helps to empower individuals and families to take charge of disease management through goal-setting, planning, problem-solving, and follow-up. The goal of delivery system design is to deliver efficient, effective, evidence-based and culturally competent clinical and self-management care, including regular follow-up with the care team. Decision support helps to ensure that clinical care is based on patient and family preferences and values, in addition to evidence-based practice. Finally, clinical information systems help to organize patient data in order to achieve effective, individualized care planning, including open communication among the stakeholders (e.g., patient, family, providers) and timely reminders for follow-up care.

Application to Vulnerable Populations

The CCM is the only population-focused model presented in this chapter. Providers working in a community setting can use the elements of this model to design delivery systems within their practices that help to ensure patients and families receive care that supports self-management of chronic disease. For vulnerable populations, the assurance of timely, continued follow-up care is critical. Transportation issues, lack of ability to communicate with patients and families outside of office visits (e.g., lack of a phone), and language barriers can impede effective care delivery. Designing clinical information systems that address vulnerable populations' barriers to follow-up care is important. Open communication, using the primary language preference of the patient and family, and decision support incorporating a patient's and family's values may strengthen self-management of chronic disease.

Research Example

Adams et al. (2007) conducted a systematic review of the implementation of the CCM in the prevention and management of chronic obstructive pulmonary disease (COPD) among adults. Adams and colleagues identified 32 research studies in the literature that examined the use of the CCM in preventing or treating COPD. Adams et al. found that researchers who reported using two or more CCM elements noted lower rates of hospitalizations for COPD exacerbations, fewer emergency room or unscheduled office visits, and shorter lengths of hospital stays for patients who were readmitted to the hospital for a COPD exacerbation.

Practice Application

A family nurse practitioner (FNP) who runs a community clinic serving uninsured adults is concerned about the number of patients with type 2 diabetes who cancel their follow-up appointments. He determines that transportation issues, financial issues, and language barriers are three most common obstacles to follow-up care. The FNP uses the CCM to institute the following changes: (1) incorporation of goal-setting and problem-solving during office visits (self-management support), (2) assurance of the presence of an interpreter during office visits and routine use of prescription assistance plans to enable patients/families to afford medications (delivery system design and decision support), (3) partnering with a local charitable agency who will provide bus vouchers for patients (clinical information systems), and (4) reminder phone calls the day before the appointments (clinical information systems).

CONCLUSION

Eight middle-range concepts and theories were presented in this chapter. Key concepts and relevant studies are summarized in Appendix 7.1 at the end of this chapter. The middle-range concepts and theories were contextualized for the care of vulnerable populations. Examples of the use in research and clinical practice were given for each concept or model.

REFERENCES

Adams, S. G., Smith P. K., Allan, P. F., Anzueto, A., Pugh, J. A., & Cornell, J. E. (2007). Systematic review of the chronic care model in chronic obstructive pulmonary disease prevention and management. *Archives of Internal Medicine, 167*, 551–561.

Agency for Healthcare Research and Quality. (2008). *National healthcare disparities report 2008.* Retrieved from www.ahrq.gov/qual/nhdr08

Ahern, N. R. (2006). Adolescent resilience: An evolutionary concept analysis. *Journal of Pediatric Nursing, 21*, 175–185.

Bandura, A. (1977). Self-efficacy: Toward a unifying theory of behavioral change. *Psychological Review*, *84*, 191–215.

Bandura, A. (1986). *Social foundations of thought and action*. Englewood Cliffs, NJ: Prentice Hall.

Bandura, A. (1995). *Self-efficacy in changing societies*. New York: Cambridge University Press.

Bandura, A., Blanchard, E. B., & Ritter, B. (1969). Relative efficacy of desensitization and modeling approaches for inducing behavioral, affective, and attitudinal changes. *Journal of Personality and Social Psychology*, *13*, 173–199.

Bandura, A., & Perloff, B. (1967). Relative efficacy and self-monitored and externally imposed reinforcement systems. *Journal of Personality and Social Psychology*, *7*, 111–116.

Blair, S. N., Haskell, W. L., Ho, P., Paffenbarger, R. S., Farquhar, J. W., & Wood, P. (1985). Assessment of habitual physical activity by a 7-day recall in a community survey and controlled experiments. *American Journal of Epidemiology*, *122*, 794–804.

Bowlby, J. (1971). *Attachment*. London: Pelican.

Cassel, J. (1974). Psychosocial process and "stress:" Theoretical perspectives. *International Journal of Health Services*, *4*, 471–482.

Cohen, S. M. (2009). Concept analysis of adherence in the context of cardiovascular risk reduction. *Nursing Forum*, *44*, 25–36.

Colbert, A. M., Sereika, S. M., & Erlen, J. A. (2012). Functional health literacy, medication-taking self-efficacy and adherence to antiretroviral therapy. *Journal of Advanced Nursing*, *68*, 295–304.

Coleman, K., Austin, B. T., Brach, C., & Wagner, E. H. (2009). Evidence on the chronic care model in the new millennium. *Health Affairs*, *28*, 75–85.

Crosby, R. A., Kegler, M. C., & DiClemente, R. J. (2009). Theory in health promotion practice and research. In R. J. DiClemente, R. A. Crosby, & M. C. Kegler (Eds.), *Emerging theories in health promotion practice and research* (2nd ed., pp. 4–17). San Francisco, CA: Jossey-Bass.

Fahrenwald, N. L., & Shangreaux, P. (2006). Physical activity behavior of American Indian mothers. *Orthopaedic Nursing*, *25*(1), 22–29.

Fair, A. M., Monahan, P. O., Russell, K., Zhao, Q., & Champion, V. L. (2012). The interaction of perceived risk and benefits and the relationship to predicting mammography adherence in African American women. *Oncology Nursing Forum*, *39*, 53–60.

Finfgeld-Connett, D. (2005). Clarification of social support. *Journal of Nursing Scholarship*, *37*, 4–9.

Haase, J. E., & Peterson, S. J. (2013). Resilience. In S. J. Peterson & T. S. Bredow (Eds.) *Middle range theories: Application to nursing research* (3rd ed., pp. 256–284). Philadelphia: Wolters Kluwer Health, Lippincott Williams & Wilkins.

Im, Y. J., & Kim, D. H. (2011). Factors associated with the resilience of school-aged children with atopic dermatitis. *Journal of Clinical Nursing*, *21*, 80–88.

Institute of Medicine. (2003). *Unequal treatment: Confronting racial and ethnic disparities in healthcare*. Washington: National Academies Press.

Janis, I. L., & Mann, L. (1977). Decision-making: *A psychological analysis of conflict, choice, and commitment*. New York: The Free Press, Macmillan.

Kornhaber, R. A. (2011). Building resilience in burns nurses: A descriptive phenomenologic inquiry. *Journal of Burn Care & Research*, *32*, 481–488.

Lee, G. E. (2010). Predictors of adjustment to nursing home life of elderly residents: A cross-sectional survey. *International Journal of Nursing Studies, 47*, 957–964

Marcus, B. H., Rakowski, W., & Rossi, J. S. (1992). Assessing motivational readiness and decision making for exercise. *Health Psychology, 11*, 257–261.

Marcus, B. H., Selby, V. C., Niaura, R. S., & Rossi, J. S. (1992). Self-efficacy and the stages of exercise behavior change. *Research Quarterly for Exercise and Sport, 63*, 60–66.

McBride, C., Bryan, A., Bray, M., Swan, G., & Green, E. (2012). Health behavior change: Can genomics improve behavioral adherence? *American Journal of Public Health, 102*, 401–405.

McCurry, M. K., Hunter Revell, S. M., & Roy, S. R. (2010). Knowledge for the good of the individual and society: Linking philosophy, disciplinary goals, theory, and practice. *Nursing Philosophy, 11*, 42–52.

Nokes, K., Johnson, M. O., Webel, A., Rose, C. D., Phillips, J. C., Sullivan, K., . . . Holzemer, W. L. (2012). Focus on increasing treatment self-efficacy to improve human immunodeficiency virus treatment adherence. *Journal of Nursing Scholarship, 44*, 403–410.

Nutting, P. A., Dickinson, W. P., Dickinson, L. M., Nelson, C. C., King, D. K., Crabtree, B. F., & Glasgow, R. E. (2007). Use of chronic care model elements is associated with higher-quality care for diabetes. *Annals of Family Medicine, 5*(1), 14–20.

Ohlendorf, J. M. (2012). Stages of change in the trajectory of postpartum weight self-management. *Journal of Obstetric, Gynecologic, and Neonatal Nursing, 41*, 57–70.

Ozanne, A. G. O., Strang, S., & Persson, L. I. (2011). Quality of life, anxiety and depression in ALS patients and their next of kin. *Journal of Clinical Nursing, 20*, 283–291

Pender, N. (1996). *Health promotion in nursing practice* (3rd ed.). Stamford, CT: Appleton & Lange.

Pender, N., Murdaugh, C. L., & Parsons, M. A. (2010). *Health promotion in nursing practice* (6th ed.). Upper Saddle River, NJ: Prentice Hall.

Prochaska, J. O. (1979). *Systems of psychotherapy: A transtheoretical analysis.* Homewood, IL: Dorsey Press.

Prochaska, J. O., & DiClemente, C. C. (1982). Transtheoretical therapy: Toward a more integrative model of change. *Psychotherapy: Theory, Research, & Practice, 19*, 276–288.

Prochaska, J. O., & DiClemente, C. C. (1983). Stages and processes of self-change of smoking: Toward an integrative model of change. *Journal of Consulting and Clinical Psychology, 51*, 390–395.

Prochaska, J. O., Redding, C. A., & Evers, K. E. (1997). The Transtheoretical model and stages of change. In K. Glanz, B. K. Rimer, & F. M. Lewis (Eds.), *Health behavior and health education: Theory, research, and practice* (2nd ed., pp. 60–84). San Francisco, CA: Jossey-Bass.

Prochaska, J. O., Velicer, W. F., DiClemente, C. C., & Fava, J. L. (1988). Measuring the processes of change: Application to the cessation of smoking. *Journal of Consulting and Clinical Psychology, 56*, 520–528.

Richardson, G. E. (2002). The metatheory of resilience and resiliency. *Journal of Clinical Psychology, 58*(3), 307–321.

Richardson, L. D., & Norris, M. (2010). Access to health and health care: How race and ethnicity matter. *Mount Sinai Journal of Medicine, 77*, 166–177.

Risjord, M. (2010). *Nursing knowledge: Science, practice, and philosophy*. Chichester, West Sussex: Wiley-Blackwell.

Rosario, R., Araujo, A., Oliveira, B., Padrao, P., Lopes, O., Teixeria, V., . . . Moreira, P. (2013). Impact of an intervention through teachers to prevent consumption of low nutrition, energy-dense foods and beverages: A randomized trial. *Preventive Medicine*, 57(1), 20–25.

Sandau, K. E., Bredow, T. S., & Peterson, S. J. (2013). Health-related quality of life. In S. J. Peterson & T. S. Bredow (Eds.), *Middle range theories: Application to nursing research* (3rd ed., pp. 210–223). Philadelphia: Wolters Kluwer Health, Lippincott Williams & Wilkins.

Sharoni, S. K. A., & Wu, S. V. (2012). Self-efficacy and self-care behavior of Malaysian patients with type 2 diabetes: A cross-sectional survey. *Nursing and Health Sciences*, 14, 38–45.

Sjolander, C., & Ahlstrom, G. (2012). The meaning and validation of social support networks for close family of persons with advanced cancer. *BMC Nursing*, 11, 17. Retrieved from http://www.biomedcentral.com/1472-6955/11/17

Spiker, B. (1996). Three levels of quality of life. In B. Spiker (Ed.), *Quality of life and pharmacoeconomics in clinical trials* (2nd ed., p. 2). Philadelphia: Lippincott-Raven.

Stark, M., Chase, L., & DeYoung, A. (2010). Barriers to health promotion in community dwelling elders. *Journal of Community Health Nursing*, 27, 175–186.

Sut, H. K., Kaplan, P. B., Sut, N., & Tekbas, S. (2012). The assessment of quality of life in female Turkish patients with overactive bladder. *International Journal of Nursing Practice*, 18, 20–27.

van der Bijl, J. J., van Poelgeest-Eeltink, A., & Shortridge-Baggett, L. M. (1999). The psychometric properties of the diabetes management self-efficacy scale for patients with type 2 diabetes mellitus. *Journal of Advanced Nursing*, 30, 352–359.

Walker, S. N., Pullen, C. H., Hertzog, M., Boeckner, L., & Hageman, P. A. (2006). Determinants of older rural women's activity and eating. *Western Journal of Nursing Research*, 28, 449–468.

Walsh, J. C., Mandalia, S., & Gazzard, B. G. (2002). Responses to a 1-month self-report on adherence to antiretroviral therapy are consistent with electronic data and virological treatment outcomes. *AIDS*, 25, 269–277.

Wilson, I. B., & Cleary, P. D. (1995). Linking clinical variables with health-related quality of life. *Journal of the American Medical Association*, 273, 60.

APPENDIX 7.1

Summary Table

Concept/Theory	Authors	Topic	Notes
Self-Efficacy	Walker, Pullen, Hertzog, Boeckner, & Hageman (2006)	Impact of perceived self-efficacy on healthy eating among rural Midwestern women	A clinical trial of 179 women was conducted; greater self-efficacy predicted higher intake of fruits, vegetables, and whole grains, and lower fat intake.
Adherence	Nokes et al. (2012)	Increasing treatment self-efficacy to improve adherence to antiretroviral medications	Descriptive survey study of 1,414 United States adults diagnosed with human immunodeficiency virus on antiretroviral treatment; self-efficacy was a strong predictor of adherence to antiretroviral medications.
Change	Ohlendorf (2012)	Stages of change and postpartum weight management among adult postpartum women in the Midwest United States	Descriptive survey study of 191 adult postpartum women; 80% of the women reported higher stages of change (action or maintenance phases) 8 weeks after birth than in the immediate postpartum period.
Social Support	Lee (2010)	Social support as a predictor of adjustment to skilled nursing facilities among elderly residents in South Korean skilled nursing facilities	Descriptive cross-sectional study of 156 skilled nursing facility residents; successful adjustment to nursing home life was predicted by emotional support from staff and fellow residents.

Concept/Theory	Authors	Topic	Notes
Health-Related Quality of Life (HRQOL)	Sut, Kaplan, Sut, & Tekbas (2012)	The effect of overactive bladder on HRQOL among Turkish women	Descriptive, cross-sectional study of 280 pre- and post-menopausal women; women with overactive bladder reported significantly lower levels of HRQOL in the domains of coping, concern, sleep, and social than women without overactive bladder.
Health Promotion	Rosario et al. (2013)	Impact of an elementary school-based intervention on the consumption of low nutrition, energy-dense foods and beverages among 6–12 year old children	Randomized controlled trial of 464 children aged 6–12 years from seven Portuguese elementary schools; children in the intervention group who received a 6-month program based on the Health Promotion Model reported a reduced consumption of low nutrition, energy-dense foods compared to the control group.
Resilience	Im & Kim (2011)	Identification of factors associated with resilience among 7–15-year-old children diagnosed with atopic dermatitis	Descriptive survey of 102 children and their parents; children who reported higher levels of resilience reported shorter illness duration, lower symptom severity, and better relationships with parents, teachers, and friends.

Concept/Theory	Authors	Topic	Notes
Chronic Care	Nutting et al. (2007)	Association of using the chronic care model with diabetes outcomes among 30 United States small primary care practices	Descriptive survey of 90 primary care providers; providers that used elements of the chronic care model reported lower patient glucose values and lower ratios of total cholesterol to high-density lipoprotein cholesterol.

Chapter 8

The Utility of Leininger's Culture Care Theory with Vulnerable Populations

Rick Zoucha

OBJECTIVES

At the end of this chapter, the reader will be able to

1. Explain Leininger's culture care theory.
2. Describe how Leininger's theory can be applied to nursing practice with vulnerable populations.
3. Propose at least two research projects in which Leininger's theory might serve as the conceptual framework.

INTRODUCTION

In the ever evolving healthcare environment in the United States, there are a variety of people who have access to services that promote health and well-being and reduce the effects of illness. Similarly, there are people who are not afforded the same access to healthcare services because of their vulnerability.

For an individual, group or community to be vulnerable is to be susceptible to harm (Adger, 2006). According to Campos-Outcalt et al. (1994), vulnerable populations can be defined as groups of people who experience physical disabilities, mental disabilities, cultural differences, geographic separation, and limited economic resources, and, due to these barriers, might be unable to become integrated into the mainstream health services and delivery system. The authors include as vulnerable the urban and rural poor (especially ethnic and racial minorities), Native Americans, chronically disabled children and adults, the frail elderly, homeless individuals, and undocumented immigrants. Vulnerable populations can also be defined in terms of subpopulations or subgroups who, because of their position in the social strata, are exposed to certain contextual conditions that are different from those experienced by the rest of the population (Frohlich & Potvin, 2008). Shi and Stevens (2010) define vulnerable populations as racial and ethnic minorities, the uninsured, children, the elderly, the poor, the chronically ill, people with AIDS, alcohol or substance abusers, homeless individuals, underserved rural and urban groups, people who do not speak English or have difficulties in communicating in healthcare settings, those who are poorly educated or illiterate, low-income individuals, and members of minority groups. Vulnerable populations in the United States have greater health needs and the overall the number of vulnerable people is increasing (Shi & Stevens, 2010). In addition, people who are victims of violence are at risk of being vulnerable (Zoucha, 2006).

Leininger (1996a) contended that, regardless of economic, political, and even genetic differences, everyone has a culture. This chapter discusses Leininger's culture care theory and the utility of the theory in working with vulnerable populations defined by their cultural differences in the research and practice settings.

LEININGER'S THEORY OF CULTURE CARE DIVERSITY AND UNIVERSALITY

Leininger defined care as "those assistive, supportive and enabling experiences or ideas towards others with evident or anticipated needs to ameliorate or improve human conditions or lifeways" (Leininger & McFarland, 2006, p. 12). Leininger (1996b) further described culture as learned values, beliefs, rules of behavior, and lifestyle practices of a particular group of people. Andrews and Boyle (2011) determined that culture has four basic characteristics. Culture is not a thing, but rather a process of discovery of ideas that are socially transmitted. Culture gives meaning to ideas that shape behavior and perceptions (Locke & Bailey, 2014). According to Leininger (1991b) and Andrews and Boyle (2011), humans exist within a culture, and culture is viewed as a universal phenomenon.

Leininger combined the concept of culture and an ethical orientation of caring to develop a theory appropriate for nursing practice, research, and education (Zoucha & Husted, 2000). She also contended that individuals, families, and communities must be viewed in the context of culture (Zoucha & Husted, 2002).

Leininger's Culture Care Diversity and Universality: A Worldwide Nursing Theory (McFarland & Wehbe-Alamah, 2015) is the product of more than 6 decades of research and development, during which she studied over 60 cultures and identified at least 172 care constructs for use by nursing and other healthcare professionals. The sunrise model (McFarland & Wehbe-Alamah, 2015) depicts Leininger's theory as having seven cultural and social structure dimensions: (1) technological, (2) religious and philosophical, (3) kinship and social, (4) political and legal, (5) economic, (6) educational, and (7) cultural values, beliefs, and lifeways. The theory describes diverse healthcare systems as ranging from folk beliefs and practices to nursing and other healthcare professional systems often utilized by people around the world.

Leininger described two systems of caring that exist in every culture she studied (Leininger & McFarland, 2006). The first system of caring is generic and is considered the oldest form of caring or nurturing. Generic caring consists of culturally derived interpersonal practices and is considered essential for health, growth, and survival of humans (Reynolds & Leininger, 1993). Generic caring is often referred to as *folk practices* and is defined culturally (Leininger, 1996b).

The second type of caring is considered therapeutic, cognitively learned, practiced, and transmitted through formal and informal means of professional education such as schools of nursing, medicine, and dentistry (Leininger & McFarland, 2006). Professional learning can and does include concepts and techniques to enhance professional practices, as well as interpersonal communication techniques and holistic aspects of care. Historically, professional care has not always included ideas about folk care, because such beliefs may not have been valued by nurses and other healthcare professionals (Leininger & McFarland, 2002).

In her theory, Leininger contended that if professional and generic care practices do not fit together, this discordance might affect client/patient recovery, health, and well-being, and result in care that is not culturally congruent with the beliefs of the person, family, or community (Leininger & McFarland, 2006). To provide culturally congruent care, Leininger asserted that professionals must link and synthesize generic and professional care knowledge to benefit the client (Leininger & McFarland, 2002). This link is a bridge, where a bridge is appropriate, between the professional and folk healthcare systems.

According to this theory (Clarke, McFarland, Andrews, & Leininger, 2009), three predictive modes of care may be derived from and based on the use of generic (emic) care knowledge and professional (etic) care knowledge, obtained from research and experience using the sunrise model. The three modes of action are: (1) cultural care preservation/maintenance, (2) cultural care accommodation/negotiation, and (3) cultural care repatterning/restructuring.

Cultural care preservation/maintenance refers to assistive, supportive, facilitative, or enabling professional actions and decisions that help individuals, families, and communities from a particular culture to retain and preserve care values so that they can maintain well-being, recover from illness, or face possible handicap or death (McFarland & Wehbe-Alamah, 2015). Leininger described *cultural care accommodation/negotiation* as assistive, facilitative, or enabling creative professional actions and potential decisions that can help individuals, families, and communities of a particular culture to adapt to or to negotiate with others, for the purpose of satisfying healthcare outcomes with professional caregivers (Leininger & McFarland, 2002). *Cultural care repatterning/restructuring* is described as the assistive, supportive, facilitative, and enabling activities by nurses and other healthcare professionals that promote actions and decisions that may help the person, family, or community to change or modify behaviors affecting their lifeways in order to achieve a new and different health pattern. This repatterning/restructuring (Leininger, 2002b) is done while respecting the individual's, family's, and community's cultural values and beliefs, while still providing and promoting a healthier lifeway than before the changes were coestablished with the person, family, and community. Leininger (2002a) asserts in her theory that these three predicted modes of action serve to guide judgments, decisions, and actions, and ultimately culminate in the delivery of culturally congruent care.

Leininger (2002a) describes culturally congruent care as beneficial, satisfying, and meaningful to the individuals, families, and communities served by nurses. In contrast, cultural imposition occurs when nurses and other healthcare professionals impose their own beliefs, practices, and values on another culture because they believe their ideas are superior to those of the other person or group (Leininger, 2002a). Leininger uses the concepts of cultural congruence and cultural imposition to focus on acceptable (caring) and unacceptable (noncaring) behavior by nurses in the practice, education, and research arenas.

UTILITY OF THE THEORY IN NURSING RESEARCH AND PRACTICE

In addition to the development of the theory of culture care, Leininger (1991a) developed a research method that is very useful in understanding the phenomenon of culturally based care for vulnerable populations. As described earlier, vulnerability includes culture differences. Leininger's qualitative ethnonursing research method was created to work in conjunction with the theory (and the sunrise model) as a guide for research. According to Leininger and McFarland (2006), the ethnonursing research method is described as "a qualitative nursing research method focused on naturalistic, open discovery, and largely inductive (emic) modes to document, describe, explain, and interpret informants' worldview, meaning and symbols, and life experiences as they bear on actual or potential nursing care phenomena" (p. 21). Leininger (2002a) suggests that this method can be used in conjunction with research enablers such as: (1) Leininger's Observation–Participation–Reflection Enabler, (2) Leininger's Stranger to Trusted Friend Enabler, (3) the Sunrise Model Enabler, (4) the Specific Domain of Inquiry Enabler, and (5) Leininger's Acculturation Enabler.

These enabler guides can also be used in the clinical setting in an attempt to move from stranger to trusted friend in the new relationship between the nurse and client. The notion of being viewed as a friend can promote culturally congruent care in many cultures (Zoucha & Reeves, 1999). Such a friend-like or personal relationship between the nurse and the client/patient can decrease the cultural difference vulnerability of the person, as it permits the cultural care needs of the client to become known to the nurse. The nurse is then able to promote care that is congruent with the person's culture and, essentially, to promote the health and well-being needs of the person, family, and community.

The connection between theory, research, and practice is addressed by using the identified enablers to promote a deeper understanding of the cultural phenomenon of interest, regardless of the context (research or clinical practice). This allows for a holistic and comprehensive view of the domain of inquiry and the particular culture being studied. As transcultural nurse researchers and clinicians seek to understand the phenomena of interest for vulnerable populations, it becomes possible to decrease the aspect of vulnerability described as cultural differences. If transcultural nurses do utilize the findings from relevant studies in their actual clinical practice, then each nurse's understanding of the person, family, and community can be viewed from a cultural care perspective, thereby not only increasing the understanding of the cultural care needs but also exposing the vulnerability related to being culturally different.

The concern with personal, family, and community vulnerability regarding cultural differences is that if nurses pursue an understanding of culture in relation to health and well-being, then they have an ethical motivation to promote care that is culturally congruent. This motivation might potentially decrease the vulnerability of the individual, family, and community. Zoucha and Husted (2000) contend that cultural caring should consider the person, family, and community in the context of their culture, and that this perspective will result in the promotion of ethical and culturally congruent care. In agreement with Leininger's theory, Zoucha and Husted (2000) believe that it is the ethical responsibility and duty of the nurse to promote, provide, and encourage care that is culturally based and congruent with the values, beliefs, and traditions of the individual, family, and community.

Leininger's theory provides a holistic and emic view of those factors that describe culture and those cultural values and beliefs that are meaningful to individuals, families, and communities. However, the theory does not explicitly state, in the context of either the sunrise model or the theory, the related factors of racism, poverty, and history of oppression that are commonly encountered among people from cultures other than the dominant culture in the United States. Leininger did consider these issues in her writing and presentations but does not make them clear in her explication of the theory and sunrise model in relationship to research and clinical practice. Adding the factors of racism, poverty, and history of oppression to the sunrise model as part of the experience for people of different cultures (other than the dominant culture) may assist nurses and other healthcare professionals in better understanding the meaning of vulnerability. Through the use of such theory, nurses and other healthcare professionals can promote health and well-being while decreasing the experience of being vulnerable.

CONCLUSION

In summary, individuals, families, and communities that are identified as vulnerable due to cultural differences can be understood in a manner that seeks to expose the source of that vulnerability and focuses on the cultural care needs. Leininger's Theory of Culture Care Diversity and Universality promotes a deep and clear understanding of the individual, family, and community from a unique cultural perspective. Using this theory and the identified enablers for research and clinical practice allows nurses to view the individual, family, and community from the perspective of the seven cultural factors identified in the sunrise model (religion, kinship, technology, education, economic, political and legal, and cultural lifeways). By adopting this viewpoint, nurses and other healthcare professionals can decrease the vulnerability of the individual, family, and community by uncovering the concerns that derive from cultural difference and promoting ethical practice that is congruent with the cultural beliefs of those in the caring relationship with nurses and other healthcare professionals.

REFERENCES

Adger, W. N., (2006). Vulnerability. *Global Environmental Change, 16,* 268–281.

Andrews, M. M., & Boyle, J. S. (Eds.). (2011). *Transcultural concepts in nursing care* (6th ed.). Philadelphia: Wolters Kluwer Health.

Campos-Outcalt, D., Fernandez, R., Hollow, W., Lundeen, S., Nelson, K., & Schuster, B. (1994). Providing quality health care to vulnerable populations. Retrieved from http://www.primarycaresociety.org/1994d.htm

Clarke, P. N., McFarland, M. R., Andrews, M. M., & Leininger, M. (2009). Caring: Some reflections on the impact of the culture care theory by McFarland & Andrews and a conversation with Leininger. *Nursing Science Quarterly, 22*(3), 233–239.

Frohlich, K. L., & Potvin, L. (2008). Transcending the known in public health practice: The inequality paradox: The population approach and vulnerable populations. *American Journal of Public Health, 98*(2), 216–221.

Leininger, M. M. (1991a). Ethnonursing: A research method with enablers to study the theory of culture care. *NLN Publishing, 15*(2402), 73–117.

Leininger, M. M. (1991b). The theory of culture care diversity and universality. *NLN Publishing, 15*(2402), 5–68.

Leininger, M. (1996a). Culture care theory, research, and practice. *Nursing Science Quarterly, 9*(2), 71–78.

Leininger, M. (1996b). Response to Swendson and Windsor: Rethinking cultural sensitivity. *Nursing Inquiry, 3*(4), 238–241.

Leininger, M. (2002a). Culture care theory: A major contribution to advance transcultural nursing knowledge and practices. *Journal of Transcultural Nursing, 13*(3), 189–192.

Leininger, M. (2002b). Madeleine Leininger on transcultural nursing and culturally competent care. Interview by Mary Agnes Seisser. *Journal of Healthcare Quality, 24*(2), 18–21.

Leininger, M., & McFarland, M. (2002). *Transcultural nursing: Concepts, theories, research and practice.* New York: McGraw Hill.

Leininger, M., & McFarland, M. (2006). *Culture care diversity and universality: A worldwide nursing theory* (2nd ed.). Sudbury, MA: Jones and Bartlett.

Locke, D., Bailey, D. F., (2014). *Increasing multicultural understanding* (3rd ed.). Los Angeles, CA: Sage.

McFarland, M. R., & Wehbe-Alamah, H. B., (2015). *Leininger's culture care diversity and universality: A worldwide nursing theory* (3rd ed.). Burlington, MA: Jones and Bartlett.

Reynolds, C. L., & Leininger, M. M. (1993). *Madeline Leininger, culture care diversity and universality theory.* Newbury Park, CA: Sage.

Shi, L., & Stevens, G. (2010). *Vulnerable populations in the United States* (2nd ed.). San Francisco: Jossey-Bass.

Zoucha, R. (2006). Considering culture in understanding interpersonal violence. *Journal of Forensic Nursing, 2*(4), 195–196.

Zoucha, R., & Husted, G. L. (2000). The ethical dimensions of delivering culturally congruent nursing and health care. *Issues in Mental Health Nursing, 21*(3), 325–340.

Zoucha, R., & Husted, G. L. (2002). The ethical dimensions of delivering culturally congruent nursing and health care. *Review Series Psychiatry, 3*, 10–11.

Zoucha, R. D., & Reeves, J. (1999). A view of professional caring as personal for Mexican Americans. *International Journal for Human Caring, 3*(3), 14–20.

Chapter 9

Application of the Health Belief Model in Women with Gestational Diabetes

Janeen S. Amason and Shih-Yu (Sylvia) Lee

OBJECTIVES

At the end of this chapter, the reader will be able to

1. Explain the main variables of the Health Belief Model.
2. Evaluate the usefulness of the Health Belief Model in pregnant women diagnosed with gestational diabetes.
3. Apply the Health Belief Model to research in women diagnosed with gestational diabetes during pregnancy and postpartum.

GESTATIONAL DIABETES AND RISK OF TYPE 2 DIABETES

Gestational diabetes (GD) has been recognized as a common complication of pregnancy that will resolve after childbirth, but recent research has shown that this diagnosis may signify a lifetime of health issues including the development of type 2 diabetes (DM) (Baptiste-Roberts et al., 2009; Bellamy, Casas, Hingorani, & Williams, 2009; Feig, Zinman, Wang, & Hux, 2008; Lee, Hiscock, Wein, Walker, & Permezel, 2007; Lee, Jang, Park, Metzger, & Cho, 2008; Reece, Leguizamon, & Wiznitzer, 2009). In the United States, approximately 10.8% of women (12.6 million) who are aged 20 years or older have been diagnosed with type 2 diabetes, with higher rates identified in minority groups including Hispanics, non-Hispanic Blacks, and Asian Americans (Centers for Disease Control and Prevention [CDC], 2011). The World Health Organization (WHO,

2010) predicts that if no action is taken, deaths associated with DM will double by the year 2030. Additionally, DM may shorten an individual's life expectancy by one-third (CDC, 2008)) and is the seventh leading cause of death in the United States (CDC, 2011). The most common complications of DM include cardiovascular disease, kidney failure, neuropathy, and retinopathy (CDC, 2008; National Institutes of Health [NIH], 2008; WHO, 2010). Obesity, sedentary lifestyles, sleep disturbance, and stress have been associated with the development of type 2 diabetes (Chaput, Despres, Bouchard, & Tremblay, 2007; Gunderson et al., 2008; Knutson & Cauter, 2008). Early prevention strategies, such as weight loss, increase in physical activity, and healthy diet, will decrease the incidence of DM and the associated complications in populations at risk for developing DM (CDC, 2011; Knowler et al., 2002; NIH, 2008), therefore specific populations, such as women with a history of GD, should adopt health behavior strategies to prevent or delay DM.

Gestational diabetes is defined as a form of diabetes that begins or is first recognized during pregnancy. GD occurs because of pancreatic beta cells' inability to produce sufficient insulin for increased demands during the third trimester of pregnancy (American Diabetes Association [ADA], 2008; Agency for Healthcare Research and Quality [AHRQ], 2009; Pridjian & Benjamin, 2010). Each year, this disorder affects approximately 4–10% of pregnant women in the United States (ADA, 2010; AHRQ, 2009; Pridjian & Benjamin, 2010). Research has shown that women diagnosed with GD are at risk of developing DM after childbirth (Feig et al., 2008; Knowler et al., 2002; Lee et al., 2007; Lee et al., 2008; Ratner et al., 2008). A landmark epidemiological study, the Diabetes Prevention Program (Knowler et al., 2002), which evaluated men and women's risk of developing DM, found that women with a history of GD had a 71% higher incidence rate of developing DM than those without a history of GD (Ratner et al., 2008). Maternal body mass index (BMI) was positively correlated with the risk of DM. Women with GD who engaged in healthy lifestyle behaviors decreased the risk of DM by 50%. However, compared to women with no diagnosis of GD, women with GD were less able to sustain the weight loss and physical activity as compared to women with no diagnosis of GD, thus increasing risk of DM.

Risk Factors Contributing to Development of DM

There are additional risk factors that contribute to the development of DM such as overweight/obesity (BMI > 25), sedentary lifestyles, use of insulin during pregnancy, an early diagnosis of GD (< 24 weeks' gestation), and inappropriate nocturnal sleep time (Baptiste-Roberts et al., 2009; Chaput, Despres, Bouchard, Astrup, & Tremblay, 2009; Jarvela et al., 2006; Krishnaveni et al., 2007; Ogonowski & Miazgowski, 2009). The incidence rates of DM are higher in women with GD who had increased severity of gestational diabetes (defined by insulin use, neonatal hypoglycemia, and recurrent GD), required insulin therapy during pregnancy, and had early diagnosis (< 24 weeks' gestation) of GD during the pregnancy (Jarvela et al., 2006; Ogonowski & Miazgowski, 2009; Russell, Dodds, Armson, Kephart, & Joseph, 2008). In addition, a relationship has been identified between sleep duration (≤ 6 hours per night or ≥ 9 hours per night) and impaired glucose tolerance (Chaput et al., 2009; Knutson & Cauter, 2008; Knutson, Spiegel, Penev, & Cauter, 2007; Tasali, Leproult, & Spiegel, 2009). Insulin sensitivity and pancreatic beta cell function are influenced by sleep, with glucose levels remaining stable through the sleep cycle and glucose metabolism and insulin production increasing during the waking hours. The quantity and quality of sleep affects glucose tolerance by affecting the normal homeostasis of the mechanisms that maintain and stabilize glucose levels (Ip & Mokhlesi, 2007), leading to impaired glucose tolerance if sleep patterns are altered. Shorter sleep (≤ 6 hours) and longer sleep (≥ 9 hours) duration decreases insulin sensitivity and glucose tolerance, thus increasing risk of DM.

Prevention of DM: Healthy Lifestyle Behaviors

Prevention of DM through adoption of healthy behaviors has been well established in the literature (Knowler et al., 2002; Tuomilehto et al., 2001). The International Diabetes Federation has developed a three-step plan for prevention of DM through: (1) identification of those at higher risk for developing type 2 diabetes, (2) use of a measurement of that risk, and (3) interventions to prevent the disease (Alberti, Zimmet, & Shaw, 2007).

As described above, there are modifiable risk factors associated with the development of DM, which include obesity, unhealthy diet, and physical inactivity. Studies have shown that obesity, which is a BMI > 25, leads to poor insulin secretion and sensitivity, thus increasing the risk of DM. A simple weight loss (through healthy diet) of 10% of body weight can improve glycemic control (Case, Willoughby, Haley-Ziltin, & Maybee, 2006; Costacou & Mayer-Davis, 2003). The prevention strategies seem simple, but changing behaviors takes time and can only be achieved when individuals are engaged in the process (Saunders & Pastors, 2008; Yun, Kabeer, Zhu, & Brownson, 2007). Modifiable life behaviors and prevention strategies are important concepts to prevent or delay the development of DM (Yun et al., 2007). The clinical trial Diabetes Prevention Program (DPP) identified a 58% reduction of risk of DM when weight loss, exercise, and healthy diet were implemented (Knowler et al., 2002). The DPP used individualized training for nutrition, weight loss and weight management, and physical activity to assist with the participant's health behavior modifications. Participants (3,234) were randomly assigned into three groups: lifestyle intervention group, metformin intervention group, and placebo group. In a cumulative incidence of diabetes review, individuals assigned to the lifestyle intervention group (4.8/100 person) had lower incidence of DM with greater weight loss and physical activity than the other groups (7.8/100 person for metformin group; 11.0/100 person for placebo group). In a subsequent review of the DPP (Ratner et al., 2008), the researchers focused on 350 women with a history of GD specifically and found that lifestyle modifications (healthy diet and exercise) decreased their DM risk by 50%. Women in the placebo group with a history of GD had a greater incidence of DM (15.2/100 person).

It has been suggested that when individuals are identified as at risk for DM, they should be counseled by healthcare providers, therefore women with GD should be provided with information on the long-term effects of GD and DM preventive care including diet, exercise, and weight reduction (Ratner, 2007). Available data from intervention studies have identified that general strategies of healthy diet, exercise, and modest weight loss lowers the risk of DM. According to the American Diabetes Association (ADA, 2010) and American College of Obstetricians and Gynecologists (ACOG, 2009), women with GD should be counseled to lose weight, eat a healthy diet, and engage in moderate exercise after delivery and to continue these behaviors for a lifetime. These recommendations are consistent with the information provided to the general public for people who are at risk for developing DM. Studies such as the DPP show that women with GD had similar reduction of DM risk when compared with women with no GD diagnosis when diet and exercise interventions were followed (Ratner, 2007), thus demonstrating that these behaviors are appropriate for women with GD. However, research is limited in addressing the best approach to engage women with GD to adopt these healthy lifestyle behaviors. Furthermore, women who are caring for a newborn have unique needs and are more likely to have a difficult time participating in multiple counseling sessions; therefore, modification of known lifestyle intervention strategies to fit the busy lifestyle of a new mother is necessary (England et al., 2009).

THE HEALTH BELIEF MODEL

The Health Belief Model (HBM) was first introduced in the 1950s to explain the lack of participation in screening and health promotion programs and was one of the first theories that focused on health behaviors (National Cancer Institute [NCI], 2005; Rosenstock, 1974). The public health service at the time noted that although free or low-cost screenings and preventive services were available for tuberculosis, cervical cancer, dental disease, influenza, and other prevalent diseases, there was an extensive failure in use of the services (NCI, 2005; Rosenstock, 1974). The HBM was influenced by the theories of Kurt Lewin and was developed by a group of social psychologists (Dr. Hochbaum, Dr. Kegles, Dr. Leventhal, and Dr. Rosenstock) in order to explain preventive health behavior, especially in individuals who were asymptomatic (Rosenstock, 1974).

The HBM is one of the most widely used theories to examine the barriers and foundation of a person's participation in programs that focus on prevention of disease and promotion of a healthy lifestyle (NCI, 2005). Over the years, the framework has evolved to be used in a variety of health promotion and illness prevention studies and programs to assist in developing meaningful strategies that will decrease illness. The HBM provides a framework for understanding why some people take action to avoid illness, while others do not. The basis of this framework is that health behavior is related to a person's perceptions about a disease and the interventions necessary to decrease the incidence of the disease. In this context, there is a belief that people will act judiciously to promote their own health and avoid an illness, thus health motivation is the principal focus (Maiman & Becker, 1974; Rosenstock, 1974).

The premise of the model is that an individual's health behavior is based on his or her beliefs or perceptions about a disease and prevention of the illness using strategies that are available. The core assumptions of the HBM are based on the thought that a person will adopt a health behavior to avoid disease if the individual believes that he or she is susceptible to the disease, believes the consequence of the disease would be serious, believes that the disease occurrence can be avoided, believes the benefit of taking action to reduce a health threat exceeds any associated cost, and believes that he or she can effectively implement the recommended health behavior (Janz & Becker, 1984; Rosenstock, 1974; Rosenstock, Strecher, & Becker, 1988). The health behavior also depends on the value of the goal and the probability that an action will be successful in achieving the goal (Janz & Becker, 1984).

The HBM has been used to explain and predict participation in long-term and short-term health behaviors including smoking cessation (Schofield, Kerr, & Tolson, 2007), condom use (Macintyre, Rutenberg, Brown, & Karim, 2004; Sayles et al., 2006; Zak-Place & Stern, 2004), exercise (Fallon, Wilcox, & Ainsworth, 2005; Schwarzer et al., 2007) and breast cancer screening (Janz & Becker, 1984; Lee-Lin et al., 2007; Wu, West, Chen, & Hergert, 2006). The application of the HBM is a useful tool to examine commonalities that influence people to adhere to health promotion activities. Compliance of healthcare regimens has been widely evaluated with dietary, medication compliance, use of contraceptives, and dental hygiene.

The HBM (see **Figure 9-1**) is organized into three categories that include individual perceptions, modifying behaviors, and likelihood of action to show relationships of the concepts to an individual's motivation to participate in a health action or behavior. The original model had four main concepts that included perceived susceptibility, perceived severity, perceived benefits, and perceived barriers (Maiman & Becker, 1974; Rosenstock, 1974). In recent years, cues to action and self-efficacy have been added to the framework to meet the challenge of habitual unhealthy behaviors such as overeating, sedentary lifestyle, and smoking (NCI, 2005). For this discussion, the updated model will be reviewed

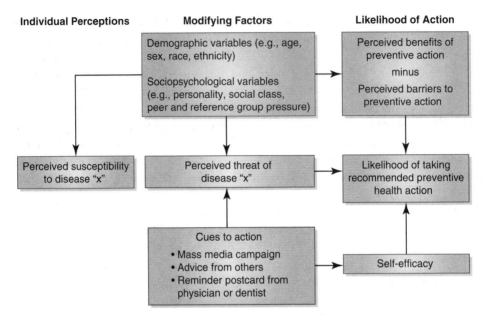

Figure 9-1 Health Belief Model
Reproduced from Rosenstock, I. (1974). Historical origins of the health belief model. *Health Education Monographs, 2*(4), 328–335. HEALTH EDUCATION MONOGRAPHS by SOCIETY FOR PUBLIC HEALTH EDUCATION; SOCIETY OF PUBLIC HEALTH EDUCATORS. Reproduced with permission of SOCIETY FOR PUBLIC HEALTH EDUCATION in the format Republish in a book via Copyright Clearance Center.

using six main concepts that include: perceived susceptibility and perceived severity (two variables together imply perceived threat of an illness), perceived benefits, perceived barriers (Maiman & Becker, 1974; Rosenstock, 1974), cues to action, and self-efficacy (NCI, 2005). Self-efficacy was added to the model to examine an adherence component that is essential in engaging in health behaviors. All of the concepts influence a person's decision making about whether or not he or she will engage in prevention, screening, and measures to control for an illness (Family Health International [FHI], 2002; NCI, 2005; Rosenstock et al., 1988).

Major Concepts and Definitions of the Health Belief Model

Perceived susceptibility is a person's belief (perception) of his or her chance of developing a disease and influences the adoption of health behaviors. The greater the perception of risk, the greater the likelihood that a person will engage in behaviors to decrease their risk for a disease (Rosenstock, 1974). If a person does not perceive themselves at risk for DM, then the individual will not grasp the importance of screening and health behavior modifications. This is especially important when symptoms may not be exhibited, although a disease process is present. According to the model, women with GD will have an increased perception of susceptibility for developing DM, will be more likely to request that healthcare providers perform postpartum testing and will be advocates for blood glucose screening throughout their lifetime. These women will also be more likely to adopt healthy lifestyle behaviors (e.g., weight loss, healthy diet, and exercise) to prevent or delay the development of DM.

Perceived severity is the person's opinion of how serious the condition is or will be and the consequences of that disease (Rosenstock, 1974). The individual will evaluate how this disease will affect her life if she develops the condition or if the illness is left untreated. The concerns are not only focused on the medical aspects, but also the psychological and social consequences as well (FHI, 2002; Rosenstock, 1974). The physical complications associated with DM include cardiovascular disease, kidney disease, blindness, and amputations (Diabetes Research Institute [DRI], 2010). The individual will also evaluate the consequences of the disease and how the consequences will affect their family. A childbearing-age woman will weigh the consequences of the disease on how she will take care of her children and family. A person's perception may be different if a family member has DM and if that member has had complications from the disease process. An individual who has observed the devastating consequences of poor DM management that resulted in amputation or kidney failure is more likely to perceive the severity. Also, direct knowledge of the daily activities of diet management and glucose monitoring will influence the person regarding the management regimen necessary to prevent associated complications. In addition, a woman who had to take insulin during her pregnancy because of GD may comprehend the severity of the disease more than a woman who managed insulin intolerance with diet alone and had no complications.

Perceived benefits are the person's beliefs that the proposed strategy will reduce the illness threat (Rosenstock, 1974). This is a key component in adapting prevention strategies such as glucose screening. The benefits of a healthy lifestyle for the woman are that she will have more energy, may prevent complications of the disease, and may have a longer life. In addition, the health benefit will prevent complications in future pregnancies and harmful affects to the fetus such as macrosomia, congenital anomalies, and increased risk of obesity and DM in her offspring (Kitzmiller, Dang-Kilduff, & Taslimi, 2007).

Perceived barriers are the person's perception of the cost of implementing the proposed health behavior—that is, the possible negative consequences of implementing a health strategy. The person weighs the benefits against the barriers and may determine the barriers are outweighed by the benefits (Maiman & Becker, 1974; NCI, 2005). There are many obstacles that may interfere with instituting a behavior, which may include physical, psychological, and financial demands of the strategy. The person may consider whether the benefits outweigh the consequences of the old behavior (Rosenstock, 1974). Some of the perceived barriers for postpartum women include role changes, time constraints, fatigue, lack of childcare, and the financial cost of procedures if they have no insurance coverage for laboratory testing.

Cues to action address the influences of a person's environment to make changes. Rosenstock (1974) believed that some type of cue was essential in the decision-making process. The cues make the individual aware of his or her own feelings about a problem, thus assisting in the readiness to make a change or adopt a health action (Janz & Becker, 1984; Rosenstock, 1974). An important component of a cue to make it effective is that the person must want to make a change. Cues to action may be external, which may include advice from family members, friends, or the media. The prompting of action may also be from the encouragement by healthcare providers to perform a certain action. Internal cues may be derived from life experiences, uncomfortable symptoms, or thoughts about a condition that have been conceptualized by symptoms associated with the condition (Maiman & Becker, 1974). A woman who has a family member with DM may be more likely to initiate change than one who has had no contact with the illness or with an individual who is a strong proponent to be their own healthcare advocate. For studies in women with GD, an external cue in the form of advice from a healthcare provider or structured counseling sessions may trigger actions of the decision-making process to make healthy lifestyle behavior choices, including adoption of health behaviors such as diet, exercise, and obtaining recommended glucose screening postpartum.

Self-efficacy is a person's belief or confidence in his or her own ability to take an action that is required to meet the desired outcome. Rosenstock et al. (1988) believed that self-efficacy contributes to the HBM for initiating and maintaining behavioral change by highlighting the importance of a person feeling competent. Human beings generally do not try new things unless they believe they can successful (NCI, 2005); therefore, the confidence to implement healthcare strategies will have an influence on the likelihood of implementing the health action. Self-efficacy is influenced by past experiences as well as the positive reinforcement provided. With the knowledge of the risk of developing DM and the recommended postpartum glucose screening guidelines, women are encouraged to become active participants in their own health care. The individual must also feel confident that she can engage in healthy lifestyle behaviors, such as diet and exercise. Even if a person believes a behavior is useful, but does not believe that she is capable of performing the behavior, the likelihood of a health behavior change is low.

Modifying factors, which include demographic variables (e.g., age, sex, race, ethnicity), sociopsychological variables (e.g., personality, social class), and structural variables (e.g., knowledge of disease, previous contact with disease) affect a person's perceptions about the health threat and perceived benefits of health actions that prevent disease (Roden, 2004; Rosenstock, 1974). The individual characteristics have an influence on perceptions, thus influencing health behaviors.

The Health Belief Model Adapted for Women with Gestational Diabetes

In studies of women's health issues, the HBM has been used primarily to address breast cancer screening (Janz & Becker, 1984; Lee-Lin et al., 2007; Wu et al., 2006). The application of the HBM is a useful tool to examine commonalities that influence people to adhere to health promotion activities.

The adapted HBM (see **Figure 9-2**) is organized into three categories that include individual perceptions, modifying behaviors, and likelihood of action. Figure 9-2 shows relationships of the concepts to an individual's motivation to participate in a health action or behavior and focuses on the key concepts of perceived risk, demographic and structural variables, cues to action, perceived barriers, and self-efficacy.

Theoretical Assumptions

The premise of the model is that an individual's health behavior is based on his or her beliefs or perceptions about a disease and prevention of the illness by available strategies. As discussed in the previous section, the core assumptions of the HBM are based on the thought that a person will adopt a health behavior to avoid disease if the individual believes that he or she is susceptible to a disease, believes the consequence of the disease

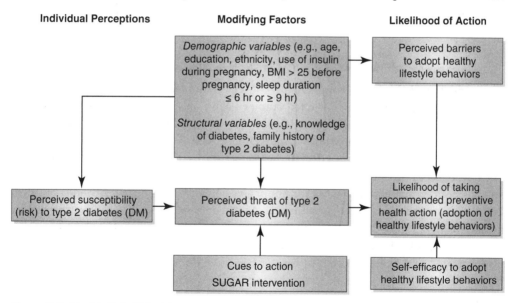

Figure 9-2 Health Belief Model

Modified from Rosenstock, I. (1974). Historical origins of the health belief model. *Health Education Monographs,* *2*(4), 328–335. HEALTH EDUCATION MONOGRAPHS by SOCIETY FOR PUBLIC HEALTH EDUCATION; SOCIETY OF PUBLIC HEALTH EDUCATORS. Reproduced with permission of SOCIETY FOR PUBLIC HEALTH EDUCATION in the format Republish in a book via Copyright Clearance Center.

would be serious, believes that the disease occurrence can be avoided, believes the benefit of taking action to reduce a health threat exceeds any associated cost, and believes that he or she can effectively implement the recommended health behavior (Janz & Becker, 1984; Rosenstock, 1974; Rosenstock et al., 1988). The behavior depends also on the value of the goal and the probability that an action will be successful in achieving the goal (Janz & Becker, 1984).

Concepts for the Adapted Health Belief Model

The concepts of the model have been discussed previously in this chapter. For the study in women with GD, specific modifying factors for this population are important to focus on due to the associated risk factors for developing DM. Modifying factors, which include demographic variables (use of insulin during pregnancy, BMI > 25 before pregnancy, sleep duration) and structural variables (knowledge of diabetes, family history of type 2 diabetes), affect a person's perceptions about the health threat and perceived barriers of health actions that prevent disease (Roden, 2004; Rosenstock, 1974). A GD woman's individual characteristics have an influence on her perceptions, thus will influence her adoption of healthy lifestyle behaviors to prevent the development of DM after childbirth. For example, a woman with a greater knowledge of DM will have a higher perceived risk of developing DM, thus impacting behavioral change.

Use of the Health Belief Model to Guide Study in Women with Gestational Diabetes

Although, the HBM framework has been used in numerous studies associated with adoption of healthy behaviors, limited studies have focused on the adoption of health behaviors in women with GD (Jones, Roche, & Appel, 2009). This model is useful for the vulnerable population of women with GD because its focus on the health beliefs and attitudes of individuals and the effect on health behaviors. This model has been viewed as one of the most influential in relation to health promotion, has strong empirical support, and has been evaluated thoroughly for use in a variety of health behavior studies (Roden, 2004). In relation to this model, women with a history of GD who perceive themselves at risk for developing DM will more likely advocate to be screened for the disease and implement healthy behaviors to decrease their risk for developing DM. Studies have demonstrated that women with a history of GD often do not perceive themselves at risk for developing DM (Jones et al., 2009; Kim et al., 2007; Malcolm, Lawson, Gaboury, & Keely, 2009).

This framework is useful to guide the development of interventions designed to increase knowledge about GD and long term risks of DM, recommended follow-up glucose screening postpartum, and healthy lifestyle strategies to prevent or delay the development of DM (Amason, Lee, Hewell, & Aduddell, 2013). According to the HBM, women with a higher perceived threat and higher self-efficacy to adopt healthy behaviors are more likely to engage in positive health behaviors. Interventions can also be implemented to increase women's perceived susceptibility of DM and self-efficacy to adopt healthy lifestyle behaviors. Specific barriers can be identified which hinder adoption of behaviors and lead to development of essential resources that assist woman with GD to adopt healthy lifestyle behaviors. Also, demographic and structural variables have an influence on perceived risk of the woman. Research has indicated that women with a family history of diabetes, who are obese, have impaired sleep, and who used insulin during pregnancy are more likely to develop DM after GD. According to the HBM, these types of variables will influence the perception of risk of developing DM in a woman with a history of GD. The goal is for women with GD to adopt healthy lifestyle behaviors (e.g., weight loss, healthy diet, and exercise) to prevent the development of DM, and obtain blood glucose screening as indicated, therefore identification of these influences is important to develop effective intervention strategies. The development of an educational intervention based on known influences on behavior will be beneficial in helping women with GD adopt healthy behaviors to prevent DM.

Evaluation of the Health Belief Model

As discussed previously in this chapter, research has shown that concepts of the HBM are significantly associated with health behaviors such as smoking cessation (Schofield et al., 2007), condom use (Macintyre et al., 2004; Sayles et al., 2006; Zak-Place & Stern, 2004), exercise (Fallon et al., 2005; Schwarzer et al., 2007) and breast cancer screening (Janz & Becker, 1984; Lee-Lin et al., 2007; Wu et al., 2006), and thus strengthen the use of the model in a study focused on adoption of healthy lifestyle behaviors in women with GD. The HBM has been used extensively in research and in a variety of settings, populations, and health conditions to predict health practices (Janz & Becker, 1984; Smith & Stasson, 2000). This theory has been criticized for not providing guidelines as to how individual variables predict behavior, but some authors believe that the lack of structure gives more flexibility, thus making the theory more adaptable to predict behaviors in a variety of situations (Nejad, Wertheim, & Greenwood, 2005).

The HBM also has known weaknesses. The theory does not provide operational definitions of the variables, thus leading to diverse methodology in various studies (Armitage & Conner, 2000). A major weakness of the model is that other variables that influence behaviors of individuals are not addressed in this theory. The HBM is a psycho-social model, and therefore limits the explanation for health behavior to be only attitudes and beliefs, and excludes other factors (Janz & Becker, 1984; Munro, Lewin, Swart, & Vomink, 2007). For example, the model does not take into consideration that some behaviors are habitual, which interferes with the decision-making process for adoption of a behavior (Munro et al., 2007). In addition, some health behaviors are adopted for other reasons than health; for example, dieting to lose weight for appearance and not weight loss for health reasons (Janz & Becker, 1984).

CONCLUSIONS AND IMPLICATIONS

Although there are limited studies that focus specifically on women with GD and the adoption of health behaviors, research does indicate that women do not perceive them-selves at risk for developing DM (Kim et al., 2007; Malcolm et al., 2009; Morrison, Lowe, & Collins, 2010). Using the HBM, healthcare providers can implement effective strategies, such as client education, that will increase the perceived risk and increase knowledge of GD and the related risk of developing DM within their lifetime. Also, in determining the perceived barriers to adopting healthy lifestyles, healthcare providers can assist with education and resources to break down those barriers. Once education is provided, healthcare providers must then focus on the self-efficacy component of the theory. Healthcare providers can assist in increasing a woman's self-efficacy by allowing her to be part of the decision-making process and work to develop a plan that will fit her life and family dynamics.

Acknowledgments

The author would like to extend a special thank you to Kathie Aduddell, EdD, RN and Sandra Hewell, PhD, MN, WHNP-BC.

REFERENCES

Agency for Healthcare Research and Quality (AHRQ). (2009). *Gestational diabetes: A guide for pregnant women.* [Brochure]. Eisenberg Center at Oregon Health and Science University.

Alberti, K. G., Zimmet, P., & Shaw, J. (2007). International Diabetes Federation: A consensus on type 2 diabetes prevention. *Diabetic Medicine, 24,* 451–463.

Amason, J., Lee, S., Hewell, S., & Aduddell, K. (2013). The effect of an educational intervention in women with gestational diabetes: A pilot study. Unpublished manuscript. Byrdine F. Lewis School of Nursing and Health Professions, Georgia State University, Atlanta, GA.

American College of Obstetricians and Gynecologists (ACOG). (2009). Postpartum screening for abnormal glucose tolerance in women who had gestational diabetes mellitus. *Obstetrics & Gynecology, 113*(6), 1419–1421.

American Diabetes Association (ADA). (2008). For Mother's Day, fighting a disease in mothers: Gestational diabetes. *Diabetes Forecast, 61*(5), 61–63.

American Diabetes Association (ADA). (2010). *Gestational Diabetes.* Retrieved from http://www .diabetes.org/diabetes-basics/gestational/what-is-gestational-diabetes.html

Armitage, C., & Conner, M. (2000). Social cognition models and health behaviour: A structured review. *Psychology and Health, 15,* 173–189.

Baptiste-Roberts, K., Barone, B. B., Gary, T. L., Golden, S. H., Wilson, L. M., Bass, E. B., & Nicholson, W. K. (2009). Risk factors for type 2 diabetes among women with gestational diabetes: A systematic review. *The American Journal of Medicine, 122,* 207–214.

Bellamy, L., Casas, J. P., Hingorani, A. D., & Williams, D. (2009). Type 2 diabetes mellitus after gestational diabetes: A systematic review and meta-analysis. *Lancet, 373,* 1773–1779.

Case, J., Willoughby, D., Haley-Ziltin, V., & Maybee, P. (2006). Preventing type 2 diabetes after gestational diabetes. *The Diabetes Educator, 32*(6), 877–886.

Centers for Disease Control and Prevention (CDC). (2008). *National diabetes fact sheet, 2007: General information and national estimates on diabetes in the United States.* Retrieved from http://www.cdc.gov/diabetes/pubs/pdf/ndfs_2007.pdf

Centers for Disease Control and Prevention (CDC). (2011). *National diabetes fact sheet, 2011: Fast facts on diabetes.* Retrieved from http://www.cdc.gov/diabetes/pubs/pdf/ndfs_2011.pdf

Chaput, J., Despres, J., Bouchard, C., & Tremblay, A. (2007). Association of sleep duration with type 2 diabetes and impaired glucose tolerance. *Diabetologia, 50,* 2298–2304.

Chaput, J., Despres, J., Bouchard, C., Astrup, A., & Tremblay, A. (2009). Sleep duration as a risk factor for the development of type 2 diabetes or impaired glucose tolerance: Analyses of the Quebec Family Study. *Sleep Medicine, 10,* 919–924.

Costacou, T., & Mayer-Davis, E. J. (2003). Nutrition and prevention of type 2 diabetes. *Annual Review of Nutrition, 23,* 147–170.

Diabetes Research Institute (DRI). (2010). *Diabetes fact sheet.* Retrieved from http://www.diabetesresearch.org/Page.aspx?pid=484

England, L. J., Dietz, P. M., Njoroge, T., Callaghan, W. M., Bruce, C., Buus, R. M., & Williamson, D. F. (2009). Preventing type 2 diabetes: Public health implications for women with a history of gestational diabetes mellitus. *American Journal of Obstetrics & Gynecology, 200,* 365e1–365e8.

Fallon, E. A., Wilcox, S. W., & Ainsworth, B. E. (2005). Correlates of self-efficacy for physical activity in African American women. *Women & Health, 41*(3), 47–62.

Family Health International (FHI). (2002). *Behavior change: A summary of four major theories.* Retrieved from http://ww2fhi.org/en/aids/aidscap/aidspubs/behres/bcr4theo.html

Feig, D. S., Zinman, B., Wang, X., & Hux, J. E. (2008). Risk of development of diabetes mellitus after diagnosis of gestational diabetes. *Canadian Medical Association Journal, 179*(3), 229–234.

Gunderson, E., Rifas-Shiman, R., Oken, E., Rich-Edwards, J., Kleinman, K., Taveras, E., & Gillman, M. (2008). Association of fewer hours of sleep at 6 months postpartum with substantial weight retention at 1 year postpartum. *American Journal of Epidemiology, 167*(2), 178–187.

Ip, M., & Mokhlesi, B. (2007). Sleep and glucose intolerance/diabetes mellitus. *Sleep Medicine Clinics, 2*(1), 19–29.

Janz, N. K., & Becker, M. H. (1984). The health belief model: A decade later. *Health Education Quarterly, 11*(1), 1–47.

Jarvela, I. Y., Juutinen, J., Koskela, P., Hartikainen, A. L., Kulmala, P., Knip, M., & Tapanainen, J. S. (2006). Gestational diabetes identifies women at risk for permanent type 1 and type 2 diabetes in fertile age. *Diabetes Care, 29*(3), 607–612.

Jones, E. J., Roche, C. C., & Appel, S. J. (2009). A review of the health beliefs and lifestyle behaviors of women with previous gestational diabetes. *Journal of Obstetric, Gynecologic & Neonatal Nursing, 38*(5), 516–526.

Kim, C., McEwen, L. N., Piette, J. D., Goewey, J., Ferrara, A., & Walker, E. A. (2007). Risk perception for diabetes among women with histories of gestational diabetes mellitus. *Diabetes Care, 30*(9), 2281–2286.

Kitzmiller, J., Dang-Kilduff, L., & Taslimi, M. (2007). Gestational diabetes after delivery. *Diabetes Care, 30*(Supplement 2), S225–S235.

Knowler, W. C., Barrett-Conner, E., Fowler, S. E., Hamman, R. F., Lachin, J. M., Walker, E. A., & Nathan, D. M. (2002). Reduction in the incidence of type 2 diabetes with lifestyle intervention or metformin. *The New England Journal of Medicine, 346*(6), 393–403.

Knutson, K. & Cauter, E. (2008). Associations between sleep loss and increased risk of obesity and diabetes. *Annals of the New York Academy of Sciences, 1129*, 287–304.

Knutson, K., Spiegel, K., Penev, P., & Cauter, E. (2007). The metabolic consequences of sleep deprivation. *Sleep Medicine, 11*, 163–178.

Krishnaveni, G. V., Hill, J. C., Veena, S. R., Geetha, S., Jayakumar, M. N., Karat, C. L., & Fall, C. (2007). Gestational diabetes and the incidence of diabetes in the 5 years following the index pregnancy in South Indian women. *Diabetes Research and Clinical Practice, 78*, 398–404.

Lee, A., Hiscock, R., Wein, P., Walker, S., & Permezel, M. (2007). Gestational diabetes mellitus: Clinical predictors and long-term risk of developing type 2 diabetes. *Diabetes Care, 30*(4), 878–883.

Lee, H., Jang, H. C., Park, H. K., Metzger, B. E., & Cho, N. H. (2008). Prevalence of type 2 diabetes among women with a previous history of gestational diabetes mellitus. *Diabetes Research and Clinical Practice, 81*, 124–129.

Lee-Lin, F., Menon, U., Pett, M., Nail, L., Lee, S., & Mooney, K. (2007). Breast cancer beliefs and mammography screening practices among Chinese American immigrants. *Journal of Obstetrics, Gynecologic & Neonatal Nursing, 36*, 212–221.

Macintyre, K., Rutenberg, N., Brown, L., & Karim, A. (2004). Understanding perceptions of HIV risk among adolescents in kwazulu-natal. *AIDS and Behavior, 8*(3), 237–250.

Maiman, L., & Becker, M. (1974). The health belief model: Origins and correlates in psychological theory. *Health Education Monographs, 2*(4), 336–353.

Malcolm, J., Lawson, M. L., Gaboury, I., & Keely, E. (2009). Risk perception and unrecognized type 2 diabetes in women with previous gestational diabetes mellitus. *Obstetric Medicine, 2*, 107–110.

Morrison, M. K., Lowe, J. M., & Collins, C. E. (2010). Perceived risk of type 2 diabetes in Australian women with a recent history of gestational diabetes mellitus. *Diabetic Medicine, 27*(8), 882–886.

Munro, S., Lewin, S., Swart, T., & Vomink, J. (2007). A review of health behaviour theories: How useful are these for developing interventions to promote long-term medication adherence for TB and HIV/AIDS? *BMC Public Health, 7*(104), 1–16.

National Cancer Institute (NCI). (2005). *Theory at a glance: A guide for health promotion practice (second edition).* Retrieved from http://www.cancer.gov/PDF/481fd53-63df-41bc-bfaf-5aa48ee1da/TAAG3.pdf

National Institutes of Health (NIH). (2008). *Fact sheet: Type 2 diabetes.* Retrieved from http://diabetes.niddk.nih.gov/dm/pubs/statistics/index.htm#prevention

Nejad, L., Wertheim, E., & Greenwood, K. (2005). Comparison of the health belief model and the theory of planned behaviour in the prediction of dieting and fasting behaviour. *Journal of Applied Psychology, 1*(1), 63–74.

Ogonowski, J., & Miazgowski, T. (2009). The prevalence of 6 weeks' postpartum abnormal glucose tolerance in Caucasian women with gestational diabetes. *Diabetes Research and Clinical Practice, 84,* 239–244.

Pridjian, G., & Benjamin, T. (2010). Update on gestational diabetes. *Obstetrics and Gynecology Clinics of North America, 37*(2), 255–267.

Ratner, R. (2007). Prevention of type 2 diabetes in women with previous gestational diabetes. *Diabetes Care, 30*(2), S242–S245.

Ratner, R. E., Christophi, C. A., Metzger, B. E., Dabelea, D., Bennett, P. H., Pi-Sunyer, X., Fowler, S., & Kahn, S. E. (2008). Prevention of diabetes in women with a history of gestational diabetes: Effects of metformin and lifestyle interventions. *Journal of Clinical Endocrinology & Metabolism, 93,* 4774–4779.

Reece, E. A., Leguizamon, G., & Wiznitzer, A. (2009). Gestational diabetes: The need for a common ground. *Lancet, 373,* 1789–1797.

Roden, J. (2004). Revisiting the health belief model: Nurses applying it to young families and their health promotion needs. *Nursing and Health Sciences, 6,* 1–10.

Rosenstock, I. (1974). Historical origins of the health belief model. *Health Education Monographs, 2*(4), 328–335.

Rosenstock, I., Strecher, V., & Becker, M. (1988). Social learning theory and the health belief model. *Health Education Quarterly, 15*(2), 175–183.

Russell, C., Dodds, L., Armson, B., Kephart, G., & Joseph, K. (2008). Diabetes mellitus following gestational diabetes: Role of subsequent pregnancy. *BJOG: An International Journal of Obstetrics & Gynaecology, 115,* 253–260.

Saunders, J. T., & Pastors, J. G. (2008). Practical tips on lifestyle management of type 2 diabetes for the busy clinician. *Current Diabetes Reports, 8,* 353–360.

Sayles, J. N., Pettifor, A., Wong, M. D., MacPhail, C., Lee, S. J., Hendriksen, E., … Coates, T. (2006). Factors associated with self-efficacy for condom use and sexual negotiation among South African youth. *Journal of Acquired Immune Deficiency Syndromes, 43*(2), 226–233.

Schofield, I., Kerr, S., & Tolson, D. (2007). An exploration of the smoking-related health beliefs of older people with chronic obstructive pulmonary disease. *Journal of Clinical Nursing, 16,* 1726–1735.

Schwarzer, R., Schuz, B., Ziegelmann, J. P., Lippke, S., Luszczynaska, A., & Scholz, U. (2007). Adoption and maintenance of four health behaviors: Theory guided longitudinal studies on dental flossing, seat belt use, dietary behavior, and physical activity. *Annals of Behavioral Medicine, 33*(2), 156–166.

Smith, B., & Stasson, M. (2000). A comparison of health behavior constructs: Social psychological predictors of AIDS-preventive behavioral intentions. *Journal of Applied Social Psychology, 30*(3), 443–462.

Tasali, E., Leproult, R., & Spiegel, K. (2009). Reduced sleep duration or quality: Relationships with insulin resistance and type 2 diabetes. *Progress in Cardiovascular Diseases, 51*(5), 381–391.

Tuomilehto, J., Lindstrom, J., Eriksson, J. G., Valle, T. T., Hamalaninen, H., Ilanne-Parikka, P., ... Uusitupa, M. (2001). Prevention of type 2 diabetes mellitus by changes in lifestyle among subjects with impaired glucose tolerance. *The New England Journal of Medicine, 344*(18), 1343–1350. http://www.unmc.edu/nursing/Health_Promoting_Lifestyle_Profile_II.htm

World Health Organization (WHO). (2010). *Diabetes.* Retrieved from http://www.who.int/mediacentre/factsheets/fs312/en/print.html

Wu, T. Y., West, B., Chen, Y. W., & Hergert, C. (2006). Health beliefs and practices related to breast cancer screening in Filipino, Chinese and Asian Indian women. *Cancer Detection and Prevention, 30,* 58–66.

Yun, S., Kabeer, N., Zhu, B., & Brownson, R. (2007). Modifiable risk factors for developing diabetes among women with previous gestational diabetes. *Preventing Chronic Disease: Public Health Research, Practice, and Policy, 4*(1), 1–5.

Zak-Place, J., & Stern, M. (2004). Health belief factors and dispositional optimism as predictors of STD and HIV preventive behavior. *Journal of American College Health, 52*(5), 229–236.

Chapter 10

Common Sense Model of Illness Behavior: Older Adults Diagnosed with Acute Myocardial Infarction

Deonna S. Tanner

OBJECTIVES

At the end of this chapter, the reader will be able to

1. Describe the key concepts of the Common Sense Model of Illness Behavior.
2. Evaluate the effectiveness of the Common Sense Model of Illness Behavior in older adults diagnosed with acute myocardial infarction.
3. Apply the concepts of the Common Sense Model of Illness Behavior to guide future research.

INTRODUCTION

Cardiovascular disease (CVD) is a significant, preventable health problem and, since 1990, has been responsible for more deaths worldwide than any other health problem (World Health Organization [WHO], 2008). In the United States, even though overall mortality rates from CVD have to some extent decreased, CVD remains the number one cause of death for both men and women (American Heart Association [AHA], 2012; Xu, Kochanek, Murphy, & Tejada-Vera, 2007). Although CVD indicates a variety of acute coronary events, it commonly manifests as an acute myocardial infarction (AMI).

An AMI is a serious, life-threatening medical event and approximately every 60 seconds, at least one person in the United States dies from complications related to AMI. Most often an AMI occurs when the coronary blood flow is obstructed, usually from a blood clot, resulting in ischemia to the myocardial tissue. (AHA, 2009). AMI symptoms are individualized, but typical symptoms of AMI are classified as, but not limited to, chest, arm, or jaw pain/discomfort; shortness of breath (with or without chest pain/discomfort); diaphoresis; nausea; and may also include lightheadedness. After a diagnosis of AMI is confirmed, treatment requires timely medical interventions such as thrombolytic and reperfusion therapies to restore the coronary blood flow (AHA, 2010). The type of intervention depends on the patient's physical manifestations, as well as the extent and features of the AMI, but all medical interventions work to restore perfusion and minimize damage to the myocardial tissue.

Despite major advances in technology resulting in innovative medical reperfusion therapies to effectively treat this serious health threat, a majority of individuals with AMI symptoms, particularly older adults, do not seek professional medical treatment in a timely manner. This delay, known as treatment seeking delay (TSD) significantly contributes to the disability and death associated with AMI (AHA, 2010). Clinical research, a process which helps to develop new nursing knowledge, has focused on TSD for many years as it is a global problem. As clinical research often uses a theoretical perspective to guide the study design, the purpose of this chapter is to discuss the key concepts of the Common Sense Model of Illness Behavior (CSM) as well as to evaluate the effectiveness of this theoretical framework. An example will also be offered from recent research that used the CSM to examine the decision-making process of older adults experiencing symptoms of AMI that demonstrates the applicability of the CSM for future research.

THE COMMON SENSE MODEL OF ILLNESS BEHAVIOR

Formerly known as the Theory of Self-Regulation (SRT), the CSM conceptualizes an individual as a capable and effective problem solver who has common sense beliefs that guide behavior in response to a health threat (Difenbach & Leventhal, 1996; Hagger & Orbell, 2003; Leventhal, Leventhal, & Contrada, 1998; Leventhal, Meyer, & Nerenz, 1980; Leventhal, Nerenz, & Steele, 1984). These common sense beliefs are known as illness representations or illness responses and are based largely on internal and external influencing sources which assist an individual to make sense of and cope with health as well as illness (Difenbach & Leventhal, 1996; Leventhal et al., 1980; Leventhal et al., 1984).

Since the 1980s this theory has been extensively used to understand how individuals perceive, manage, and cope with a broad range of illnesses. Previous studies using the CSM as a theoretical framework include, but are not limited to, research on kidney disease, pulmonary illness, diabetes mellitus, venous thrombosis, and certain types of cancer (Fowler, Kirchner, Kuiken, & Baas, 2007; Hagger & Orbell, 2003; Kapstein et al., 2007; Kelly et al., 2005; McAndrew et al., 2008; O'Neill, 2002). This model has also been used as a theoretical framework for previous nursing research in an attempt to understand the decision-making process related to seeking treatment for AMI symptoms for individuals of all ages (Dracup et al., 1995; Dracup et al., 2009; Goff et al., 1999; Harralson, 2007; King & McGuire, 2007; McKinley, Moser, & Dracup, 2000; Meischke, Eisenberg, Shaeffer, & Henwood, 2006; Meischke et al., 1999; Ryan & Zerwic, 2003; Tullman, Haugh, Dracup, & Bourguignon, 2007; Zerwic, 1998, 1999; Zerwic, King, & Wlasowicz, 1997; Zerwic, Ryan, DeVon, & Drell, 2003). Overall, these research studies utilized qualitative and quantitative research designs to determine factors that influence the patient's decision-making process when experiencing symptoms of AMI. However, very few studies have used the CSM with a focus solely on older adults.

CONCEPTS OF THE COMMON SENSE MODEL OF ILLNESS BEHAVIOR

The major concepts of CSM are the cognitive and emotional illness representations and subsequent coping processes. Within the model, these coping processes are followed by the concept of *appraisal*, which is the evaluation of the coping processes in order to control or manage a health threat. According to the theory, the systematic process begins when an individual perceives a threat to health through the experience of physical manifestations of illness, known as symptoms. When a health threat is perceived, an individual progresses through three stages: (1) mental representations of the health threat (cognitive and emotional aspects), (2) coping actions/behaviors designed in an attempt to manage the health threat, and (3) appraisal of how well the coping procedures managed the health threat (Difenbach & Leventhal, 1996; Leventhal et al., 1980; Leventhal et al., 1984). In order to explain the relationships among the major concepts, an illustration of the CSM is included (see **Figure 10-1**).

Overview of the Illness Representations

The cognitive and emotional illness representations are the crux of the CSM and are defined as an individual's perceived susceptibility of the health threat and subsequent mental interpretation of the illness (Leventhal & Cameron, 1987; Leventhal et al., 1998). Illness representations are individualized and are made up of simultaneous cognitive and emotional responses to the health threat. The cognitive element of illness representation has five major concepts which are identified within the CSM. These concepts include: identity, cause, controllability, timeline, and consequences of the illness. Simultaneous with the development of these representations are the individualized emotional representations experienced by the individual (**Figure 10-1**).

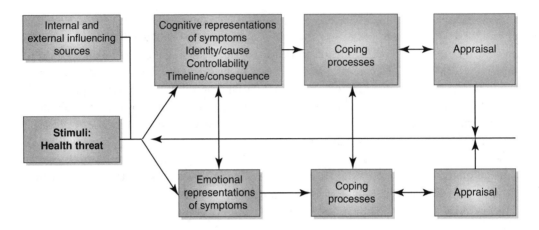

Figure 10-1 Illustration of the Common Sense Model of Illness Behavior

Reprinted from Patient Education & Counseling, 10, Leventhal, H., & Cameron, L., Behavioral theories and the problem of compliance, Pages 117–138, Copyright 1987, with permission from Elsevier.

According to the CSM, illness representations are influenced by internal and external influencing sources that assist an individual in making sense of and coping with health and illness (Difenbach & Leventhal, 1996). Internal influencing sources may include sociodemographic and clinical factors, previous experience with health and illness, as well as objective knowledge, expectations, and beliefs about the health threat (Difenbach & Leventhal, 1996). Another internal source within the model that may influence how a person responds to a health threat is an individual's cultural/social role. External influencing sources within the context of the model include one's social network including, but not limited to, spouses or significant others, family, friends, and even healthcare providers (HCP). These sources may be positive influences helping to prompt action in an attempt manage a health threat or negative influences impeding action against a threat (Leventhal & Cameron, 1987).

Cognitive Illness Representations: The Concepts of Identity and Cause

Identity is the first concept of the cognitive illness representations. Identity is not only the name or label of the health threat, it also includes the perceived relationship between the health threat and the associated physical symptoms (Difenbach & Leventhal, 1996). Labeling the illness is based on previous experience and expectations regarding illness or disease. Cause is the concept which is linked to identity. This concept relates to the individual's belief about the probable origin of the health threat. Probable causes of illness may include biological, emotional, environmental, and/or psychological factors (Fowler et al., 2007; Hagger & Orbell, 2003).

Identity and cause are recognized within the literature as being important in explaining the decision-making process related to seeking treatment for AMI. Identifying symptoms associated with AMI is difficult because symptoms are individualized; many persons, particularly older adults, do not experience typical symptoms. As stated, typical symptoms may include chest, arm, and/or jaw pain; shortness of breath (with or without chest discomfort); diaphoresis; nausea; and may also include lightheadedness (AHA, 2010). There is scientific evidence that suggests older adults (older women in particular) are more likely to experience atypical AMI symptoms. These atypical symptoms may include, but are not limited to, abdominal pain, confusion, nausea and/or vomiting, chest tightness (not described as pain), dizziness, dyspnea, shoulder/back pain, headache, and weakness (Gregoratos, 2001; Johansson, Stromberg, & Swahn, 2004; McSweeney Cody, & Crane, 2001; McSweeney et al., 2003; McSweeney, Lefler, & Crowder, 2005; Sjostrom-Strand & Fridlund, 2008; Song, Yan, Yang, Sun, & Du, 2010; Tullman et al., 2007; Xanthos et al., 2010). Experiencing atypical AMI symptoms may make it difficult for individuals to identify symptoms as heart-related, which may delay the decision to seek treatment (Moser et al., 2006). There is also empiric evidence that has been consistent over time, that demonstrates individuals whose physical symptoms of AMI match their perceived expectations, make the decision to seek treatment sooner than those whose expectations and symptoms do not match (Horne, James, Petrie, Weinman, & Vincent, 2000; Johnson & King, 1995; McKinley et al., 2000; Noureddine, Arevian, Adra, & Puzantian, 2008; Ruston, Clayton, & Calnan, 1998). On the other hand, when discrepancies between expected AMI symptoms and experienced symptoms occur, individuals are more likely to delay seeking treatment (Albarran, Clarke, & Crawford, 2007; Banks & Malone, 2005; Hwang, Ryan, & Zerwic, 2006; Johansson et al., 2004; Kentsch et al., 2002; King & McGuire, 2007; Lovelin, Schei, & Hole, 2007; Martin et al., 2004; McSweeney et al., 2001; McSweeney et al., 2003; Moser, McKinley, Dracup, & Chung, 2005; Zerwic et al., 2003).

Cognitive Illness Representations: The Concept of Controllability

Controllability is also known as the cure/control concept within the cognitive illness representations. This concept refers to the individual's beliefs of personal and medical control over the prevention, progression, and/or recovery from a health threat (Difenbach & Leventhal, 1996; Hagger & Orbell, 2003). These perceptions are influenced by the responsiveness to interventions initiated to manage a health threat. According to the CSM, if the intervention does not have the desired effect and symptoms are not cured or controlled (noted during the appraisal process), individuals are prompted to implement a new strategy to manage or recover from the health threat (Leventhal & Cameron, 1987). Empiric evidence demonstrates that individuals who attempt to control or cure their symptoms delay seeking treatment for AMI significantly longer than those who do not (Clark, 2001; Leslie, Urie, Hooper, & Morrison, 2000; Lovelin et al., 2007; Turis, 2009). Furthermore, having the ability to control symptoms is noted as a significant predictor of prolonged pre-hospital delay for individuals with AMI symptoms (Lesneski, 2009).

Cognitive Illness Representations: The Concepts of Timeline and Consequence

Timeline is related to one's beliefs about the expected duration and course of the illness as well as expected recovery time (Leventhal et al., 1998). This concept includes the individual's perception about whether the health threat is acute (short term or temporary), chronic (long term), or cyclic (long term with acute exacerbations). Timeline is linked to consequence within the model. Consequence is the belief about the repercussions of the health threat on the physical, economic, and/or social aspects of an individual's daily life. Examples of consequences of health threats may include loss in one's social role, economic hardship, disability, and even death (Difenbach & Leventhal, 1996). Within the context of AMI and delay, evidence from previous studies demonstrates that individuals who perceive AMI symptoms to be temporary or without life-threatening consequences delay seeking treatment longer than those who do not (Banks & Dracup, 2006; Moser et al., 2005; Taylor, Garewal, Carter, Bailey, & Aggarwal, 2005). In addition, not taking symptoms seriously is noted as a significant predictor for delay in the decision to seek treatment for AMI (Johansson et al., 2004; Kentsch et al., 2002).

Emotional Illness Representations

Emotional representations are parallel to the cognitive representations within the CSM (Figure 10-1). Emotional representations are essential elements that also guide decision making by invoking emotional reactions in response to the health threat. These emotional reactions are highly individualized and may include emotions such as worry, anxiety, uncertainty, anger, stress, and/or fear (Difenbach & Leventhal, 1996). According to the model, if the emotional element is accompanied by some type of action plan, individuals are motivated to take action against a health threat. If the emotional element becomes too overwhelming, emotions may consume the cognitive illness representation, which results in minimal or no coping processes (Difenbach & Leventhal, 1996).

Coping Processes

In order to manage a health threat, the individual uses coping processes, also known as symptom management strategies. These processes are relative to the perceived susceptibility of the health threat and involve taking action to manage cognitive and emotional illness representations (McAndrew et al., 2008). Cognitive coping processes are used to diminish the perceived susceptibility of the health threat, while emotional coping processes are intended to diminish emotional reactions in response to a health threat.

The Concept of Appraisal

The final concept of the CSM is the concept of appraisal. In this phase of the process, an individual evaluates the effectiveness of his or her coping strategies against the health threat (Difenbach & Leventhal, 1996). Although it is described as the final concept of the model, this phase actually acts as a feedback loop. As such, if the coping strategies are appraised by the individual to be ineffective, the representations will be altered, which leads to new coping strategies in an attempt to manage or recover from the health threat (Figure 10-1). Then again, if the strategies for coping are appraised to be effective, these strategies may influence the illness representations and could be used as coping efforts by the individual when faced with future health threats (Difenbach & Leventhal, 1996).

THE COMMON SENSE MODEL OF ILLNESS BEHAVIOR ADAPTED FOR OLDER ADULTS DIAGNOSED WITH AMI

There is no theoretical model to date that solely focuses on the decision-making process related to seeking treatment for symptoms of AMI for older adults. However, the CSM has been tested over many years of scientific research in an attempt to explain how individuals cognitively and emotionally respond to a health threat. This theory is well-established and is the framework most often used to guide research to examine the decision-making process related to seeking treatment for AMI symptoms (Byrne, Walsh, & Murphy, 2005; Dracup et al., 2009; Dracup et al., 1995; Goff et al., 1999; Harralson, 2007; King & McGuire, 2007; McKinley et al., 2000; Meischke et al., 2006; Meischke et al., 1999; Ryan & Zerwic, 2003; Tullman et al., 2007; Walsh, Lynch, Murphy, & Daly, 2004; Zerwic, 1998, 1999; Zerwic et al., 1997; Zerwic et al., 2003).

Concepts for the Adapted Model

Although the CSM is a useful framework to guide research regarding decision making, an adapted version of the CSM was used to study the decision-making process of older adults when experiencing symptoms of AMI. The modified CSM is presented in **Figure 10-2**. As one can see, the original model and the adapted model are quite similar. However, within the context of this research, the health threat or stimuli that begins the systematic process is specifically defined as physical symptoms of AMI. In the adapted version of the CSM, cognitive representations are reflected by an individual's symptom interpretation, the perceived level of control over symptoms, and perceived level of seriousness of symptoms.

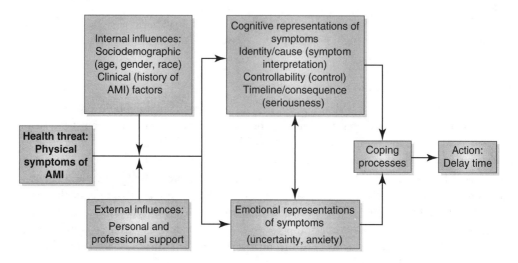

Figure 10-2 Adapted Common Sense Model of Illness Behavior for Study on the Examination of Factors That Influence Treatment Seeking Delay Among Older Adults Diagnosed with Acute Myocardial Infarction

Modified from Leventhal, H., Leventhal, E., & Contrada, R. J. (1998). Self-regulation, health and behavior: A perceptual cognitive approach. *Psychology & Health, 13,* 717–734. Psychology & Health by ROUTLEDGE. Reproduced with permission of ROUTLEDGE in the format reuses in a book/textbook via Copyright Clearance Center.

Internal influencing sources such as sociodemographic (age, gender, race), clinical factors (history of previous AMI), and external influencing sources (personal and professional support) are also specifically defined and included in the adapted model. As noted in the original model, the cognitive representations are parallel to the emotional representations in the adapted model. However, in the original model, the emotional representations describe more general, emotional reaction(s) when an individual experiences symptoms of an illness or disease. Although there are many emotional responses that may be experienced in response to AMI symptoms for older adults, feelings of uncertainty and anxiety are the focus in the adapted model because these emotions are the ones most commonly described in the literature regarding AMI (Banks & Malone, 2005; Henriksson, Lindahl, & Larsson, 2007; Khraim, Scherer, Dorn, & Carey, 2009; Lesneski, 2009; Moser et al., 2005; Pattenden, Watt, Lewin, & Stanford, 2002; Taylor et al., 2005). Anxiety regarding AMI symptoms is also identified as a significant predictor of reduced delay time (Khraim et al., 2009; McKinley et al., 2000). In contrast, uncertainty regarding AMI symptoms significantly adds to delay in seeking treatment for AMI symptoms (Kentsch et al., 2002; McKinley et al., 2000; Pattenden et al., 2002; Taylor et al., 2005).

The next phase of the adapted CSM is the coping processes (symptom management strategies), which are determined by the cognitive and emotional representations of symptoms. Lastly, the desired outcome or action by the individual is seeking timely treatment for AMI symptoms, measured in minutes from the onset of symptoms to presentation to the emergency department. Appraisal and the subsequent feedback loop were not included in the adapted model. Appraisal was not included in the adapted model as it is not relevant because individuals in the study had already experienced an AMI and sought treatment. An illustration of the adapted model is included (Figure 10-2).

THEORETICAL ASSUMPTIONS

In general, the CSM assumes that decision making occurs within several systematic stages and has many influences. The primary basis of the CSM is that individuals are capable problem solvers with the ability to make rational, effective decisions in response to a health threat (Hagger & Orbell, 2003). The model also assumes individuals have control over their own actions and behavior. In addition, the model suggests individuals have implicit beliefs about health and illness and when illness is perceived to be enough of a health threat, some type of coping response will be initiated by the individual. Lastly, it is believed that emotional responses may alter an individual's perception of the importance of seeking treatment in response to a health threat (Leventhal et al., 1980).

EVALUATION OF THE COMMON SENSE MODEL

Although the CSM is not exclusive to the decision-making process of seeking treatment for AMI for older adults, it has been used extensively as the theoretical framework for previous research. This research includes how individuals perceive, manage, and cope with a broad range of illnesses in many different settings which demonstrates its flexibility and strength as a theoretical model. Furthermore, it adds to the strength of the model that evidence from empiric studies has demonstrated treatment-seeking behavior is consistently predicted by the five illness representations which comprise the major concepts within the CSM (Byrne et al., 2005; Horne et al., 2000; King & McGuire, 2007; McKinley et al., 2000; Meischke et al., 1999; Walsh et al., 2004; Zerwic et al., 2003).

Although the CSM has many strengths that support its use in future research, no model is without limitations. For example, the literature on TSD consistently examines the importance of the influence that others have on the decision-making process (Keenan, 2001; Kentsch et al., 2002; Quinn, 2005; Thuresson et al., 2007). However, the CSM only acknowledges "others" as an external influencing source, but this influence is not emphasized as a major concept within the original model, and as such, this may be considered a limitation (Dracup et al., 1995). Some scholars argue that the CSM is too complex, with numerous concepts. Even so, the theory and its concepts are not difficult to understand.

CONCLUSIONS AND FUTURE DIRECTIONS

A theoretical framework or model is simply a tool to guide the study design of research. The CSM is a framework that has been used over the past 3 decades to explain the process of self-regulated decision making in response to a health threat and therefore, it is considered a well-established model of health behavior. Although the major concepts of this model are well supported and it is one of the most commonly used models used to attempt to explain the decision-making process to seek treatment for AMI symptoms, it is not limited within this context. Previous research has provided support that the relationships within the model are useful for the study of cognitive as well as emotional responses to a wide variety of acute and chronic health threats (Hagger & Orbell, 2003). This demonstrates the applicability of the model to be used in future research in the study of health behavior for a number of illnesses.

By the year 2030, it is projected one in every five Americans will be over the age of 65 and currently, older adults are the chief consumers of healthcare resources. As this population continues to increase, it is imperative for research related to prolonged delay in seeking treatment for AMI to focus on this vulnerable group because early intervention has the potential to decrease the mortality and morbidity associated with AMI (AHA, 2010; Ryan & Zerwic, 2003). At present, few studies focus solely on older populations (Alexander et al., 2005; Dodd, Saczynski, Zhao, Goldberg, & Gurwitz, 2011; Halon, Adawi, Dobrecky-Mery, & Lewis, 2004) even though risk for AMI is higher and overall prognosis is worse for people older than age 65 compared with younger populations (Dodd et al., 2011; Hwang et al., 2006; Maheshwari, Laird-Fick, Cannon, & DeHart, 2000; Popitean et al., 2005; Ryan & Zerwic, 2003). In fact, those at highest risk for AMI are older adults as the incidence of AMI increases with age (AHA, 2010). Although most CVD studies focus on younger populations, older age has been identified as a sociodemographic variable that is significantly associated with delay of treatment for an AMI (Gibler et al., 2002; Goff et al., 1999; Goldberg et al., 2009; Johansson et al., 2004). In addition, age greater than 65 years is reported to be an independent predictor for TSD related to AMI (Blohm, Hartford, Karlsson, & Herlitz, 1998; Kentsch et al., 2002; Ryan & Zerwic, 2003). However, results are contradictory; other studies have found no association between older age and prolonged prehospital delay time (Lesneski, 2009; Rasmussen, Munck, Kragstrup, & Haghfelt, 2003; Thuresson et al., 2007). Inconsistent findings indicate a need for additional research that focuses on older adults with AMI.

REFERENCES

Albarran, J. W., Clarke, B. A., & Crawford, J. (2007). 'It wasn't chest pain really, I can't explain it!' An exploratory study on the nature of symptoms experienced by women during their myocardial infarction. *Journal of Clinical Nursing, 16,* 129–1301.

Alexander, K. P., Roe, M. T., Chen, A. Y., Lytle, B. L., Pollack, C. V., Foody, J. M., & Petersen, E. D. (2005). Evolution in cardiovascular care for elderly patients with non-ST segment elevation acute coronary syndromes. *Journal of the American College of Cardiology, 46*(8), 1479–1487.

American Heart Association. (2009). Heart disease and stroke statistics: 2009 update. Retrieved from http://circ.ahajournals.org/content/119/3/e21

American Heart Association. (2010). Heart disease and stroke statistics: 2010 update. Retrieved from http://circ.ahajournals.org/content/121/7/e46

American Heart Association. (2012). Heart and stroke statistics: 2012 update. Retrieved from http://www.heart.org/HEARTORG/General/Heart-and-Stroke-Association-Statistics_UCM_319064_ SubHomePage.jsp

Banks, A. D., & Malone, R. E. (2005). Accustomed to enduring: Experiences of African-American women seeking care for cardiac symptoms. *Heart & Lung, 34*(1), 13–21.

Banks, A. D., & Dracup, K. (2006). Are there gender differences in the reason why African Americans delay in seeking medical help for symptoms of an acute myocardial infarction? *Ethnicity & Disease, 17*, 221–227.

Blohm, M. B., Hartford, M., Karlsson, T., & Herlitz, J. (1998). Factors associated with pre-hospital and in-hospital delay time in acute myocardial infarction: A 6-year experience. *Journal of Internal Medicine, 243*(3), 243–250.

Byrne, M., Walsh, J., & Murphy, A. W. (2005). Secondary prevention of coronary heart disease: Patient beliefs and health-related behavior. *Journal of Psychosomatic Research, 58*, 403–415.

Clark, A. (2001). Treatment decision-making during the early stages of heart attack: A case for the role of body and self in influencing delays. *Sociology of Health & Illness, 23*(4), 425–446.

Difenbach, M. A., & Leventhal, H. (1996). The common sense model of illness representations: Theoretical and practical considerations. *Journal of Social Distress and the Homeless, 5*(1), 11–38.

Dodd, K. S., Saczynski, J. S., Zhao, Y., Goldberg, R. J., & Gurwitz, J. H. (2011). Exclusion of older adults and women from recent trials of acute coronary syndromes. *Journal of the American Geriatrics Society, 59*(3), 506–511.

Dracup, K., McKinley, S., Riegel, B., Moser, D. K., Meischke, H., Doering, L. V., & Pelter, M. (2009). A randomized clinical trial to reduce patient prehospital delay to treatment in acute coronary syndrome. *Circulation Cardiovascular Quality and Outcomes, 2*, 524–532.

Dracup, K., Moser, D. K., Eisenberg, M., Meischke, H., Alonzo, A. A., & Braslow, A. (1995). Causes of delay in seeking treatment for heart attack symptoms. *Journal of Social Science Medicine, 40*, 379–392.

Fowler, C., Kirchner, M., Kuiken, D. V., & Baas, L. (2007). Promoting self-care through symptom management: A theory-based approach for nurse practitioners. *Journal of the American Academy of Nurse Practitioners, 19*, 221–227.

Gibler, W. B., Armstrong, P. W., Ohman, E. M., Weaver, W. D., Stebbins, A. L., Gore, J. M., & Topler, E. J. (2002). Persistence of delays in presentation and treatment for patients with acute myocardial infarction: The GUSTO-I and GUSTO-III experience. *Annals of Emergency Medicine, 39*(2), 123–145.

Goff, D. C., Feldman, H. A., McGovern, P. G., Goldberg, R. J., Simons-Morton, D. G., Cornell, C. E., & Hedges, J. R. (1999). Pre-hospital delay in patients hospitalized with heart attack symptoms in the United States: The REACT trial. *American Heart Journal, 138*(6), 1046–1057.

Goldberg, R. J., Spencer, F. A., Fox, K. A., Brieger, D., Steg, G., Gurfinkel, E, & Gore, J. M. (2009). Pre-hospital delay in patients with acute coronary syndromes (from the global registry of acute coronary events [GRACE]). *American Journal of Cardiology, 103,* 598–603.

Gregoratos, G. (2001). Clinical manifestations of acute myocardial infarction in older patients. *The American Journal of Geriatric Cardiology, 10*(6), 345–347.

Hagger, M. S., & Orbell, S. (2003). A meta-analytic review of the common-sense model of illness representations. *Psychology and Health, 18*(2), 141–184.

Halon, D. A., Adawi, S., Dobrecky-Mery, I., & Lewis, B. S. (2004). Importance of increasing age on the presentation and outcome of acute coronary syndromes in elderly patients. *Journal of the American College of Cardiology, 43*(3), 346–352.

Harralson, T. L. (2007). Factors influencing delay in seeking treatment for acute ischemic symptoms among lower income, urban women. *Heart & Lung, 36,* 96–104.

Henriksson, C., Lindahl, B., & Larsson, M. (2007). Patients' and relatives' thoughts and actions during and after symptom presentation for acute myocardial infarction. *European Journal of Cardiovascular Nursing, 6,* 280–286.

Horne, R., James, D., Petrie, K., Weinman, J., & Vincent, R. (2000). Patients' interpretation of symptoms as a cause of delay in reaching hospital during acute myocardial infarction. *Heart, 83,* 388–393.

Hwang, S. Y., Ryan, C., & Zerwic, J. J. (2006). The influence of age on acute myocardial infarction symptoms and patient delay in seeking treatment. *Progress in Cardiovascular Nursing, 21*(1), 20–27.

Johansson, I., Stromberg, A., & Swahn, E. (2004). Ambulance use in patients with acute myocardial infarction. *Journal of Cardiovascular Nursing, 19*(1), 5–12.

Johnson, J. A., & King, K. B. (1995). Influence of expectations about symptoms on delay in seeking treatment during an acute myocardial infarction. *American Journal of Critical Care, 4,* 29–35.

Kapstein, A. A., Van Korlaar, I. M., Cameron, L. D., Vossen, C. Y., Van Der Meer, F., & Rosendaal, F. R. (2007). Using the Common-Sense Model to predict risk perception and disease-related worry in individuals at increased risk for venous thrombosis. *Health Psychology, 26*(6), 807–817.

Keenan, J. (2001). Illness behavior in acute myocardial infarction. *Primary Health Care Research, 2,* 249–260.

Kelly, K., Leventhal., H., Andrykowski, M., Toppmeyer, D., Much, J., Dermidy, J., . . . Levine, A. A. (2005). Using the Common Sense Model to understand perceived cancer risk in individuals testing for BRCA1/2 mutations. *Psycho-Oncology, 12,* 34–48.

Kentsch, M., Rodemerk, U., Muller-Esch, G., Schnoor, U., Munzel, T., Ittel, T. H., . . . Mitusch, R. (2002). Emotional attitudes toward symptoms and inadequate coping strategies are major determinants of patient delay in acute myocardial infarction. *Clinical Research in Cardiology, 91,* 147–155.

King, K. B., & McGuire, M. A. (2007). Symptom presentation and time to seek care in women and men with acute myocardial infarction. *Heart & Lung, 36*(4), 235–243.

Khraim, F. M., Scherer, Y. K., Dorn, J. M., & Carey, M.G. (2009). Predictors of decision to delay to seeking healthcare among Jordanians with acute myocardial infarction. *Journal of Nursing Scholarship*, *41*(3), 260–267.

Leslie, W. S., Urie, A., Hooper, J., & Morrison, C. E. (2000). Delay in calling for help during myocardial infarction: Reasons for delay and subsequent pattern of accessing care. *Heart*, *84*, 137–141.

Lesneski, L. (2009). Factors influencing treatment delay for patients with acute myocardial infarction. *Applied Nursing Research*, *23*(4), 185–190.

Leventhal, H., & Cameron, L. (1987). Behavioral theories and the problem of compliance. *Patient Education & Counseling*, *10*, 117–138.

Leventhal, H., Leventhal, E., & Contrada, R. J. (1998). Self-regulation, health and behavior: A perceptual cognitive approach. *Psychology & Health*, *13*, 717–734.

Leventhal, H., Meyer, D., & Nerenz, D. R. (1980). The common sense representation of illness danger. In S. Rachman (Ed.), *Contributions to Medical Psychology* (pp. 7–30). New York: Pergamon Press.

Leventhal, H., Nerenz, D. R., & Steele, D. J. (1984). Illness representations and coping with health threats. In A. Baum, S. E. Taylor, & J. E. Singer (Eds.), *Handbook of Psychology and Health* (Vol. *4*, pp. 219–252). Hillsdale, NJ: Lawrence Erlbaum Associates.

Lovelin, M., Schei, B., & Hole, T. (2007). Pre-hospital delay, contributing aspects and responses to symptoms among Norwegian women and men with first time acute myocardial infarction. *European Journal of Cardiovascular Nursing*, *6*, 308–313.

Maheshwari, A., Laird-Fick, H. S., Cannon, L. A., & DeHart, D. J. (2000). Acute MI. *Geriatrics*, *55*(2), 32–39.

Martin, R., Lemos, K., Rothrock, N., Russell, D., Tripp-Reimer, T., Lounsbury, P., . . . Gordon, E. (2004). Gender disparities in common sense models of illness among MI victims. *Health Psychology*, *23*(4), 345–353.

McAndrew, L. M., Musumeci-Szabo, T. J., Mora, P. A., Vileikyte, L., Burns, E., Halm, A. E., & Leventhal, H. (2008). Using the common sense model to design interventions for the prevention and management of chronic illness threats: From description to process. *British Journal of Health Psychology*, *13*, 195–204.

McKinley, S., Moser, D. K., & Dracup, K. (2000). Treatment seeking behavior for acute myocardial infarction symptoms in North America. *Heart & Lung*, *29*(4), 237–247.

McSweeney, J. C., Cody, M., & Crane, P. B. (2001). Do you know them when you see them? Women's prodromal and acute symptoms of myocardial infarction. *Journal of Cardiovascular Nursing*, *15*(3), 26–38.

McSweeney, J. C., Cody, M., O'Sullivan, P., Elberson, K., Moser, D. K., & Garvin, B. J. (2003). Women's early warning symptoms of acute myocardial infarction. *Circulation*, *108*, 2619–2623.

McSweeney, J. C., Lefler, L. L., & Crowder, B. F. (2005). What's wrong with me? Women's coronary heart disease diagnostic experiences. *Progress in Cardiovascular Nursing*, *20*(2), 48–57.

Meischke, H., Eisenberg, M., Shaeffer, S., & Henwood, D. K. (2006). The 'Heart Attack Survival Kit' project: An intervention designed to increase seniors' intentions to respond appropriately to symptoms of acute myocardial infarction. *Health Education Research*, *15*(3), 317–326.

Meischke, H., Yasui, Y., Kuniyuki, A., Bowen, D. J., Andersen, R., & Urban, N. (1999). How women label and respond to symptoms of acute myocardial infarction: Responses to hypothetical scenarios. *Heart & Lung*, *28*(4), 261–269.

Moser, D. K., Kimble, L. P., Alonzo, A., Dracup, K., Go, A. S., Kothari, R. U., & Zerwic, J. J. (2006). AHA scientific statement: Reducing delay in seeking treatment by patients with acute coronary syndrome and stroke. *Circulation*, *114*, 168–182.

Moser, D. K., McKinley, S., Dracup, K., & Chung, M. L. (2005). Gender differences in reasons patients delay in seeking treatment for acute myocardial infarction symptoms. *Patient Education and Counseling*, *56*, 45–54.

Noureddine, S., Arevian, M., Adra, M., & Puzantian, H. (2008). Response to signs and symptoms of ACS: Differences between Lebanese men and women. *American Journal of Critical Care*, *17*, 26–35.

O'Neill, E. S. (2002). Illness representations and coping of women with chronic obstructive pulmonary disease. *Heart & Lung*, *31*(4), 295–302.

Pattenden, J., Watt, I., Lewin, R. J., & Stanford, N. (2002). Decision making processes in people with symptoms of acute myocardial infarction: A qualitative study. *British Medical Journal*, *324*, 1006–1009.

Popitean, L., Barthez, O., Rioufol, G., Zeller, M., Arveux, I., Dentan, G., . . . Cottin, Y. (2005). Factors affecting the management of outcome in elderly patients with acute myocardial infarction particularly with regard to reperfusion. *Gerontology*, *51*, 109–415.

Quinn, J. R. (2005). Delay in seeking care for symptoms of acute myocardial infarction: Applying theoretical model. *Research in Nursing & Health*, *28*, 283–294.

Rasmussen, C. H., Munck, A., Kragstrup, J., & Haghfelt. (2003). Patient delay from onset of chest pain suggesting acute coronary syndrome to hospital admission. *Scandinavian Cardiovascular Journal*, *37*, 183–186.

Ruston, A., Clayton, J., & Calnan, M. (1998). Patients' action during their cardiac event: Qualitative study exploring differences and modifiable factors. *British Medical Journal*, *316*, 1060–1064.

Ryan, C. J., & Zerwic, J. J. (2003). Perceptions of symptoms of myocardial infarction related to health care seeking behaviors in older adults. *Journal of Cardiovascular Nursing*, *18*(3), 184–196.

Sjostrom-Strand, A., & Fridlund, B. (2008). Women's descriptions of symptoms and delay reasons in seeking medical care at the time of a first myocardial infarction: A qualitative study. *International Journal of Nursing Studies*, *45*, 1003–1010.

Song, L., Yan, H., Yang, J., Sun, Y., & Du, H. (2010). Impact of patients' symptom interpretation on care-seeking behaviors of patients with acute myocardial infarction. *Journal of Chinese Medicine*, *123*, 1840–1844.

Taylor, D. McD., Garewal, D., Carter, M., Bailey, M., & Aggarwal, A. (2005). Factors that impact upon the time to hospital presentation following onset of chest pain. *Emergency Medicine Australasia*, *17*, 204–211.

Thuresson, M., Jarlov, M. B., Lindahl, B., Svennson, L., Zedigh, C., & Herlitz, J. (2007). Thoughts, actions, and factors associated with pre-hospital delay in patients with acute coronary syndrome. *Heart & Lung*, *36*, 398–409.

Tullman, D. F., Haugh, K. H., Dracup, K. A., & Bourguignon, C. (2007). A randomized controlled trial to reduce delay in older adults seeking help for symptoms of acute myocardial infarction. *Research in Nursing and Health*, 30, 485–497.

Turis. S. A. (2009). Women's decision to seek treatment for symptoms of potential cardiac illness. *Journal of Nursing Scholarship*, 41, 5–12.

Walsh, J. C., Lynch, M., Murphy, A. W., & Daly, K. (2004). Factors influencing the decision to seek treatment for symptoms of acute myocardial infarction. *Journal of Psychosomatic Research*, 56, 67–73.

World Health Organization. (2008). *The Atlas of Heart Diseases and Stroke*. Retrieved from http://www.who.int/cardiovascular_diseases/en/cvd_atlas_14_deathHD.pdf

Xanthos, T., Pantazopoulos, I., Vlachos, I., Stroumpoulis, K., Barouxis, D., Kitsou, V., & Papadimitriou, L. (2010). Factors influencing arrival of patients with acute myocardial infarction at emergency departments: Implications for community nursing interventions. *Journal of Advanced Nursing*, 66(7), 1469–1477.

Xu, J., Kochanek, K. D., Murphy, S., & Tejada-Vera, B. (2007). *National vital statistics report: Final data for 2007. Centers for Disease Control*. Retrieved from http://www.cdc.gov/nchs/data/nvsr/nvsr58/nvsr58_19.pdf

Zerwic, J. J. (1998). Symptoms of acute myocardial infarction: Expectations of a community sample. *Heart & Lung*, 27(2), 75–81.

Zerwic, J. J. (1999). Patient delay in seeking treatment for acute myocardial infarction symptoms. *Journal of Cardiovascular Nursing*, 13(3), 21–32.

Zerwic, J. J., King, K. B., & Wlasowicz, G. S. (1997). Perceptions of patients with cardiovascular disease about the causes of coronary artery disease. *Heart & Lung*, 26(2), 92–98.

Zerwic, J. J., Ryan, C. J., DeVon, H. A., & Drell, M. J. (2003). Treatment seeking for acute myocardial infarction symptoms. *Nursing Research*, 52(3), 159–167.

II

Research

Chapter 11

Research with Vulnerable Populations: Implications for Developed and Developing Countries

Maria da Gloria M. Wright and Mary de Chesnay

OBJECTIVES

At the end of this chapter, the reader will be able to

1. Discuss the historical antecedents for current legislation.
2. Identify the key studies that violated human rights and led to modern protections.
3. Apply ethical principles to study vulnerable populations.

INTRODUCTION

In this chapter, we provide a historical context for modern legislation to guarantee the rights of participants in research. Early attention to the rights of humans led to focused attention on the rights of animals. While nurses do conduct research with animals, the vast majority of studies involve human participants. Previous editions of this book have focused on the research process and how to incorporate ethical principles and practices into research (de Chesnay, Murphy, Wilson, & Taualii, 2012). Here we shift to an international focus to conceptualize research ethics as an international concern and to discuss some of the issues that separate the developing world from the developed world. Some of the following studies are commonly discussed in methods classes, but others are less famous. All show a marked lack of empathy for the human subjects in the interest of science, personal glory, or public interest at the expense of individual rights.

HISTORICAL BACKGROUND FOR RESEARCH WITH VULNERABLE POPULATIONS

In the evolution of medical science through research, many unethical situations occurred that became inconvenient to the medical profession and some governments. These unethical clinical medical studies usually were performed using vulnerable populations and occurred in developed as well as developing countries. These situations forced the development of more restrictive national and international ethical code recommendations on how to conduct research with vulnerable populations.

The Syphilis Study: Experiments in the United States in Tuskegee, Alabama and in Guatemala

Study of Untreated Syphilis in Negro Males in Tuskegee, Alabama (1932–1972)

During 1932–1972, the U.S. Public Health Services (PHS), in collaboration with Tuskegee Institute (now Tuskegee University) in Macon County, Alabama, carried out a syphilis study on Negro males. The objective of the study was to record the natural history of syphilis in male blacks. Most of these black men were poor and illiterate. Although penicillin became available to treat syphilis in 1947, the participants in the study did not receive it. In July of 1972, the study was denounced to the public—the story of 40 years of nontherapeutic experiments entitled "Tuskegee Study of Untreated Syphilis in the Negro Male." After this publication, the international community reacted strongly and many actions were initiated by U.S. government agencies. An ad hoc advisory panel was organized to review the study. The panel concluded the study was "ethically unjustified" and in October of 1972 the study was officially ended. The panel found the following misconduct: (a) the scientific research protocols were either ignored or deeply flawed and did not ensure the safety and well-being of the black men involved in the study; (b) the participants in the study were never told about or offered informed consent; (c) researchers had not informed the black men of the actual name of the study; (d) the participants never knew about the debilitating and life-threatening consequences of the treatments they received, the impacts on their wives, girlfriends, and children they may have conceived once involved in the study; and (e) there were no choices given to the participants to quit the study when penicillin became available (Reverby, 2012).

Those responsible for the study published more than 13 articles in peer reviewed journals about the findings. The outcome of this situation included: (a) a class-action suit, successfully won; (b) institution of federal rules on informed consent and human subject protections; and (c) in 1997, President Bill Clinton offered a formal apology. The

"US/Tuskegee/Alabama Study" became the prime example of racism in research, misconduct in implementing research, and misconduct of government (Reverby, 2012; Tuskegee University, 2014).

The Sexual Transmissible Diseases Inoculation Studies in Guatemala (1946–1948)

During 1946–1948, the Guatemala inoculation studies were implemented by the U.S. Venereal Disease Research Laboratory (VDRL), together with the PHS, the Pan American Sanitary Bureau (today the Pan American Health Organization), with funds from the National Institutes of Health (NIH), and the support of Government of Guatemala. The objectives were: (a) to obtain information about methods of prophylaxis against syphilis, gonorrhea, and chancroid; (b) to increase understanding of the effects of penicillin in the treatment of syphilis; (c) to assist in better understanding of the question of false positive serology tests for syphilis; and (d) to enhance knowledge of the biology and immunology of syphilis in man (Reverby, 2012). Sex workers, prisoners, mental patients, children, and soldiers were the sample population for these studies. Participants were inoculated with STD agents. The researchers did not obtain informed consent. The outcomes of this situation included: (a) the records of the study were discovered in the University of Pittsburgh archives by Dr. Reverby; (b) the article she prepared regarding this study was presented to a former director of the Centers for Disease Control (CDC) and this information was passed on to the authorities of the CDC and then to the White House; (c) a federal apology was presented on October 1, 2010; (d) the worldwide media covered the story; (e) in 2011, the Presidential Commission for the Study of Bioethical Issues reported about the investigation; and (f) the Guatemalan survivors presented a lawsuit to the U.S. Federal Court, but it was not approved. In 2012, however, the survivors appealed and the CDC offered some compensation to the government of Guatemala for STD care and bioethics research. The "US/PHS STD Inoculations Studies in Guatemala" became an example of exploitation of a vulnerable population in developing countries, misconduct in implement a research study in a developing country.

The Nazi Human Experiments

During World War II, several German physicians performed painful and often deadly experiments on thousands of prisoners, mostly Jews, but also some Romani, ethnic Poles, Soviet POWs, and disable non-Jewish Germans without their consent. These experiments can be divided into three categories (Gomes, 2010; U.S. Holocaust Memorial Museum, 2013).

1. Experiments aimed at facilitating the survival of military personnel
2. Experiments aimed at developing and testing pharmaceuticals and treatment methods for injuries and illness
3. Experiments to advance the racial and ideological tenets of the Nazi worldview

After WWII, many Nazi war criminals fled to South America. It has been documented that the famous German doctor Josef Mengele, who was responsible for the experiments to advance the racial and ideological tenets of the Nazi worldview, continued his genetic experiments with twins in Brazil, in a city called Candido Godoi (Hall, 2012). The ethical implications of these experiments indicated that Nazi German ideology and practice were guided by utilitarian moral principles, and they believed they did not need to use informed consent. The researchers published the findings of the experiments in a number of postwar scientific journals.

There is a controversy regarding using the findings of the Nazi studies as evidence-based for research today (Bekier, 2010). The outcome of these situations included: (a) after WWII several international codes, rules, and declarations were established on how to conduct research on human being and protect them from harm; and (b) international courts were established to judge the persons responsible for these atrocities. These experiments demonstrated the exploitation, racism, and lack of humanitarian practice in conducting research with vulnerable populations.

The Human Radiation Experiments

During the Cold War that followed WWII, the United States prepared for a possible nuclear attack by performing several experiments on human subjects to test the effects of radiation exposure and different treatments. These experiments were performed by different U.S. agencies (Cantwell, 2001). Some of the experiments in United States included: (a) exposing people to biological and chemical weapons; (b) human radiation experiments including: radioactive iodine, uranium, plutonium, other radioactive materials, fallout research, and irradiation; and (c) surgical experiments. In general, these tests were performed on children, sick people, mine workers, mentally disabled individuals, prisoners, or other vulnerable populations (Kaye, 2001). Some of these experiments were also performed abroad in the Marshall Islands (Skoog et al., 2002), the Orinoco basin of Venezuela, and in the Amazon forest in Brazil with indigenous populations (Hume, 2001a, b).

Most of these experiments were considered unethical in that they were performed illegally—without the knowledge, consent, or informed consent of the individuals included in the experiments. Though supposedly in the public interest, the researchers violated the public trust. The outcomes of these situations included: (a) the implications for ethical, professional and legal aspects of these situations were very strong among the U.S. medical and scientific community; (b) a commitment to ethical research was reinforced; and (c) many congressional investigations and hearings were opened about the experiments. In 1994, President Bill Clinton formed the Advisory Committee on Human Radiation Experiments (ACHRE, 1995) to investigate and prepare a report regarding the use of human subjects as test subjects for experiments on ionizing radiation that use federal funds.

The Thalidomide Tragedy

Thalidomide, an immune-modulatory and anti-angiogenic drug, became available in 1956 in West Germany. It gained popularity in Europe and Canada in the late 1950s and early 1960s for the treatment of nausea in pregnant women and as a sedative. It could be purchased without prescription (Moos et al., 2003). In early 1960, it became apparent that thalidomide treatment was responsible for birth defects in thousands of children and it was banned in the United States (Kim, 2011).

However, the use of thalidomide had spread to developing countries. In South America, thalidomide is still a current teratogenic problem. In Brazil, today there are babies born with thalidomide embryopathy because of leprosy prevalence, availability of thalidomide, and deficiencies in the control of the drug in the market (Vianna et al., 2011). Thalidomide is the most infamous tetratogen in history (Greek, Shanks, & Rice, 2011). Because of findings indicating the consequences of thalidomide use in humans, the U.S. Food and Drug Administration (FDA) did not approve its use.

The thalidomide disaster has implications today. Despite its tragic history, thalidomide has found its place in the treatment of leprosy, HIV/AIDS, and cancer (Greenstone, 2001). The issues that are raised by this situation include: (a) dangerous use of pharmaceutical agents without proper analysis and adequate testing by the laboratory companies; (b) the need to establish continuing monitoring and regulation of drugs, especially those with teratogenic potential; (c) all pharmaceutical companies should be compliant and release all of the data about their drugs, including the studies with negative results; and (d) physicians should be able to reevaluate a drug in the face of significant adverse reactions. This situation reinforces the importance and role of regulatory agencies for the production, distribution, and monitoring of the sale and use of drugs in the marketplace in both developed and developing countries.

The Milgram Study

In the early 1960s, the American social psychologist, Stanley Milgram, conducted at Yale University and other places, a series of psychological studies to determine the influence of authority on people's willingness to commit acts that harm another human being. The publication of the findings of these experiments aroused several ethical and methodological critiques (Russell, 2014). According to Benjamin and Simpson (2009), the Milgram study answered the big and important question about blind obedience—about how far a person will go to inflict pain on a stranger when instructed to do so by an authority figure. Haslam and Reicher (2012) indicated that the individual's willingness to follow authorities is conditional on identification with the authority in question and an associated belief that the authority is right. Haslam, Loughnan, and Perry (2014) examined the ambiguity of the situation and apparent skepticism about the experiment set-up questions regarding blind obedience to authority. Although the findings originated by Milgram's different experiments produced answers to many issues that were never before studied in psychology, they also raised serious concerns. The outcomes of these experiments included: (a) the Milgram Shock Experiment raised questions about research ethics in studies that cause extreme emotional stress, and (b) the legacy of Milgram obedience studies produced dramatic changes in the fields of personality and social psychology. These kinds of experiments indicated that, in the implementation of ethical scientific research, there should be a balance between studies that contain higher versus lower experimental realism.

The Willowbrook Hepatitis Study

During mid 1950s to early 1970s, hepatitis studies were conducted at the Willowbrook State School in Staten Island, NY, an institution for mentally retarded children. The hepatitis study had the following goals: (a) to study the natural history of hepatitis A, and (b) to study the effectiveness of gamma globulin as a preventive measure for this disease. New children admitted to the school were infected with live viruses (Krugman & Ward, 1958; Krugman, 1986). The ethical implications of these studies were: (a) parental consent by group method, (b) use of retarded children as experimental subjects, (c) experiments built upon social deprivation, and (d) studies were not directly therapeutic to those children (Rothman, 1982). The Willowbrook hepatitis studies are good examples of stigmatization of retarded children in society and their use as subjects for experimentation in research studies.

The Jewish Chronic Diseases Study

In the early 1960s, studies were undertaken at Brooklyn's Jewish Chronic Disease Hospital with chronically mentally ill Jewish patients (Layman, 2009). The objective of these studies was to determine how a weakened immune system influenced in the spread of cancer. To evaluate this situation the researchers injected live cancer cells into the bloodstream of each participant in the studies (Howard-Jones, 2009). Ethical implications regarding these studies included: (a) patients were not informed they would receive cancer cells; (b) the physician responsible for the patients' care had not been consulted; (c) no committee reviewed the protocol prior to implementation of the studies; (d) informed consent was deceptive, inadequate, and not translated into the patients' language (Katz, 1992; Langer, 1966). These studies are another good example of discrimination and stigmatization of disabled patients in the process of doing medical research.

San Antonio Contraceptive Study

During early 1970s, an oral contraceptive study was implemented among poor Mexican American women to evaluate the efficacy of different kinds of female contraceptive pills. Half of the participants in the study received a contraceptive and the other half a placebo.

In the middle of the study the two halves were switched (Kim, 2012). Ethical implications included: (a) the women were not informed they would be receiving inactive medication, and (b) large numbers of the participants in the placebo group became pregnant during the study. This is another example of exploitation of a vulnerable population.

Tearoom Trade Study

During 1965–1968 a social researcher conducted a study of anonymous male homosexual encounters in public men's rooms. The researcher, without identifying himself as such, acted as a "watchqueen" for two men to have sexual activity. Then he wrote the license plate numbers of the men whom he had observed and traced them to their homes, where he would ask them to fill out a questionnaire, indicating that it was for a general "social health survey" (Kim, 2012). In some cases the men had not "come out of the closet" and their wives learned about their sexual orientation through the researcher's approach. The ethical implications of this study include: (a) the subjects of the study were never informed they were participating in a study about male homosexuality; (b) the subjects did not sign a consent form to participate in the study; (c) the author used their license plate numbers to track down the subjects illegally; and (d) there were violations of their privacy and deceit, both in the initial setting and in the follow-up interviews (Kim, 2012; Lenza, 2004). This situation indicated the stigma of homosexuality in the society and the violation of people's privacy.

The Havasupai Study

At the end of the 1980s and beginning of the 1990s, researchers from Arizona State University (ASU) developed a partnership with the Havasupai Tribe called the Diabetes Project with the Havasupai Tribe. The members were suffering with high rates of type 2 diabetes (American Indian and Alaska Native Genetics Resource Center [AIANGRC], 2014). This tribe was living in a remote part of the Grand Canyon area of northern Arizona. As part of the study, the tribal participants agreed to collection of blood samples, handprints, and fingerprints (Santos, 2008). After several years of study, the researchers did not find a genetic link to type 2 diabetes. However, they used the blood samples that contained DNA to proceed with other unrelated studies: schizophrenia, migration, and inbreeding (Sterling, 2011). In 2003, the Havasupai became aware that the analysis of their blood samples had been used for further studies on schizophrenia, tribeal origin, and degree of inbreeding (Lowenberg, 2010). In 2004, the Havasupai Tribe filed a lawsuit against Arizona Board of Regents and the ASU researchers for misuse of their DNA samples. The lawsuit included the following complaints: lack of informed consent, violation of civil rights through mishandling of blood samples, unapproved use of the data, and violation of medical confidentiality (AIANGRC, 2014). In 2010, a settlement between Arizona Board of Regents and the Havasupai Tribe was reached, in which

41 tribal members received $700,000 for compensation, funds for a clinic and school, and return of the DNA samples (Mello & Wolf, 2010). This is another example of ethical misconduct and exploitation of a vulnerable population.

Ethics Foundations

The above summary indicates that these studies, conducted with vulnerable populations, violated ethical protocols in their implementation and reinforces the urgent need to establish rigorous standards to conduct research with human subjects. In the following section, we present the development of ethics research codes—principles on how to conduct ethical research with human subject.

CODES AND PRINCIPLES

The Nuremberg Code

The Nuremberg Code was created in 1947, after the Nazi doctors trial in Nuremberg, Germany. A close look at the code indicated it was based on the *Guidelines for Human Experimentation 1931* (Ghooi, 2011). The Nuremberg Code is considered the blueprint for today's principles of the rights of subjects participating in medical research (Shuster, 1997). The code is composed of 10 principles. The highlights of the code are:

- Voluntary and informed consent
- Experiments scientifically necessary and conducted by qualified personnel
- Benefits outweigh risks
- Subjects must have the ability to withdraw from the research (Layman, 2009; Kim, 2012).

It is the first internationally recognized code of research ethics.

Amendments to the Federal Food, Drug, and Cosmetic Act

As a consequence of the thalidomide tragedy, the Kefauver-Harris Amendment was passed in the U.S. Congress in 1962 to ensure efficacy and drug safety before distribution to consumers (Food and Drug Administration [FDA], 2014). This law revolutionized the drug development industry by empowering the FDA to require the drug industry to conduct extensive animal pharmacological and toxicological tests before a drug can be tested in humans. The new law also required the drug industry present proof of effectiveness of the new drugs (Benjamin, 2002). Following these initiatives, more rules were created regarding ethics and research such as: National Research Act (1974); Common Rule (1991); International Conference on Harmonisation (1996); Presidential Commission for the Study of Bioethical Issues (1979); Council for International Organizations of Medical Sciences (CIOMS) guidelines; National Bioethics Advisory Commission (NBAC); other professional codes of ethics: e.g., Hippocratic oath; government agency codes of ethics for: NIH, NSF, FDA, EPA, USDA; and private organization codes of ethics: e.g., Public Responsibility in Medicine and Research (PRIM&R), American Psychological Association (APA); Association of Clinical Research Professionals (ACRP), International Committee of Medical Journal Editors, American Chemical Society, American Society for Clinical Laboratory Science, American Anthropological Association, American Association of University Professors, and Nuffield Council on Bioethics (Hart, 2012; Ketupanya, 2009).

Declaration of Helsinki

The World Medical Association (WMA) in 1964 developed the Declaration of Helsinki, in Finland which received several amendments over the years. It is a Code of Ethics on Human Experimentation for the medical community (Abraham, Grace, Parambi, & Pahuja, 2008). The Declaration gives central emphasis on informed consent as a requirement for ethical research and standard of care. It also mentions ethical review, risk/benefit aspects, research with vulnerable groups, and other issues regarding the protection of autonomy, rights and welfare of subjects (WMA, 2001; Tyebkhan, 2003). The Declaration of Helsinki has helped the development of similar codes around the world.

Belmont Report

In 1974 the U.S. Congress passed the National Research Act creating the National Commission for the Protection of Human Subjects of Biomedical and Behavior Research. The primary responsibility of the National Commission was to identify the ethical principles that would guide all research involving human subjects. To carry out these responsibilities, the commission considered: (a) the boundaries between biomedical and behavior research and the distinction between medical practice (treatment) and research, (b) the role of assessment of risk-benefit criteria in determining the appropriateness of research involving human subjects, c) appropriate guidelines for the selection of human subjects to participate in the studies, d) the nature and definition of informed consent in different settings of research implementation (Department of Health and Human Services [HHS], 1979). *The Belmont Report* was published in 1979 with the key provisions: (a) *respect for persons*: individual autonomy and protection of individuals with reduced autonomy; (b) *beneficence*: maximize benefits and minimize harms; and (c) *justice*: equitable distribution of research costs and benefits. This report was important for the development of the bioethics field of study and practice in the United States and abroad and is an essential reference for institutional review boards (IRBs; Kim, 2012).

CROSS-CUTTING ISSUES IN INTERNATIONAL RESEARCH WITH VULNERABLE POPULATIONS

The globalization process has facilitated moving an increased number of clinical trials conducted by the pharmaceutical industry, academics, and private research centers from the developed world to developing countries using vulnerable populations for their trials (Glickman et al., 2009). This situation has brought financial benefits for those who are responsible for the clinical trials and other types of research, but not necessarily to the specific vulnerable populations in those countries (Clark, 2002; Lo & Bayer, 2003; Varnus & Satcher, 1997).

Conducting international research between developed and developing countries provides challenges for the ethical review process and for the protection of human subjects. Review of past research with unethical issues and research conducted with vulnerable populations in developed countries has prevented new abuses, but abuses continue to be perpetrated in developing countries that do not have the infrastructure to protect their citizens from unethical researchers (McIntosh et al., 2008; Mabunda, 2001).

According to Muwonge and Sembajwe (2013), the distribution of the research burdens in the developing world such as, sub-Saharan Africa, Southeast Asia, Latin America, and Eastern Europe have increased drastically. The vulnerable population participants in the different studies have been exploited due to poverty, illiteracy, limited resources, education, and access to health care, resulting in uneven distribution of risks. The framework used to conduct collaborative international research is generally based on U.S. government regulations, and it is operationalized in the form of institutional review boards and the use of informed consent documents (London, 2002; Schwenzer, 2008; Bhat & Hegde, 2006).

Informed consent is the cornerstone of all research with human subjects, and it is based on the fundamental ethical principles of respect for persons and for human dignity (Wolitz, Emmanuel, & Shah, 2009). However, obtaining an informed consent signed by members of a vulnerable population in developing countries has many challenges. According to Buchanan (2008), Bhat and Hegde (2006), and Mystakidou et al. (2009), some of the challenges are: (a) cultural barriers; (b) language difficulties or inadequate information; (c) absence of local institutional review boards; (d) how to develop a definition of "informed" and criteria for assessing its attainment; (e) cultural aspects of the individual decision-making processes used in the studies; (f) how individual priority, autonomy, and privacy are considered over moral considerations; (g) how to make understandable and show the utility of individual informed consent; and (h) how to demonstrate the purpose of informed consent requirements.

If international, collaborative research continues to exist, researchers from developed countries must apply ethical principles in each of the research studies they conduct abroad. The European Commission (2009) prepared some considerations about ethics in research and international cooperation: (a) the studies need to address and answer the needs of the country where the research is carried out, which involves adding value to the health and welfare of the participants, their community, and/or their country; (b) the studies should follow the basic principles of scientific merit as well as adherence to ethical principles; and (c) the studies must adhere to relevant European Union, national legislation, and international guidelines.

These same ethical considerations should be applied when universities send health professions students abroad. In many cases, the students are not equipped to work in the developing countries. Sometimes, researchers use graduate students to collect data and in these situations, the distribution of benefits can be considered exploitation of the students as well as the subjects (Bhat, 2008).

The big challenge for the researchers is to establish procedures that are both ethically sound and culturally sensitive (Dowdy, 2006). It is critical to develop partnerships and collaborations with local counterparts to guarantee the share of power, interest, knowledge, and leadership for the success of the study and the benefit for all of the parties involved (Wright, 2000).

CONCLUSION

In this chapter, we reviewed key studies in the historical evolution of research ethics. It is clear that the developed world has made great strides in providing protocols for the protection of human subjects, but these same protections need to apply to research conducted abroad regardless of whether or not the local communities have their own rules and regulations. While the challenges of conducting cross-cultural research are many, the common denominator must be respect for the rights of participants.

REFERENCES

Abraham, S., Grace, D., Parambi, T., & Pahuja, S. (2008). Milestones in development of good clinical practice. Retrieved from http://ispub.com/ISH/9/1/11621

Advisory Committee on Human Radiation Experiments (ACHRE). (1995). Executive summary of final report. Retrieved from http://biotech.law.Isu.edu/research/reports/ACHRE/summary.html

American Indian and Alaska Native Genetics Resource Center. (2014). Havasupai Tribe and the lawsuit aftermath. Retrieved from http://genetics.ncai.org/case-study/havasupai-Tribe.cfm

Bekier, M. (2010). The ethical considerations of medical experimentation on human subjects. [Chapter 7: Human Experimentation, Section 4, readings.]. Retrieved from http://www.qcc.cuny .edu/socialscincies/ppcorino/MEDICAL_ETHICS_TEXT/Chapter_7_Human_Experimentation/ Reading-Nazi-experimentation.htm

Benjamin, D. (2002). Drug development and testing. Retrieved from http://www.doctorbenjmin .com/drugdev/drugdev/html

Benjamin, J. A., & Simpson, J. A. (2009). The power of the situation: The impact of Milgram's obedience studies on personality and social psychology. *American Psychology Association, 64*(1), 12–19.

Bhat, S. B. (2008). Ethical coherence when medical students work abroad. *Lancet, 372,* 1133–1134.

Bhat, S. B., & Hegde, T. T. (2006). Ethical international research on human subjects research in the absence of local Institutional Review Boards. *Journal of Medical Ethics, 32,* 535–536.

Buchanan, D. (2008). Assuring adequate protections in international health research: A principled justification and practical recommendation for the role of community oversight. *UMass Institute for Global Health Faculty Publications* (Paper 2). Retrieved from http://scholar works.umass .edu/umigh_faculty_pubs/2

Cantwell, A. (2001). The human radiation experiments: How scientists secretly used US citizens as guinea pigs during the Cold War. Retrieved from http://www.whale.to/cantwell9.html

Clark, P. A. (2002). AIDS research in developing countries: Do the ends justify the means? *Medical Science Monitor, 8*(9), ED5–ED16.

De Chesnay, M., Murphy, P., Wilson, L., & Taualii, M. (2012). Research with vulnerable populations. In M. de Chesnay & B. Anderson (Eds.), *Caring for the vulnerable* (pp. 185–201). Sudbury, MA: Jones and Bartlett.

Department of Health and Human Services. (1979). Ethical principles and guidelines for the protection of human subjects of research: The National Commission for the Protection of Human Subjects of Biomedical and Behavioral Research. Retrieved from http://www.hhs.gov/ohrp/ humansubjects/guidance/Belmont.html

Dowdy, D. W. (2006). Partnership as an ethical model for research in developing countries: The example of the "implementation trial." *Journal of Medical Ethics, 32*(6), 357–360.

European Commission. (2009). Ethics in research and international cooperation. *Research Directorate–General–Unit L3–Governance and Ethics.* Belgium. Retrieved from ftp://ftp.cordis .europa.eu/pub/fp7/docs/developing-countries_en.pdf

Food and Drug Administration. (2014). Consumer information. Retrieved from www.fda.gov/ consumer/.../ucm322856.htm

Greek, R., Shanks, N., & Rice, M. J. (2011). The history and implications of testing thalidomide on animals. *The Journal of Philosophy, Science, & Law, 11,* 1–19.

Greenstone, G. (2011). The revival of thalidomide: From tragedy to therapy. *BC Medical Journal, 53*(5), 230–233.

Ghooi, R. B. (2011). Nuremberg Code: A critic. *Perspective in Clinical Research, 2*(2), 72–76.

Glickman, S. W., McHutchison, J. G., Peterson, E. D., Cairns, C. B., Harrington, R. A., Califf, R. M., & Schulman, K. A. (2009). Ethical and scientific implications of the globalization of clinical research. *The New England Journal of Medicine, 360*(8), 816–823.

Gomes, T. (2010). Nazi experiments. *Hohonu, 8,* 13–16.

Hall, A. (2012). Secret files reveal 9,000 Nazi war criminals fled to South America after WWII. *Nexus Community Forum.* Retrieved from http://nexusnow.info/forum/archive/indexphp/t-10968.html

Hart, O. (2012). Ethics review: Ethical considerations of the past and present. University of South Florida Research & Innovation Conference. [Paper presented.] Retrieved from www.Research .usf.edu/...ethical-considerations – of-the

Haslam, N., Loughnan, S., & Perry, G. (2014). Meta-Milgram: An empirical synthesis of the obedience experiments. *Public Library of Science—ONE, 9*(4), 1–9.

Haslam, A., & Reicher, S. D. (2012). Contesting the "nature" of conformity: What Milgram and Zimbardo's studies really show. *Public Library of Science—Biology*, 10(11), 1–7.

Howard-Jones, N. (1982). Human experimentation in historical and ethical perspectives. *Social Science and Medicine*. 16(5), 1429–1448.

Hume, D. W. (2001). Darkness in El Dorado. [archived document]. Anthropological niche of Douglas W. Hume. Retrieved from http://anthroniche.com/darkness_documents/052.htm; http://www.thebulletin.org/issues/2001/jf01/jf01sea.html

Katz, J. (1992). Abuse of human beings for the sake of science. In A. L. Caplan (Ed.), *When medicine went mad: Bioethics and the Holocaust* (pp. 233–270). Totowa, NJ: Humana Press.

Kaye, J. (2001). Documentary on early US radiation experiments on black children. Retrieved from http://my.firedoglake.com/valtin/2011/05/25/documentary-on-erly-u-s-radiation-experiments-onbalck-children-video-trailes/.firedoglake

Ketupanya, A. (2009). History of research ethics: Origin of international guidelines. Retrieved from www.tm.mahidol.ac.th/jitmm.../JITMM - 3-12-2009 - C41 – Ketupanya.pdf

Kim, J. H. (2011). Thalidomide: The tragedy of birth defects and the effective treatment of disease. *Toxicological Sciences*, 122(1), 1–6.

Kim, W. O. (2012). Institutional Review Board (IRB) and ethical issues in clinical research. *Korean Journal of Anesthesiology*, 62(1), 3–12.

Krugman, S. (1986). The Willowbrook hepatitis studies revisited: Ethical aspects. *Reviews of Infectious Diseases*, 8(1), 157–162.

Krugman, S., & Ward, R. (1958). Clinical and experimental studies on infectious hepatitis. *Pediatrics*, 22, 1016.

Langer, E. (1966). Human experimentation: New York verdict affirms patient's right. *Science* 151(3711), 663–666.

Layman, E. J. (2009). Human experimentation: Historical perspective of breaches of ethics in US health care. *The Health Care Management*, 28(4), 354–374.

Lenza, M. (2004). Controversies surrounding Laud Humphreys' tearoom trade: An unsettling. *Sociology and Social Policy*, 24(3/4/5), 20–31.

Lo, B., & Bayer, R. (2003). Establishing ethical trials for treatment and prevention of AIDS in developing countries. *British Medical Journal*, 2003(327), 337–339.

London, L. (2002). Ethical oversight of public health research: Can rules and IRBs make a difference in developing countries? *American Journal of Public Health*, 92(7), 1079–1084.

Lowenberg, L. (2010). The Havasupai case and how to make consent forms better. *The Center for Law and Biosciences*, 23(1), 1–3.

Mabunda, G. (2001). Ethical issues in HIV research in poor countries. *Journal of Nursing Scholarship*, 33(2), 111–114.

Mello, M. M., & Wolf, L. E. (2010). The Havasupai Indian Tribe case: Lessons for research involving stored biologic samples. *The New England Journal of Medicine*, 363(3), 204–207.

McIntosh, S., Sierra, E., Dozier, A., Diaz, S., Quinones, Z., Primack, A., Chadwick, G., & Ossip-Klein, D. (2008). Ethical review issues in collaborative research between US and low-middle income country partners: A case example. *Bioethics*, 22(8), 414–422.

Moos, R., Stolz, R., Cerny, T., & Gillessen, S. (2003). Thalidomide: From tragedy to promise. *Swiss Medical Weekly*, 133, 77–87.

Muwonge, H., & Sembajwe, L. F. (2013). Incentive use in research: Protecting vulnerable populations from exploitation. *Archives Medical Review Journal, 22*(3), 408–417.

Mystakidou, K. et al (2009). Ethical and practical challenges in implementing informed consent: HIV/AIDS clinical trials in developing or resource-limited countries. *Journal of Social Aspects of HIV/AIDS, 6*(2), 46–57.

Reverby, S. M. (2012). Ethical failures and history lessons: The U.S. Public Health Service Research Studies in Tuskegee and Guatemala. *Public Health Reviews, 34*(1), 1–18.

Rothman, D. (1982). Were Tuskegee and Willowbrook Studies in nature? *Hasting Center Report, 12*(2), 5–7.

Russell, N. (2014). Stanley Milgram's obedience to authority "relationship" condition: Some methodological and theoretical implications. *Social Science, 3*, 194–214.

Santos, L. (2008). Genetic research in native communities. *Progress in Community Health Partnerships, 2*(4), 321–327.

Schwenzer, K. J. (2008). Protecting vulnerable subjects in clinical research: Children, pregnant women, prisoners, and employees. *Respiratory Care, 53*(10), 1342–1349.

Shuster, E. (1997). Fifty years later: The significance of the Nuremberg Code. *The New England Journal of Medicine, 337*(20), 1436–1440.

Skoog, K., Clestial, R., Satris, S., Spennermann, D., Underwood, R., & Wyttenbach-Santo, R. (2002). U.S. nuclear testing on the Marshall Islands 1946–1958: Teaching ethics. *The Journal of the Society for Ethics across the Curriculum, 3*(2), Retrieved from Ethics.iit.edu/eelibrary/node/8503

Sterling, R. L. (2011). Genetic Research among the Havasupai: A cautionary tale. *American Medical Association Journal of Ethics–Virtual Mentor, 13*(2), 113–117. Retrieved from http://virtualmentor.ama.assn.org/2011/02/hlaw1-1102.html

Tuskegee University. (2014). *Centers of excellence.* Retrieved from http://www.tuskegee.edu/about_us/centers_of_excellence/bioethics_center/about the_usphs_syphilis_study.aspx

Tyebkhan, G. (2003). Declaration of Helsinki: The ethical cornerstone of Humana clinical research. *Indian Journal of Dermatology, Venereology and Leprology, 69*(3), 245–247.

Wright, M. G. M. (2000). A critical-holistic paradigm for an interdependent world. *American Behavioral Scientist, 43*(5), 808–823.

Wolitz, R., Emmanuel, E., & Shah, S. (2009). Rethinking the responsiveness requirement for international research. *Lancet, 374*, 847–849.

World Medical Association. (2001). Declaration of Helsinki. *Bulletin of the World Health Organization, 79*(4), 373–374.

Varnus, H., & Satcher, D. (1997). Ethical complexities of conducting research in developing countries. *The New England Journal of Medicine, 337*, 1003–1005.

Vianna, F.S.L., Lopez-Camelo, J., Leite, J., Sanseverino, M., Dutra, M., Castilla, E., & Schuler-Faccini, L. (2011). Epidemiological surveillance of birth defects compatible embryopathy in Brazil. *Public Library of Science—ONE, 6*(7), e21735.

United States Holocaust Memorial Museum (2013). Nazi medical experiments. Retrieved from http://www.ushmm.org/wlc/en/article.php?ModuleId=10005168

Chapter 12

Sample Qualitative Research Proposal: A Study to Develop a Disclosure to Children Intervention for HIV/AIDS-Infected Women

Tommie Nelms

OBJECTIVES

At the end of this chapter, the reader will be able to

1. How to use the literature to build a compelling case for the need for a research study.
2. How qualitative methodology can be used to frame a research study.
3. How to design a qualitative study from beginning to end.

Author's note: The following is an actual research proposal that was developed and carried out. The literature upon which it was based is not current.

ABSTRACT

Disclosing their diagnosis of HIV/AIDS to their children is one of the most difficult issues for women. Literature supports the notion that interventions are needed to support women in the distressing task of disclosing their HIV diagnosis to their children and to give them directions for how to do it (Black & Miles, 2002). The purpose of this study is to develop an intervention to help and support women in disclosing an HIV/AIDS diagnosis to their children. Phenomenological methodology will guide data gathering from several sources: (1) HIV/AIDS-infected women who have disclosed to children will be interviewed about their experiences, (2) HIV/AIDS nurses and counselors will be interviewed about their experiences of working with women who have disclosed their diagnoses to children, (3) literature will be gathered regarding best practices for disclosure of such information to children, and (4) an expert in the psychology of mothering will be consulted periodically. Data sets will be qualitatively analyzed separately, then together to create the written intervention. Directions for disclosure of their diagnosis would release women from the burden of keeping a secret from their children and allow them more time to educate, process with, and comfort children while their health is still good.

PURPOSE OF THE STUDY

Literature related to mothers' experiences of having HIV/AIDS reveals that disclosure of their diagnosis to their children is one of the most difficult issues women face (Andrews Williams, & Neil, 1993; Faithfull, 1997; Lather & Smithies, 1997; Mellins & Ehrhardt, 1994; Moneyham et al., 1996; Niebuhr, Hughes, & Polland, 1994; Pilowsky, Sohler, & Susser, 1999; Semple et al., 1993). Consequently, most women don't disclose their diagnosis unless or until it becomes absolutely necessary. Findings from ongoing research with HIV-infected mothers of dependent children by this researcher confirm this finding. Failure to disclose to children results in a number of consequences for the mother and her children. Living with a diagnosis of HIV/AIDS is a profound experience for women and the amount of work and energy required to hide the diagnosis from children is a burden that negatively impacts a woman's health and well-being, things she must work hard to safeguard with a diagnosis of HIV/AIDS. Hiding the diagnosis from children also leaves the children open to feelings of betrayal, anger, and uncertainty when they do learn the diagnosis. Current literature supports the notion that interventions are needed to support women with the distressing task of disclosing their HIV diagnosis to their children and to give them directions for how to do it (Black & Miles, 2002). The purpose of this study is to develop an intervention to help and support women in disclosing a diagnosis of HIV/AIDS to their children. Background information will be sought from a number of sources relevant to the development of such an intervention. First, HIV/AIDS-infected women who have disclosed to their children will be interviewed about their experiences of disclosure. Second, HIV/AIDS counselors, case managers, and nurses will be consulted about their experiences of working with women who have chosen to disclose to children, as well as those who have not. Recommendations for best practices in this area will also be sought from these individuals. Third, literature will be gathered regarding knowledge and best practices regarding the disclosure of difficult information to others, especially children. And finally, an expert in the psychology of mothering will be consulted about knowledge upon which to build such an intervention. Disclosing a diagnosis of HIV/AIDS to one's children, while a difficult task, has the potential to strengthen maternal–child communication and relational patterns that would support both mothers and their children should the mother become ill and die.

SIGNIFICANCE

While advances in drug treatment are changing the course of HIV/AIDS for many individuals, AIDS remains the leading cause of death among women between ages of 25 and 44, and the incidence of HIV in women is increasing at a rate four times that of men in the United States. The ages of 16 to 44, the prime childbearing and child rearing ages for women, are also the ages when the largest numbers of women are diagnosed with HIV/AIDS (Centers for Disease Control [CDC], 2001). Many HIV-infected women with dependent children are living and mothering day-to-day with HIV/AIDS and must consider the possibility that end-of-life preparations need to be made for the time when their disease progresses and death becomes a reality. Of the 4 million babies born in the United States each year, 70,000 have HIV-positive mothers (CDC, 1996). It is impossible to count the numbers of children whose mothers become HIV positive while their children are growing up (Lather & Smithies, 1997). It was estimated that by the end of the 20th century, 80,000 children and adolescents in the United States would be orphaned by parental death caused by HIV (American Academy of Pediatrics, 1999).

While mothers with other diseases such as breast and ovarian cancer must also contemplate end-of-life and leaving dependent children, the stigma associated with HIV/AIDS causes HIV-infected mothers to face issues that are unique, and one of these issues is disclosure of the diagnosis to their children. Little nursing research addresses end-of-life issues faced by dying or terminally ill parents of dependent children and no nursing research addresses how mothers prepare themselves and their children for their own deaths. Nor is there literature about how mothers disclose their diagnoses of a life-threatening illness, like HIV/AIDS, to their children, although experts in both mothering and HIV/AIDS care advocate this practice early in a woman's diagnosis. Literature does reveal, however, that HIV-infected mothers struggle with whether or not to disclose their HIV status to their children. Disclosure to children was a major concern to participants in a study by Moneyham et al. (1996). Although women believed children should be told, many had not disclosed because of the negative effect it would have on children, along with the fear children would not keep the information confidential. By not disclosing, however, participants feared children would find out their HIV status by other means. In interviews with predominately white, well-educated HIV-positive women (68% mothers), Semple et al. (1993) found that disclosure to children was the most stressful aspect of their diagnoses. Disclosure to young children was associated with developmentally regressive behavior, acting out, and fear and anxiety about family stability and loss of the parent, as well as unwanted disclosure to neighbors, friends, and acquaintances, consequences also noted by other researchers (Mellins & Ehrhardt, 1994; Niebuhr et al., 1994). Positive HIV status disclosed to adolescents was linked to negative reactions like anger, hostility, disrespect, and runaway behaviors.

Andrews et al. (1993) found mothers were bound to children in secrecy and struggled with whether to disclose their diagnosis to young children. Most decided not to disclose, saying young children couldn't understand or deal with the anxiety of knowing their mother may die within a few years. If children were HIV positive, mothers feared how they would be treated. Where both mother and child(ren) were HIV positive there was a double burden of secrecy. Mothers had to reassure children and themselves about their health when both were vulnerable to decline. Mothers were concerned about the time when their physical condition would make it impossible not to disclose they had a terminal illness and whether it would be preferable to discontinue contact with children before their condition got too bad for children to bear.

Faithfull (1997) found that disclosure to children varied according to the developmental needs of the child, the state of health of the mother, and the differing abilities of the women to tolerate the painful feelings involved. Some women waited for the children to take the lead with disclosure. Sowell and Misener (1997) found family members to whom women disclosed their conditions most often were their mother and a child who lived with them. They concluded that a number of minor children were providing support to HIV-infected mothers. Lather & Smithies (1997) advocate getting honest with children who are old enough to understand. And according to Pilowsky et al. (1999) parental disclosure to children facilitates planning for guardianship of children and is essential if children are to be included in the planning.

It should be noted that some of the literature presented here is at least 10 years old and during that time period the outlook for those diagnosed with HIV/AIDS has drastically improved. In an ongoing qualitative study by this researcher with 16 HIV-infected mothers of dependent children about their mothering and end-of-life issues, several reasonably healthy women who had been infected with the virus for 18 to 20 years were interviewed. Although most of the women interviewed were reasonably healthy; others, diagnosed for 8 to 10 years, were in poor health and had experienced several critical AIDS-related illnesses. While increasingly characterized as a chronic disease to be managed, much like diabetes, HIV/AIDS is still a life-threatening, highly stigmatized, potentially fatal disease.

Findings from the researcher's study also revealed that disclosure to children was a major issue for the women, and the majority had not done so. While all women were distressed and burdened by the diagnosis of HIV/AIDS, those who were hiding their diagnosis from children were further burdened by trying to keep a secret from their children and from feelings they were lying to their children by not being honest. The few women who had disclosed their diagnosis to their children expressed relief at not having to keep the secret from their children and reported strengthened mother–child bonds and support from their children. Women who had not revealed to children expressed fear about children's reactions and said they wanted their children to have happy childhoods. They did not want to "burden" their children with knowing their mother had a life-threatening illness.

A few women wanted to tell their children, but didn't know the best way to do it and others were planning to tell their children at some point in the future if the women remained healthy (Nelms, 2004). Because disclosure was not the focus of the study, those who had disclosed were not asked specifically about that experience. While it seems reasonable that children might have reactions to disclosure such as acting out or running away, as was found in some studies, an HIV/AIDS counselor consulted by the researcher said she had never had a client experience such a reaction by her children in her 13 years of encouraging mothers to disclose to children early in their diagnosis.

One factor that has changed little in the more than 20 years of HIV/AIDS is the stigma. Stigma is still a pervasive part of the HIV/AIDS experience and one that continues to impact women's decisions about disclosure to children and others. In a study of 48 HIV-infected African American mothers of young children, Black and Miles (2002) found that stigma was still very much a part of mothers' disclosure decisions. Disclosure to children was said to be distressing and women had few directions about how to do it. They also noted that nurses had an important role in supporting women in disclosure decisions. While the literature supports the notion that disclosure to children is a major and distressing issue for HIV/AIDS-infected women, there are no directions for how women should to do it, nor are there directions for how nurses and other HIV/AIDS care workers educate and support women through the process. The proposed study would fill that gap in the literature by giving nurses and other HIV/AIDS care workers an intervention to use when facilitating the disclosure of a diagnosis of HIV/AIDS to one's children.

Women report being burdened by a diagnosis of HIV/AIDS and their efforts to keep their diagnosis a secret from their children. Hiding the diagnosis forces women to lie to their children about medicines, doctor visits, and illnesses and most report that lying to their children is something they dislike doing. Working to keep a secret from children can also cause women to withdraw from their children, thereby setting up the possibility of poor communication and relational patterns, which are detrimental to both women and their children. Disclosure of their diagnosis to children would release women from the burden of keeping a secret from their children, giving them more energy to devote to their health and well-being, and that of their children. Disclosure to children would also afford women the support and understanding from those who love them the most, their children. Disclosure early in the diagnosis would allow women and children an extended period of adjustment when women are reasonably healthy and prevent them from having to disclose to children when they are sick or prevent children from having to find out about their mother's diagnosis from others, when they are more likely to feel betrayed, angry and uncertain. Disclosure to children when women are healthy would allow them more time to educate, process with, and comfort children while energy levels are still high and there is time to strengthen bonds and build good memories for what HIV-infected women characterize as an uncertain future (Nelms, 2004).

Women also report the isolating and burdensome nature of mothering with HIV/AIDS and their lack of resources for support and relief in this area. Partnering with nurses and HIV/AIDS care workers in disclosing their diagnosis to their children could diminish women's senses of isolation and burden and give them a sense that others recognize and support them in their struggles. Stigma is still a pervasive part of the HIV/AIDS experience and women further perpetuate that stigma by failing to disclose the diagnosis to their children. An intervention for disclosure to children would give women, along with HIV/AIDS care nurses and counselors, an opportunity to partner to decrease the stigma associated with a diagnosis of HIV/AIDS.

While HIV/AIDS care nurses and other healthcare professionals and counselors encourage HIV-infected women to disclose to their children early in the diagnosis, there are no directions for how to go about this distressing task. The development of an intervention would give this group a concrete process to share with women, in addition to their encouragement. A disclosure intervention could also be used by HIV/AIDS-infected women, as well as men, when disclosing the diagnosis to other family members, friends, and associates.

Given the human tendency to deny death, along with cultural fears about death and dying, it is not surprising that little nursing research addresses end-of-life issues faced by dying or terminally ill parents of dependent children or how mothers prepare themselves and their children for their own deaths. Clearly one of the first actions in such preparations would have to be disclosure of the life-threatening condition to children. Development of an intervention for the disclosure of a life-threatening disease like HIV/AIDS to children and the presentation of that process could lead to both methodological and theoretical knowledge about how to develop other, similar interventions for mothers and parents faced with disclosing distressing, traumatic information to children of all ages.

SPECIFIC AIMS

This research will gather data from various sources in order to develop an intervention to give HIV-infected women knowledge, directions, and support related to disclosing their HIV/AIDS diagnosis to their children. It is anticipated that the intervention will be in a written format that could be read and discussed with, then given to HIV-infected women early in their diagnosis of HIV to acquaint them with the best knowledge and practices regarding how to disclose their diagnosis to their children. The materials will have information related to the burdens of not revealing to children for themselves and their children, the benefits of revealing to children for themselves and their children, the earliest age(s) at which to disclose to children, along with the best strategies for disclosure. There will also be information about what reactions women might expect from children given their developmental stages, along with ways of dealing with the reactions in developmentally appropriate ways. There will also be information about how to support children during AIDS-related illnesses the mother may experience. It is also anticipated that the materials will give directions for women to work in partnership with HIV/AIDS care nurses, counselors, or other healthcare providers for support throughout the disclosure process and beyond.

RATIONALE

The rationale guiding the development of the intervention is that disclosure of the diagnosis to children is a good thing for HIV/AIDS-infected women and their children, and with knowledge, direction, and support many women will disclose the diagnosis to their children early in their diagnosis. The literature clearly verifies the notion that issues of disclosure are important to HIV-infected women with children and actions to hide the diagnosis burden women in many ways. Many women recognize that they should tell their children, but are unsure how to go about the disclosure process and are fearful of the reactions they might receive from their children. HIV/AIDS care nurses, case managers, and counselors advocate women's disclosure to children early in their diagnosis, but lack clear direction for how women should go about disclosure. A combination of the experiences of women who have disclosed their HIV/AIDS diagnosis to their children, the knowledge and experience of HIV/AIDS care nurses, case managers, and counselors, the knowledge of an expert in the psychology of mothering, and the best knowledge and practices regarding disclosure of difficult information found in the literature should provide a comprehensive foundation for the development of a sound disclosure intervention.

LITERATURE REVIEW

(see *Background in Significance* section)

Author's note: Some formats use a separate section for literature review prior to the study. In this proposal it is assumed that the primary literature review will be performed when the concepts emerge from the data.

METHODS

The methodological approach that undergirds this study is phenomenology. This type of research lends itself to questions concerned with understanding everyday human experiences. The focus of research in this paradigm is everyday lived experience, which can only be obtained from those who live the experience (Heidegger, 1927/1962; Benner & Wrubel, 1989). Through phenomenologic inquiry, insights and understandings of shared human experiences can be developed. And from these insights and understandings, comprehensive overviews of phenomena can be framed, from which nursing interventions and strategies can be developed for implementation and evaluation. This study will take the phenomenologic research process through to the intervention development stage. A comprehensive overview of the phenomenon of HIV/AIDS-infected women's experiences of disclosure of their diagnosis to their dependent children will be explicated and from that, an intervention for disclosure of HIV status to children will be developed. Two groups who live this experience, one directly and the other indirectly, will be interviewed in-depth about their experiences of the phenomenon. HIV-infected women who have disclosed their diagnosis to their children will be interviewed about their experiences, and HIV/AIDS care nurses, case managers, and counselors will be interviewed about their experiences of working with and encouraging women to disclose to their children. The knowledge and understandings gained from these two groups will be combined with information gathered from literature on disclosure of distressful information, along with input gathered from an expert in the psychology of mothering to develop the HIV disclosure intervention.

There are two target populations in this study. The first is HIV/AIDS-infected women who have disclosed their diagnosis to their dependent children and the second is HIV/AIDS care nurses, case managers, and counselors. Participants for the study will be drawn from HIV/AIDS-infected women served by an AIDS Service Organization (ASO) in a south central state and HIV/AIDS care workers employed by ASO and XXX House, an agency serving HIV/AIDS-affected families in the same area.

HIV/AIDS-infected women served by the ASO are white, African American, African, and Hispanic women with an average of three dependent children. Approximately half are single and half are married/partnered. The majority of the women are middle to low socioeconomic status. Many work to support themselves and their children, in addition to receiving benefits for which they qualify through the ASO and other government agencies. In some cases, health status prevents the women from working.

The researcher has been conducting research with HIV/AIDS-infected women served by the ASO for 3 years and volunteers weekly in the agency's well-being clinic. A counselor at the ASO has indicated that there are as many as 16 women served by the agency that have disclosed their HIV status to their dependent children. (Most HIV-infected women served by the agency have not disclosed, but are encouraged to do so.) The counselor has invited the researcher to attend a monthly women's support group, led by her, to recruit women who are willing to be interviewed about their experience of disclosure to children. It is anticipated eight to ten HIV-infected women will be interviewed. According to Lincoln and Guba (1985), this number of participants is generally adequate to illuminate a phenomenon.

There is one LVN, one master's prepared nurse practitioner, one counselor, and two medical case managers at the ASO. Each of these individuals will be asked to participate in an interview with the researcher about their experiences of working with women regarding their issues of disclosure to dependent children. These individuals will be asked for experiential knowledge they believe would contribute to a disclosure intervention for women. HIV/AIDS care nurses and counselors from XXX House will also be contacted by the researcher and asked to participate in an interview about their experiences of disclosure with HIV-infected women. While very few clients at ASNT have HIV/AIDS-infected children, all families served by XXX House have HIV/AIDS-infected mothers and/or fathers and children. This difference should add a broader range of HIV/AIDS care worker knowledge and experience to the phenomenon. It is anticipated 8 to 10 HIV/AIDS care workers (nurses, case managers, and counselors) will be interviewed.

Instruments

In-depth, open-ended interviews will be conducted with HIV-infected women and HIV/AIDS healthcare workers. The focus of interviews with infected women will be their experiences of disclosing their HIV diagnosis to their children. Women will be asked about how they came to disclose, who may have been instrumental in their decision, strategies they used, their children's reactions, the impact of disclosure on their relationship with their children, their health, and they and their children's day-to-day lives. Women will be asked to share any other aspects of the experience of disclosure they believe relevant to the discussion. The focus of interviews with nurses, case managers, and counselors will be their experiences of working with HIV-infected women who have disclosed to their children, their beliefs about the benefits and burdens of disclosure, the degree to which they encourage and support women in disclosure to children, and knowledge they believe relevant to a disclosure intervention for women.

Procedures

HIV/AIDS-infected women who have disclosed their diagnosis to their dependent children will be recruited through counselors, nurses, and case managers at the ASO. The researcher will share the purposes of the project with counselors, nurses, and case managers and ask their help in identifying and recruiting HIV-infected women who have disclosed to participate. Given the stigma and sensitive nature of HIV infection, it has worked well in the past to have an ASO healthcare worker make the first contact about the investigator's research purposes with HIV-infected women and assess their willingness to participate in the project prior to contact by the researcher. The researcher will also recruit women at monthly women's support group sessions at the ASO, with the counselor's permission. Any HIV/AIDS-infected woman who has disclosed her diagnosis to a dependent child(ren) will be asked to share her experience of disclosure in a face-to-face interview with the researcher. (See **Appendix 12.1.**)

HIV/AIDS counselors, nurses, and case managers will be approached in person or telephoned by the researcher and asked for their participation in a face-to-face interview about their experiences of working with HIV-infected women who have disclosed their diagnosis to dependent children. (See Appendix 12.1.) Participants from both groups will be asked for permission to audiotape the interview for transcription purposes. A professional transcriptionist will transcribe the interviews verbatim. Any identifying information about participants will be removed from tapes by the researcher prior to transcription.

Plan for Data Management/Analysis

Data for the study will consist of texts from the interviews with HIV-infected mothers, interviews with HIV/AIDS care workers, and information gathered from literature related to disclosure of distressful information, especially to children. All data will be entered into The Ethonograph computer data management program. Each set of data will be qualitatively analyzed separately for patterns, themes, and exemplars. The patterns, themes, and exemplars from each data set will then be merged and organized into a structure that outlines and supports a disclosure intervention. Each set of data, as well as the merged data set will be analyzed using the phenomenologic method developed by Giorgi (1970). The procedural steps are: (a) naïve description of the phenomenon is accomplished via interviews with participants, (b) the researcher reads the entire description to get a sense of the whole, (c) the researcher rereads the descriptions a number of times and identifies individual units (patterns and themes), (d) the researcher eliminates redundancies in the units, clarifying or elaborating the meanings of the units by relating them to each other and to the whole, (e) the researcher reflects on the given units and transforms the meanings from concrete language into the language or concepts of the science, and (f) the researcher then integrates and synthesizes the insights into a descriptive structure communicated to others. All interviews are analyzed using this process until all data are integrated into the final descriptive structure, which in this case will form the basis of the disclosure intervention.

As the data are organized and developed into an intervention, they will be submitted for ongoing review and discussion with the consultant, an expert in the psychology of mothering. Prior to finalization of the intervention, HIV/AIDS care counselors, case managers, and nurses will be asked for their review and critique, along with a sample of HIV-infected women who disclosed to their dependent children. The critique and feedback from these groups will be incorporated into the final structure of the intervention.

Limitations

While the researcher has conducted a number of qualitative studies in which participants with various experiences were interviewed in-depth, and while she has conducted qualitative data analysis in each case that lead to implications and recommendations for nursing practice, she has not specifically taken qualitative data about the same topic from three different sources and analyzed it with the intention of developing a specific nursing/healthcare intervention. While the researcher feels confident that following the same systematic data analysis process she has used in the past will serve the purpose of this study, inexperience in a process of this exact nature may serve as a limitation.

Human Subjects Use

IRB approval for the study has been obtained. Potential participants will be assured anonymity and confidentiality. Participants will be asked to sign an informed consent prior to study participation. Women served by the ASO will be assured that study participation is voluntary and refusal to participate will in no way affect the care and service they receive from the agency. Participants will not be personally identified in any data or intervention outcomes of the study.

Time Frame

August–December: Recruit and interview HIV/AIDS-infected women who disclosed to their children, recruit and interview HIV/AIDS care workers, conduct ongoing research of disclosure and child development literature, share early insights with consultant.

January–April: Analyze data sets separately and merged, share analysis with consultant.

May–July: Develop disclosure intervention and get feedback from consultant and selected participants. Finalize written disclosure intervention for publication and pilot testing.

Support

1. *Facilities/Resources*: XXX University is a comprehensive public university, primarily for women, offering baccalaureate, masters, and doctoral degree programs. XXX University, a teaching and research institution, is the largest university for women in the United States. It offers high quality education in the liberal arts and sciences and

professional studies, especially in the health sciences and conducts research to enhance the progress and welfare of the people of the state, the nation, and the world.

The Office of Information Technology Services is the primary technology service provider for XXX University providing effective, efficient, and high-quality information technology support. Computing and communication services include multimedia services, communications design and engineering, support for the communications infrastructure, help desk services, operations services and systems programming.

The XXX University library offers students and faculty access to print and electronic information. The library has holdings of 549,116 print volumes and 10,000 e-book volumes, 8,287 current periodical and serial publications, 1,532,563 microforms, and 84,120 audiovisual materials to support all major areas of study at the university. The Integrated Library Information System includes both an online catalog that is capable of printing out searches of materials within the library and an online circulation and reserve system. The system is available throughout the University's mainframe computer for access on or off campus.

The investigator has a high capacity personal computer networked to the university mainframe and the Internet. The investigator has word processing and a qualitative data management program, The Ethonograph, installed on her personal computer. Both the principal investigator and the consultant are faculty at XXX University with individual faculty offices.

2. *Collaborative Arrangements*: Participants (both HIV-infected women and HIV/AIDs healthcare employees) will be recruited through two ASOs. One ASO serves six counties in a south central state. The researcher has received permission from the agency's research committee to conduct the proposed study within the facility. The CEO/director of the ASO will provide a letter upon request attesting to this agreement. Offices are available at locations of the ASO in two different counties for interviews with participants. HIV/AIDS care workers from XXX House, the second ASO, will be recruited by the program director. Potential participants will be telephoned by the researcher to arrange a face-to-face interview in a designated office within the ASO.

3. *Consultative Support*: A faculty member in the philosophy and psychology department at XXX University will provide consultation for the project. She has expertise in the psychology of mothering and has consulted with the primary researcher on research findings related to mothering and end-of-life issues experienced by HIV-infected women with dependent children. The consultant teaches a course in the psychology of mothering and conducts research related to spirituality in HIV-infected persons and psychological issues in postpartum women.

Table 12-1 Budget and Budget Justification

Item	Cost
Personnel	0
Secretarial	0
Typing costs	$1,620
Research assistants	0
Consultants	$150
Supplies	$368
Equipment	0
Computer costs	0
Travel expenses	$350
TOTAL	$2,488

Budget justification:
Typing costs: Transcription of audiotapes. The projected amount of $1,620 covers 18 1.5 hour tapes = 27 hours requiring 4 hours/hour to transcribe at $15 per hour.
Consultants: The projected amount of $150 covers 3 hours of consultation at $50 per hour.
Supplies: The projected amount of $368 includes audiotapes and batteries ($68), duplicating ($150), and general supplies such as computer disks, printer cartridges, paper, along with envelopes and postage for mailing results to some participants ($150).
Travel expenses: The projected amount of $350 is for travel for data collection in three counties in south central state, 1,000 miles at $.35 per mile

Budget

Table 12-1 shows the budget and budget justification for the study. No personnel costs were required since the researcher was able to conduct the study using existing resources. It should be noted that qualitative research is highly cost-effective in that minimal equipment is required. The major cost is time of the investigator, which can be subsidized by the University in terms of the requirement for scholarly productivity.

REFERENCES

American Academy of Pediatrics. (1999). Committee on Pediatric AIDS. *Pediatrics, 103*(2), 509–511.

Andrews, S., Williams, A., & Neil, K. (1993). The mother-child relationship in the HIV-positive family. *IMAGE: Journal of Nursing Scholarship, 25*, 193–198.

Benner, P., & Wruble, J. (1989). *The primacy of caring: Stress and coping in health and illness.* Menlo Park, CA: Addison-Wesley.

Black, P., & Miles, M. (2002). Calculating the risks and benefits of disclosure in African American women who have HIV. *Journal of Obstetric, Gynecologic, and Neonatal Nursing, 31*(6), 688–697.

Centers for Disease Control and Prevention. (1996). National Center for HIV, STD, and TB Prevention. *HIV/AIDS surveillance report*, *8*(2), Atlanta, GA.

Centers for Disease Control and Prevention. (2001). National Center for HIV, STD, and TB Prevention. *HIV/AIDS surveillance report*, *12*(2). Atlanta, GA.

Faithfull, J. (1997). HIV-positive and AIDS-infected women: Challenges and difficulties of mothering. *American Journal of Orthopsychiatry*, *67*(1), 144–151.

Giorgi, A. (1970). *Psychology as a human science: A phenomenologically based approach.* New York: Harper & Row.

Heidegger, M. (1962). *Being and time* (J. Macquarrie & E. Robinson, Trans.). New York: Harper & Row. (Original work published 1927).

Lather, P., & Smithies, C. (1997). *Troubling the angels: Women living with HIV/AIDS.* Boulder, CO: Westview Press.

Lincoln, Y., & Guba, E. (1985). *Naturalistic inquiry.* Beverly Hills, CA: Sage.

Mellins, C., & Ehrhardt, A. (1994). Families affected by pediatric acquired immunodeficiency syndrome: Sources of stress and coping. *Journal of Developmental and Behavioral Pediatrics*, *15*, S54–S76.

Moneyham, L., Seals, B., Demi, A., Sowell, R., Cohen, L., & Guillory, J. (1996). Experiences of disclosure in women infected with HIV. *Health Care for Women International*, *17*, 209–221.

Nelms, T. (2004). Burden: The phenomenon of mothering in HIV-infected women with dependent children. Unpublished article.

Niebuhr, V., Hughes, J., & Polland, R. (1994). Parents with human immunodeficiency virus infection: Perceptions of their children's emotional needs. *Pediatrics*, *93*, 421–426.

Pilowsky, D., Sohler, H., & Susser, E. (1999). The parent disclosure interview. *AIDS Care*, *11*(4), 447–452.

Semple, S., Patterson, T., Temoschok, L., McCutchan, J., Straits-Troster, K., Chandler, J., Grant, I., & HNRC Group. (1993). Identification of psychobiological stressors among HIV positive women. *Women and Health*, *20*(4), 15–36.

Sowell, R., & Misener, T. (1997). Decisions to have a baby by HIV-infected women. *Western Journal of Nursing Research*, *19*(1), 56–70.

APPENDICES

Appendix 12.1: Interview Formats

HIV-Infected Mother Interview Guide

Talk to me about your experience of disclosing your HIV diagnosis to your children.
What individuals, if any, were instrumental in your decision to disclose to your children?
What strategy(ies) did you use to disclose to your children?
What were your children's reactions to your disclosure?
What has been the impact of your disclosure on your relationship with your children?
What has been the impact of your disclosure on your health?
What has been the impact of the disclosure on your and your children's day-to-day lives?
What would you say to other women about disclosing to their children?

HIV/AIDS Care Nurses, Case Managers, and Counselors Interview Guide

Talk to me about your experiences of working with HIV-infected women who have disclosed their diagnosis to their children.
What have been your experiences of the benefits and burdens of women's disclosure to their children?
To what degree do you encourage women to disclose their diagnosis to their children?
To what degree do you support women in their disclosure of their diagnosis to their children?
What knowledge do you believe is most relevant regarding women's disclosure of HIV to their children?
What would you say to other nurses, case managers, or counselors working with women to disclose their HIV diagnosis to their children?

Appendix 12.2: Consent Form

I, _____, agree to participate in the research project entitled, Implementation and Evaluation of a Disclosure to Children Intervention for HIV-infected Women, which is being conducted by Tommie Nelms, Kennesaw State University, 1000 Chastain Road #1601, Kennesaw, GA, 30144, 678-797-2088. I understand that participation is entirely voluntary; I can withdraw my consent at any time and have the results of the participation returned to me, removed from the experimental records, or destroyed.

The following points have been explained to me;

1. The reason for the research is to learn about telling my children my diagnosis and the best ways to do it. The benefits I may expect from it are less stress from no longer keeping a secret from my children and a closer, more honest relationship with my children.

2. The procedures are as follows:

- An agreement was made with the agency contact person that a meeting between me and the researcher could be arranged at a place of my choice.
- At the first meeting I will be asked some questions about myself and my children and some questions that will help me decide if I am ready to tell my children my diagnosis or not. This meeting may last about 1 hour.
- If I decide I am NOT ready I will be given a brochure and asked to contact the agency or the researcher in the future if I decide to tell my children my diagnosis.
- If I decide I am ready I will be given a brochure and have a discussion with the researcher about the information in the brochure about telling my children my diagnosis.
- Shortly after I tell my children my diagnosis I will contact the researcher to talk about the experience. This will be a second meeting/talk and should last about 30 minutes.
- Three months after I tell my children I will be contacted by the researcher and asked to talk about how things are going between me and my children as a result of telling them my diagnosis. This talk should last about 30 minutes.
- Six months after I tell my children I will be contacted by the researcher and asked to talk about how things are going between me and my children as a result of telling them my diagnosis. This talk should last about 30 minutes.

3. The discomforts or stresses that may be faced during this research are: I may feel stress or anxiety from thinking about telling my children my diagnosis or from telling my children my diagnosis.

4. Participation entails the following risks:

- There is a risk of the release of confidential, embarrassing, or private information. My confidentiality will be protected and I am free to withhold embarrassing or private information. Only the researcher will have access to my information, no names or identifying information will be included in publications or presentations that result from the study. All information will be destroyed within 5 years.

- There is a risk I will feel stress or anxiety from thinking about or telling my children my diagnosis. Counseling is available to me through the AIDS Service Organization.
- There is a risk my children may feel sad, angry, afraid, depressed or misbehave as a result of telling them my diagnosis. Counseling is available to my children through the AIDS Service Organization.

5. The results of this participation will be anonymous and will not be released in any individually identifiable form without the prior consent of the participants unless required by law.

_____

Signature of Investigator, Date

_____

Signature of Participant, Date

PLEASE SIGN BOTH COPIES, KEEP ONE AND RETURN THE OTHER TO THE INVESTIGATOR

Research at XXX University that involves human participants is carried out under the oversight of an Institutional Review Board. Question or problems regarding these activities should be addressed to Dr. XX, Chairperson of the Institutional Review Board, [address, phone.]

Chapter 13

Sample Quantitative Research Proposal: Effect of Video-Based Education on Knowledge and Perceptions of Risk for Breast Cancer Genes *BRCA1* and *BRCA2* in Urban Latinas

Janice B. Flynn and Janice M. Long

OBJECTIVES

At the end of this chapter, the reader will be able to

1. Use the outline from Chapter 13 to propose a quantitative study that can be conducted with urban Latinas at risk for breast cancer.
2. Describe the ethical implications of conducting quantitative research with this particular vulnerable population.

Author's note: This chapter is a shortened version of a sample outline of a quantitative research proposal for a dissertation. The study has not been conducted.

CHAPTER I: STUDY OVERVIEW

The purpose of this study is to determine the effect of a video-based educational intervention for knowledge and perceptions of risk for *BRCA1* and *BRCA2* (*BRCA1/2*) in an urban Latina population. It is hypothesized that the intervention will increase knowledge about risk for inherited breast cancer (IBC) associated with *BRCA1/2* and increase awareness of the risk of having a mutation in *BRCA1/2*.

Research Questions

1. What is the effect of a video-based educational intervention on knowledge of *BRCA1/2* testing among Latinas?
2. What is the effect of a video-based educational intervention on perception of risk for a gene mutation in *BRCA1/2* for Latinas?

Null Hypothesis

1. There are no significant differences in pre- and post-test scores for knowledge about *BRCA1/2* between intervention and control groups.
2. There are no significant differences in pre- and post-test scores for perception of risk of *BRCA1/2* between intervention and control groups.

Background

Among all breast cancers, 5–10% have been linked to genetic mutations in two identified breast cancer genes, *BRCA1/2* (Campeau, Foulkes, & Tischkowitz, 2008). Germline genetic mutations in *BRCA1/2* have been linked to an 85% lifetime risk of developing breast cancer at an average age of 30 to 40 years (King, Marks, & Mandell, 2003; Schwartz et al., 2009). Development of gene sequencing technology led to the commercial availability of deoxyribonucleic acid (DNA) testing for *BRCA1/2*. This kind of DNA testing (also referred to as genetic testing) for *BRCA1/2* is not considered a population screening tool. Instead, individuals with preliminary risks for IBC should be identified and referred for further analysis of risk, including detailed pedigree development. Research is needed to identify best practices for teaching women about the risks for IBC related to *BRCA1/2*. Women need to know and understand their own risk for IBC to decrease their anxiety and worry if they are not at high risk of carrying the mutations in *BRCA1/2*. Knowledge of risk can inform decision making related to genetic testing for the abnormal genes.

In the sparse literature related to knowledge and perceptions about genetic testing, some researchers have found that Latinas have low knowledge (Honda, 2003; Kinney, Gammon, Coxworth, Simonsen, & Arce-Laretta, 2010; Ramirez, Aparicio-Ting, de Majors, & Miller, 2006) and negative perceptions of genetic testing (Thompson,

Valdimarsdottir, Jandorf, & Redd, 2003). In contrast, other researchers have identified positive attitudes in this population, including increased interest in participating in cancer genetics services and testing (Ramirez et al., 2006; Ricker et al., 2007; Sussner, Jandorf, Thompson, & Valdimarsdottir, 2013). Ramirez et al. (2006) concluded that high interest in genetic testing may be driven by lack of knowledge of risk factors for IBC. Kinney et al. (2010) concluded there was a need for bilingual media to increase awareness about IBC. Further study is needed to describe knowledge and perceptions of IBC linked to *BRCA1/2* status in Latinas.

Theoretical Framework

The theoretical base for the study is Health Belief Model (HBM), as defined in **Table 13-1**. Using constructs of the HBM, this study will describe the effectiveness of an educational intervention as the modifying factor (knowledge about *BRCA1/2*) and the individual perception of perceived risk of having an altered breast cancer gene. From these variables, the study will explore knowledge and perceptions about *BRCA1/2* in Latinas.

Assumptions

For this study, the following assumptions are identified:

1. Subjects are capable of understanding the instruments.
2. The subjects' responses to the instruments represent their perceptions.
3. Knowledge about *BRCA1/2* and perceptions of risks of inherited breast cancer can be measured in women.

Table 13-1 Organizational Constructs of the Health Belief Model Applied to Genetics

Individual perceptions	Modifying factors	Cues to action	Likelihood of action
Breast cancer susceptibility	Age, race	Genetic testing awareness	Intent to obtain testing for breast cancer genes
Altered gene susceptibility	Knowledge of *BRCA1/2*		
Breast cancer seriousness	Breast cancer family history		
Genetic testing—benefits, barriers	Personal breast cancer risks		

Sources: Data from: Flynn, J. B. (2001). Health beliefs about inherited breast cancer and genetic testing for *BRCA1* and *BRCA2* in women who have never been diagnosed with breast cancer and who use mammography services. Doctoral dissertation. Retrieved from CINAHL (2003135289); Champion, V., & Scott, C. (1997). Reliability and validity of breast cancer screening beliefs scales in African American women. *Nursing Research, 46,* 331–338; Lerman, C., Biesecker, B., Benkendorf, J., Kerner, J., Gomez-Caminero, A., Hughes, C., & Reed, M. M. (1997). Controlled trial of pretest education approaches to enhance informed decision-making for *BRCA1*. *Journal of the National Cancer Institute, 89*(2), 148–157; Rosenstock, I. (1966). Historical origins of the health belief model. In M. Becker (Ed.), *The health belief model and personal health behavior* (pp. 1–8). Thorofare, NJ: Slack.

4. Women who have mutations in *BRCA1/2* are at higher risk for developing breast cancer at an earlier age.
5. Acculturation in Latina immigrants to the United States may have an effect on these women's knowledge of *BRCA1/2* and perceptions of risk for IBC.

Definitions

1. Breast cancer genes (*BRCA1/2*)

Theoretical definition: BRCA1/2 are tumor suppressor autosomal dominant genes that are carried in paternal and maternal blood lines (Schwartz et al., 2009; Turnpenny & Ellard, 2005). *BRCA1* is located on the long arm of chromosome 17 (q12–21), while *BRCA2* is on the long arm of chromosome 13. *BRCA1* is thought to account for 30–40% of breast cancer in families with a high incidence of breast cancer and as much as 90% of combined breast and ovarian cancer (Schwartz et al., 2009; Yarbro, Frogge, & Goodman, 2005). *BRCA2* is considered to be responsible for 35% of early-onset breast cancer, but also has been linked with other cancers such as pancreatic, fallopian tube, and uterine cancers, male breast cancer, and adult leukemia (Turnpenny & Ellard, 2005). Multiple mutations of both genes have been reported. While the two genes are modestly different in molecular characteristics, *BRCA1/2* are commonly grouped together given that their similarities outweigh the differences.

Operational definition: Risk factors for both genes include the client or a first-degree blood relative with early-onset breast cancer; the client or a first-degree blood relative with ovarian cancer; bilateral breast cancer in the client or a first-degree blood degree relative; both ovarian and breast cancer in the client or a first-degree blood relative; the client or a blood relative known to have a *BRCA1* or *BRCA2* mutation; Ashkenazi Jewish women who have breast or ovarian cancer or a family history of one or both diseases; and breast cancer in a male family member (Narod, 2006; Schwartz et al., 2009; Turnpenny & Ellard, 2005).

2. Knowledge about inherited breast cancer and *BRCA1*

Theoretical definition: An understanding of inheritance of breast–ovarian cancer susceptibility and genetic testing (Flynn, 2001; Lerman et al., 1996).

Operational definition: Knowledge about inherited breast cancer and *BRCA1/2* based on the score on the Knowledge About Inherited Breast Cancer and *BRCA1/2* Questionnaire (Lerman et al., 1996). The 11-item true/false scale measures knowledge of inheritance patterns and risk factors for *BRCA1/2*.

3. Health beliefs

Theoretical definition: An individual's feelings of personal vulnerability to a specific health problem and the conviction that the benefits of taking action to protect health outweigh the barriers that will be encountered. Beliefs about personal susceptibility and seriousness of disease combine to produce the degree of threat or negative valence of a particular disease (Rosenstock, 1966).

Operational definition: Perceived risk of having a *BRCA1/2* mutation is the score on the Perceived Risk of Having a *BRCA1* Mutation Scale (Lerman et al., 1996).

4. Latino culture: The attitudes and behavior that are characteristic of the Latino population.
5. Promotores de salud: Hispanic/Latino community health workers who advocate for healthy lifestyles, serve as lay health educators, and act as communicators between health consumers and providers.
6. Faith-based settings: A group of individuals united on the basis of religious or spiritual beliefs (Ransdell & Rehling, 1996).

Limitations

1. Caution must be exercised in making inferences from the results of this study to Latinas outside the geographic region or to Latinas from ethnic groups other than those included in the study.
2. Subjects may be reluctant to answer questions related to genetics due to a lack of knowledge or understanding of the meanings of the terms. They may also be fearful or uncertain about the implications for their own family.
3. Data provided by the participants are expected to consist of their own perceptions of their risk for inherited breast cancer and their own knowledge of the condition. Some participants may have past experience with *BRCA1/2* and may have communicated with other subjects.

Significance to Latinas

In the United States, breast cancer is the second leading cause of death from cancer in women, and the most frequently diagnosed cancer in women. In general, women living in the United States have a 12.3% chance of developing breast cancer in a lifetime, with the average onset between 60 and 70 years of age (American Cancer Society [ACS], 2013). Among Latinas, breast cancer is the most frequently diagnosed cancer and leads to higher mortality in this group. While the breast cancer incidence rate in Latinas is lower than that in non-Hispanic white women, breast cancer among Latinas is more likely to be underdiagnosed (ACS, 2007). For those Latinas who are diagnosed with breast cancer, more are likely to have reached a late-stage breast cancer level compared with non-Latina whites (Shavers, Harlan, & Stevens, 2003; Vanderpool, Kornfeld, Rutten, & Squiers, 2009).

In general, Latinos have not been found to have a significantly higher rate of carrying the *BRCA1/2* genes than other ethnic groups; however, in a recent study of 746 Hispanic women with personal or family history of breast or ovarian cancer, 25% had a *BRCA* gene mutation (Chung So, 2013). Another ethnic group that has been identified as having a higher incidence of *BRCA1/2* is Ashkenazi Jews. Early haplotype studies suggest a founder effect between Ashkenazi Jews and individuals of Mexican descent; however, this linkage has not been broadly confirmed in the literature (Weizel et al., 2005). It is important to reach the Latina population early to identify risk and implement education programs on the urgency for comprehensive screening for at-risk Latinas and, early recognition and treatment of breast cancer.

Feasibility and Application

Examining the effects of a video-based educational intervention on knowledge and perception of risk for *BRCA1/2* among Latinas appears to be a feasible, researchable study. It can be measured quantitatively and is easily implemented. Exploring this research question may provide information useful to nurses in diverse settings, ranging from public health and home care to acute care settings. The findings could also prove helpful for nurse practitioners and other healthcare providers who are uniquely positioned to provide education on breast health and cancer prevention for Latinas. If educational videos are effective in increasing the knowledge and awareness of risk for *BRCA1/2*, it is possible that more Latinas will be better informed about their personal risk for *BRCA1/2*.

CHAPTER II: REVIEW OF THE RESEARCH LITERATURE *BRCA1* AND *BRCA2*

Four genetic mutations have been linked to breast cancer: *BRCA1, BRCA2,* p53 (associated with Li-Fraumeni syndrome), and *CD1* (associated with Cowden syndrome and possibly ataxia telangiectasia [ATM]). Of these genetic mutations, the *BRCA1/2* set has been implicated more directly in causation of breast and ovarian cancers (Schwartz et al., 2009). *BRCA1* and *BRCA2* were identified with positional cloning in 1994 and 1995, respectively (Futreal et al., 1994; Miki et al., 1994; Wooster et al., 1995). Schwartz and colleagues (2009) also concluded that familial breast cancers in clients who test negative for the *BRCA1/2* genes are presumably due to other, as yet unidentified, high-penetrance genes.

Soon after the cloning of *BRCA1/2*, multiple studies of high-risk families identified risk factors associated with mutation in *BRCA1* and *BRCA2* (Frank et al., 1998; Narod, 2006). Those findings have held up throughout the past 15 years and were reaffirmed by Schwartz and colleagues (2009) at the International Consensus Conference on Breast Cancer Risk, Genetics, and Risk Management. Risks for *BRCA1/2* include the following:

- Client or first-degree blood relative with early-onset breast cancer
- Client or first-degree blood relative with ovarian cancer
- Bilateral breast cancer in client or first-degree blood relative
- Both ovarian and breast cancer in client or first-degree blood relative
- Client or blood relative known to have a *BRCA1* or *BRCA2* mutation

- Ashkenazi Jewish women who have breast or ovarian cancer or a family history of one or both diseases
- Breast cancer in a male family member

Because mutations in *BRCA1/2* are rare, screening for these mutations in the general population is unwarranted. However, in this information age, news of genetic advances is instantly available to the general public through media and the Internet and may increase expectations, anxiety, and worry about genetic testing (Lerman et al., 1996; Wang, Gonzalez, Janz, Milliron, & Merajver, 2007). One of the greatest challenges in the immediate future will be for healthcare providers to assist individuals with the interpretation of genetic advances and applications of these advances in the diagnosis and treatment of genetically linked adult-onset disease.

Most scientists agree that testing for the genetic alterations *BRCA1/2* should include extensive genetic counseling. Contrary to that recommendation, the reality is that biotechnology companies are offering genetic testing for the breast cancer genes to healthcare providers and to the general public (Turnpenny & Ellard, 2005). Studies in the literature of women's knowledge and perceptions about genetic testing for breast cancer are few in number and mostly limited to women in high-risk populations (Lerman et al., 1997; Lerman et al., 1996; Ramirez et al., 2006).

Studies on genetic testing for cancer susceptibility suggest that the motivation for genetic testing may diminish as individuals at low to moderate risks receive education about the limits and risks of testing. Following a study of families with high-risk kindreds, Lerman and colleagues (1997) concluded that standard educational approaches may be equally effective as expanded counseling approaches in enhancing knowledge for decision making about genetic testing. Confirming Lerman et al.'s earlier findings, Ramirez et al. (2006) concluded that culturally sensitive educational materials are needed to inform Hispanics about hereditary risk for breast cancer. Descriptions of the systematic study of what women in the general population know and think about inherited breast cancer and associated genetic testing are extremely limited in the literature, and this topic clearly warrants further study. Reports on the implementation of educational programs for women who may not be at high risk for IBC are absent in the literature. Additionally, further study is needed to determine whether individuals outside identified high-risk kindreds have an inflated view of their personal risk of having a genetic mutation in *BRCA1/2*.

Health Belief Model

The HBM was originally proposed as a theoretical framework for explaining why some people who are free of disease or illness take actions to avoid illness, whereas others fail to take protective actions (Rosenstock, 1966). The intention of the model was to predict who would or would not use preventive measures to maintain health as well as to recommend interventions that might increase the predisposition of resistant individuals to adopt health-protecting behaviors. The HBM is based on the assumption that behavior is determined by the individual's subjective perception of the environment (Rosenstock, 1974). Cues or stimuli to health behavioral action may be internal, such as a symptom, or external, such as interaction with others or the mass media (Maiman & Becker, 1974). Other assumptions of the HBM include the premise that health is a valued goal for most individuals and that people can accept the possibility that they may have a serious illness in the complete absence of symptoms.

Based on the social–psychological work of Lewin (1935), HBM reflects health protection as avoidance of negatively valence regions of illness and disease (Davidhizar, 1983). To further explain a negative valence region, Lewin (1935) described the life space in which an individual exists as being composed of regions—some having negative valence, some having positive valance, and others being relatively neutral. Illness is conceived to exist in the region of negative valence, and has the potential to move an individual from neutral or positive valence to negative valence.

Becker (1974) modified the HBM to further define variables that predict the likelihood of taking recommended preventive health actions. Variables proposed as directly affecting predisposition to take action include the perceived threat to personal health and the belief that the benefits of preventive action outweigh the perceived barriers to action.

In analyzing this model's utility for health protective behaviors, Pender (1996, pp. 35–36) summarized it as including the following propositions:

1. Beliefs about personal susceptibility and the seriousness of a specific disease combine to produce the degree of threat or negative valence of a particular disease.
2. Perceived susceptibility reflects individuals' feeling of personal vulnerability to a specific health problem.
3. Perceived seriousness or severity of a given health problem can be judged either by the degree of emotional arousal created by the thought of having the disease or by the medical and clinical or social difficulties (family and work) that individuals believe a given health condition would create for them.
4. Perceived benefits are beliefs about the effectiveness of recommended actions in preventing the health threat.
5. Perceived barriers are perceptions concerning the potential negative aspects of taking action, such as expense, danger, unpleasantness, inconvenience, and time required.
6. Modifying variables such as demographic, sociopsychologic, and structural variables, as well as cues to action, only indirectly affect action tendencies through these variables' relationship with the perception of threat.

After reviewing a 10-year period of HBM research, Janz and Becker (1984) concluded that perceived barriers are the most powerful of the HBM dimensions in explaining or predicting health behavior. These authors also noted the implication that perceived susceptibility is an important variable in understanding protective health behaviors. Pender (1996) credits the HBM as being foundational to the development of the health promotion model, in which she defines health protection as "decreasing the probability of experiencing health problems by active protection against pathologic stresses or detection of health problems in the asymptomatic stage. Health protection focuses on efforts to move away from or avoid the negatively valenced states of illness" (p. 34).

While not a formal part of the HBM, the concepts of primary, secondary, and tertiary prevention have been used to describe health protection activities. According to Fensler and Miller (1997), the HBM has been used "extensively as a framework for the identification of individuals who engage in behaviors relevant to primary and secondary prevention" (p. 82). *Primary prevention* is the specific protection against a disease to prevent its occurrence. Examples include mass immunizations to prevent disease, reductions in risk factors, and control of air, water, and noise pollution so as to prevent chronic diseases. *Secondary prevention* is defined as organized, direct screening efforts or education of the public to promote early case finding of individuals with disease so that treatments can be implemented to halt pathologic process and limit disability. Examples include use of home kits for detection of occult blood in the stool and public education to promote health behaviors such as mammography and breast self-examination. *Tertiary prevention* is aimed at minimizing residual disability from disease and promoting a productive life, within the limitation of the residual effects. Examples include cardiac rehabilitation and stroke rehabilitation (Pender, 1996).

In cancer research, the HBM has been used extensively as a theoretical framework for identifying behaviors relevant to primary and secondary prevention. Specific to breast cancer, this model has been used to study breast self-examination practices (Champion, 1994, 1995; Rutledge & Davis, 1998; Sensiba & Stewart, 1995) and mammography screening for breast cancer (Champion, 1994; Fischera & Frank, 1994; Johnson & Meischke, 1994).

The utility of the HBM in cancer research and screening is well established. Health motivation and perceived barriers have been validated as strong predictors of individuals' intentions and behaviors related to cancer prevention and screening (Champion, 1995; Cody & Lee, 1990; Johnson & Meischke, 1994; Kelly, Zyzanski, & Alenagno, 1991; Sensiba & Stewart, 1995; Wyper, 1990).

Use of the HBM in genetic testing for breast cancer has been primarily limited to women in high-risk populations (Lerman et al., 1997; Lerman et al., 1996). In an effort to evaluate health beliefs about *BRCA1/2* in a more general population, Flynn (2001) studied 270 women with no prior diagnosis of breast cancer. The results revealed that perceived susceptibility to breast cancer, intent to obtain genetic testing, and the numbers of first-degree relatives with ovarian cancer were significant predictors of perceived risk of having an altered breast cancer gene. In 2007, Wang et al. surveyed 205 women prior to their genetic counseling appointments, and then completed a chart audit to determine genetic testing decisions. A significant three-way interaction existed between perceived susceptibility, perceived severity, and worry about being a *BRCA1/2* carrier that affected testing decisions. McGarvey et al. (2003) used the HBM to investigate differences among ethnically diverse, low-income women. This study concluded that barriers and health beliefs differ among ethnic groups and that clients should not be collapsed into general categories, but rather grouped according to country of origin.

Methods of Education for Latinas

No studies were found that provided evidence for effective health education methods for teaching Latinas about genetic testing for *BRCA1/2*. However, a few studies did suggest that Latinos might benefit from video-based education. A study conducted by Gordon and Iribarren (2008) found that participants who were dominant Spanish speakers preferred education in video form or in their homes on television. Another study conducted with Latinos regarding end-of-life decision making supported the concept that videos were a useful teaching strategy but must be culturally sensitive to the ethnic group's beliefs and practices (Volandes, Ariza, Abbo, & Paasche-Orlow, 2008). Murphy et al. (2007) used culturally sensitive video vignettes that were specific to the patient's own ethnic group to teach a variety of health topics. These educational vignettes were found to be more effective in communicating health messages compared to the usual brochure.

CHAPTER III: METHODOLOGY

Design

An experimental, comparison design will be used to examine participant knowledge and perception of risk for *BRCA1/2* before and after exposure to a culturally sensitive, Spanish-language video. To control for testing bias, a randomly selected sample of participants will receive the same pre- and post-testing over an identical time frame as the participants who view the video education program. It is anticipated that the intervention group results will demonstrate significantly higher knowledge level and awareness of *BRCA1/2* compared to the control group. The researchers are fluent in the Spanish language, and promotores de salud from the two faith-based settings will be trained as research assistants for each of the on-site groups. This project proposal will be sent to the institutional review board (IRB) for approval prior to implementation of the actual study.

Sample

A convenience sample of approximately 50 Latinas from 18 to 50 years of age will be recruited for participation in the study through a partnership with two local promotores de salud faith-based programs. The two faith-based settings have Latino memberships numbering more than 2,000, and each has from six to eight promotores de salud who work with the congregations.

Once candidates demonstrate an interest in participating, they will be invited to a meeting at a designated community setting. All participants will initially gather into one room, where each will receive a copy of the consent form for participation. Consent forms will be written in Spanish and English. The consent form will include the following information: (1) the purpose of the study, (2) description of the intervention, (3) length of time involved, (4) descriptions of the risks and benefits, (5) strategies for maintaining confidentiality, and (6) contact information for the primary researcher and the IRB. A researcher will read the consent form aloud and answer questions. All participants will be asked to complete a demographic questionnaire.

The Knowledge About Inherited Breast Cancer and *BRCA1* Questionnaire and the Perception of Risk for *BRCA1/2* instruments (pre- and post-tests, respectively) will be administered to all participants. Once the consent forms are read and signed, and the pre-tests collected, 25 participants who are randomly assigned to the intervention group will leave the room with one researcher and promotore de salud research assistant. A total of 25 participants will be present in each of the two locations. Participants remaining in the control group setting will not be subjected to the intervention.

Setting

The study will take place at a community meeting site where two rooms are available, one of which can accommodate as many as 50 participants. The two rooms will be isolated from each other to assure that no sound from either can be overheard.

Instrumentation

Two instruments (pre- and post-tests) and a demographic form will be used for the study:

- *Knowledge About Inherited Breast Cancer and* BRCA1 *Questionnaire.* The Knowledge About Inherited Breast Cancer and *BRCA1* Questionnaire is an 11-item true/false scale used to assess knowledge of inherited breast–ovarian cancer susceptibility and genetic testing. It is scored based on the number of correct responses (range = 0–11). Permission is not necessary for use this instrument, which was developed by the National Center for Human Genome Research Cancer Studies Consortium (Lerman et al., 1996) as a part of a set of core instruments. This document is in the public domain.
- *Perception of Risk for* BRCA1 *and* BRCA2. Perception of Risk for *BRCA1* and *BRCA2* is the score on the Perceived Risk of Having a *BRCA1* Mutation Scale. Permission is not necessary for use this instrument, which was developed by the National Center for Human Genome Research Cancer Studies Consortium (Lerman et al., 1996) as a part of a set of core instruments. This document is in the public domain.

Demographic Data (Investigator Developed)

A demographic questionnaire developed by the investigator will be used to gather descriptive data for subjects. Demographic data will include age, marital status, geographical origin of ancestors, ethnic background, education (highest level), occupation, employment status, ethnic background, family income, family background (e.g., adopted), and number of children.

Data Analysis

The data from each demographic, pre-test, and post-test will be entered into a statistical program for analysis using unique identification codes for each participant. Two researchers will examine the data independently to assure accuracy.

Frequency distributions will be examined for central tendencies and for possible outliers and missing variables. A two-variable analysis of variance (ANOVA) will be conducted to examine differences between participants' pre- and post-test scores on each of the two instruments. Both within-group and between-group analysis will provide a means to determine whether either the control group or the intervention group achieves statistically significant improvement between the predictor variable or pre-test of knowledge and awareness of *BRCA1* and *BRCA2* compared to the post-test awareness and knowledge.

Validity and Reliability

The Knowledge About Inherited Breast Cancer and *BRCA1/2* Questionnaire has been tested in previous studies and found to be reliable (alpha = .74) and valid (Flynn, 2001; Lerman et al., 1997; Lerman et al., 1996). Reliability and validity cannot be determined for the Perception of Risk for *BRCA1* because it is a one-item scale.

Procedures

1. Funding to conduct the study will be obtained.
2. Community partners will be identified.
3. The IRB application will be submitted to the university IRB committee.
4. An advisory board will be formed and will include a representative from the university and other community partners, and one promotore de salud from each of the faith-based settings.
5. Once IRB approval is obtained, computer software (SPSS) will be purchased and forms for data collection printed.
6. Flyers will be developed explaining the intent of the study, the date and time, and the location for each setting. Each flyer will be written in both Spanish and English.
7. Promotores de salud at each setting will be trained on the purpose of the study, the methods involved in recruiting, and their role in recruiting participants. Flyers will

be given to each promotore de salud to distribute on a designated date to that individual's congregation.

8. With the help of the promotores de salud, two rooms will be reserved at a central location that is convenient for participants from each of the two faith-based settings.

9. A database will be created using the list of participants provided by each promotore de salud from each location.

10. A 2-hour meeting will be held at the designated setting. At the start of the meeting, the researchers will introduce the participants to the study and explain and obtain informed consent from all participants. The purpose of the study will be explained as well as participants' right to leave if they do not wish to participate. The participants will be asked to complete three forms: one covering demographics, the Knowledge About Inherited Breast Cancer and *BRCA1/2* Questionnaire, and the Perceptions of Risk for *BRCA1* instrument. All participants will hear the same instructions. Once the initial forms are completed, a randomly selected group (Group 1) will be asked to move to a second room, where they will receive the video education intervention on *BRCA1/2*. All other participants will be designated as Group 2.

11. While Group 1 is viewing the video, Group 2 will view a general health and wellness video. After watching the video, the participants will be asked to complete the post-test.

12. The group randomized to view the video education program will view the video vignette education on *BRCA1/2*. They will then be provided with refreshments and the post-tests will be completed.

13. The participants will be thanked for their participation and the meeting will be dismissed at least 2 hours from the time it began.

14. The data will be entered by the two researchers into SPSS, and analysis conducted using SPSS. Data will then be presented to the advisory board for discussion and determination of next steps.

15. The research findings will be prepared in a final report to the funder, the advisory committee, and the community partners including the promotores de salud. The findings will then be disseminated through poster and/or oral presentations.

Timeline

After funding is secured, it is expected that the study will take place over 6 months with the meeting itself occurring in one 2-hour time frame (Appendix 13.1). This timeline may be adjusted depending on the availability of promotores de salud to recruit participants and adequate space to conduct the meetings.

Budget

Refer to Appendix 13.2 for a summary of the proposed budget with justifications.

REFERENCES

American Cancer Society (ACS). (2007). *Cancer facts and figures for Hispanic/Latinos 2006–2008.* Atlanta, GA: Author.

American Cancer Society (ACS). (2013). *Facts and figures 2013–2014.* Atlanta, GA: Author.

Becker, M. (Ed.). (1974). *The health belief model and personal health behavior.* Thorofare, NJ: Slack.

Campeau, P. M., Foulkes, W. D., & Tischkowitz, M. D. (2008). Hereditary breast cancer: New genetic developments, new therapeutic avenues. *Human Genetics, 124*(1), 31–42.

Champion, V. (1994). Beliefs about breast cancer and mammography by behavioral stage. *Oncology Nursing Forum, 21,* 1009–1014.

Champion, V. (1995). Results of a nurse delivered intervention on proficiency and nodule detection with self breast examination. *Oncology Nursing Forum, 22,* 819–824.

Champion, V., & Scott, C. (1997). Reliability and validity of breast cancer screening beliefs scales in African American women. *Nursing Research, 46,* 331–338.

Chung So, H., (January 11, 2013). Genetic tests may miss *BRCA* mutations in Latinas. In *City of Hope: Breakthroughs.* Retreived from http://breakthroughs.cityofhope.org/latinas-breast-cancer-genetics

Cody, R., & Lee, C. (1990). Behaviors, beliefs and intentions in skin cancer prevention. *Journal of Behavioral Medicine, 13,* 373–389.

Davidhizar, R. (1983). Critique of the health belief model. *Journal of Advanced Nursing, 8,* 46–72.

Fensler, J., & Miller, M. (1997). Factors affecting health behavior. In S. Groenwald, M. Frogge, M. Goodman, & C. Yarbro (Eds.), *Cancer nursing: Principles and practices* (4th ed., pp. 77–93). Sudbury, MA: Jones and Bartlett.

Fischera, S. D., & Frank, D. I. (1994). The health belief model as a predictor of mammography screening. *Health Values: The Journal of Health Behavior, Education & Promotion, 18*(4), 3–9.

Flynn, J. B. (2001). *Health beliefs about inherited breast cancer and genetic testing for BRCA1 and BRCA2 in women who have never been diagnosed with breast cancer and who use mammography services.* Doctoral dissertation. Retrieved from CINAHL (2003135289).

Frank, T., Manley, S., Olopade, O., Cummings, S., Garber, J., Bernhardt, B., ... Thomas, A. (1998). Sequence analysis of *BRCA1* and *BRCA2*: Correlations of mutations with family history and ovarian cancer risk. *Journal of Clinical Oncology, 17*(7), 2417–2425.

Futreal, P., Liu, Q., Shattuck-Eidens, D., Cochran, C., Harshman, K., Tavigian, S., ... Miki, Y. (1994). *BRCA1* mutations in primary breast and ovarian carcinomas. *Science, 266,* 120–122.

Gordon, N. P., & Iribarren, C. (2008). Health-related characteristics and preferred methods of receiving health education according to dominant language among Latinos aged 25 to 64 in a large northern California health plan. *BMC Public Health, 8,* 305.

Honda, K. (2003). Who gets the information about genetic testing for cancer risk? The role of race/ethnicity, immigration status, and primary care clinicians. *Clinical Genetics, 64*(2), 131–136.

Janz, N., & Becker, M. (1984). The health belief model: A decade later. *Health Education Quarterly, 11,* 1–47.

Johnson, J., & Meischke, H. (1994). Factors associated with adoption of mammography screening: Results of a cross-sectional and longitudinal study. *Journal of Women's Health, 3,* 97–105.

Kelly, R., Zyzanski, S., & Alenagno, S. (1991). Prediction of motivation and behavior change following health promotion: Role of health beliefs, social support, and self efficacy. *Social Science Medicine, 32,* 311–320.

King, M., Marks, J., & Mandell, J. (2003). Breast and ovarian cancer risks due to inherited mutations in *BRCA1* and *BRCA2. Science, 302*(5645), 643–646. Retrieved from MEDLINE with Full Text database.

Kinney, A. Y., Gammon, A., Coxworth, J., Simonesen, W. E., & Arce-Laretta, M. (2010). Exploring attitudes, beliefs, and communication preferences of Latino community members regarding *BRCA1/2* mutation testing and preventive strategies. *Journal of Genetics in Medicine, 12*(2), 105–115.

Lerman, C., Biesecker, B., Benkendorf, J., Kerner, J., Gomez-Caminero, A., Hughes, C., & Reed, M. M. (1997). Controlled trial of pretest education approaches to enhance informed decision-making for *BRCA1. Journal of the National Cancer Institute, 89*(2), 148–157.

Lerman, C., Narod, S., Schulman, K., Hughes, C., Gomez-Caminero, A., Bonney, G., … Lynch, H. (1996). *BRCA1* testing in families with hereditary breast–ovarian cancer: A prospective study of patient decision making. *Journal of the American Medical Association, 24,* 1885–1892.

Lewin, K. (1935). *A dynamic theory of personality: Selected papers.* New York: McGraw-Hill.

Maiman, L., & Becker, M. (1974). The health belief model: Origins and correlates in psychological theory. In M. Becker (Ed.), *The health belief model and personal health behavior* (pp. 9–26). Thorofare, NJ: Slack.

McGarvey, E., Clavet, G., Johnson, J., Butler, A., Cook, K., & Pennino, B. (2003). Cancer screening practices and attitudes: Comparison of low-income women in three ethnic groups. *Ethnicity and Health, 8*(1), 71–82.

Miki, Y., Swensen, J., Shattuck-Eidens, D., Futreal, P. A., Harshman, K., Tavtigian, S., … Ding, W. (1994). A strong candidate for the breast and ovarian cancer susceptibility gene *BRCA1. Science, 266*(5182), 66–71.

Murphy, D., Balka, E., Poureslami, I., Leung, D. E., Nicol, A. M., & Cruz, T. (2007). Communicating health information: The community engagement model for video production. *Canadian Journal of Communication, 32,* 383–400.

Narod, S. (2006). Modifiers of risk of hereditary breast cancer. *Oncogene, 25*(43), 5832–5836. Retrieved from MEDLINE database.

Pender, N. (1996). *Health promotion in nursing practice* (3rd ed.). Stamford, CT: Appleton & Lange.

Ramirez, A. G., Aparicio-Ting, F. E., de Majors, S. S., & Miller, A. R. (2006). Interest, awareness, and perceptions of genetic testing among Hispanic family members of breast cancer survivors. *Ethnicity & Disease, 16*(2), 398–403.

Ransdell, L. B., & Rehling, S. L. (1996). Church-based health promotion: A review of the current literature. *American Journal of Health Behavior, 20*(4), 195–207.

Ricker, C. N., Hiyama, S., Fuentes, S., Feldman, N., Kumar, V., Uman, G. C., … Weitzel, J. N. (2007). Beliefs and interest in cancer risk in an underserved Latino cohort. *Preventive Medicine, 44*(3), 241–245.

Rosenstock, I. (1966). Historical origins of the health belief model. In M. Becker (Ed.), *The health belief model and personal health behavior* (pp. 1–8). Thorofare, NJ: Slack.

Rosenstock, I. (1974). Why people use health services. *Milbank Memorial Fund Quarterly, 44,* 94–127.

Rutledge, D., & Davis, G. (1998). Breast self-examination compliance and the health belief model. *Oncology Nursing Forum, 15,* 175–179.

Schwartz, G. F., Hughes, K. S., Lynch, H. T., Fabian, C. J., Fentiman, I. S., Robson, M. E., … Untch, M. (2009). Proceedings of the International Consensus Conference on Breast Cancer Risk, Genetics & Risk Management. *Breast Journal, 15*(1), 4–16.

Sensiba, M., & Stewart, D. (1995). Relationship of perceived barriers to breast self-examination in women of varying ages and levels of education. *Oncology Nursing Forum, 22,* 1265–1268.

Shavers, V. L., Harlan, L. C., & Stevens, J. L. (2003). Racial, ethnic variation in clinical presentation, treatment, and survival among breast cancer patients under age 35. *Cancer, 97*(1), 134–147.

Sussner, K. M., Jandorf, L., Thompson, H. S., & Valdimarsdottir, H. B. (2013). Barriers and facilitators to *BRCA* genetic counseling among at-risk Latinas in New York City. *Psychooncology, 22*(7), 1594–1604.

Thompson, H. S., Valdimarsdottir, H. B., Jandorf, L., & Redd, W. (2003). Perceived disadvantages and concerns about abuses of genetic testing for cancer risk: Differences across African American, Latina and Caucasian women. *Patient Education & Counseling, 51*(3), 217–227.

Turnpenny, P., & Ellard, S. (2005). *Emery's elements of medical genetics.* London: Elsevier Churchill Livingston.

Vanderpool, R. C., Kornfeld, J., Rutten, L. F., & Squiers, L. (2009). Cancer information-seeking experiences: The implications of Hispanic ethnicity and Spanish language. *Journal of Cancer Education, 24*(2), 141–147.

Volandes, A. E., Ariza, M., Abbo, E. D., & Paasche-Orlow, M. (2008). Overcoming educational barriers for advance care planning in Latinos with video images. *Journal of Palliative Medicine, 11*(5), 700–706.

Wang, C., Gonzalez, R., Janz, N. K., Milliron, K. J., & Merajver, S. D. (2007). The role of cognitive appraisal and worry in *BRCA1/2* testing decisions among a clinic population. *Psychology and Health, 22*(6), 719–736.

Weizel, J., Langos, V., Blazer, K., Nelson, R., Ricker, C., Herzog, J., … Neuhausen, S. (2005). Prevalence of *BRCA* mutations and founder effect in high-risk Hispanic families. *Cancer Epidemiology, Biomarkers and Prevention, 14*(7), 1666–1671.

Wooster, R., Bignell, G., Lancaster, J., Swift, S., Seal, S., Mangion, J., … Micklem, G. (1995). Identification of the breast cancer susceptibility gene *BRCA2. Nature, 378*(6559), 789–792.

Wyper, M. (1990). Breast self-examination and the health belief model: Variations on a theme. *Research in Nursing Health, 13,* 421–428.

Yarbro, C., Frogge, M., & Goodman, M. (2005). *Cancer nursing principles and practice* (6th ed.). Sudbury, MA: Jones and Bartlett.

APPENDICES

Appendix 13.1: Detailed Timeline

Activities	Months					
	1	**2**	**3**	**4**	**5**	**6**
Identify community partner(s) Establish advisory committee	X					
Prepare and submit IRB application	X					
Recruit co-investigator, promotores de salud	X					
Orient project team to roles Train promotores de salud in on-site research assistant role		X				
Develop flyers for recruitment of participants and provide them to promotores de salud		X				
Print forms in Spanish (demographic forms, pre-tests, and post-tests)			X			
Recruit participants			X			
Secure the meeting location			X			
Formally invite participants to the meeting date and time				X		
Prepare random assignment numbers using SPSS				X		
Conduct the meeting				X		
Enter data in SPSS					X	
Analyze data					X	
Discuss findings with advisory committee and determine implications for the population and next steps					X	
Prepare reports to the advisory committee and other community partners (including promotores de salud)					X	
Prepare manuscripts						X
Disseminate results to providers and nurses through department meetings, publications, and presentations						X

Appendix 13.2: Proposed Budget and Budget Justification

Proposed Budget

A.	**Personnel**	**$46,580**
	1. Principal investigator: Dr. Jan Flynn	
	Academic year salary (sample salary = 50,000)	
	Stipend requested (25% effort year 50,000) =	12,500
	Fringe benefits (30% of salary year 50,000) =	3,750
	2. Co-principal investigator: Dr. Janice Long	
	Academic year salary (sample salary = 50,000)	
	Stipend requested (25% effort year 50,000) =	12,500
	Fringe benefits (30% of salary year 50,000) =	3,750
	3. Promotores de Salud	
	2 positions (@ 50% effort): $10/hr year 20 hr/week × 26 weeks =	10,400
	Fringe benefits (30% year 20,000) =	3,120
	4. Graduate research assistant	
	$14/hr for 40 hr total	
	No fringe benefits	560
B.	**Project operating expenses**	**$1,600**
	1. Video *BRCA1/2* (Spanish and English versions)	1,250
	2. Office supplies	200
	3. Travel	150
	Total funding request	**$48,180**

Budget Explanation/Justification

A. Personnel

1. Principal Investigator: Dr. Jan Flynn has expertise in genetic research and testing and in teaching patients about inherited breast cancer risk. Dr. Flynn's role in the study is to oversee the general operations of the study, including the budget and assurance of human subjects' protection. She will lead the research advisory committee.

2. Co-principal Investigator: Dr. Janice Long has expertise in working with the Latino population and has conducted research and oversight of a faith-based promotores de salud program where the study subjects will be recruited. Dr. Long will be responsible for recruiting two promotores de salud to work with the study and for training the two promotores de salud as research assistants in collaboration with Dr. Flynn. Consent forms will be read to participants in Spanish.

Drs. Flynn and Long will collaborate on writing the final reports and dissemination of study findings.

3. Promotores de Salud: Two promotores de salud who are experienced in working with the clients in the two faith-based settings will assist the researchers in coordination of activities for recruitment of study participants. They will deliver flyers to the congregants at each of the two settings and will coordinate acquisition of the location and rooms where the study will take place. The promotores de salud will also communicate with the candidates prior to and during the 2-hour study session, and each will attend the research advisory committee meetings.

4. Graduate Research Assistant: The research assistant will assist with form preparation for the study (including copying and making packets for each participant), data entry, and report writing. If a graduate research assistant cannot be recruited, an attempt will be made to recruit an undergraduate research assistant.

B. Project Operating Expenses

1. A culturally sensitive video on *BRCA1* testing in Latinos will be purchased for the study. A second copy of the same video in English will also be purchased and made available for researchers to review. The cost of the two videos is expected to be $1,250.

2. Office supplies (ink cartridges, paper, folders and binders for each participant as well as materials for duplicating the forms to be used for the study for 50 participants) are expected to cost $4/participant, for a total cost of $200.

3. Both the researchers and promotores de salud will be traveling to the research site, to research advisory committee meetings, and to investigate locations to conduct the study. Travel for the researchers and promotores de salud was calculated based on the total number of trips estimated (20 trips at 15 miles per trip) multiplied by the state rate of $0.50 per mile for 300 miles for a cost of $150.00.

Chapter 14

Life History of Jim: "I Am Not Broken"

Mary de Chesnay and Anne Batson

OBJECTIVES

At the end of this chapter, the reader will be able to

1. Describe the life history methodology as distinct from biography and autobiography.
2. Propose a methodology that can be used to collect life histories.
3. Provide an example of collecting a life history.

INTRODUCTION

The first author's life history program of research on success in overcoming adversity began with a study of successful African American adults in the Southeast and was replicated in the Northeast and western United States. This study was reported in the first edition of this book (de Chesnay, 2005). During research courses with graduate students, she found that students became excited about the methodology and several went on to complete graduate work using the life history methodology. Subsequently, an undergraduate course in vulnerable populations inspired a team of baccalaureate nursing students to collect life histories of young women who had successfully overcome addiction to drugs or alcohol. Another student in the class worked independently to collect the life history of a woman who had been sexually abused. Most recently, for a doctoral course in qualitative research, a student (Batson) used life history to tell the story of a man who personally inspired her. The story of Jim is reported in this edition. Involving students at all levels of education shows the usefulness of the design for nursing research.

Life history is a technique or method widely used in traditional ethnography to assist the ethnographer to understand the culture through the eyes of articulate representatives who are willing to relate their life stories to the researcher (de Chesnay, 2015). As ethnography developed from the traditional form of going to live in a remote community for at least a year to a highly focused way of studying culture, so life histories are evolving into a new technique for understanding aspects of a culture through the eyes of people who live it. Research on successfully transcending adversity helps nurses to provide individualized care. Though the life experiences are not necessarily generalized, at least the nurse can use what some people experience to provide care to others with similar health conditions, while continuously validating with each person the aspects of experience that are unique to that person.

Life history differs from autobiography in that the agent of interpretation is the researcher, not the person whose life is being described. The informant relates his or her story to the researcher, who then interprets the story in light of the research questions and the cultural context in which the informant lives (de Chesnay, 2005).

As nurses, social workers, and other health professionals developed research programs that focus on emic data, they adapted life history methods to better suit their own fields. However, because non-anthropologists bring diverse training and other traditions to their research, some confusion in the literature arises when authors equate life history with oral history. *Life history* is a story told by a researcher from data generated by a key informant and framing his or her life within the cultural context in which the person lived life (de Chesnay, 2015). In contrast, *oral history* focuses on the historical context and is useful when the researcher wishes to document the historical evolution of a group, such as nurses who practiced in the military during the Vietnam War or survivors of the influenza epidemic of 1919.

THE METHODOLOGY

The methods for these studies were developed by de Chesnay in an attempt to refine the traditional anthropological techniques for nursing research. In traditional life history work, framed within a year-long immersion in fieldwork, the stories can unfold over time as the ethnographer becomes part of the scene. For nursing research, the abbreviated version described here provides the nurse/researcher with direction for active intervention that may not help the person but can be used to help people with the same condition. The original study was reported in the first edition of this book (de Chesnay, 2005). It is important to note that the data derived from life histories are emic (from the person's viewpoint) rather than etic (from the researcher's viewpoint). Emic data are more powerful for the purpose of developing culturally appropriate interventions because of the increased likelihood of their relevance to the target audience.

Three methods of data collection may be used in constructing life histories, in addition to participant observation: a series of semi-structured interviews, genograms, and time lines. The research question for the study on alcohol is this: How does a person achieve success in overcoming the obstacles associated with the condition of substance abuse and the particular challenges faced by affluent teenagers?

Key informants were recruited purposively. Genograms and specific demographic data for the sample are not presented here to protect participants' privacy. The genogram was originally developed as a clinical tool in family therapy, but is now widely used as an assessment tool in nursing and medicine. Gathering genogram information involved asking questions about the family of origin and successful role models within the family. In the life history presented here, interviews included broad questions about the definition of success, facilitative factors and barriers, and stories from the informants' youth. Generally three or four interviews lasting approximately 1 to 2 hours were necessary. Interviews were audiotaped to ensure accuracy.

The timeline data collection tool is simply a horizontal line on a blank page with "birth" at the left end and "present age" at the right end. Informants were asked to indicate on the line the critical events in their lives and the ages at which the events occurred. The timeline helped to clarify the sequence of events that were important to the informant. Informants were given copies of the genograms and timelines, and were encouraged to change them as needed during the intervals between interview sessions.

The institutional review board granted approval to the Principal Investigator (PI) and approval has been renewed on an annual basis for this ongoing study, with minor changes to account for new research assistants. Once a doctoral student committed to conducting the interviews for the course, the informant was recruited, the consent form was explained and signed, and the interviews were scheduled, conducted, and analyzed. The other doctoral students in the course assisted with analysis of data by validating concepts and themes that emerged from the interviews.

THE LIFE HISTORY

In the following section, Anne Batson describes her interviews with Jim. She followed the methodology described above but only interview data are reported here in order to preserve his privacy.

The Key Informant, Jim: "I Am Not Broken"

Jim was a 34-year-old man who was born with cerebral palsy. I first met him through work with my husband and had heard his story in a casual conversation. I had only met him once. I knew what he had done with his life to overcome his adversity, and he agreed to be interviewed for my class project. Little did I know he also had been a victim of sexual and physical abuse by his father and that he had been sexually abused in a Catholic safe house.

Results

Six main concepts emerged from this interview: vulnerability, autonomy, support, normalcy, fortitude, and fighting back. The concepts emerged somewhat chronologically; the first being vulnerability. Jim was aware of his vulnerability since infancy because he had been told of the cardiac and apnea alarms that were needed once he was home from the hospital. He seemed to have periods in his life when he felt very vulnerable: exercises in his childhood were painful, he required a walker, he was advised by his teachers not to climb the jungle gym, and his father physically mistreated him as a young boy to the point where Jim had to defend himself. Jim underwent multiple surgeries during his developmental years that intermittently reminded him that he needed medical intervention to correct his defects. Jim also had periods of feeling invincible and indestructible that conflicted with his vulnerability. At times, he should have respected his limitations to avoid injury. Jim argues this notion, claiming that the injuries made him who he is today and that he would have engaged in those dangerous activities if he had to live those years over again.

People think I'm broken. I am not broken.

A subconcept of vulnerability is fragility. Jim aggravated his joints by using crutches too early in his bone development, thus contributing to chronic pain later in life. He was injured while wrestling in high school. He placed himself and others at risk when trying to drive. He is more fragile than an able-bodied person and when an opponent broke his back, he had to decide what his capabilities were. The sexual assault at the group home exposed his vulnerability and fragility more than the wrestling injury. Jim was harmed and violated because he could not defend himself. His only protection was to leave that environment. From that point forward, he never knowingly placed himself in a dangerous situation.

The second concept was autonomy. Jim was raised by parents who gave him the right to be heard from a very young age. He made some of the decisions regarding the timing of his surgeries. He argued for a place at Space Camp in 6th grade, and he was a spokesperson for a national service organization for his disability. Jim became a leader at a young age because of his involvement with the organization. His parents granted him independence and, at times, later in his life, forced his independence upon him. His mother did not let him return home after he flunked out of college his first semester. His anger toward her at that time made him more autonomous. In an effort to move as far away as possible, he left Ohio for Alaska and found great happiness. Jim had the freedom to live his life as he chose. He involved himself with certain activities in high school against his father's wishes. He owned his mortality during his suicide attempts. Smaller examples of autonomy include refusing to get a handicap parking permit. Jim's mother permitted her son to decide his destiny and to take responsibility for what he has become.

When I was 5 years old I met a state senator, who called me Little Jimmy. I said: "That's fine if I am allowed to call you Little ....

His parents encouraged him to speak up to people, and for that respect from his parents who encouraged his autonomy, he is very grateful.

The third concept is support. As a young child, Jim claimed that he was "never without a net." He felt his parents' support through his early years. He understood the support of the national service organization with which he became so involved. Although he was their spokesperson and embraced the teachings and offerings of the organization, they instilled in him the ideal of being a "fighter" rather than be a victim of his disability. As Jim aged, he realized that the support from his father was not as solid as that from his mother. This might be considered a subconcept of partial support. His father supported some of Jim's decisions. He did not support the decision to wrestle, an activity that caused a lumbar fracture and a separated shoulder. Jim's father was an alcoholic and died when Jim was only 17, leaving Jim with the decision to remove life support. Jim lost the support of his father in his formative years but continued to have his mother's full support. Parental support gave way to support from friends and coworkers. Their encouragement ultimately led to Jim's decision to go to culinary school and find his career path.

I was allowed to do my own thing but never without a net.

The fourth concept is normalcy. Jim, at the age of 4, remembers wanting to cast off the walker because "other kids did not use walkers." He wanted to go to Space Camp and summer camp because his friends went. He participated in sports through his primary school years to obtain a sense of belonging and normalcy. He joined a fraternity to do what other college students were doing. Jim used the word *normal* throughout the interview. He referred to his mother's reaction to events in his childhood as normal. She grounded him like normal mothers do. She permitted him to climb the jungle gym with the other kids to allow normalcy. Jim referred to his teenage years as being normal. He got in trouble as normal kids do. Jim defined himself not as special or handicapped or disabled. He defined himself as normal throughout the interview. When asked if he saw his disability, he responded that he only sees it when it benefits him. He can use the disability to his advantage if needed; otherwise, he disregards it and wishes others would, too.

The fifth concept is fortitude. There are several moments in Jim's life when he had a choice. He could have given in to the pain—emotional or physical—or, he could push through the difficult time. He chose to wrestle on the high school team. Jim chose to continue a 4-year term as the (service organization) poster child. He chose to become employed rather than receive disability checks as his sole source of income. He chose to fight to go to camps and culinary school. He chose to live rather than commit suicide. These events take great fortitude to overcome the emotional damage that potentially results from each of these events, let alone the series of traumas in Jim's life. He mentally pushes through the pain and challenges that face him daily. He invites additional hurdles into his life: athletics, fencing, and using a regular wheelchair instead of an electric chair. He does not back down from these barriers. He fights for his accomplishments.

Fighting back is the final concept. Jim has had numerous moments where he physically or verbally fought an opponent. He knocked out his father in self-defense. He reprimanded a Senator for patronizing him; he argued to go to Space camp and had to fight for a place at summer camp. His photograph on the (service organization) poster showed him standing with his walker wearing boxing gloves. He was nicknamed "tiger" by his mother. Jim had to fight for his summer jobs in Alaska and convince the dean at culinary school to let him stay. He verbally reprimands people who say insensitive things to him and at times corrects them, so that "they won't say anything stupid to someone else." He fights to make himself seen as a person and not just a disability. He fights the ignorant and he fights the well-meaning but misinformed. Jim's life has been a struggle and he fights back to achieve the things he believes he should be permitted to do. He was given the support and autonomy to be a fighter by those in his early life, and he engages in this fight on many levels. He is steadfast in the notion that he does not consider himself to be broken and anyone who does see him that way is in for a fight.

CONCLUSION

In this chapter we outlined the methodology for life history used by the first author and provided an example of the actual conduct of the study with a person from a traditionally vulnerable group. That he does not consider himself "broken" is the lesson we might all take away from this interview. To use the term *vulnerable* as a political mechanism to obtain services is appropriate, but to label individuals as vulnerable might be seen as depriving them of autonomy and treating them disrespectfully—it might be an "unkind kindness." This quote captures the doctoral student's sentiment about labeling people:

> There was one moment in the interview where he paused, and I wondered if he thought I was one of the insensitive people. Yet, he taught me as much as I have learned from all my education. I had to check my own insensitivity at the door about 10 minutes into this interview. When I started the interview I treated him like a patient—wanting to take care of him. He set me straight right away that I should not have that attitude. He was offended by my sympathy. It was discourteous to him. He would not allow it.

REFERENCES

de Chesnay, M. (2005). *Caring for the Vulnerable*. Sudbury, MA: Jones and Bartlett.

de Chesnay, M. (2015). *Springer Series on Qualitative Nursing Research: Using Life History*. New York: Springer Publishing Co.

Chapter 15

The Use of Community-Based Participatory Research to Understand and Work with Vulnerable Populations

Ellen F. Olshansky and Robynn Zender

OBJECTIVES

At the end of this chapter, the reader will be able to

1. Discuss community-based participatory action research as a methodology.
2. Describe how community action research meets the ethical standards for research with vulnerable populations.

INTRODUCTION

Health disparities and lack of access to health care among some disadvantaged populations have received increasing attention and concern among healthcare providers and health policy makers (Minkler & Wallerstein, 2010; Department of Health and Human Services, 2014). As healthcare providers and policy makers have become more concerned about the health of vulnerable populations, more research has been developed to better understand their plight. The goal of these research studies is to determine the most effective interventions. These studies, however, often fail to present the perspective of those who are vulnerable, resulting in less than optimal interventions. This chapter presents an overview of community-based participatory research (CBPR)—a more effective approach to learning about and working effectively with vulnerable populations.

Vulnerable populations encompass those groups with both decreased access to care and increased risk for illness and accidents. In trying to intervene with various vulnerable populations, it is imperative that healthcare providers understand their perspectives rather than imposing on them what we believe to be their experiences. Without such understanding, we may unwittingly exacerbate problems; moreover, community members who are vulnerable may feel that they are being given edicts, feel disempowered, and lack a voice in deciding on a solution to their problems. An example is the exclusion of women from clinical trials, which has often had the disastrous result that findings related to men were simply applied to women—without scientific evidence for the clinical significance of these findings. Women as a population became vulnerable by virtue of being excluded from research. Today, however, the National Institutes of Health (NIH) mandates the inclusion of women in such investigations unless there is an obvious rationale for excluding them. Unfortunately, even the inclusion in clinical trials does not always guarantee that the perspectives and voices of women will be taken into account in the research. Improvements in the inclusion or reporting of sex or race/ethnicity in clinical trials have not been achieved (Geller, Koch, Pellettieri, & Carnes, 2011), and the concern of appropriate recognition of women's issues continues to be argued and debated (Polit & Beck, 2012).

Many researchers use open-ended approaches to understanding the experiences of others, including asking open-ended questions without imposing variables a priori. This approach yields important data that would not otherwise be generated. However, such research, even if it used open-ended questions, is often conceptualized as being done *on* the participants. CBPR takes a different approach, by actively involving the participants as co-researchers. This approach fills an unmet need; Montoya and Kent (2011), for example, addressed the need for community members themselves to contribute to identifying the needs within their communities. This chapter presents an overview of the CBPR method and then describes why it is appropriate for working with vulnerable populations.

OVERVIEW OF COMMUNITY-BASED PARTICIPATORY RESEARCH

CBPR is an action-oriented research method that involves a team approach, inclusive of all participants. *All participants* means that the researchers and the researched exist as equal members of the research team, all with an important voice in the research. Rather than referring to the process of doing research *on* people, this approach refers to doing research *with* people. The people are those members of a community of interest, those who are most directly affected by the phenomenon being studied. The members of a community also work in tandem with the researchers, leading to a collegial research effort within an environment of collaboration, rather than the traditional hierarchical environment. One important goal of CBPR is to empower those who have not been empowered (e.g., those who are vulnerable) by helping them to eliminate oppressive situations or conditions that are contributing to their marginalization and vulnerability.

CBPR engages community members as active participants in the research. An important aim of this research is to generate an understanding of the community members' perspectives and needs, in order to develop interventions that more effectively meet the needs of the community members. The concept of action is integral to CBPR (in fact, some refer to this kind of research as "participatory action research" or "action research") because the overt goal of this research is to take constructive action. CBPR is most appropriate for addressing the needs of vulnerable populations because it encourages the direct and active involvement of the members of those populations. Such an approach seeks to mitigate inequalities and oppression among vulnerable groups.

In recent years, CBPR has received increasing attention. Israel, Eng, Schulz, and Parker (2012), Jagosh et al. (2012), and Minkler and Wallerstein (2010) have all addressed the importance of this approach to research in better understanding the nuances and complexities in communities of interest. Olshansky and colleagues (2005) described how CBPR can be used to understand and alleviate health disparities. At the Eastern Nursing Research Society (ENRS), a research interest group was recently formed with a specific focus on CBPR, reflecting the increasing interest in this approach to research.

Israel, Schulz, Parker, and Becker (1998) have aptly described eight key principles of CBPR:

1. Recognizing that the community is the unit of study
2. Building on the strengths already present in the community
3. Continually facilitating collaboration and partnership in each phase of the research
4. Integrating knowledge and action (e.g., knowledge alone is not enough; it must be coupled with action for social change)
5. Promoting the alleviation of social inequality by co-learning
6. Using an iterative process
7. Focusing on wellness and an ecological perspective of health
8. Partnering in the dissemination of research findings

This chapter uses the framework presented by Israel and colleagues (1998, 2012). The next section takes an in-depth look at each of these principles, followed by a focus on the applicability of each to working with vulnerable populations.

PRINCIPLES OF CBPR: APPLICABILITY TO VULNERABLE POPULATIONS

Recognizing That the Community Is the Unit of Study

This principle addresses the central focus of CBPR: the community and the factors that influence the community must be understood and addressed to understand the issues of the individual within the community. This concept is consistent with the ecological framework that addresses social, political, economic, environmental, and sociological factors as part of the community context and as contributors to the experience of individuals within the community. Although the experiences of each individual are important and each individual is unique, the focus is on the community, which is the context under which the individual experiences situations and problems. Individual differences within communities are taken into account to develop a comprehensive understanding of the complexities within communities.

Building on the Strengths Already Present in the Community

This principle embraces the attitude that members of the community already have strengths, despite the fact that they are vulnerable by virtue of unequal access to care and perhaps oppression by other dominant groups. In the spirit of empowerment, it is important to learn from these individuals how they view their strengths, how they would like to use their strengths to tackle the problems identified, and how they can improve on present strengths. It is imperative that the community members articulate these strengths and explain why they view them as strengths. They may need assistance in recognizing their strengths because traditionally this has not been a focus, particularly when researchers approach community members to conduct research. Researchers are usually focused on the problems and deficits. It must be emphasized, however, that despite taking a perspective of strengths, this research does focus on defining problems that need to be alleviated. The important point is that the problems of the community be addressed through a perspective of how the strengths of the community members can serve as the foundation for the interventions to address the community problems identified. Conversely, it is imperative that the members of the research team truly listen to and hear the community members' descriptions of how they cope with situations, how they have managed in the past, and what their views are in regard to how to continue to manage and move forward despite the vulnerabilities that they experience on a daily basis.

Focusing on strengths encourages empowerment among the members of the community. They feel that they have something to offer rather than being told what they should do by the researchers or health professionals. In addition, the researchers can learn from the community participants. Rather than imposing their views on the community participants (the traditional approach), the researchers can begin to understand what works best for the community participants.

Continually Facilitating Collaboration and Partnership in Each Phase of the Research

Collaboration and partnership are signature aspects of CBPR. To develop a collaborative partnership with the members of a vulnerable community requires much planning (de Chesnay, Murphy, Harrison, & Taualii, 2008; Ganann, 2013). It takes time to develop a true partnership with members of the community, particularly when vulnerable community members have traditionally had a lack of trust of researchers from an academic or other institution. Taking the time initially to develop trust, thereby enabling the entree of the traditional researcher into the community, is crucial to the success of the research. Strategies for achieving this trusting relationship include going into the community and conducting focus groups on site (as opposed to having the community members travel to the location of the researcher). Lakes and colleagues (2014) conducted a qualitative study of the process of building trust between faith leaders in a community and academic researchers. They discovered that finding common ground was essential as well as sharing a commitment to open and ongoing communication.

It is important that the researchers venture out of their "ivory towers." Community members, likewise, need to know that they have an open invitation to visit the researcher's location. Nevertheless, the point of overriding importance is for the researchers to enter the context of the community members. By doing so, they strive to understand the context and to reverse the often stereotypical view of the ivory towers of academia. Gaining entree into the community and developing trust among the community members are only the beginning of this collaboration and partnership, however. Community members are considered equal partners in the research. They have an active voice in determining the research question, in designing the research method, in contributing to the data collection and analysis, and in disseminating the research results. They work in partnership as equal members of the research team.

It is important to recognize the unique skills and contributions made by each member of the research team. The community members are the experts in the actual phenomenon under study. The traditional researchers are the experts in research methodology, including collection and analysis of data, and writing up or presenting research results (often with community members as authors due to their contributions to the research process). Therefore, each member of the research team contributes to the overall effort based on his or her area of expertise, but all members of the research team are involved in all the steps of the research process to greater or lesser degrees.

Focus groups are commonly used in CBPR as a way to involve all members of the research team and to elicit perspectives from the various members of the research team.

Focus groups are a way of facilitating discussion within an atmosphere of openness, where the goal is to hear the various perspectives and views of community members and the traditional research members. The focus group serves several purposes. First, it helps members of the team get to know one another and allows them to hear each person's perspectives and description of his or her own experiences. Second, it helps the members come together in a collaborative manner as they begin to understand each person's experiences, focusing on the differences among them while also looking for and eventually being able to define commonalities. Third, the focus group allows the members to more clearly define the research problem, establish the focus of the research, and identify the goals and outcomes of the research.

Integrating Knowledge and Action

A crucial component of CBPR is action, in the form of developing and implementing interventions within the community that will help to alleviate the problems identified by the research group. CBPR is a form of research with the overt purpose of making social change to alleviate disparities, oppression, and other factors that lead to vulnerability. CBPR is true *translational research*, in that the translation into practice occurs in an immediate and ongoing fashion from the moment the research commences and throughout the entire process. By working closely and collaboratively with community members who desire constructive social change, the emphasis on action to achieve this constructive change is paramount in CBPR. This approach is especially germane to nursing education, as nursing students are a strong voice for social change necessary to improve health disparities among vulnerable populations (Boutain, 2011).

Promoting the Alleviation of Social Inequality by Co-Learning

The principles discussed in the previous subsections contribute to alleviating social inequality. The principle of promoting the alleviation of social inequality by co-learning is directly related to the principle of integrating knowledge and action. To alleviate social inequality, it is imperative that constructive social change leads to social emancipation and alleviation of oppression. Such social change will truly be useful only if those less fortunate (those who are vulnerable) are empowered. Integrating this principle into CBPR reflects the complexity of this research approach. This research process encompasses developing collaborative partnerships, involving all members of the community actively in the research project, overtly seeking to make social change in a constructive manner, and doing all of this while empowering those less fortunate. In fact, without such empowerment, the other aspects of the research will not be achieved. Muhammad and colleagues (2014) have aptly described the importance of the involvement of the community members as a means to address unequal power relationships.

Using an Iterative Process

An iterative process is one in which each of the phases of a study is conducted in a circular, as opposed to a linear, fashion. A phase is not a discrete part of the process; rather, each phase informs the next phase, and subsequent phases may lead to returning to previous phases to make changes based upon continuous learning throughout the CBPR process. This iterative process is central to all qualitative research. CBPR employs qualitative research methods through focus groups (and sometimes individual interviews), eliciting perspectives of informants in their own words, and approaching data in an interpretive manner.

The research begins in an inductive manner, as the research question is open-ended and the goal is to learn the perspectives of the members of the community without imposing preconceived variables on the investigation. As the research continues, certain variables that are generated through the research process receive greater focus based on the presence of continuing data to support these variables. In qualitative terms, this practice is referred to as saturation of data (Strauss & Corbin, 1998). At this point, data collection becomes more deductive—that is, focused on looking for further evidence of both predetermined (from initial data, in this case) and emerging variables. Previously collected data are reanalyzed with the explicit purpose of looking for data or evidence to support the existence of these variables. This iterative process involves going back and forth, a process in which data collection influences data analysis, which then influences furthers data collection.

Focusing on Wellness and an Ecological Perspective of Health

CBPR proposes that multiple and interacting factors within the social context influence and are influenced by health. This ecological perspective embraces the notion that context is a key factor in understanding how to promote wellness. The context includes biological, psychological, environmental, social, and interpersonal factors. Health and wellness occur within this context. Using CBPR, the research team seeks to understand the factors in this ecological perspective. These factors are uncovered by open-ended questions and participant observation.

Partnering in the Dissemination of Research Findings

As noted earlier, in CBPR all members of the research team are involved in all aspects of the research process, including the dissemination of research findings. Traditionally, the dissemination of research has consisted of researchers writing for publication or presenting their findings at conferences. These publications and conferences are typically refereed—that is, reviewed by a panel of experts who are also researchers and scholarly peers. In CBPR, those peer reviews continue, but research findings are also disseminated in magazines and meetings of the lay public. Those publications that are sent to peer-reviewed journals will, ideally, include the lay community members as co-authors. The research data and findings are "owned," in a sense, by all members of the research team—a key aspect of CBPR.

CBPR AND VULNERABLE POPULATIONS

Vulnerable populations often lack a voice in regard to what they need and how these needs could best be met. Traditionally, presumed "experts" from health care and other arenas have dictated solutions to vulnerable populations—a one-way flow of information. This dominant attitude, while perhaps well meaning, is usually counterproductive, because it keeps vulnerable populations in vulnerable positions, and where they lack a voice. A CBPR approach seeks to address these limitations of the traditional approach to assisting vulnerable populations. It aims to assist the vulnerable in attaining and maintaining a voice, to recognize those who are vulnerable as the true experts about the issues they are experiencing, and to ultimately enable them to forge a partnership in social change (Brownson, Roux, & Swartz, 2014).

Implementing a CBPR Approach with Vulnerable Populations

Even after establishing the critical need for CBPR in alleviating inequalities and oppressions suffered by vulnerable groups, it remains difficult to implement such an approach. Although many barriers exist, one goal of nurses and other healthcare providers and researchers is to work actively to overcome those barriers. This section presents strategies for implementing CBPR in research and healthcare settings.

In academic research settings, support for such an approach is sorely needed. The National Institutes of Health (NIH) (2014) clearly recognizes the need for CBPR, reflected by its call for research proposals that incorporate CBPR. In educational settings, this approach should be included in research courses in undergraduate and graduate programs. As CBPR projects have become more prevalent, concerns about scientific integrity, defined as a set of professional standards and ethical obligations, of these studies have been raised (Kraemer Diaz, Spears Johnson, & Arcury, 2013). Project team members have various disciplines, cultures, and communities that inform their norms, expectations, and agendas. Inadequate or inappropriate training, and lack of access to resources (e.g., time, money, equipment, staff) have been identified as limitations to the acquisition of quality data and the performance of scientifically rigorous methods. For example, a lack of access to time, money, and appropriate research training may lead to recruiting of inappropriate participants or an inability to complete data collection as necessary, thereby compromising scientific integrity. Awareness of such concerns and taking steps to address them during the planning stages of CBPR projects may ensure scientific integrity within this research approach (Kraemer Diaz et al., 2013).

Academic researchers and healthcare clinicians should partner with one another to develop research programs that include community members. An ideal CBPR project would include academic researchers, clinicians, and community members. In addition, health policy experts and members of health insurance companies could be included in such research. Inclusion of policy makers as stakeholders is necessary to impact those most burdened by health inequities through bridging evidence and policy making (Cacari-Stone, Wallerstein, Garcia, & Minkler, 2014). Additionally, the inclusion of youth in CBPR is sorely lacking. Only 15% of CBPR studies that focused on topics important to young people actually included those young people as partners in the research process (Jacquez, Vaughn, & Wagner, 2013). Another important consideration with CBPR is the well-being of patient/community participants. In a review conducted by Attree and colleagues (2011), both positive and negative consequences of participating in CBPR were shown to exist. Negative consequences included exhaustion and stress from time and financial resources that were drained by continued participation, "consultation fatigue" and disappointment with long-term engagement in the CBPR process, and excessive struggle with physical demands reported by individuals with physical disabilities. Positive consequences included perceived benefits for the health, both mentally and physically; self-confidence; self-esteem; a sense of personal empowerment; and the development of social relationships. All participants in the research process contribute important perspectives. When the research team is expanded to include the voices of community members, those individuals then have the opportunity to voice their concerns directly to the various members of the healthcare team.

REFERENCES

Attree, P., French, B., Milton, B., Povall, S., Whitehead, M., & Popay, J. (2011). The experience of community engagement for individuals: A rapid review of evidence. *Health & Social Care in the Community*, *19*(3), 250–260.

Boutain, D. M. (2011). Social justice in nursing: A review of the literature. In M. de Chesnay & B. A. Anderson (Eds.), *Caring for the vulnerable* (3rd ed., pp. 43–57). Sudbury, MA: Jones and Bartlett.

Brownson, R. C., Roux, A. V. D., & Swartz, K. (2014). Commentary: Generating rigorous evidence for public health: The need for new thinking to improve research and practice. *Annual Review of Public Health*, *35*, 1–7.

Cacari-Stone, L., Wallerstein, N., Garcia, A., & Minkler, M. (2014). The promise of community-based participatory research for health equity: A conceptual model for bridging evidence with policy. *American Journal of Public Health*, *104*(9), 1615–1623.

de Chesnay, M., Murphy, P. M., Harrison, L., & Taualii, M. (2008). Methodological and ethical issues in research with vulnerable populations. In M. de Cehsnay & B. Anderson (Eds.), *Caring for the Vulnerable*, 155–170. Sudbury, MA: Jones and Bartlett.

Department of Health and Human Services. (2014). *Healthy people 2020*. Retrieved from http://www.healthypeople.gov/2020/default.aspx

Ganann, R. (2013). Opportunities and challenges associated with engaging immigrant women in participatory action research. *Journal of Immigrant and Minority Health, 15*(2), 341–349.

Geller, S. E., Koch, A., Pellettieri, B., & Carnes, M. (2011). Inclusion, analysis, and reporting of sex and race/ethnicity in clinical trials: Have we made progress? *Journal of Women's Health, 20*(3), 315–320.

Israel, B. A., Eng, E., Schulz, A. J., & Parker, E. A. (Eds.). (2012). *Methods in community-based participatory research for health* (2nd ed.). San Francisco, CA: Jossey-Bass.

Israel, B. A., Schulz, A. J., Parker, E. A., & Becker, A. B. (1998). Review of community-based research: Assessing partnership approaches to improve public health. *Annual Review of Public Health, 19*, 173–202.

Jagosh, J., Macaulay, A. C., Pluye, P., Salsberg, J., Bush, P. L., Henderson, J., ... & Greenhalgh, T. (2012). Uncovering the benefits of participatory research: Implications of a realist review for health research and practice. *Milbank Quarterly, 90*(2), 311–346.

Jacquez, F., Vaughn, L., & Wagner, E. (2013). Youth as partners, participants or passive recipients: a review of children and adolescents in community-based participatory research (CBPR). *American Journal of Community Psychology, 51*(1–2), 176–89

Kraemer Diaz, A. E., Spears Johnson, C. R., & Arcury, T. A. (2013). Variation in the interpretation of scientific integrity in community-based participatory health research. *Social Science & Medicine, 97*, 134–142.

Lakes, K. D., Vaughn, E., Pham, J., Tran, T., Jones, M., Baker, D., ... Olshansky, E. (2014). Community member and faith leader perspectives on the process of building trusting relationships between communities and researchers. *Clinical Translational Science Journal, 7*(1), 20–28.

Minkler, M., & Wallerstein, N. (Eds.). (2010). *Community-based participatory research for health: From process to outcomes*. San Francisco, CA: John Wiley & Sons.

Montoya, M. J., & Kent, E. E. (2011). Dialogical action: Moving from community-based to community-driven participatory research. *Qualitative Health Research, 21*(7), 1000–1011.

Muhammad, M., Wallerstein, N., Sussman, A. L., Avila, M., Belone, L., & Duran, B. (2014). Reflections on researcher identity and power: The impact of positionality on community based participatory research (CBPR) processes and outcomes. *Critical Sociology*, (in press). 0896920513516025.

National Institutes of Health (NIH). (2014). Community-based participatory research. Retrieved from http://obssr.od.nih.gov/scientific_areas/methodology/community_based_participatory_research/

Olshansky, E., Sacco, D., Braxter, B., Dodge, P., Hughes, E., Ondeck, M., ... Upvall, M. J. (2005). Participatory action research to understand and reduce health disparities. *Nursing Outlook, 53*, 121–126.

Polit, D. F., & Beck, C. T. (2012). Gender bias undermines evidence on gender and health. *Qualitative Health Research, 22*(9), 1298–1298.

Strauss, A., & Corbin, J. (1998). *Basics of qualitative research: Techniques and procedures for developing grounded theory* (2nd ed.). Thousand Oaks, CA: Sage

Chapter 16

Decreasing Vulnerability in Childbirth: Waterbirth in Military Treatment Facilities

Elizabeth Nutter

OBJECTIVES

At the end of this chapter, the reader will be able to

1. Discuss how the culture of childbirth in the United States makes childbearing women vulnerable.
2. Explain how an interdisciplinary team can facilitate a protocol change to decrease vulnerability among childbearing women and their fetuses.
3. Describe how Larrabee's Model for Evidence-Based Practice Change was used to translate evidence into clinical practice.

VULNERABILTY IN CHILDBIRTH

Childbearing women and their fetuses are considered vulnerable populations. Healthcare providers must protect these vulnerable populations by ensuring evidence-based care that promotes optimal maternal and fetal/neonatal outcomes. Currently in the United States (U.S.), intrapartum care practices frequently obstruct a mother's ability to achieve physiological childbirth (Declercq, Sakala, Corry, & Applebaum, 2006). In 2009, 6 out of 10 of the most common hospital procedures were maternity-related, including Cesarean section, repair of obstetric laceration, artificial rupture of membranes, and fetal monitoring (Wier et al., 2009). In 2010, 32.8% of American mothers underwent Cesarean birth, and 3.62% of all births were accomplished with vacuum or forceps (Martin et al.,

2012). Evidence indicates that maternal and neonatal morbidity and mortality rates vary according to route of delivery (spontaneous vaginal, operative vaginal, or Cesarean section). With operative childbirth, short-and long-term health consequences may result, including infection, hemorrhage, chronic pain, and death (Aasheim, Nilsen, Lukasse, & Reinar, 2011).

PAIN MANAGEMENT OPTIONS IN CHILDBIRTH

Women in the United States have fewer pain management options in childbirth than women in other industrialized nations, suggesting that lack of professional training in nonpharmacological pain techniques in the United States fosters a dependence on pharmacological intervention during childbirth (Marmor & Krol, 2002).

Epidural/Spinal Anesthesia

Epidural/spinal anesthesia is the most common method of pain management used during childbirth in the United States (Declercq et al., 2006). In a 2005 survey of over 1,500 women, 76% used epidural/spinal analgesia during childbirth, while 14% used nonpharmacological pain management techniques during childbirth (Declercq et al., 2006). Although providing effective pain management during childbirth, epidural analgesia is not without risk. It is associated with an increased risk of assisted vaginal birth, maternal hypotension, intrapartum fever, longer second stage of labor, oxytocin administration, and an increased risk of Caesarean section for fetal distress (Anim-Somuah, Smyth, & Jones, 2011; Caton et al., 2002; Lieberman & O'Donoghue, 2002).

Nonpharmacological Pain Management

Research suggests that nonpharmacological pain management techniques support normal spontaneous vaginal birth, with minimal to no obstetrical intervention and minimal to no risk of adverse side effects for the mother or neonate (Leslie, Romano, & Woolley, 2007; Simkin & Bolding, 2004). Waterbirth and water labor are examples of effective nonpharmacological pain management that promote physiological childbirth (American College of Nurse-Midwives [ACNM], 2014; Nutter, Meyer, Shaw-Battista, & Marowitz, 2014). *Waterbirth* is the delivery of a neonate entirely underwater. *Water labor* is the use of immersion during some portion of the labor, with birth into air. Delineation of these terms is essential given evidence that benefits and potential risks differ between labor and birth in water (Nutter et al., 2014).

Current waterbirth research suggests that the potential benefits of waterbirth outweigh morbidity and mortality. Neonatal mortality rates are low and similar to those of uncomplicated vaginal birth (Nutter et al., 2014). Complications appear to be rare among low-risk women and neonates (ACNM, 2014; Nutter et al., 2014). An integrative analysis of peer-reviewed literature demonstrates that waterbirth is associated with:

- High levels of maternal satisfaction with both pain relief and the experience of childbirth
- Increased likelihood of an intact perineum
- Decreased incidence of episiotomy and severe perineal lacerations
- Reduced potential for postpartum hemorrhage
- No difference in maternal or neonatal infection rates or nursing admissions (Nutter et al., 2014).

Despite this evidence, waterbirth is not frequently offered to childbearing women in U.S. hospitals. The current political climate in the United States may place obstetric providers in a litigious position as the general population is not well educated about this option and may have concerns about safety. In 2009, only 229 U.S. hospitals offered this option (Nutter et al., 2014).

POSITIONS OF PROFESSIONAL ORGANIZATIONS ON WATERBIRTH

The American Congress of Obstetricians and Gynecologists (ACOG) and the American Academy of Pediatrics (AAP) published a committee opinion *against* the routine use of waterbirth:

> *The safety and efficacy of immersion in water during the second stage of labor have not been established, and immersion in water during the second stage of labor has not been associated with maternal or fetal benefit. Given these facts and case reports of rare but serious adverse effects in the newborn, the practice of immersion in the second stage of labor should be considered an experimental procedure that only should be performed within the context of an appropriately designed clinical trial with informed consent.*

(ACOG/AAP, 2014, p. 912)

The American College of Nurse-Midwifes (ACNM) published a position statement *supporting* waterbirth:

> *Researchers indicate that women who experience uncomplicated pregnancies and labors with limited risk factors and evidence-based management have comparable maternal and neonatal outcomes whether or not they give birth in water. Professional liability carriers, hospital administrators, health care insurers, and regulatory entities should not prevent or disallow maternity care providers or facilities with maternity services from providing immersion hydrotherapy for labor and birth with trained attendants who follow evidence-based guidelines.*

(ACNM, 2014, p. 1)

In contrast to the obstetrical culture in the United States, waterbirth is offered routinely in the United Kingdom, where evidence-based guidelines support waterbirth as a clinical practice for low-risk women. In a joint statement, the Royal College of Obstetricians and Gynaecologists (RCOG) and the Royal College of Midwives (RCM) stated that a review of the limited data on waterbirth is reassuring, despite documentation of potentially rare but serious neonatal complications. The statement affirms that women have the right to make an informed choice on location of birth, including in water. To achieve best practice, women must be involved in planning their own care with information, advice, and support from professionals (Alfirevic & Gould, 2006).

AN EVIDENCE-BASED APPROACH TO PRACTICE CHANGE

The purpose of this chapter is to discuss the use of translational research to develop a waterbirth protocol for healthcare providers supporting childbearing women in U.S. Military Treatment Facilities (MTFs). This research is based the Model for Evidence-Based Practice Change (Larrabee, 2009). According to Larrabee (2009), an evidence-based project can be prompted by a variety of factors, including a new "hot topic" or a new standard from the Joint Commission or a professional organization. Interest may arise from publication of new research that impacts clinical practice, the occurrence of a sentinel event, or complaints from patients or healthcare providers.

Examining a clinical problem involves consideration of risk, number of clients impacted, anticipated reimbursement and alignment with an organization's mission, vision, and values. Individuals with unique expertise or interest or a charter team can spearhead practice change within an organization. A multidisciplinary approach using physicians, nurses, organizational leaders, and other healthcare disciplines increases the likelihood of identifying key stakeholders.

Structured brainstorming and teamwork, led by a designated team leader, are key components of the model (Larrabee, 2009; Melnyk & Fineout-Overholt, 2011). Because evidenced-based projects are resource- and time-sensitive, a team should reach consensus on the priority of clinical topics and review internal data, benchmarking this data with external data (Larrabee, 2009). Standardized language organizes and links knowledge with clinical decisions and facilitates communication and understanding of terms within a multidisciplinary team. Potential interventions, outcome indicators, and expected patient outcomes can be identified and linked to relevant systems and economic outcomes (Larrabee, 2009).

The ultimate goal of this process is an evidence-based program that improves or promotes optimal patient outcomes. This can be achieved through use of multiple tools such as protocols, policy, procedures, care maps, or guidelines. A new practice is more likely to be adopted if five key attributes are considered:

- Relative advantages of change
- Observable benefits of change
- Simplicity of change
- Augmented support for technology
- Innovation/system fit (Larrabee, 2009)

Innovations are most likely to succeed when there is representation and participation, education of participants, use of social networks, and performance feedback (Larrabee, 2009; Melnyk & Fineout-Overholt, 2011).

WATERBIRTH PROTOCOL IN THE U.S. ARMY

This translational doctor of nursing practice (DNP) capstone project developed an evidence-based waterbirth protocol for healthcare providers supporting childbearing women in MTFs. In 2011, the U.S. Army consultant to the Surgeon General for Obstetricians and Gynecologists and the consultant to the Surgeon General for Women's Health Advance Practice Nurse requested a multicenter clinical trial to examine maternal and neonatal outcomes with waterbirth in Army MTFs. At the time, few MTFs offered waterbirth and each practice followed its own protocol. Without a standardized approach to waterbirth in Army MTFs, a multicenter clinical trial would not be possible.

As the team leader, the author, a DNP student who is a commissioned officer in the Army, identified and contacted key stakeholders—obstetrical leaders in MTFs offering waterbirth. A team was established to develop an evidence-based, standardized approach to waterbirth in Army MTFs globally. The author interviewed nurse-midwife chiefs, OB/GYN department chiefs, key obstetrical leaders in the Army, and intrapartum nurses at MTFs that offered waterbirth. An assessment revealed that each MTF followed a different waterbirth protocol. All nurse-midwife chiefs interviewed supported waterbirth. The majority of intrapartum nurses reported that they liked helping women to labor and give birth in water, although some nurses were apprehensive about caring for patients without a provider's direct presence in overseeing the care. The literature supported this finding. Stark and Miller (2009) studied labor and delivery nurses' perceptions of the use of water during childbirth. Intrapartum nurses in facilities where certified nurse midwives (CNMs) do most of the deliveries were more likely to support use of water during childbirth. Nurses working in facilities with higher rates of epidurals perceived more barriers to the use of hydrotherapy during childbirth. Stark and Miller (2009) concluded, "Providing hydrotherapy requires a supportive environment, adequate policy, staffing, and a collaboration relationship among the healthcare team" (p. 667). The internal data from these interviews were compared with external data for benchmarking. Clinical protocols at civilian facilities also revealed a lack of uniformity, confirming the need for evidence-based protocols and standard operating procedures to guide waterbirth practice.

To guide the literature review, the author used a hierarchy of evidence to evaluate the creditability and quality of the evidence, per Melnyk and Fineout-Overholt (2011). The author used the Matrix Method (Garrard, 2011) to create a detailed literature matrix, organizing the literature thematically and indexing content by level of evidence. A total of 1,121 articles were accessed with the removal of 187 duplicates. After review of abstracts, 844 articles were excluded on the basis of the inclusion criteria. A total of 84 articles met criteria for inclusion in the review. These articles included:

- Three randomized controlled studies
- One systematic review of descriptive studies
- Sixty observational studies
- Three qualitative studies
- Seventeen case reports

After the exclusion of subjects described in multiple publications, the experience of 48,679 subjects who were reported to have waterbirth was included. The studies examined *maternal outcomes* (episiotomy, perineal outcomes, infection, analgesia, pain perception, complications, labor length, satisfaction, and medical intervention), *fetal-neonatal outcomes* (Apgar scores, neonatal intensive care unit [NICU] admission, infection, complications, morbidity and mortality), and *protocol variables* (inclusion criteria, exclusion criteria, fetal monitoring, timing of immersion, and water temperature. Waterbirth literature demonstrated a rate of cord avulsion of approximately 2.4 per 1,000 births. No data exist to compare this rate with conventional birth (Nutter et al., 2014).

Foster (2007) conducted a study using mixed methods. She demonstrated that the majority of participants who delivered in water reported positive experiences and believed that waterbirth was safe. Ninety percent of participants strongly believed that waterbirth tubs should be available during childbirth in MTFs. Foster's study helped to confirm that military beneficiaries desire the option for water labor and waterbirth in MTFs. Her study also revealed a need for obstetric providers to provide information and education about waterbirth allowing women to make informed decisions about the use water during childbirth (Foster, 2007).

Most published waterbirth research consists of simple descriptive or case-control observational studies performed outside of the United States; results are heterogeneous. Current nonexperimental waterbirth research provides the best available data on outcome and safety, despite appropriate critique of the limitations of this evidence. Current evidence supports that outcomes of waterbirth are likely equivalent, if not improved, among healthy women with low-risk pregnancies, compared to conventional birth (Nutter et al.,

2014). The literature review served as the foundation for the development of an evidence-based protocol to guide the clinical practice of waterbirth in MTFs.

Because MTFs already offer waterbirth, facilitating a standardized evidence-based approach was feasible. The clinical protocol included the following pieces: a standardized operating protocol (SOP); staff education in the form of a CE workshop; CE pre-test and post-test; and patient education in the form of a lecture, educational handout, consent form, provider waterbirth patient screening tool, waterbirth clinical audit tool, and staff competency assessment.

The protocol was implemented in four phases at one of the Army MTFs offering waterbirth. The first phase included a CE workshop for all intrapartum providers (CNMs, obstetricians, family medicine physicians, pediatricians, and registered nurses). The CE provided information on waterbirth theory, evidence-based practice, and SOP overview. Before and immediately after delivery of the CE workshop, the team administered a 15-item, 3-option, multiple-choice questionnaire to all CE attendees. The question measured provider knowledge of waterbirth, and the team analyzed the data to determine the effectiveness of CE in increasing the intrapartum provider's knowledge of waterbirth.

The second phase included patient education. Patients received written education on hydrotherapy use in labor and birth. The team used chart audits of waterbirths to ensure documentation that the patient received education on the risks, benefits, and alternatives to waterbirth. When staff education was completed, phase three commenced, including the implementation of the SOP to guide clinical practice. Overall compliance of the protocol is monitored by periodic review of components of the SOP. Upon completion of the pilot study, the team solicited verbal and written feedback from individuals using the new practice protocol and made minor adjustments to the protocol. The team emailed the proposed plan to key Army leaders, who disseminated the information accordingly.

CONCLUSION

An evidence-based, standardized approach to waterbirth will foster support for the use of water during childbirth in MTFs. We expect that this project will increase intrapartum providers' knowledge in caring for mothers who use water during childbirth. We also expect that this protocol will provide mothers with the information needed to determine if they wish to use waterbirth. Finally, we expect that a standardized, evidence-based approach to caring for mothers using waterbirth will provide intrapartum providers with the skills to optimize maternal and neonatal outcomes among mothers opting for waterbirth in MTFs. Continuous use of the protocol throughout the Army will sustain this project, including ongoing patient and staff education, monthly chart audits to evaluate compliance with the protocol, and audits of patient outcomes.

The U.S. Army plans to conduct a clinical trial analyzing maternal and neonatal outcomes after waterbirth. The Army MTF standardized evidence-based waterbirth protocol provides the fundamental skills and knowledge required to facilitate a multicenter trial. This protocol will guide each MTF in the clinical practice of waterbirth and in data collection to allow the maternal and neonatal outcome data to be evaluated and disseminated within the Army and through peer-reviewed journals.

The future of waterbirth in promoting physiological birth in the United States depends on the beliefs and experiences of providers CNMs, obstetricians, pediatricians, labor and delivery nurses, and hospital administrators). When professionals use evidence-based practice guidelines in relation to infection control, management of cord rupture, and strict adherence to eligibility criteria, the risk of poor outcome for the woman and her neonate after a waterbirth is uncommon (ACNM, 2014; Alfirevic & Gould, 2006).

This evidence-based waterbirth program, based on Larrabee's Model for Evidence-Based Practice Change, fosters a birth culture within MTFs promoting waterbirth as a way to support women desiring physiological childbirth. As a result, vulnerability for women and their fetuses during childbirth is reduced.

REFERENCES

Aasheim, V., Nilsen, A. B. V., Lukasse, M., & Reinar, L. M. (2011). Perineal techniques during the second stage of labour for reducing perineal trauma. *Cochrane Database of Systematic Reviews (Online)*, (12), CD006672.

Alfirevic, Z., & Gould, D. (2006). *Immersion in water in labour and birth (RCOG /Royal College of Midwives Joint Statement No.1)*. Retrieved from http://www.rcog.org.uk/womens-health/clinical-guidance/immersion-water-during-labour-and-birth

American College of Nurse-Midwives. (2014). *Position statement: Hydrotherapy during labor and birth*. Retrieved from http://www.midwife.org/acnm/files/ccLibraryFiles/Filename/000000004048/Hydrotherapy-During-Labor-and-Birth-April-2014.pdf

American College of Obstetricians and Gynecologists and American Academy of Pediatrics [ACOG/AAP]. (2014). Immersion in water during labor and delivery. Committee Opinion No. 594. *Obstetrics and Gynecology*, *123*, 912–915.

Anim-Somuah, M., Smyth, R., & Jones, L. (2011). Epidural versus non-epidural or no analgesia in labour. *Cochrane Database of Systematic Reviews*, *12*, CD000331.

Caton, D., Corry, M. P., Frigoletto, F. D., Hopkins, D. P., Lieberman, E., Mayberry, L., ... Young, D. (2002). The nature and management of labor pain: Executive summary. *American Journal of Obstetrics and Gynecology*, *186*(5 Suppl Nature), S1–S15.

Declercq, E. R., Sakala, C., Corry, M. P., & Applebaum, S. (2006). Listening to mothers II: Report of the Second National US Survey of Women's Childbearing Experiences. New York: Childbirth Connection. Retrieved from https://childbirthconnection.org/listeningtomothers/

Foster, T. M. (2007). *Patient perceptions, attitudes, and barriers to using water for comfort in labor and birth*. Unpublished master's thesis. Seattle, WA: University of Washington.

Garrard, J. (2011). *Health science literature review made easy: The research matrix* (3rd ed.). Sudbury, MA: Jones & Bartlett Learning.

Larrabee, J. (2009). *Nurse to nurse evidence-based practice: Expert interventions*. New York: McGraw Hill Medical.

Leslie, M. S., Romano, A., & Woolley, D. (2007). Step 7: Educates staff in nondrug methods of pain relief and does not promote use of analgesic, anesthetic drugs: The coalition for improving maternity services. *The Journal of Perinatal Education, 16*(Suppl 1), 65S–73S.

Lieberman, E., & O'Donoghue, C. (2002). Unintended effects of epidural analgesia during labor: A systematic review. *American Journal of Obstetrics and Gynecology, 186*(5 Suppl Nature), S31–S68.

Marmor, T. R., & Krol, D. M. (2002). Labor pain management in the United States: Understanding patterns and the issue of choice. *American Journal of Obstetrics and Gynecology, 186*(5 Suppl), S173–S180.

Martin, J., Hamilton, B., Ventura, S., Osterman, M., Wilson, E., & Mathews, T. J. (2012). Births: Final data 2010. *US Department of Health and Human Services: National Vital Statistics Reports, 61*(1), 1–21.

Melnyk, B. M., & Fineout-Overholt, E. (2011). *Evidence-based practice in nursing and healthcare: A guide to best practice* (2nd ed.). Philadelphia, PA: Lippincott Williams & Wilkins.

Nutter, E., Meyer S., Shaw-Battista J., & Marowitz A. (2014). Waterbirth: An integrative analysis of peer reviewed literature. *Journal of Midwifery & Women's Health, 59*(3), 286–319.

Simkin, P., & Bolding, A. (2004). Update on nonpharmacologic approaches to relieve labor pain and prevent suffering. *Journal of Midwifery & Women's Health, 49*(6), 489–504.

Stark, M. A., & Miller, M. G. (2009). Barriers to the use of hydrotherapy in labor. *Journal of Obstetric, Gynecologic, and Neonatal Nursing, 38*(6), 667–675.

Wier, L., Pfunter, A., Maeda, J., Strangers, E., Ryan, K., Jagadish, P., … Elixhauser, A. (2009). HCUP facts and figures: Statistics on hospital-based care in the United States. Rockville, MD: Agency for Healthcare Research and Quality. Retrieved from http://www.hcup-us.ahrq.gov/reports/factsandfigures/2009/TOC_2009.jsp

Chapter 17

Women of Oman: A Systematic Review of Health Issues

Christie Emerson, Genie E. Dorman, Mary de Chesnay, Diane Wilson, Bethany Francis, and Lisa McMasters

OBJECTIVES

At the end of this chapter, the reader will be able to

1. Provide a brief description of the country of Oman.
2. Describe the nature of the studies conducted to date on health issues of women in Oman.
3. Describe the gaps in the literature and specify new directions for research on the topic.

INTRODUCTION

Bordered by Saudi Arabia to the west, Yemen to the south, the United Arab Emirates to the north, and flanked by the Arabian Sea and Gulf of Oman, the Sultanate of Oman comprises about 300,000 square kilometers (about the size of Kansas). The terrain is mostly desert but there are also mountains and the coastline is long. The sultan is the hereditary ruler who may seek the advice of a group of individuals elected as an advisory council. Two of these council members are women. In 2003, universal suffrage was established for those over age 21 (Sultanate of Oman, n.d.). According to 2010 Omani census data, immigrants make up just over 30% of the population of Oman, which totals 2,773,479 (Oman Census, 2010).

The purpose of this chapter is to review the research literature on the health of the women of Oman in a systematic way that captures the best available research on a topic. The paper was prepared as an oral presentation for an international conference held at Kennesaw State University (Emerson, 2014) attended by Omani scholars and American faculty and students. We realize that systematic reviews generally require a hypothesis to examine the strength of the clinical literature, but we maintain that when the literature is only beginning to be established, a review can be written only at a beginning level.

PURPOSE

To prepare for a joint U.S. and Oman conference, the authors conducted a comprehensive literature review to describe the state of current research on the women of Oman and their health issues. The systematic literature review covered the period from 2000–2014 by using an all-database search through GALILEO, the University System of Georgia. This systematic review was a collaborative effort among three faculty members and three student coauthors. The students' contribution constituted fieldwork for their nursing elective in vulnerable populations, for which this book serves as the required text.

METHODOLOGY

Search Strategy

The keywords used for the first round of searching were *Omani* and *women*. A surprising number of health-related articles were found that included Omani samples or that referred to aspects of Omani culture. Almost 1,600 articles were reviewed and most were excluded because they were not articles based on data. When *health* was added as a search term, almost 600 articles were found. These were narrowed down to 65 articles that represented research based on data, included Omani participants, and included adult women. However, because many of these articles included men and women from other Middle Eastern countries, we narrowed the selection further to 34 quantitative and qualitative studies that included only adult women of Oman and related to their health issues.

Inclusion Criteria

1. Articles based on data and published in refereed journal literature
2. Qualitative or quantitative research
3. Adult women of Oman as sample population (note that women of Oman and Omani women may not mean the same thing because many women who live in Oman are immigrants and the studies did not differentiate indigenous women from immigrants)
4. Predominant theme of study related to health status or health issues

Exclusion Criteria

1. Studies that included Omani men or children
2. Studies in which women of Oman were included with women from other countries
3. Unpublished studies such as dissertations

Limitations

A systematic review is always limited by the ability of the researchers to capture all of the relevant research. Since GALILEO is widely used, the team feels confident that we reviewed all studies in the refereed literature to which we had access. The main medical journal of Oman is published in English, but there are always translation issues that should be considered. However, because the journal is refereed, we will trust the translations.

RESULTS

Thirty-four research studies met the criteria and were included in this review (**Table 17-1**). The studies were sorted into seven categories: complications of pregnancy ($n = 8$), pregnancy co-morbidities ($n = 7$), gynecology ($n = 4$), mental health ($n = 4$), Caesarian section ($n = 4$), ectopic pregnancy ($n = 3$), genetics ($n = 3$), and breast cancer ($n = 1$). Several themes emerged from the review of the literature.

Theme 1: Studies Were Retrospective and Predominately Quantitative Research Methodology

Of the 34 studies reviewed, 26 used a quantitative research methodology:

- 23 retrospective
- 1 quasi-experimental
- 2 prospective correlational

The remaining eight studies used a qualitative methodology. Six of these were case reports (Alkaabi et al., 2012; Dhar, 2009, 2012; Mathew, 2002; Nayar, Zanak, & Ahmed, 2003; Waad-Allah et al., 2014) and two, both related to mental health, were phenomenological studies (Al-Azri, Al-Awisi, Al-Rasbi, & Al-Moundhri, 2013; McDermott-Levy, 2011).

Theme 2: Studies Were Largely Conducted at Single Sites

Of the 34 studies reviewed, 18 were conducted at single sites. The two predominant sites were Sultan Qaboos University Hospital, a primary hospital and regional referral center in Muscat, the capital of Oman, and Nizwa Hospital, a regional referral center for the Al-Dakhilya central region (Tashfeen & Hamdi, 2013). Two of the studies used data from a randomized community-based intervention study entitled, "Delaying the Development of Diabetes Mellitus Type 2 in Oman," which was conducted in Bidbid, a city with a homogeneous population located about 30 km west of Muscat (Al-Farsi et al., 2010). In two other studies, (Al Riyami, Afifi, & Fathalla, 2005; Mabry, Al-Riyami, & Morsi, 2007), data from the 2000 National Health Survey were used.

Theme 3: Studies Were Predominately Related to Pregnancy and Reproductive Health

Twenty-two of the 34 studies were related to pregnancy, the topic focus that made up four of the seven categories into which the studies were divided. These categories included pregnancy co-morbidities, pregnancy complications, Caesarian section, and ectopic pregnancy. In addition, four of the studies were related to gynecology (Al-Riyami et al., 2005; Al-Shukri et al., 2014; Gowri & Krolikowski, 2001; Mabry et al., 2007).

Theme 4: Studies Were Predominately Done from the Medical Perspective Only

The studies were largely conducted from the medical perspective, which commonly focuses on disease management. However, a few studies did draw conclusions that included health promotion, such as nutrition counseling, health education, and health screening. Health promotion, through early detection and counseling, was recommended in five of the studies (Al-Azri et al., 2013; Al Busaidi, Al-Farsi, Ganguly, & Gowri, 2012; Al Hinai & Al Hinai, 2014; Al Riyami et al., 2005; Alshishtawy, 2008). Al-Hinai, Al-Muqbali, Al-Moqbali, Gowri, & Al-Maniri (2013) recommended that there should be more nutrition counseling offered by healthcare professionals at prenatal visits. It is of significance to note that none of the studies were conducted by nurses or incorporated a nursing perspective.

DISCUSSION

A preponderance of the studies (26) that met the criteria employed a quantitative research methodology. Of these, all but three were retrospective. Generally, retrospective study designs are considered to be inferior to prospective study designs for a number of reasons, including the reliance on the accuracy of the medical record and the difficulty of controlling bias (Hess, 2004). In order to gain a broader understanding of women's health issues in Oman, a variety of research methodologies should be used including quantitative studies with a prospective focus. In addition, the implementation of more qualitative-based research studies would serve to achieve a better understanding of the opinions, feelings, and experiences of women about health care.

The use of multiple locations in clinical research allows for better generalizability study results (Sprague, Matta, & Bhandari, 2009). Considering that almost half of the studies in this review were conducted at single sites, more research needs to be done using multicenter collaboration. The two primary sites, Sultan Qaboos University Hospital and Nizwa hospital, both serve urban populations, which potentially skewed the research samples. With the exception of two studies (Alshishtawy, 2008; McDermott-Levy, 2011), every study sample was selected from patients who sought health care from and were treated by healthcare providers. This highlights the need for more research on the health issues of women of Oman to include subjects who have not sought health care, whether due to lack of access or attitudes toward health care.

Because the authors examined studies related to health issues of adult women in Oman, it is not surprising that many of the studies were related to pregnancy and reproductive health. It is notable that only one of the studies (Mabry et al., 2007) addressed the use of contraception, even though the results of the 2008 National Reproductive Health Survey indicate that 53.8% of Omani women have used family planning methods (Oman Ministry of Health [MOH], 2008). In 2014, the Oman Ministry of Health identified health research priorities in the area of women's health to include:

- Study on rates and determinants of early marriage, early and late pregnancy, short birth spacing, and methods of birth spacing, unmet needs, and lost pregnancies
- Prevalence and causes of infertility and its social and psychological consequences
- Study of hypertension, diabetes, urinary tract infection, toxemia, obesity, and anemia among pregnant women, and in relation to perinatal morbidity and mortality (also maternal morbidity and mortality)
- Study on the quality and adequacy of maternity care services, counseling before marriage/pregnancy; during pregnancy, childbirth, and after birth; and in relation to the outcome of pregnancies and labor (comparison between rural and urban and governorates)
- Prevalence, determinants, and outcomes of intrauterine growth retardation (IUGR)
- Identifying the signs of pregnancy complications, health education/counseling, and advice provided from the viewpoint of a pregnant woman, and communication between service providers and pregnant women
- Study to determine the rates of dystocia and caesarean delivery (voluntary and mandatory), and its impact on the health of the newborn and mother
- Study to determine the ability of those who are responsible for obstetrics (doctor or nurse/midwife) to identification, referral, and registration of different birth defects and the genetic disorders of newborns
- Comparison between doctors and nurses/midwives regarding the outcomes of pregnancies and deliveries of women (antenatal and natal care) in primary care

- Study of the health status of women after menopause (in terms of psychological state, osteoporosis, female hormones, early screening for cancer, etc.)
- Study of the maternal mortality, physical and psychological health status (particularly depression), and health service utilization of mothers in the post-partum period (6 weeks) and policy implication
- Study on the prevalence rate of low birth weight (causes and prevention methods) (MOH, 2014)

The fact that most of the studies included in the review were conducted from the medical perspective, suggests the need for research related to the women of Oman from all members of the healthcare team. There was an obvious void in studies involving nursing science as well as other allied health professions. This offers many opportunities for studies to add to the body of knowledge of the health care of the women of Oman.

REFERENCES

Al-Ajmi, K., Ganguly, S. S., Al-Ajmi, A., Al-Mandhari, Z., & Al-Moundhri, M. S. (2012). Insulin-like growth factor 1 gene polymorphism and breast cancer risk among Arab Omani women: A case-control study. *Breast Cancer: Basic and Clinical Research*, 6, 103–112.

Al-Azri, M., Al-Awisi, H., Al-Rasbi, S., & Al-Moundhri, M. (2013). Coping with a diagnosis of breast cancer amongst Omani women. *Journal Of Health Psychology*, 19(7), 836–846.

Al-Busaidi, I., Al-Farsi, Y., Ganguly, S., & Gowri, V. (2012). Obstetric and non-obstetric risk factors for cesarean section in Oman. *Oman Medical Journal*, 27(6), 478–481.

Al-Farsi, Y., Brooks, D., Werler, M., Cabral, H., Al-Shafei, M., & Wallenburg, H. (2010). Effect of high parity on the occurrence of prediabetes: A cohort study. *Acta Obstetricia Et Gynecologica Scandinavica*, 89(9), 1182–1186.

Al-Farsi, Y., Brooks, D., Werler, M., Cabral, H., Al-Shafei, M., & Wallenburg, H. (2011). Effect of high parity on occurrence of anemia in pregnancy: A cohort study. *BMC Pregnancy and Childbirth*, 117, 289–293.

Al-Hinai, F., & Al-Hinai, S. (2014). Prospective study on prevalence and risk factors of postpartum depression in Al-Dakhlyia Governorate in Oman. *Oman Medical Journal* 29(3), 198–202.

Al-Hinai, M., Al-Muqbali, M., Al-Moqbali, A., Gowri, V., & Al-Maniri, A. (2013). Effects of pre-pregnancy body mass index and gestational weight gain on low birth weight in Omani infants: A case-control study. *Sultan Qaboos University Medical Journal*, 13(3), 386–391.

Alkaabi, J., Alkindi, S., Riyami, N., Zia, F., Balla, L., & Balla, S. (2012). Successful treatment of severe thrombocytopenia with romiplostim in a pregnant patient with systemic lupus erythematosus. *Lupus*, 21(14), 1571–1574.

Al-Riyami, A., Afifi, M., & Fathalla, M. (2005). Reliability of Omani womens self-reporting of gynaecologic morbidities. *Medical Principles & Practice*, 14(2), 92–97.

Al-Riyami, N., Al-Ruheili, I., Al-Shezawi, F., & Al-Khabori, M. (2013). Extreme preterm premature rupture of membranes: Risk factors and feto-maternal outcomes. *Oman Medical Journal*, *28*(2), 108–111.

Alshishtawy, M. (2008). Strategic approach to improving maternal survival in Oman. *Oman Medical Journal*, *23*(3), 179–186.

Al-Shukri, M., Mathew, M., Al-Ghafri, W., Al-Kalbani, M., Al-Kharusi, L., & Gowri, V. (2014). A clinicopathological study of women with adnexal masses presenting with acute symptoms. *Annals of Medical and Health Sciences Research*, *4*(2), 286–288.

Bhat, S., Hamdi, I., & Bhat, S. (2004). Placenta previa in a referral hospital in Oman. *Saudi Medical Journal*, *25*(6), 728–731.

Clark, C. J., & Simmonds, J. V. (2011). An exploration of the prevalence of hypermobility and joint hypermobility syndrome in Omani women attending a hospital physiotherapy service. *Musculoskeletal Care*, *9*, 1–10.

Dhar, H. (2009). Colloid cyst of third ventricle presenting as pseudoeclampsia. *Archives of Gynecology & Obstetrics*, *280*(6), 1019–1021.

Dhar, H. (2012). Ruptured rudimentary horn at 22 weeks. *Nigerian Medical Journal, 53*(3), 175–177.

Dhar, H., Hamdi, I., & Rathi, B. (2011). Methotrexate treatment of ectopic pregnancy: Experience at Nizwa hospital with literature review. *Oman Medical Journal*, *26*(2), 94–98.

Emerson, C. (2014, November). *Health issues of Omani women: An integrative review.* Presented at Women of Oman: Changing Roles and Transnational Influence Conference at Kennesaw State University, Kennesaw, GA.

Gowri, V., & Krolikowski, A. (2001). Chronic pelvic pain. Laparoscopic and cystoscopic findings. *Saudi Medical Journal*, *22*(9), 769–770.

Hamdi, I., Karri, K., & Ghani, E. (2002). Pregnancy outcome in women with sickle cell trait. *Saudi Medical Journal*, *23*(12), 1455–1457.

Hess, D. (2004). Retrospective studies and chart reviews. *Respiratory care*, *49*(10), 1171–1174.

Mabry, R., Al-Riyami, A., & Morsi, M. (2007). The prevalence of and risk factors for reproductive morbidities among women in Oman. *Studies in Family Planning*, *38*(3), 121–128.

Machado, L., Gowri, V., Al-Riyami, N., & Al-Kharusi, L. (2012). Caesarean myomectomy: Feasibility and safety. *Sultan Qaboos University Medical Journal*, *12*(2), 190–196.

Mathew, M. M. (2002). Recurrent EP in the ipsilateral fallopian tube. *Fertility Weekly*, *6*(4), 17–18.

Mathew, M., Kumari, R., Vaclavinkova, V., & Krolikowski, A. (2002). Caesarean sections at Sultan Qaboos University Hospital: A three-year review. *Journal for Scientific Research. Medical Sciences/Sultan Qaboos University*, *4*(1–2), 29–32.

McDermott-Levy, Ruth. (2011). The lived experience of female Arab-Muslim nurses studying in the United States. 2009. CINAHL Plus with Full Text, EBSCOhost (accessed May 23, 2014).

Ministry of Health, Oman (MOH). (2002). *National reproductive health survey 2008.* Oman: Author.

Ministry of Health, Oman (MOH). (2014). *Health research priorities.* Oman: Author.

Mohan, A., Mathew, M., & Rizvi, S. (2008). Use of intravenous sulprostone for the termination of pregnancy with fetal death in second and early third trimester of pregnancy. *Sultan Qaboos University Medical Journal, 8*(3), 306–309.

Nayar, R. C., Zanak, S. R., & Ahmed, S. M. (2003). Hysterical stridor: A report of two cases. *ENT: Ear, Nose & Throat Journal, 82*(1), 46.

Oman Census. (2010). Retrieved from http://www.ncsi.gov.om/NCSI_website/documents/Census_2010.pdf

Sprague, S., Matta, J., & Bhandari, M. (2009). Multicenter collaboration in observational research: Improving generalizability and efficiency. *The Journal of Bone and Joint Surgery: American Volume, 91*(3), 80–86.

Sultanate of Oman. Retrieved from http://www.omansultanate.com/

Tashfeen, K., & Hamdi, I. (2013). Polyhydramnios as a predictor of adverse pregnancy outcomes. *Sultan Qaboos University Medical Journal, 13*(1), 57–62.

Thomas, A., Kaur, S., & Somville, T. (2002). Abnormal glucose screening test followed by normal glucose tolerance test and pregnancy outcome. *Saudi Medical Journal, 23*(7), 814–818.

Waad-Allah, S., Mula-Abed, F. B., Pambinezhuth, M. K., Al-Kindi, N. B., Al-Busaidi, H., Al-Muslahi, N., & Al-Lamki, M. A. (2014). Congenital Adrenal Hyperplasia due to 17-alpha-hydoxylase/17,20-lyase deficiency presenting with hypertension and pseudohermaphroditism: First case report from Oman. *Oman Medical Journal, 29*(1), 55–59.

Zaidan, Z., Burke, D., Dorvlo, A., Al-Naamani, A., Al-Suleimani, A., Al-Hussaini, A., ... Al-Adawi, S. (2002). Deliberate self-poisoning in Oman. *Tropical Medicine & International Health, 7*(6), 549–556.

APPENDIX

Appendix 17.1: Summary of Included Studies

Table 17-1 Summary of Included Studies

Category	Design	Sample	Limitations	Conclusions
Pregnancy co-morbidities *n* = 7				
Al-Hinai et al. (2013)	Retrospective case-control study (both cases and controls identified by computerized hospital information system.	150 Omani women who delivered low birth weight (LBW) infants and 300 Omani women who delivered normal birth weight infants at Sultan Qaboos University Hospital (SQUH)	**Selection bias, misclassification, and unmeasured cofounders Single site	Underweight women and those with less-than-recommended gestational weight gain were at a higher risk of delivering LBW infants. More nutrition counseling should be offered by healthcare providers during prenatal visits.
Alkaabi et al. (2012)	Case report Good	34-year-old Omani woman, 27 weeks' pregnant with systemic lupus erythematosus who developed severe thrombocytopenia	Case report	Pt. did not respond to traditional treatment modalities, but did respond to a less common medication used to treat SLE. The case supports the use of the less common drug in pregnancy where immunosuppressive therapy is limited because of potential teratogenicity.
Dhar (2009)	Case report Good	32-year-old Omani woman, 39 weeks' pregnant	Case report	In cases of eclampsia with persistent symptoms, healthcare providers should get a CT scan to r/o intracranial tumors.

(Continues)

Category	Design	Sample	Limitations	Conclusions
Hamdi, Karri, and Ghani (2002)	Retrospective case-control study Good	319 pregnant women with sickle cell trait (SCT) treated at Nizwa Hospital, surrounding hospitals and health centers	Small experimental group (319)	Special care is needed for pregnancy, labor, puerperium, and surgery for women with SCT to prevent complications such as anemia, infection, and fetal wastage.
Machado, Gowri, Al-Riyami, and Al-Kharusi (2012)	Retrospective cohort study Good	Eight pregnant women with myomas which resulted in pregnancy complications and underwent myomectomy at the time of C-section at SQUH	Small sample; eight cases over 11-year time period	Caesarean myomectomy in selected patients in well-equipped tertiary settings is recommended because it could have positive bearing on future reproductive outcomes.
Thomas, Kaur, and Somville (2002)	Retrospective cohort study Good	200 pregnant women who delivered at SQUH July 1999–June 2000. Half with abnormal glucose screening test and half with normal glucose screening test	One site only	Even minor abnormalities of glucose metabolism w/out gestational diabetes are a significant risk factor for fetal overgrowth and associated problems.

Category	Design	Sample	Limitations	Conclusions
Pregnancy complications *n* = 8				
Al-Farsi et al. (2011)	Retrospective population-based cohort study Good	1,348 pregnancies among 341 women enrolled in AMAL study (Delaying Development of Diabetes Mellitus Type 2 in Oman–Omani residents between 18 and 60 randomly selected from the residents of Bidbid)	Selection bias (participants self-selected; self-reported data); also (**) selection bias–pregnancies with missing maternal health cards (MHCs) were excluded **Assumption: may be flawed by assuming that only pregnancies reaching the 12th week as action for parity; single site	Increasing parity increases the risk of occurrence of anemia in pregnancy (AIP) in a dose-response fashion.
Al-Farsi et al. (2010)	Retrospective population-based cohort study Good	3196 pregnancies among 532 women enrolled in AMAL study (Delaying Development of Diabetes Mellitus Type 2 in Oman–Omani residents between 18 and 60 randomly selected from the residents of Bidbid)	Selection bias (participants self-selected; self-reported data); also (**) selection bias–pregnancies with missing maternal health cards (MHCs) were excluded **Assumption: may be flawed by assuming that only pregnancies reaching the 12th week as action for parity; single site	High parity by itself does not increase the risk of developing prediabetes in later life despite the temporary diabetogenic effect of pregnancy.

(Continues)

Category	Design	Sample	Limitations	Conclusions
Al Hinai et al. (2014)	Quantitative, prospective instruments: Edinburgh Postnatal Depression Scale (Arabic version) administered 1-week post-delivery consisting of 10 questions regarding mother's feeling over the past 7 days; Second questionnaire to identity possible risk factors of PND administered at 2 weeks post-delivery and at 8 weeks post-delivery. Good	Arabic speaking Omani women who gave birth to a normal healthy child and attended the postnatal clinic and child vaccination clinic of the primary healthcare facilities at 2 and 8 weeks post-delivery.	**Use of unvalidated version (Arabic) of Edinburgh Postnatal Depression Scale; selection bias; assessment tool regarding risk factors associated with PND did not include all possible predictors.	Among few studies looking at postnatal depression (PND) in the Middle East. On average 12% of Omani women are at high risk of developing PND. Early detection and management of at risk mothers is necessary due to negative and long-term consequences.
Al Riyami, Al-Ruheili, Al-Shezawi, and Al-Khabori (2013)	Retrospective cohort study Good	44 women who delivered at SQUH with preterm premature rupture of membranes (PPROM) before 26 weeks' gestation and had a normal fetal anatomy scan and delivered at SQUH	One site; small sample (44)	Concurrent infection rate was high among patients with PPROM. No baseline maternal factors predicted the need for c-section–likely due to small sample size.

Category	Design	Sample	Limitations	Conclusions
Alshishtawy (2008)	Retrospective analysis of published and unpublished data Good	Oman Ministry of Health data on maternal deaths in or outside health facilities 1990–2007 were reviewed.	Selection bias; sample only represented those who sought medical care	The maternal mortality rate in Oman is high compared with other Gulf and developed countries. This poses a challenge to meeting the fifth Millennium Development Goal (MDG) to be achieved by 2015. Recommendations are: · Insure access and use of quality skilled care for all women and their newborns · Health education interventions · Strengthening monitoring of maternal deaths
Bhat, Hamdi, and Bhat (2004)	Retrospective case control study (medical records) Good	Pregnant women with placenta previa from Oct 1998 to Sept 2002 at Nizwa Hospital, Al-Dakhliya region, Oman	Selection bias (one hospital over 4-year time period); single site	In spite of higher maternal age, parity, and previous abortions having high odds of presenting pregnancies with major placenta previa, no significant statistical association could be proven. Also, no statistically significant difference in premature delivery could be established between pregnancies presenting with major or minor placenta previa. Antepartum hemorrhage irrespective of severity was a strong predictor of preterm outcome.

(Continues)

Category	Design	Sample	Limitations	Conclusions
Mohan, Mathew, and Rizvi. (2008)	Observational cohort study with retrospective data collection and analysis Good	97 women with a gestational age from 12–30 weeks and fetal death confirmed by ultrasound treated at SQUH, Muscat, Oman. 86.7% were Omani nationals and the remainder were from various other countries	One site only	IV use of sulprostone (PGE2 analogue) was both safe and effective in the termination of pregnancy with fetal death in second and early third trimester of pregnancy; however it requires continuous IV access and close monitoring of maternal VS.
Tashfeen and Hamdi (2013)	Retrospective cohort (477 with 900 in control group) Instrument: abdominal ultrasound Good	477 women with polyhydramnios and 900 with normal amniotic fluid levels selected randomly, with singleton pregnancies who delivered at Nizwa Hospital Jan 2002–Dec 2007.	One site	Polyhydramnios is associated with an increased risk of adverse perinatal outcomes, and there is significant positive relation with maternal age, diabetes, fetal anomalies, and fetal macrosomia

Category	Design	Sample	Limitations	Conclusions
Gynecology *n* = 4				
Al Riyami et al. (2005)	Retrospective study of survey fieldwork Instrument: National Health Survey (a multistage, stratified probability-sampling design Good	1,364 ever-married women aged 15–49 who completed the questionnaire and underwent gynecological exam and lab tests as part of the 2000 National Health Survey	Validity of questionnaire (*) assumptions regarding sexual activity based on religious beliefs	Self-report of vaginal discharge coupled with clinical exam could be used in community diagnosis of reproductive tract infections (RTIs). Self-report of symptoms of vaginal prolapse could also be used for community diagnosis of genital prolapse. A urinary culture should supplement self-reports of symptoms of UTI to enhance specificity, although the presence of a positive culture in the absence of symptoms is of no clinical significance in nonpregnant women or women without renal disease.
Al-Shukri et al. (2014)	Retrospective descriptive study Good	57 women who had surgical intervention for acute symptoms of adnexal masses from June 2007 to May 2012 at SQUH	One site; some sample (57) over 5-year period	Complications of adnexal masses such as torsion and hemorrhage are common causes of acute abdominal pain. Timely diagnosis of the adnexal pathology and surgical intervention will help preserve reproductive outcome.

(Continues)

Category	Design	Sample	Limitations	Conclusions
Gowri and Krolikowski (2001)	Nonexperimental prospective correlational study Instrument: Clinical evaluation (physical examination, lab work, pap smear, ultrasound, cystoscopy, laparoscopy) Excellent	49 Omani women with chronic pelvic pain referred to SQUH from Oct 1998–Sept 2000	One site (selection bias); small sample size (49)	Pelvic adhesions are the most common finding in Omani women presenting with chronic pelvic pain.
Mabry et al. (2007)	Retrospective study of survey fieldwork Instrument: National Health Survey (a multistage, stratified probability-sampling design	1,365 ever-married (have been married at least once, but might not be married now) nonpregnant women aged 15–49 in Oman who completed the health questionnaire and underwent gynecological exam and lab tests as part of the 2000 National Health Survey	Validity of questionnaire (*) assumptions regarding sexual activity based on religious beliefs	One in four Omani women suffers from reproductive tract infections (RTIs), 1 in 10 suffers from UTIs, and 1 in 10 suffers from genital prolapse, indicating that reproductive health services in Oman should be strengthened.

Category	Design	Sample	Limitations	Conclusions
Mental health *n* = 4				
Al-Azri et al. (2013)	Qualitative, phenomenology Excellent	19 women aged 24 to 55 (mean of 40 years and median of 39 years); time from diagnosis from few months to 3 years; patients in different modalities of treatment; all seeking treatment at SQUH Outpatient Oncology Department or Oncology Ward. All were Omani Muslims	**Not generalizable; sample all literate; hospital-based interviews; single site	Coping strategies identified: denial, optimism, withdrawal, Islamic beliefs and practices, and the support of family members and healthcare providers. Islamic beliefs and practices were the most common. Healthcare professionals should be aware of and respect women's coping strategies and encourage their use to reduce the psychological symptoms. They should also make family and friends aware of their role in supporting and encouraging coping strategies.
McDermott-Levy (2011)	Qualitative, phenomenology Excellent	12 Omani diploma nurses aged 25–37 (mean 27.5) who were in the U.S. for 16 months to complete the requirements for a Bachelors of Science in Nursing.	**Interviewer was participants' academic advisor and in a position of authority; lack of proficiency in English	Without the presence of their family, the Omani women described experiencing discrimination, exposure to different ways of thinking and living, as well as an awareness of being alone and doing things on their own. They reported finding new freedoms and independence in the U.S. that they had not experienced in Oman. These experiences enabled them to mature and grow; it was transformative as the women described the sense of increased responsibility and awareness of their personal and professional capabilities.

(Continues)

Category	Design	Sample	Limitations	Conclusions
Nayar et al. (2003)	Case report (2 cases) Good	2 women, ages 62 and 53, treated at Ibri Regional Referral Hospital in Oman	Case report	Review of two cases of hysterical stridor. Once the diagnosis was made both were successfully treated with a dose of anxiolytic.
Zaidan et al. (2002)	Retrospective, descriptive Good	Patients admitted to hospitals with acute and emergency services (A&E) in Muscat and surrounding area with drug overdose, ingestion, self-poisoning or deliberate self-harm from 1993–1998.	Data extracted from a variety of hospitals' A&E records from a 5-year period. **Data limited to what could be collected in routine monitoring; DSH more likely to be unreported (view findings with caution)	Conclusions not specific to women although all stats reported male and female separately.
C-section n = 4				
Al Busaidi et al. (2012)	Retrospective case-control correlational study; personal interviews Excellent	500 randomly selected women who delivered singlets at four hospitals in Oman: 250 vaginal deliveries and 250 c-sections	Matched according to time and place of delivery, but cannot match all potential factors influencing outcomes.	The findings of this study highlight the importance of health education throughout the antenatal period for Omani women. Health promotion can best be addressed through specialized counseling clinics, which are not yet available in Oman.

Category	Design	Sample	Limitations	Conclusions
Dhar, Hamdi, and Rathi (2011)	Retrospective descriptive correlational analysis; hospital record review Good	All women who delivered by Caesarean section at Nizwa Hospital were used to establish a rising rate of Caesarean section.	One site only; 1 year of data only	Multilevel, multidisciplinary approach and strategies are needed to reduce Caesarean sections in Oman.
Gowri and Al-Zakwani (2010)	Retrospective correlational analysis Good	94 consecutive patients admitted to SQUH with diagnosis of preeclampsia from July 2006 to Dec 2007	**Did not analyze mild and severe preecampsia separately; one site	Cesarean delivery was significantly high in patients with elevated uric acid regardless of whether they were preterm or term. Also, a significant number of babies (term and preterm) were admitted to the neonatal unit when delivered by mothers with elevated uric acid.
Mathew, Kumari, Vaclavinkova, and Krolikowski (2002)	Retrospective correlational analysis; hospital records over 3-year period Good	All patients who underwent Caesarean section at SQUH between July 1, 1998 and June 30, 2001–727 women–13% of all deliveries.	One site only	Rate of Caesarean delivery is similar to the rest of the world. Indications and nature and frequency of complications of Caesarean are similar to other academic hospitals in developed countries. The use of prophylactic antibiotics helps reduce morbidity associated with Caesarean section.

(Continues)

Category	Design	Sample	Limitations	Conclusions
Ectopic pregnancy *n* = 3				
Dhar et al. (2011)	Retrospective review of 60 cases (demographic data, clinical presentation, treatment progress, outcome, side effects, and future fertility analyzed using computer database) Good	60 patients with ectopic pregnancy treated as in-patients at Nizwa Hospital with single dose methotrexate regimen	One site; retrospective sample	Single dose methotrexate offers a safe and effective nonsurgical method of treating selected patients with ectopic pregnancy "in a society where tubal conservation is of utmost importance."
Dhar (2012)	Case report Good	Primigravida 22 weeks pregnant reported to Nizwa Hospital.	Case report	Careful uterine exam by experienced obstetrician in cases of mullerian anomaly may help avoid misdiagnosis and catastrophic hemorrhage.
Mathew (2002)	Case report (one case) Good	25-year-old Omani woman G5 P2 who presented with 3 ectopic pregnancies in the same tube within a 14-month period.	Case report	Further studies are needed regarding the obstetric performance of women after recurrent ectopic pregnancy in order to adequately counsel women who are interested in future fertility, even after their third ectopic pregnancy.

Category	Design	Sample	Limitations	Conclusions
Genetics _n_ = 3				
Clark and Simmonds (2011)	Cross-sectional case-control study (94 cases; 90 control); retrospective Good	Participant group: 94 Omani women, aged 18–50 years, attending physiotherapy (PT) for musculoskeletal complaints; Control group: 90 women similar age and ethnic origin who were staff at the hospital	Selection bias (self-selected); single site	The study confirms a high prevalence of joint hypermobility syndrome (JHS) among subjects with musculoskeletal symptoms and that re-attendance for PT is more frequent in patients with JHS than without.
Al-Ajmi, Ganguly, Al-Ajmi, Al-Mandhari, and Al-Moundhri (2012)	Case-control comparative study; retrospective Excellent	147 patients with breast cancer who were treated SQUH and the Royal Hospital. 134 control participants were recruited from women who did not have any history of benign breast disease, neoplastic disease, or other major health problems.	Sampling bias (self-selected)	This study confirmed that the most common allele was (CA)19, in keeping with other ethnic groups. However, there was no association between breast cancer and IGF1 CA repeats genotypes among Omani women in accordance with several large studies.

(Continues)

Category	Design	Sample	Limitations	Conclusions
Mula-Abed et al. (2014)	Case report Good	22-year-old Omani woman	Case report	This case study reports the first biochemically and genetically proven case of congenital adrenal hyperplasia due to 17a-hydroxylase/17,20 lypase deficiency in Oman and the Arab World.
Breast cancer *n* = 1				
Al-Rhabi et al. (2013)	Case-control comparative study; retrospective Good	20 patients with left-sided breast cancer treated between Oct 2009 and Mar 2010 at the National Oncology Center, Muscat	One site only; small sample size (20; 10 in each group)	Field-in-Field-Forward Planned Intensity Modulated Radio Therapy (FiF-FP-IMRT) is a simple and efficient planning technique for breast radiation.

Complications of Pregnancy GYN Co-Morbid with Pregnancy Psych-MH Pregnancy Health Promotion Ectopic Pregnancy C-Sections Fetal death Other-new category from articles I found Sultanate of Oman. Retrieved from http://www.omansultanate.com/ Breast Cancer

III

Practice and Programs

Chapter 18

Transcultural Aspects of Perinatal Health Care of Somali Women

Danuta M. Wojnar and Robin A. Narruhn

OBJECTIVES

At the end of this chapter, the reader will be able to

1. Explain the significance of Somali migration to the United States.
2. Identify key features of Somali cultural beliefs about health and illness.
3. Suggest appropriate nursing interventions for Somali women.

INTRODUCTION

Immigrating to a new country is a stressful process of readjustment and change (Enang, Wojnar, & Harper, 2002). For Somali immigrants the process is complicated by traumatic events many experienced because of the social and political turmoil in their homeland. Prior to sociocultural and political changes brought about by globalization, Somalia was peaceful country with a mainly pastoral economy. In the 1970s, commercial pastoralism was instituted, which negatively impacted the sustainability of small-scale nomadic herdsmen and agriculturalists (Chossudovsky, 1997). Introduction of commercial pastoralism also initiated events such as tight austerity programs and structural adjustment programs imposed by the International Monetary Fund (IMF) (Chossudovsky, 1997). It also reinforced Somalia's dependence on imported grain, and the influx of this cheap surplus grain led to displacement of traditional small-scale agriculturalists (Chossudovsky, 1997).

Shifts in food consumption patterns caused a decrease in demand for indigenous foods. Export of foods became more prominent than sustainable growth of indigenous food crops.

Exacerbating these occurrences was the neoliberal policy that instituted a devaluation of the Somali shilling (Chossudovsky, 1997). Traditional nomadic pastoralism was also negatively affected by the privatization of veterinary services for livestock pastoralists, lack of emergency animal feed during droughts, privatization of water, and environmental degradation of land and water. The World Bank instituted "herd adjustment" programs on the premise that indigenous herding was ruining the environment (Chossudovsky, 1997). According to Chossudovsky (1997), this developed into a cyclical series and the end result was a failure of the economy and reliance on the IMF and World Bank. Traditional pastoralism and agriculturalism were no longer a sustainable means of livelihood and the social fabric of the pastoralist economy was undone. The effects of these neoliberal policies are a predictable decrease in health and education infrastructures and resulting adverse outcomes. Debt service obligations overwhelmed Somalia and IMF loans were cancelled (Chossudovsky, 1997), however Somalia continued to be affected by structural adjustment programs and inadequate public infrastructures (Chossudovsky, 1997). The last legitimate government of Somalia was overthrown in 1991, and since then, Somalia has been plagued by anarchy and competing interests (Marchal, Mubarak, Del Buono, & Manzolillo 2000).

Initially, globalization came slowly to Somalia due to low rates of urbanization and low exposure to global trends. Globalization and trade practices eventually affected Somalia, which became a pawn in East-West relations (Patman, 2007). The United States prevailed over Soviet Union (USSR) absolutism and promoted the process of globalization in the 1980s (Patman, 2007). In 1992, the combination of constant civil war and drought resulted in the death of an estimated 300,000 Somalis. This episode was a pivotal event in shaping the post-Cold War security environment. Civil conflicts from weakened or failed states were now the main threat to world order. Somalia moved from being a Cold War pawn to being a new threat to world order because it was now a failed state (Patman, 2007).

After global trends led to detente between the USSR and the United States, Somalia was of less strategic importance. This caused the withdrawal of support by the USSR, which was followed by humanitarian aid by the United States. A series of insurrections began to plague the country (Marchal et al., 2000). In 1990, Siad Barre's government collapsed and civil war ensued. Former patrons of Somalia had supplied massive amounts of weaponry and this contributed to the violent warfare and banditry experienced during 1991–1992 (Marchal et al., 2000). Inter-clan warfare, amassing of personal wealth by corruption, abuse of power, and repression led to a deep distrust of government.

The United Nations (UN) intervention in Somalia from 1992 to 1995 resulted in a new influx of foreigners who worked in commerce or aid programs and brought with them a new and rapid globalization phase (Marchal et al., 2000). Globalization made the civil war more apparent in the media and the international community was able to respond to security challenges largely determined by the stance of the United States (Mac Donald, Patman, & Mason-Parker, 2007). However, the civil war and concomitant economic degradation had left Somalia in a more vulnerable position.

The global market imposed economic realities that dominated national policy and the wishes of Somali citizens (Marchal et al., 2000). The loss of sovereignty made Somalia vulnerable to issues such as illegal fishing, toxic waste dumping, undetonated landmines, and illegitimate banknote printing (Marchal et al., 2000). Additionally, the physical environment had been degraded by war, infrastructure has collapsed, and civil war had ensued (Marchal et al., 2000). Thousands of Somalis had fled their war-torn homeland and settled in refugee camps in Kenya and other neighboring countries. Many Somalis were forced to spend 10 or more years in the refugee camps while awaiting placement in various European countries, Canada, or the United States. While the environment of refugee camps offered invaluable support from family and friends; poverty, hunger, illness, exposure to violence, and lack of access to formal education, judicial systems, and unreliable access to health care made the transition to a host country for many individuals particularly challenging. Healthcare interactions with Somali clients should be viewed in that context.

SOMALIS IN THE UNITED STATES

Although the exact number of Somalis in the United States is difficult to determine, conservative estimates suggest that Somalis constitute the largest African-born Muslim group in the United States. Homeland Security indicates that between 20,000 and 30,000 Somalis immigrated to the United States from 2004 to 2006 (Homeland Security, 2007). Other sources suggest that over 50,000 Somalis fled their homeland and settled in the United States during the past decade alone (Hoefer, Rytina, & Campbell, 2006). Currently, roughly 20,000 Somali immigrants reside in the Minneapolis metropolitan area. Seattle is the second-largest Somali community with approximately 12,000 to 13,000 members. Chicago, Illinois and Columbus, Ohio follow with approximately 10,000 each (Cultural Orientation Resource Center, 2008). Smaller groups of Somalis have settled throughout the country.

Somali refugees have migrated most often because of the forces of globalization, yet upon arrival to a new country, they have too often faced xenophobia and outright discrimination (Byng, 2008). Considering the potential categories of difference between many Western healthcare providers and Somali individuals helps to illuminate the way in which the unacknowledged privilege of the healthcare provider may adversely affect the clinical encounter with a Somali individual (Narruhn & Schellenberg, 2013). Healthcare providers can provide patient and family centered care, use the premises of cultural safety, and use reflective practice as tools to counteract the manifestation of privilege. Additionally, using a more relational approach and noting the similarities in goals and humanity may assist in establishing a mutual rapport.

Significance

Several authors (Callister, 2001; Enang et al., 2002; Padela, Killawi, Forman, Demonner, & Heisler, 2012), and the National Institutes of Health (NIH), National Institute on Minority Health and Health Disparities (NIMHD), and the National Institute of Nursing Research (NINR) (2006) have long identified culturally competent care a national healthcare priority. This chapter is intended to serve as a resource guide for healthcare professionals caring for Somali clients during the perinatal period. Information presented should be used cautiously as it may not reflect the values and beliefs of the entire Somali population. While the knowledge of historical, cultural, and religious contexts can be very helpful to providing excellent care, every Somali client should be treated as a unique individual with a potentially unique set of values, beliefs, and care needs.

HEALTH AND ILLNESS

The majority of Somalis consider both wellness and illness as coming from God (Allah). They tend to seek a cure for any illness that afflicts them by using Western health care, alternative treatments, or both. If they are cured, they take it as God's will. If not, they consider it as part of God's plan and accept it with humility (Pavlish, Noor, & Brandt, 2010). Although Somalis are quite open to receiving conventional medical care, they have some healthcare restrictions based on their religious beliefs. For example, a hospitalized patient may refuse to eat pork, because it is against Islam or be treated for constipation with docusate sodium (Colace), because it contains gelatin derived from the collagen inside animals' skin and bones. Providers can play an important role in helping Somali patients to identify foods and treatment alternatives that are not offensive to their religious beliefs and, to facilitate recovery, encourage families to bring ethnic foods from home (Parve & Kaul, 2011).

For the majority of Somalis, prayer is considered a healing practice. Many people believe that a religious leader's (Imam) reciting Qur'an over the patient is one of the most effective methods of promoting cure (Abdullahi, 2001). Patients should therefore be informed of their right to receive visits from an Imam and be asked if and when they require privacy for prayers. During the Muslim holy month of Ramadan, a holiday that changes dates each year based on the lunar calendar, Somalis fast from sunrise to sundown. Although the sick are excused from fasting by Islam, some patients may choose to observe fasting. Healthcare providers should offer treatment alternatives for these patients during Ramadan. For example, whenever possible, offer long-acting medications that can be taken once a day after sundown instead of short-acting medications.

Herbs and medicinal plants are the main source of healthy well-being of more than 50% of the Somali population, and in particular, nearly 100% of those in pastoral communities, which account of nearly 70% of the country's population (Abdullahi, 2001; Carroll et al., 2007; Iman-Adan, 2012). Many Somalis seek to acquire the extracts of these plants after settling in a new country. One of the most popular herbs, black seed, called *habad sowda* or *habad al-barakah* in Somali, is used to treat conditions ranging from the common cold to skin, stomach, and intestinal disorders. Black seed is believed to offer circulatory and immune system support and to maintain and improve overall health and well-being. It is said to be a remedy recommended by the Prophet Muhammad himself and many people believe it has healing power over every ailment but death. Recent research of the chemical components and traditional uses of black seed has confirmed its positive effects on health. The aqueous and oil extracts of black seed have been shown to possess antioxidant, antiinflammatory, anticancer, analgesic, and antimicrobial activities (Gali-Muhtasib, El-Naijar, & Schneider-Stock, 2006). Other popular herbs, include likke (pronounced lea'keah in Somali), used to treat high blood pressure, control diabetes, and treat generic and maternity pain. Likke is also used for healing of wounds and swollen parts of the body. Qurac (pronounced Qu ra' in Somali) is commonly used to stop bleeding and prevent or cure infections by wrapping its fresh bark on the bleeding part of the body. Dacar (aloe vera) (pronounced Da'ar in Somali) is widely used to treat red eye, improve eyesight, prevent malaria, and treat sunburn (Iman-Adan, 2012). Because of the many and diverse use of herbs in the Somali community, it is important to ask the client if they take any traditional herbs in addition to or instead of prescribed medications.

PERINATAL HEALTH OF SOMALI WOMEN: KEY HIGHLIGHTS

Disparities

Several studies document the inequitable reproductive disparities in the Somali community (Johnson, Reed, Hitti, & Batra, 2005; Salem, Flynn, Weaver, & Brost, 2011; Small et al., 2008; Merry, Small, Blondel, & Gagnon, 2013). Merry et al. (2013) conducted a systematic review and meta-analysis of the literature regarding Cesarean delivery rates in migrant populations in Western countries and found that migrant women have consistently different rates of Caesarean than receiving-country women. These researchers conclude that there are differential Cesarean section rates in immigrants compared to receiving-country women that are not yet explained and suggest that there is a need for research on the pathways to the increased Cesarean delivery rate for migrant women. Additional findings include: Somali mothers have a higher overall Cesarean delivery rate that was indicated by fetal distress and failed induction. The most cited reasons for higher Cesarean section in migrant populations was language/communication barriers, low socio-economic status (SES), poor maternal health, gestational diabetes/high BMI, feto-pelvic disproportion, and lack of prenatal care (Merry et al., 2013).

Disparate maternal and newborn health outcomes both at the local and global level include higher Cesarean delivery rates, postdatism, and adverse neonatal outcomes including higher rates of stillbirths in six post-migration countries (Small et al., 2008). In Washington State, first-time Somali mothers were more likely to have a Cesarean delivery than black or white women in a control group, respectively (Johnson et al., 2005). At the global level Somali women were more likely to have a Cesarean delivery than host country born women (Small et al., 2008).

Postdatism, a pregnancy that goes beyond 42 weeks, is more common in women from Somalia (Johnson et al., 2005). Compared with the host-country women in six post-migration countries, women from Somalia were less likely to give birth prematurely (Small et al., 2008); although it appears that preterm birth is increasing in this population as Somali women become acculturated in Western countries (Flynn, Foster, & Brost, 2011). The problem with high prevalence of postdatism, is that it is thought that an aging placenta is less able to support the needs of the fetus. There is some evidence that postdatism is a generational phenomenon; for example, Morken, Melve, and Skjaerven (2011) found that in Norway, a mother or a father who was the product of a post-date pregnancy was more likely to have a post-date pregnancy. How this relates to the postdatism in the Somali population and the safety of carrying a pregnancy post date is unknown. More research is clearly needed to examine factors related to ethnicity and environmental influences on postdatism.

In the Somali culture, norms concerning the number of children in a family are based on Islamic traditions. Children are considered a gift from God. Birth control and family planning are not widely practiced by Somali women. For many women, it is highly important to continue having children throughout their childbearing years (Malin & Gissler, 2009; Small et al., 2008). Many individuals value having many children in accordance with their religious beliefs. The organization WellShare uses the concept of "child spacing" that promotes preconception care to improve birth outcomes and may be more culturally congruent (WellShare, 2010). Research conducted in European countries consistently suggests that Somali women feel different, misunderstood, and vulnerable in their encounters with the healthcare personnel after immigrating to a new country because of their desire to have many children. For this reason, many delay prenatal care to avoid negative encounters with providers (Berggren, Bergstrom, & Edberg, 2006; Hill, Hunt, & Hyrkas, 2012; Vangen, Johansen, Sundby, Traeen, & Stray-Pederson, 2004).

Research conducted in the United States produced somewhat inconsistent findings. Several U.S.-based studies (Johnson et al., 2008; Wojnar, 2011) produced findings consistent with European reports. Other reports suggest that Somali women are satisfied with their care during the perinatal period and appreciate the respect shown by healthcare professionals regarding their reproductive choices (Gurnah, Khoshnood, Bradley, & Yuan, 2011). Narruhn (2008) suggests that for many Somalis, the benefit of prenatal care or testing may not be apparent because few women were accustomed to receiving preventive care in their homeland. Hence, they may intentionally delay their first visit with a midwife or obstetrician for fear that unnecessary testing will be performed (Narruhn, 2008). Likewise, Hill et al. (2012) reported that many Somali women don't seek prenatal care as long as everything appears "normal" in pregnancy to avoid unnecessary testing that may interfere with natural childbirth. It is therefore important to discuss the benefits of prenatal care and screening, acknowledge concerns, and respect the patients' decisions.

Communication

Effective verbal communication and understanding nonverbal social cues is invaluable when providing care to Somali clients. Somali women may speak with a soft voice, ask few questions, and avoid direct eye contact with the provider and other members of the healthcare team. They may be eager to shake hands with a female provider but not with a male. This is a sign of modesty, not disrespect (Wojnar, 2011).

A husband/partner, who is widely considered the head of a household in the Somali culture, may act as the spokesperson for his wife. When confronted with important healthcare decisions many women from Somalia use a relational type of autonomy that is congruent with the more communitarian style of decision making, than with that of many Western healthcare providers (Narruhn & Schellenberg, 2013). It is important to respect the patient and her husband/partner's wishes and provide a qualified health interpreter to ensure accuracy of understanding between the practitioner and the woman and her husband/partner (Hill et al., 2012). Honoring women's choices and keeping communication lines open is imperative to building trust and improving pregnancy outcomes for this population of women (Dundek, 2006; Johnson et al., 2005; Vangen et al., 2004). Considering the potential categories of difference between many Western healthcare providers and Somali individuals helps illuminate the way in which the unacknowledged privilege of healthcare provider may adversely affect the clinical encounter between the Somali individual and the healthcare provider (Narruhn & Schellenberg, 2013). Healthcare providers can provide patient and family centered care, use the premises of cultural safety, and use reflective practice as tools to counteract the manifestation of privilege. Additionally, using a more relational approach and noting the similarities in goals and humanity may assist in establishing a mutual rapport.

Although receiving care from a male provider is not prohibited, it is strongly preferred that a pregnant woman receives care from a female provider and, if necessary, interpretation services from a female interpreter. The modesty of women must be considered at all times. Only the necessary body parts should be exposed for procedures (Enang et al., 2002). If a male provider is present during the exam, the patient may want to keep her head covered with a scarf to maintain modesty. The patient may have several support persons present at all times during hospitalization or at an outpatient appointment. If male family members, including the husband, accompany the patient to hospital, they may prefer to leave the room when direct care is provided. It is a sign of respect for the woman that may be mistaken as indifference. Male providers who are not conducting the exam may want to demonstrate the same culturally accepted sign of respect. It is therefore important to check with the patient whom she wishes to be present in the room during the assessments or procedures to avoid incorrect assumptions.

Prenatal Care

Because many Somalis had no access to the conveniences of formal health care while growing up in Somalia or refugee camps, prenatal care and education regarding women's physical health, nutritional needs during pregnancy and lactation, home safety, as well as self- and infant care are essential for this population of women. Healthcare providers should be aware that female genital cutting (FGC), performed on over 90% of Somali girls in their home country, and is a taboo topic in the Somali community. It is imperative that providers who care for a woman with FGC become familiar with the types of FGC and related health risks, and establish trusting relationship before they have a conversation about FGC with their client (Ahmed & Abushama, 2005). Neglecting to learn how to properly care for a woman with FGC may lead to adverse birth outcomes, including unnecessary Cesarean section, prolonged second stage of labor, and low Apgar scores (Vangen, Johansen, Sandby, Traen, & Stray-Pedersen, 2004).

Findings of recent qualitative research (Wojnar, 2011) suggest that perinatal experiences of Somali clients may be improved by establishing a trusting relationship, seeking to understand women's perspectives, acknowledging concerns, increasing patient knowledge about pregnancy and childbirth care in the American healthcare system, and respecting decisions that may not be congruent with the provider's beliefs. Participants (15 women and 11 men) in Wojnar's (2011) study consistently expressed a desire for a trusting relationship and good communication with the provider, as well as prenatal education offered to both genders that is culturally acceptable. Participants described the ideal physical environment for prenatal classes as one that offers separate spaces for women and men and is free of anatomical figures and drawings that can be seen as offensive to Muslim religion. They also expressed desire for on-site interpretation services and daycare facilities for older children. Consistent with prior reports (Herrel et al., 2004; Narruhn, 2008) all study participants expressed anxiety with regard to Cesarean delivery. They feared severe complications such as hysterectomy or even death. Thus, Narruhn (2008) recommends assessing of women's knowledge and discussing the range of indications as well as associated risks, well in advance of childbirth.

Key points to consider:

- Prenatal care offers the opportunity to address nutritional needs during pregnancy and lactation and self- and infant care.
- Patients should be offered anticipatory guidance, encouraged to ask questions, and develop a birth plan to communicate their wishes and desires for childbirth and post-natal care.
- Prenatal classes should be offered to both genders in a culturally appropriate environment.
- A trusting relationship must be developed for a woman to feel open to discuss FGC with a healthcare professional.
- Providers must learn how to safely assist with vaginal birth for a woman with FGC.
- Neglect of FGC may lead to adverse birth outcomes including unnecessary Cesarean section, prolonged second stage of labor, and low Apgar scores.
- Reconstructive surgery to alleviate or minimize the bodily damages caused by FGC is a taboo topic in the Somali community.
- It is acceptable to raise the topic of reconstructive surgery with a woman who has experienced considerable perineal damage post-FGC, once a trusting relationship is established.
- Women with extensive FGC must be assured that the conversation and the surgery, if so desired, will be kept in strictest confidentiality.

Labor and Delivery

The quality of care provided during labor and delivery is of great importance in every culture. For Somali immigrants, the situation is such that laboring women may meet with the Western healthcare system and its institutional culture and practices for the first time. When labor and delivery care is provided to Somali women, several social, psychological, and biological factors need to be considered.

First, it is apparent that many Somali have high parity and thus, have more pregnancy and birth-related risk factors than women with fewer pregnancies (Parve & Kaul, 2011). A Somali patient may be conservative when making decisions about using common western treatments during labor such as induction of labor or epidural analgesia for pain in fear of interfering with the natural labor process that may result in Cesarean section (Herrel et al., 2004).

Pain Control

The concept of pain and pain expression during labor has different meanings for women from different cultures. Women may experience labor pain in varied degrees of intensity which is influenced by physiological, psychosocial, and cultural factors (Callister, Khalaf,

Semenic, Kartchner, & Vehvilainen-Julkunen, 2003). Research suggests that poor pain management in childbirth may result from the caregiver's inability to accurately assess patient's pain, miscommunication, or beliefs about cultural norms regarding the experience and expression of pain among various ethnic groups. Finnstrom and Soderhamn (2006) note that in the Somali language the word for *pain* is the same as the word used for *illness*. They argue that the different meanings of the word may complicate pain assessment and lead to inadequate treatment during labor. Others (Ness, 2009) suggest that some Somali women may be stoic about pain to demonstrate their overall acceptance of the pain and suffering in life. Moreover, women in Wojnar's (2011) study recalled fear of epidural analgesia to treat labor pain in order to prevent stalling of labor, Cesarean section, and chronic pain. The majority ($n = 9$) preferred traditional methods of pain control such as support of family and friends, herbal remedies, walking, frequent position changes, and prayer. Consistent with prior research (Dundek, 2006), some women in Wojnar's study expressed doula support as an appropriate method of coping with pain in labor ($n = 4$), while others ($n = 2$) were enthusiastic about receiving epidural analgesia in labor.

Key points to consider:

- Discuss pain management in labor prenatally.
- Use qualified interpreter to communicate about pain as needed.
- Don't assume that the woman is not in pain or doesn't want epidural just because she copes with pain in silence.
- Offer and support culturally accepted forms of pain relief.
- Assess for pain frequently.

Postpartum Care Needs

Somali women are highly regarded in Somali society for their roles as mothers. The woman's need for rest during the postpartum period is recognized and supported by other women in the family and community. Other women in the family take over household duties and care for older children while the postpartum woman is encouraged to rest, eat nutritious foods, and breastfeed her newborn. Many women in the Somali community are less available to provide support for new mothers because of employment obligations due to changes in the traditional social structure that came with immigration. Postpartum women stay at home and refrain from sexual activity for 40 days. At the end of 40 days, there is a celebration at the house of a relative or friends. This typically marks the first time the baby and mother have left home since delivery. Participants in the Wojnar's (2011) study were consistently nostalgic about the "40-days rule," and the care and support they received from others from their homeland during the postpartum period.

They expressed dissatisfaction with having to provide newborn care right from birth and not being able to rest.

Nearly 98% of women in Somalia initiate breastfeeding and many breastfeed for extended periods of time (Dundek, 2006). When the newborn is awake but not breastfeeding, other women take care of the baby to facilitate the mother's rest. Many women from Somalia do not practice exclusive breastfeeding because of concerns about malnutrition. Ironically, the best practice to alleviate malnutrition according to UNICEF is exclusive breastfeeding. Some women in Wojnar's (2011) study desired to "top up" their breastfed newborns with formula to make them sleep longer and thereby get adequate rest. Healthcare professionals should discuss the risks of mixed (breast and formula) feedings prenatally and talk about ways to facilitate maternal rest with the baby.

Key points to consider:

• Acknowledge the absence of postpartum support typical in Somali culture.
• Offer support in hospital similar to the support Somali women are accustomed to during the postpartum period.
• Encourage family members and friends to visit and participate in the postpartum care of the mother and newborn.
• Discuss the risks of mixed feedings (breast and formula) prenatally to help the women make informed choices about infant feeding and care during the postpartum period.
• Encourage doula support.

Death, Pregnancy Termination, and Miscarriage

In the Somali culture, consistent with the Islamic tradition, death is considered a natural part of the life cycle. *Inshallah,* which means in the Somali language "by Allah's will" suggests that everything happens according to God's plan. There is a deeply shared belief that the afterlife in paradise is quite pleasant, which helps the bereaved family with the grieving process. Traditional death rites include the reading of the Quran at the time of death and burial. Typically, the body is bathed, laid out straight, perfumed, and is often wrapped in a white cloth. Consistent with the Islamic religion, it is important that the body is buried within 24 hours after death (Roble, 2008). For many, an equally important consideration of burial is given to a body part that is lost, for example, during surgery. Some women and men in Wojnar's (2011) study expressed fears about the possibility of hysterectomy during complicated childbirth and equal distress about not being able to take the uterus home for proper burial.

Because children are considered a gift from God, Somali women don't terminate pregnancy voluntarily. One report about birth and infant mortality rates in Somalia (Omar, Hogberg, & Bergstrom, 1994) suggested that over 65% of women over the age of 45 years had six or more births, 33% had at least one miscarriage, and 20% had at least one stillbirth, while 80% of Somali women have experienced the death of at least one child (Omar et al., 1994). In spite the high neonatal mortality rates, women in Wojnar's (2011) study talked about losing their children in pregnancy, childbirth, and infancy calmly, explaining that miscarriage, fetal demise, and neonatal death are the will of God. One woman explained: "Children are gift from Allah and Allah can take them if he wishes." Hence, Somali women typically deal with the loss of a child with stoicism and deep faith that the child is in a better place and that they, as a mother, will be rewarded with more happiness for enduring the pain of losing a child.

Key points to consider:

- Having perinatal loss for Somali women and men represents the will of God.
- They grieve the loss of their child deeply but express it stoically to demonstrate their faith in God.
- Healthcare professionals caring for Somali families who are experiencing perinatal loss should recognize that the stoic acceptance of loss is not an expression of indifference but rather a deep faith that the child has gone to a better place prepared for him or her by God.

FREQUENTLY EATEN FOOD CHOICES

Halal Diet

Somali cuisine varies from region to region and is a mixture of traditional, native dishes and foreign-influenced cuisine. But all Somali foods are *halal*. In Arabic, the word *halal* means permitted or lawful under Islamic dietary guidelines. According to these guidelines from the Qu'ran, Muslim followers cannot consume the following foods:

- Pork or pork byproducts
- Animals that were dead prior to butchering
- Animals not slaughtered properly or not slaughtered in the name of Allah
- Blood and blood byproducts

Tea/Chai

Guests to any Somali home are offered spiced tea, known as *shaah hawash*. Strong black tea leaves, preferably from Kenya or southern India, are typically infused in a large metal kettle called a *kildhi*. Almost every tea/chai recipe includes ginger, cinnamon, cloves, a pinch of sugar, black tea, and milk (preferably goat milk). All of these are considered healthy ingredients. The various ingredients are introduced one into the boiling water one after another with the tea leaves going in first. Sugar is also added directly to the boiling infusion along with the milk. Somali tea/chai is a combination of spices with tea and milk that makes a delicious, healthy beverage. The tea is served hot and it is a drink of choice for women during the postpartum period.

Diet During Pregnancy and Postpartum

Traditionally, during pregnancy, Somali women tend to decrease the size of their meals to promote an easier delivery and to prevent Cesarean section. The diet usually improves during the third trimester but even then small meals are consumed. Most women do not take prenatal vitamins even when vitamins are prescribed because they see it as an intervention that may disturb the normal pregnancy process. Women believe that sufficient vitamins can be obtained from a regular diet.

Postpartum Practices

The common diet during the postpartum period is *sorghum*—porridge with butter and sugar—milk and meat. The meat is boiled with onions, potatoes, cabbage, and tomatoes, and served as a meat soup. Sometimes meat is cut into small pieces and cooked in butter and aromatic herbs. For special occasions, such as the birth of a baby, dried meat may be fried in butter and offered to family and guests.

REFERENCES

Abdullahi, M. D. (2001). *Culture and customs of Somalia.* Westport, CT: Greenwood Press.

Ahmed, B., & Abushama, M. (2005). Female genital mutilation and childbirth. *Saudi Medical Journal, 26*(3), 376–378.

Berggren, V., Bergstrom, S., & Edberg, A. K. (2006). Being different and vulnerable: Experiences of immigrant African women who have been circumcised and sought maternity care in Sweden. *Journal of Transcultural Nursing, 17*(1), 50–57.

Byng, M. D. (2008). Complex inequalities: The case of Muslim Americans after 9/11. *American Behavioral Scientist, 51*(5), 659–674.

Callister, L. (2001). Culturally competent care of women and newborns: Knowledge, attitude, and skills. *Journal of Obstetrical Gynecologic and Neonatal Nursing, 30*(2), 209–215.

Callister, L., Khalaf, I., Semenic, S., Kartchner, R., & Vehvilainen-Julkunen, K. (2003). The pain of childbirth: Perceptions of culturally diverse women. *Pain Management Nursing, 4*(4), 145–154.

Carroll, J., Epstein, R., Fiscella, K., Volpe, E., Diaz, K., & Omar, S. (2007). Knowledge and beliefs about health and preventive health among Somali women in the United States. *Health Care for Women International, 28*(4), 360–380.

Chossudovsky, M. (1997). *The globalization of poverty and the new world order.* Pincourt, Quebec: Center for Research on Globalization.

Cultural Orientation Resource Center. (2008). US refugee program statistics. Retrieved from http://www.cal.org/refugee/statistics/index.html

Dundek, L. H. (2006). Establishment of a Somali doula program at a large metropolitan hospital. *Journal of Perinatal and Neonatal Nursing, 20*(2), 128–137.

Enang, J., Wojnar, D., & Harper, F. (2002). Childbearing among diverse populations: How one hospital is providing multicultural care. *Lifelines* 4(5), 153–158.

Finnstrom, B., & Soderhamn, O. (2006). Conceptions of pain among Somali women. *Journal of Advanced Nursing 54*(4), 418–425.

Flynn P., Foster E. M., & Brost, B. (2011). Indicators of acculturation related to Somali refugee women's birth outcomes in Minnesota. *Journal of Immigrant Minority Health, 13,* 224–31.

Gali-Muhtasib, H., El-Naijar, N., & Schneider-Stock, R. (2006). The medicinal potential of black seed (Nigella sativa) and its components. *Advances in Phytomedicine, 2,* 133–153.

Gurnah, K., Khoshnood, K., Bradley, E., & Yuan, C. (2011). "They get a c-section ... they gonna to die": Somali women's fears of obstetrical interventions in the United States. *Journal of Midwifery and Women's Health, 56*(4), 340–346.

Herrel, N., Olevitch, L., DuBois, D. K., Terry, P., Thorp, D., Kind, E., & Said, A. (2004). Somali refugee women speak out about their needs for care during pregnancy and delivery. *Journal of Midwifery and Women's Health, 49,* 345–349.

Hill, N., Hunt, E., & Hyrkas, K. (2012). Somali immigrant women's health care experiences and beliefs regarding pregnancy and birth in the United States. *Journal of Transcultural Nursing, 23*(1), 72–81.

Hoefer, M., Rytina, N., & Campbell, C. (2006). Estimates of the unauthorized immigrant population residing in the United States: January 2006. *DHS Office of Immigration Statistics,* 1–6.

Homeland Security. (2007). *Refuges and asylees: 2007—US Department of Homeland Security,* retrieved from www.dhs.gov/xlibrary/assets/statistics/.../ois_rfa_fr_2007.pdf

Iman-Adan, M. (2012). Herbal medicinal plants in Somalia. Retrieved from http://www.keydmedia .net/en/article/article/herbal_medical_plants_in_somalia_-_part._3

Johnson, C., Shipp, M., Ali, S., Mues, K., Bashir, S., & Forman, J. (2008). *Barriers to reproductive health care use among Somali immigrants with female genital cutting.* Abstract: American Congress of Obstetricians and Gynecologists (ACOG): Annual Clinical Meeting.

Johnson, E., Reed, S., Hitti, J., & Batra, M. (2005). Increased risk of adverse pregnancy outcome among Somali immigrants in Washington State. *American Journal of Obstetrics & Gynecology, 193*(2), 475–482.

Mac Donald, D., Patman, R. & Mason-Parker, B. (2007). The Ethics of Foreign Policy. Burlington, VT: Ashgate Publishing Co.

Malin, M., & Gissler, M. (2009). Maternal care and birth outcomes among ethnic minority women in Finland, *BMC Public Health, 20*(9), 84.

Marchal, R., Mubarak, J., Del Buono, M., & Manzolillo, D. L. (2000). *Globalization and its impact on Somalia.* United Nations Development Programme (UNDP)/United Nations Documentation Office for Somalia: Nairobi. Retrieved from http://www.reliefweb.int/rw/rwb.nsf/AllDocsByUNID/ e715f9667b301a1fc125689c004b547c

Merry, L., Small, R., Blondel, B. & Gagnon, A. (2013). International migration and Caesarian birth: A systematic review and meta-analysis. *BMC Preganncy and Childbirth, 30,* 13–27.

Morken, N., Melve, K., & and Skjaerven, R. (2011). Recurrence of prolonged and post-term gestational age across generations: maternal and paternal contribution. *British Journal of Obstetrics and Gynecology, 118.*

Narruhn, R. A. (2008). *Perinatal profile for women from Somalia.* Retrieved from http://ethnomed .org/clinical/mother-and-infant-care/perinatal-profile-for-patients-from-somalia

Narruhn, R., & Schellenberg, I. R. (2013). Caring ethics and a Somali reproductive dilemma. *Nursing Ethics, 20*(4), 366–381.

National Institutes of Health (NIH), National Institute on Minority Health and Health Disparities (NIMHD), and the National Institute of Nursing Research (NINR). (2006). *Examining the health disparities research plan of the National Institutes of Health: Unfinished business.* Washington, DC: National Academies Press.

Ness, S. (2009). Pain expression in the perioperative period: Insights from a focus group of Somali women. *Pain Management in Nursing, 10*(2), 65–75.

Omar, M. M., Hogberg, U., & Bergstrom, B. (1994). Fertility, infertility and child survival of Somali women. *Scandinavian Journal of Social Medicine, 22*(3), 194–200.

Padela, A. I., Killawi, A., Forman, J., Demonner, S., & Heisler, M. (2012). American Muslim perceptions of healing: Key agents in healing and their roles. *Qualitative Health Research, 22*(6), 846–858.

Parve, J., & Kaul, T. (2011). Clinical issues in refugee healthcare: The Somali Bantu population. *The Nurse Practitioner, 36*(7), 48–53.

Patman, R. G. (2007). *Globalization, the demise of the cold war, and the disintegration of the Somali state.* Paper presented at the annual meeting of The International Studies Association 48th Annual Convention, Chicago, IL. Retrieved from http://www.allacademic.com/meta/p178461_ index.html

Pavlish, C. L., Noor, S., & Brandt, J. (2010). Somali immigrant women and the American health care system: Discordant beliefs, divergent expectations, and silent worries. *Social Science and Medicine, 71*(2), 353–361.

Roble, M. A. (2008). *Somali funeral traditions.* Retrieved from http://ethnomed.org/clinical/ end-of-life/somali-funeral-traditions

Salem, W., Flynn, P., Weaver, A., & Brost, B. (2011). Fertility after cesarean delivery among Somali-Born women resident in the USA. *Journal of Immigrant Minority Health, 13*(3), 494–499.

Small, R., Gagnon, A., Gissler, M., Zeitlin, J., Bennis, M., Glazier, R., ... Vangen, S. (2008). Somali women and their pregnancy outcomes post emigration: Data from six receiving countries. *An International Journal of Obstetrics and Gynecology, 115*(13), 1630–1640.

Vangen, S., Johansen, R. E., Sundby, J., Traeen, B., & Stray-Pedersen, B. (2004). Qualitative study of perinatal care experiences among Somali women and local health care professionals in Norway. *European Journal of Obstetrics, Gynecology and Reproductive Biology, 112,* 29–35.

WellShare. (2010). Why Childspacing? Retrieved from http://www.wellshareinternational.org/ why-child-spacing

Wojnar, D. (2011). *Perinatal care needs of first generation Somali immigrants in the USA.* Abstract: Western Institute of Nursing, Communicating Nursing Research Conference: Portland, OR.

Chapter 19

Navy Nurses: Vulnerable People Caring for Vulnerable Populations

Captain (Retired) Mary Anne White

OBJECTIVES

At the end of this chapter, the reader will be able to

1. Describe the work of Navy nurses and how they are vulnerable.
2. Compare and contrast the issues related to Navy nurses working in high-risk areas versus nurses in other types of disaster conditions.
3. Identify a researchable problem that involves military nurses based on the chapter.

INTRODUCTION

Imagine the vulnerability of a wife and mother of two keeping her ready bag packed in the corner and waiting for the phone to ring, bringing news as to where she will be sent in support of the war that just began in Kuwait. This takes little imagination for the writer, as it was her experience as a Navy Reserve nurse during Operation Desert Storm. Nurse Corps officers in the Navy Reserves face unique challenges as they balance their military obligations with the many competing priorities imposed by their civilian careers. They could be considered vulnerable due to their multifaceted circumstances. Their stories of providing care whenever and wherever called upon beautifully illustrate several of key concepts proposed by de Chesnay and Anderson (2008) to be particularly useful in caring for people who are vulnerable: cultural competence, resilience, and advocacy.

To appreciate these accounts, it is critical to understand more fully Navy nursing and how it differs from its civilian counterpart. Therefore, these stories will be preceded with an overview of nursing in the Navy to enhance the reader's understanding. Vignettes will then be provided as vivid examples of how these nurses have applied their skills in caring for vulnerable people in an array of global environments: deployed to war in Afghanistan, aboard the U.S. hospital ship USNS Comfort (T-AH 20) during humanitarian relief in Haiti, and in medical centers in the United States and in Europe. All of the vignettes are slices from the lives of these Reserve officers.

NAVY NURSING

Mission

Each Navy Nurse Corps officer begins a career in the Navy by taking a statutory oath of office. This promise and covenant is made to the nation: "to support and defend the Constitution of the United States, against all enemies foreign and domestic." The oath implies an affirmation of the officer to be ready to deploy anytime, anywhere to meet the mission. The Navy medicine mission is constantly changing in response to evolving world events and politics. Humanitarian missions to Haiti following a devastating earthquake, wartime deployments to Iraq, nation building in Afghanistan, or counterterrorism in the horn of Africa are to name but a few of these operations. To meet these missions, Navy nurses provide nursing care beyond the scope of traditional care, treating vulnerable individuals and populations worldwide. Their career journey includes many experiences beyond the confines of a brick-and-mortar hospital or clinic.

Clinical Competence

The Navy nurse must be clinically competent to serve in hospitals, the operational theater, on humanitarian missions, and in joint environments. The global geographic environment in which these nurses serve creates the need for them to be multitalented, with cross-training for skills in disaster nursing. Disparate circumstances necessitate a certain amount of expertise in pediatrics, obstetrics, and nonbattle disease processes. Both clinical and cultural competences are essential for them to meet the healthcare needs they will encounter on their diverse assignments.

Reserve Nurses

Nurses in the Reserves have a parallel mission. They must be clinically competent in all these arenas, yet they may not necessarily perform these skills in their civilian role. They must also be ready to perform these clinical duties immediately upon recall for a mission, often with short notice. Moreover, these nurses must accomplish their clinical and operational training on a part-time basis—that is, 1 weekend per month and 2 weeks per year.

Additionally, as mentioned earlier, they face multiple challenges as they balance their military obligations with the many competing priorities imposed by their home life and civilian career. These struggles are encapsulated in one Reserve nurse officer's conclusion that being mobilized for an active-duty assignment would actually simplify her life:

> *I believe that the most difficult challenges for a reservist is that full-time active personnel fail to recognize that we do not work just 1 weekend a month and 2 weeks a year. For the most part we all have full-time jobs—plus our military commitment, family obligations, and general-life errands and tasks. Time is of the essence and requires much organization to make all this work. This allows for just 6 days off a month to manage family plus [run] errands plus [take] personal time—not to mention the time spent preparing for a drill weekend (paperwork, courses, and presentations that are a part of our weekend). I, for one, would like to have this remembered, recognized, and appreciated. Being mobilized greatly simplified time management.*

VIGNETTES

Deployed to War

Currently, Navy nurses are serving in the Iraq and Afghanistan war zones. Such a wartime mission requires evacuating the injured from the battlefield, sending the severely injured on for higher levels of definitive care, and returning the less injured to duty as soon as possible. These nurses are providing care for their own forces as well as for forces of other coalition countries, local civilians caught in the crossfire of war, and insurgents brought for care (Wynd, 2006).

This Reserve nurse's story is about caring for children caught in the chaos of war in Afghanistan:

> *One day in early October, a group of children, including two little Afghan girls, went out to play in their village, as I'm sure they had done many times before. One child stepped the wrong way, and in a split second her life was changed forever. An improvised explosive device (IED) planted by their countrymen to kill and maim the enemy had blown up two of their own innocent girls. The girls were related to each other. One was approximately 8 years old and the other 4 years old (they don't celebrate birthdays in Afghanistan). I can't use their real names, so I will call the older girl Grace and the younger one Hope.*

The nurse then recounted caring for Grace and explained how hope was instilled in the midst of pain:

> *Grace had abdominal surgery to remove shrapnel that was blown into her little belly. She survived her surgery and did quite well. Once she could breathe on her own and was stable, she was moved to the acute care ward, where she recovered for several weeks. She was incredibly stoic and never smiled at first. Our staff of nurses and corpsmen worked tirelessly to break through that wall of fear, confusion, and mistrust. She had to endure some painful dressing changes and the usual post-op pain associated with the type of surgery she had undergone.*
>
> *One day, one young female corpsman broke down the wall, and it was the beginning of a joy-filled relationship with the ward staff. Each day she became stronger and bolder in her interactions with us. Initially, she would reluctantly hold hands. Eventually her interactions expanded to the point of hugs for everyone. She*

enjoyed being carried around by the female staff and sitting on our laps as we did our work. Her smile lit up the ward and she became quite the popular young lady. She remained with us long after her recovery time because she had to wait for her cousin to work through her ongoing problems.

Her saga continued, as Grace's advocate worked closely with the father who would soon provide the child's care:

Hope is younger and smaller than Grace, and so the explosion caused her to suffer a severe head injury. The trauma team was not sure that she would survive at all, and if she did, what her quality of life would be. It is a harsh world in the villages here if you have any sort of physical disability, and chances for survival are slim.

Hope survived her initial brain surgery and went to the ICU. She was in critical condition for a long time. After several days, the decision was made to remove her breathing tube. She was able to breathe on her on own. She clearly had significant brain damage and the outlook was grim. She came to the ward for ongoing therapy and care. Her father was at her bedside throughout her hospitalization. We worked hard to get Hope to overcome her brain injury. It still didn't look good. There are no rehab centers in Afghanistan … no brain injury units … no Bryn Mawr rehabs! This little girl had a significant brain injury and had the front part of her skull removed and sewn into her abdomen for replacement later. We finally had to face the reality that this child could not survive outside of our hospital.

We had a tearful conference with the doctors and nurses and the father. It was decided that we would pull her feeding tube and see if we could get Grace to swallow any liquids or foods. Slowly, she began to swallow her own secretions, and then we were able to give her some liquids through a syringe. We taught her father how to feed her and he did a great job. Thanks to some timely donations of Jell-o, applesauce, and Pediacare formula, we advanced her diet ever so slowly and things were looking up. Hope was beginning to move her left side and already had full use of her right side. She was whispering words but nothing that made any sense. She cried every time we looked at her, let alone changed her bandages, but we could get the occasional smile.

The officer concludes with an acknowledgment of respect for all of her patients, regardless of their differences:

I was not prepared to care for the children who are victims of this war. It is not an easy balance to deliver First World care in a Third World nation. We treat all lives here as sacred and provide the finest care to all who land on our doorstep.

During wartime, nurses work in hostile environments, often in harm's way.

Humanitarian Mission

Peacekeeping, nation building, and humanitarian missions throughout the world are often additional Navy assignments. These missions may take the form of a planned medical readiness and training exercise (MEDRETE) or they may occur in response to a natural disaster, as in the deployment of the USNS Comfort. Navy Reserve nurses involved in these humanitarian activities provide medical assistance to host nations ranging from "sick call" services to assisting in advanced surgical procedures. In these missions, it is necessary to have an understanding of the country and area-specific endemic diseases. Language barriers are also a concern, so all missions require medically trained translators.

A Reserve Nurse Corps officer who volunteered to go on the Comfort to Haiti recalled:

I am extremely proud of my career as an officer in the Navy Nurse Corps. Part of the joy of being a Navy nurse has been the opportunity to serve on many different platforms, more so than my civilian counterparts. As an adult critical care nurse, I have taken care of a variety of patients, including burn, trauma, and open-heart surgery patients as well as many others. When the earthquake hit Haiti on 12 January 2010, I felt that I had to be there and had to use my experience to help take care of my people. (Etienne, 2010)

She continued:

As I reported to the very busy intensive care unit (ICU) for further instructions, I quickly realized that my close to 30 years' nursing experience was not enough to prepare me for what I would face. Wake-up call #1: There were many injured children fighting for their life in the ICU. My relationship with children is usually all about hugs and kisses, food, and fun activities. Reality #2: I was the only health professional in the ICU who understood and spoke Creole.

As I walked in the ICU that day, I was taken back by the cry of an 8-year-old boy. "I want my father! I cannot live without my father! I don't want anything except for my father!" The depth of sorrow expressed and the choice of words by this young boy would give you the impression that he was certain that he would not see his father again. Realizing that I was the only one who understood what he was saying, I was drawn to him to try to provide comfort. My offers for any comfort measures, like pain medicine, food, and liquid, were rejected by this child, who continued to repeat, "I don't want anything but my father!" I translated what was going on to the nurse who was taking care of him. (Etienne, 2010)

She recalls her role as advocate for her patients:

I was glad that I was useful the minute that I stepped foot onto the Comfort. I had many collateral duties during my month on the Comfort, and although many were unofficial, they were very necessary. I was a patient advocate for many, with limited understanding of their medical condition. As a member of the ethics committee, we discussed best approaches to challenging cases. As a Haitian American and a senior officer, I was sought after for guidance in special circumstances. I responded to codes when possible. I worked as a liaison promoting dialogue between the translators, the ICU, and medical staff. I made rounds on the wards to visit patients who were in the ICU. I guess that you can say I was a nurse by day and ethical/social support by night. (Etienne, 2010)

HOSPITAL MISSION

Much of military nursing in these settings is characterized by the independent and autonomous nature of the work. Military nurses are often the leaders of patient care teams and, therefore, must have management and organization skills.

This Reserve nurse worked in the operating room (OR) of a major military hospital in the United States during her weekend duty. She recalls:

One morning I was assessing a soldier who was having his tenth surgical procedure. He explained that no one was with him because his father had to go back to work in Pennsylvania. I immediately went into parent mode. What a difficult decision. Even though this young man, in his early 20s, was an adult, he was very vulnerable. He leg was still stabilized by an external fixation device. He was still unsure of his future due to the injury from the IED explosion to his leg. He shared that he hoped this would be his last surgery prior to being sent to a medical facility closer to home. We started talking about his hometown, and about that time the orthopedic resident walked up. The fact that our soldier and the resident had grown up in the same home town felt serendipitous. Although they hadn't attended the same high school, they were able to establish a bond that added to the caring environment.

I did get to speak with his father prior to the surgery. I know that it made me feel better that I was able to communicate our plan, answer his questions, and assure him that we would call him after the surgery to update him on his son's condition.

She continued with another encounter:

Despite my extensive experience in the OR, the greatest challenge was caring for a soldier from Texas who had, over a period of 3 month's lost all of his extremities. This patient was in the ICU on contact precautions due to the complexity of his injuries. We were going to be doing washouts and wound evacuation changes on three extremities.

We got our handoff from the ICU nurse and then went to meet the patient. He was awake. Introducing oneself and looking directly into the eyes of what had once been a strapping Marine was surreal in some ways. His eyes probed mine, and I felt an overwhelming need to say something profound that would somehow make things better. What I did was introduce myself, perform my safety check and assessment, and help transport him to the OR, thankful that the Versed had been given. The pictures on his bedside table showed him and his wife prior to his deployment. They were both smiling, as were the children in the pictures.

She concluded:

I remember what a Navy Nurse friend of mine returning from Landstuhl shared. She had a patient with a similar injury while serving in Germany. She put her heart and soul into a soldier who lost all of his extremities. She met the family and was able to share a love of horses with the patient over time. A few months after his transport stateside, she received a picture in the mail of this soldier riding a horse, held in place by a device made by his father. Life is amazing.

Another Reserve Nurse Corps officer mobilized to a hospital in Germany reported:

This has been my first deployment, as I am a "late-comer" to the Navy Nurse Corps. The team I work on is equally divided between Army, Navy, Air Force, and civilian nurses.

I would like to share one story with you that touched me during my stay here. A young officer was injured in an IED blast. His body was fine, but his head and face were badly injured, swollen, and disfigured, and he lost one eye. Through his time here (which was longer than usual, as he was Canadian), we became accustomed to his appearance so that he became normal to us. When it was time for him to leave us, we were rolling him out on the stretcher to return home. He stopped me and signed that he needed a blanket, so I ran back to the room. (He was unable to speak but could use sign language.) I wondered why he wanted the blanket and discovered that he was not asking for it for himself, but instead because he realized that he might be difficult to look at and wanted to prevent others from being upset by his appearance—so he had me cover his face. I was amazed. In his time of great pain, sacrifice, and illness, he took the time to think of others and their feelings.

I will tell you this is not an isolated incident but rather happens many, many times. Having the opportunity to provide care in Europe—I could never have imagined how wonderful it would be to serve our nation in Europe.

CONCLUSION

These personal accounts from nurses working as Reserve nurses on the battlefield, on the hospital ship, and in a hospital setting allow us to look into the reactions and concerns of nurses as they experience vulnerable individuals and populations. Their stories provide examples of cultural competence in nursing—that is, care that embraces the cultural differences that exist between the nurse and the patient while meeting the healthcare needs of culturally diverse patients. These nurses demonstrate the ability to be open to different cultures and show the utmost respect for their patients, who were different than themselves. Inherent in their care was the need to infuse hope into their patients' despairing situations and to act as an advocate by simply informing the patient and then supporting whatever decision he or she makes.

REFERENCES

De Chesnay, M., & Anderson, B. A. (2008). *Caring for the vulnerable: Perspectives in nursing theory, practice, and research*. Sudbury, MA: Jones and Bartlett.

Etienne, F. (2010). Twice the service. *The Lantern: The Journal of Nursing Stories, 2*, 2.

Wynd, C. (2006, September 30). A proposed model for military disaster nursing. *OJIN: The Online Journal of Issues in Nursing, 11*(3), Manuscript 4.

Chapter 20

Pet Therapy in Nursing

Leslie Himot and Mary de Chesnay

At the end of this chapter, the reader will be able to

1. Give examples of vulnerable populations that respond favorably to pet-assisted therapy.
2. Discuss the use of specifically selected animals as a treatment modality in health and human service settings.
3. Recognize the contributions of companion animals and their effect on the emotional well-being of people.
4. Identify the role of the nurse as it relates to recognition of pet therapy as a viable treatment modality in vulnerable populations.

INTRODUCTION

In this chapter, the use of pet-assisted therapy is explored as a concept relevant for nursing practice and care of vulnerable populations. There are several terms for this type of program (pet therapy, animal-assisted therapy, hippotherapy, etc.) but we will use the term *pet therapy* for all the cases. The human-animal bond has long existed, but has evolved substantially from exploiting animals for the sake of food and clothing, to relating to them in ways that not only respect the animal, but enhance the quality of life for the people who coexist with them. Pet owners have long known that their relationship with their pets was special and to some therapeutic, but within the later part of the 20th century, a therapeutic discipline has developed in which animals may serve a co-therapists with humans to assist the physically and mentally ill, the acutely or chronically injured and disabled and other vulnerable populations. (Beck, 1987; Friedmann & Son, 2009; Matuszek, 2010; Muschel,

I., 1984). Animals interact with unconditional love and in a nonjudgmental way, making them excellent co-therapists for some vulnerable populations.

LESSONS LEARNED

What is clear is that the emotional cost of losing a pet, even in families not in crisis, is not to be underestimated. The trauma suffered by pets and families in Hurricane Katrina and other disasters has influenced health policy in disaster situations. When Hurricane Katrina hit New Orleans, rescuers were ill prepared to deal with companion animals. People were prioritized over pets, and thousands of animals perished or were never reunited with their families. People were forced to abandon their pets, and some, refusing to do so, lost their lives alongside their animals. Soon after the disaster, Congress passed the Pets Evacuation and Transportation Standards Act, which requires that any state receiving aid from FEMA must make provisions for evacuating and sheltering people's pets (American Veterinary Medical Association, n.d.) According to a press release from the Humane Society of the United States in 2012, more than 358 million pets reside in 63 percent of American households. A Zogby International poll found that 61% of pet owners will not evacuate if they cannot bring their pets with them (American Humane Society, 2010).

In the calm before the storm, the American Society for the Prevention of Cruelty to Animals (ASPCA) and other animal organizations and agencies erected emergency shelters, and pet owners were active in getting their animal companions ID-tagged and microchipped so that history would not be repeated in the wake of oncoming Hurricane Isaac. Sites like Petfinder.com readied themselves to assist in connecting lost pets with their families. So while the tragedies of Hurricane Katrina are still heartbreaking, lessons have been learned from past disasters, and the people of New Orleans, facing the onset of Hurricane Isaac, did not have to make the decision to abandon members of their family. Instead, the animals were treated with respect and welcomed into rescuer's arms.

HISTORICAL ACCOUNTS OF THE PET–HUMAN BOND

Historical evidence has shown that the social symbiotic relationship between man and dogs and cats developed without any coercion from the side of humans. Domestication seems to be a natural process and is not one-sided. This interaction developed beneficially and has lasted for at least 10,000 years. Literature review supports evidence of the therapeutic role of companion animals among the physically and mentally handicapped, chronically ill patients, prisoners, the aged, and children. In Filan and Llewellyn-Jones (2006), a total of 18 articles on dementia and 5 on psychiatric disorders affirmed that pets were found to have positive influences on demented patients by reducing degree of agitation and improving degree and quality of social interaction. Domestic animals are found to increase patient self-control, play an "emotional mediator" role, and serve as "social facilitator" and "catalyst" for social interaction (Wilson & Netting, 1983). The most frequently employed animals for animal-assisted activities are dogs, given their training potential and typically social nature (Jofre, 2005).

USES OF PET THERAPY

The School of Medicine at Virginia Commonwealth University includes a focus on the human–animal relationship. The Mayo Clinic speaks to the value that pet therapy animals have on palliative care and hospice patients. Nursing schools such as Oakland City University and San Antonio School of Nursing are offering pet therapy in their elective curriculum (Matuszek, 2010).

In order to provide a solid methodological structure to the notion that there is a therapeutic aspect to the human-animal bond involving animal-assisted intervention (AAI) involving dogs, Bernabei et al. (2013) tested the value of dog-assisted interventions to increase quality of life in the geriatric population. Nineteen patients (men and women) with a mean age of 85 years participated in social interactions and physical therapy sessions with dogs. Measurement of cortisol levels in the saliva and depressive state were evaluated. Results showed that dog-mediated interactions affected the daily increase in cortisol levels and had an "activational effect" in contrast to the apathetic state of institutionalized elderly. The authors concluded that dog-mediated intervention programs appear to be promising tools to improve the social skills of the institutionalized elderly.

Pet therapy can relieve the fear and even the level of pain in anxious pediatric patients (Braun, Stangler, Narveson, & Pettingell, 2009) as well as adult surgery patients (Grunert, 2009). According to Matuszek (2010), pet therapy can positively alter blood pressure, heart rate, and cardiac hormones in patients with cardiac disease and motivate rehabilitation patients to work harder in physical therapy sessions.

ADHD and Pet Therapy

In children with primary diagnosis of attention deficit hyperactive disorder, physiological reactions to handling a dog were recorded for 17 children (13 males and 4 females) (Somervill, Swanson, Robertson, Arnett, & MacLin, 2009) in attempt to answer the question: Would handling a dog by children with ADD/hyperactivity disorder be calming or exciting? The major finding was a significant increase in blood pressure and pulse rate 5 minutes after holding a dog. The conclusion was that a dog used for pet therapy with children with ADHD was more likely to have an excitatory effect than a calming one.

Cerebral Palsy and Hippotherapy

One of the earliest uses of horses in therapy was for children who suffered from cerebral palsy. In a repeated-measures study, 10 children aged 3–7 and diagnosed with cerebral palsy received 10 weeks of hippotherapy. Statistically significant results showed improved motor functioning from pre-test to post-test (Casady & Nichols-Larsen, 2004). Hippotherapy or equine-assisted therapy is used in a variety of conditions from children with motor functioning impairments to trauma victims, such as abused women and children. Although not technically pets, the horses (and therapists) are specially trained to respond to vulnerable people.

CASE SCENARIOS

In this section, case examples are presented in order to convey the breadth of available circumstances in which pet therapy is useful in health care. These examples are only a small proportion of cases in which pet-assisted therapy is documented to be successful in improving physical performance, mental health symptoms, and social functioning.

The Dog As Co-Therapist

One of the authors (de Chesnay) is a family therapist whose practice has mostly comprised child victims of sexual abuse. An 8-year old girl, seen in the early 1970s, was a particularly nonverbal patient who absolutely refused to talk about anything hurtful. Yet her mother was convinced that the child's father had sexually abused her when she discovered blood in her panties. The couple was divorced with joint custody and the child had just returned from a weekend with her father. The family (mother and daughter) were referred to the family therapist by a caseworker who could not get the child to talk. The following account is what happened after weeks of trying to work with the child and failing to get her to tell the story of what her father had done to her.

> After several sessions of play therapy I just could not get the child to open up so I made one last visit to her home to meet with my client and her mother for the purpose of terminating therapy. Because the child had told me she wanted to be a veterinarian when she grew up, I brought my Airedale for her to play with while I spoke with her mother about options. When I saw how she bonded with my dog, I suggested we all take a walk around the neighborhood. The child held the lead and the mother and I walked closely behind. At one point I said to the child: 'I realize you don't know me well and it is scary to tell bad things to strangers, but Fred is a good listener. I tell him all my problems and he just listens. Would you tell him what happened to you at your Daddy's house?' To the amazement of the mother and myself, she did just that.

Although this story does not do justice to the extensive training contemporary therapy dogs and their handlers receive, it taught the therapist valuable lessons about the need to improvise in therapy and to be open to different therapeutic strategies.

Taking Man's Best Friend to Work

An Atlanta orthopedic surgeon has been taking his Labrador retriever, Jake, to his Marietta, Georgia office for 4 years. What started as a way to get Jake out of the house, has now turned into an every Wednesday occurrence. Jake has become a welcome visitor to his patients who may have to spend time in the waiting room. He recalls:

There was one particular time in cold December, that I remember a young women rushed her elderly father to my office fearing he has broken his hip. She was in such a hurry that she only had time to put on beach-thong style sandals. While she waited, Jake came from the back cubicles to the waiting room and promptly sat down right on her feet. She said that, 'In that moment, I just knew everything was going to be alright, and I did not even move my feet. The comfort I felt by having this kind, gentle dog sit with me and warm my feet was amazing.' Her father had not broken his hip, but did require some physical therapy for a few weeks. Jake continues to be a regular every Wednesday in the office and makes his rounds to everyone in the waiting room.

Hippotherapy with Sex Trafficking Survivors

Marcella was a 15-year-old Latina girl trafficked from her hometown in Mexico at the age of 11. Brought across the border to the American southwest by a *coyote*, a Spanish term used for traffickers, she was separated from her parents and sold to a brothel in a border town, where she endured 4 years of a variety of physical and sexual torture. Rescued by a police officer, she was placed in a shelter run by a group that provided equine therapy for its residents.

I was told my horse's name was Missy and she was a beautiful mare. I could not pronounce her name because my pimp had made me drink acid and I had trouble with the "s" sound, so I called her Chula which means "beautiful" in Spanish. [The acid attack was not verified but it was clear that Marcella had suffered some kind of mouth injury that prevented her from speaking clearly.] It took me a long time to trust the people at the shelter, but Missy I loved from the beginning. She just accepted me and never judged me. I learned how to brush her and feed her and I was allowed to give her treats—she loved apples. I even learned how to ride! It was scary at first but after what I went through with my pimp, I figured if I could ride a huge horse, I could handle anything.

Dementia

Mr. McCrae was a 72-year-old man showing the early signs of dementia. At times he would parade around the house naked and become violent toward his 75-year-old wife. He was admitted to a facility that included pet therapy. His wife reported his reaction:

At first, Sam was withdrawn and angry at all of us because he was frightened and disoriented. It broke my heart to place him there, but I just couldn't cope with him at home anymore. The nurses explained their program of support and structure so that he would get used to his new home and they mentioned pet therapy. Finally, I asked that they visit Sam. Joannie [a certified pet therapist] brought her golden retriever, Sandy, to visit him. At first he wanted nothing to do with them, but you know, goldens are so friendly, it's impossible to ignore them when they have so much love to give. The dog would just sit quietly by Sam's chair and gradually placed her head near his hand. She seemed to know how to get just the right distance and let Sam come to her. It wasn't long before Sam started patting her head and then talking to her and asking when they would return. After a few weeks, I couldn't believe the change in him. He even started to go out with us for short visits—but he would never leave if Joannie and Sandy were scheduled to come.

Inpatients

At a large metropolitan hospital just north of Atlanta, Chippy, the wiry, mixed breed therapy dog, is hard at work making daily rounds on inpatient hospital patients. Nurses and physicians alike stop what they are doing at the desk and relax for just a moment, all eager to pet Chippy. As one physician put it, "I guess it is a moment to shift gears from seeing life hang in the balance to seeing life engaging with a dog that does not require anything but love and in turn gives back love. It gives you the sense of hope."

A nephrologist, at the same hospital, encourages Chippy to visit his patients whenever possible.

My patients are in end-stage renal disease and often in the hospital because they are going to have to go on dialysis. They are here to have an AV shunt put in their arm to mature for hemodialysis, and are often anxious and depressed. I think when they see Chippy, they have a moment to think outside themselves—a moment to forget that they are so sick. They are happy for that moment of interaction with an animal that loves them unconditionally.

Prisoners

While there is much anecdotal evidence that programs in which prisoners train dogs for service or adoption are effective for both animals and humans, there are few studies that provide better documentation of outcomes. One qualitative study conducted in Kansas with a women's group and a men's group found that the prisoners perceived clear and profound therapeutic effects from interacting with the animals. The researchers acknowledged possible security concerns and backlash from community members opposed to doing anything to help prisoners, but the overwhelming positive results justified their support of continuing such programs (Britton & Button, 2005). Similar results were found by Turner (2007) who reported not only increases in prisoner self-esteem but also decreases in aggression among prisoners.

IMPLICATIONS FOR NURSING

Healthcare professionals have the opportunity to work with pet therapy in vulnerable populations. Presented in this chapter are vignettes and ideas for health professionals to be true advocates for "thinking outside the box" and using this alternative therapy as a means of touching patient lives in another meaningful way. Decades of studies have spoken to the power of animals and their effect on the human spirit. In addition to changing their own practices, health professionals who have been involved in the aspects of working with animals in a therapeutic setting, have the opportunity to initiate the discussion and collaborate within the healthcare system to formulate some potentially practical and successful strategies for use of pet therapies with vulnerable populations. Nurses and other interested healthcare professionals that may not be in a position to incorporate this therapy into their practice, have an opportunity to support programs in agencies in which they work because the models have been standardized and safety issues addressed through certification of therapy animals.

CONCLUSION

The historical tradition of domesticating animals for companionship has evolved into the recognition by healthcare providers that animals can serve a more important function in healing. See Appendix 20.1 for a list of helpful websites. The days of prohibiting family members from visiting patients in the hospital have given way to formal programs of pet therapy in which animals are brought in, not just for temporary respite but also to provide relationships for people with limited access to their usual social circles.

REFERENCES

American Humane Association. (2011). Retrieved from http://www.americanhumane.org/animal-welfart-news/pfizer-animal-health-and-american-humane-association.html

American Veterinary Medical Association. (n.d.). Retrieved from https://www.avma.org/KB/Resources/Reference/disaster/Pages/PETS-Act-FAQ.aspx

Beck, A. (1987). Pet therapy program in a nursing home. *Journal of the American Medical Association, 257*(6), 843–844.

Bernabei, V., De Ronchi, D., La Ferla, T., Moretti, F., Tonelli, L., Ferrari, B., & Atti, A. R. (2013). Animal-assisted interventions for elderly patients affected by dementia or psychiatric disorders: A review. *Journal of Psychiatric Research, 47*(6), 762–773.

Britton, D., & Button, A. (2005). Prison pups: Assessing the effects of dog training programs in correctional facilities. *Journal of Social Work, 9*(4), 79–95.

Braun, C., Stangler, T., Narveson, J., & Pettingell, S. (2009). Animal-assisted therapy as pain relief intervention for children. *Complementary Therapies in Clinical Practice, 15*(2), 105–109.

Casady, R. L., & Nichols-Larsen, D. S. (2004). The effect of hippotherapy on ten children with cerebral palsy. *Pediatric Physical Therapy, 16*(3), 165–172.

Filan, S. L., & Llewellyn-Jones, R. H. (2006). Animal-assisted therapy for dementia: A review of the literature. *International Psychogeriatrics, 18*(4), 597–611.

Friedmann, E., & Son, H. (2009). The human-companion animal bond: How humans benefit. *Veterinary Clinics of North America–Small Animal Practice, 39*(2), 293–326.

Grunert, J. (2009). Pet therapy dogs help patients recover faster. Retrieved from http://www.sutie101.com/content/pet-therapy-dogs-help-patients-recover-faster-a171052

Jofre, M. L. (2005). Animal-assisted therapy in health care facilities. *Review Chilena Infectology, 22,* 257–263.

Matuszek, S. (2010). Animal-facilitated therapy in various patient populations: Systematic literature review. *Holistic Nursing Practice, 24*(4), 187–203.

Somervill, J. W., Swanson, A. M., Robertson, R. L., Arnett, M. A., & MacLin, O. H. (2009). Handling a dog by children with attention-deficit/hyperactivity disorder: Calming or exciting? *North American Journal of Psychology, 11*(1), 111–119.

Turner, W. (2007). The experiences of offenders in a prison canine program. *Federal Probation, 71*(1), 38–43.

Wilson, C. & Netting, F. (1983). Companion animals and the elderly: A state of the art summary. *Journal of the American Veterinary Medical Association, 183*(12), 425–429.

APPENDIX

Appendix 20.1: Websites for Animal-Assisted Therapy

Table 20-1 Websites for Animal-Assisted Therapy

Organization/website	Mission statement	Description of services	Comments
Animal Assisted Therapy Programs of Colorado www.animalassistedtherapyprograms.org	The mission of Animal Assisted Therapy Programs of Colorado (AATPC) is to make the benefits of animal-assisted psychotherapy accessible to people of all ages, income levels, insurance statuses and life circumstances.	AATPC is one of the first counseling centers in the nation that specifically integrates teams of professional therapists and their therapy animals to facilitate in the counseling process.	
Animal Health Foundation www.animalhealthfoundation.net	Nonprofit charitable organization committed to improving the health and welfare of animals by supporting and promoting charitable, scientific, literary, and educational activities.	Therapy dogs in Southern California	Also help pet owners in other ways
Baylor Institute for Rehabilitation Animal Assisted Therapy www.baylorhealth.com	Baylor Scott & White Health exists to serve all people by providing personalized health and wellness through exemplary care, education and research as a Christian ministry of healing.	Although providing quality care is our main objective, we are always happy to offer our patients alternative types of treatment that may help them during their recovery. And sometimes, bringing our furry friends to visit (and work with) our patients does just the trick!	
Equine Assisted Growth and Learning Association http://www.eagala.org/	Our vision is that every person worldwide will have access to these services known as Equine Assisted Psychotherapy and Equine Assisted Learning.	(EAGALA) is the leading international nonprofit association for professionals using equine therapy to address mental health and human development needs.	

Organization/website	Mission statement	Description of services	Comments
HOPE Youth Ranch www.hopeyouthranch.org	The mission of HOPE Youth Ranch is to foster hope rather than despair, potential rather than limitation, healing rather than hurting, belonging rather than isolation and what the future can be rather than what the past has been. It is our greatest wish that we can help teens and their families find hope.	Transforming lives, restoring families in Hudson, Florida.	
McKenna Farms Therapy www.mckennafarmstherapy.org	To provide innovative therapy programs and resources for individuals with special needs and their families, while continuing to give back to our community.	McKenna Farms Therapy Services is a nonprofit organization that provides therapy services to individuals with special needs in Northwest Georgia.	Equine-assisted therapy
O.K. Corral Series http://okcorralseries.com/	The O.K. Corral Series educates, promotes, and supports professionals in the practice of authentic equine-assisted work. Authentic equine-assisted work honors and integrates natural horse and herd behavior as a model for human mental and emotional health using the equine-assisted philosophies developed by Greg Kersten, Founder of Equine Assisted Psychotherapy.	Equine-assisted work honors the natural behavior of horses and herds. Horses are skilled at keeping themselves safe and adept at survival; their natural behaviors are optimal for mental and physical health.	
Pet Partners (formerly Delta Society) www.petpartners.org	Pet Partners is the leader in promoting and demonstrating that positive human–animal interactions improve the physical, emotional, and psychological lives of those we serve.	Pet Partners, formerly Delta Society, is a 501(c)(3) nonprofit organization that helps people live healthier and happier lives by incorporating therapy, service and companion animals into their lives.	Bellevue, WA

Chapter 21

Undocumented Immigrants: Connecting with the Disconnected

Edwina Skiba-King

OBJECTIVES

At the end of this chapter, the reader will be able to

1. Describe the diverse composition of the undocumented immigrant population.
2. Discuss the scope of influence undocumented status has on quality of life.
3. Identify strategies that support therapeutic connections with undocumented persons.

INTRODUCTION

In this chapter, I ask you to set aside everything you think you know about undocumented immigrants. Doing so will allow you a glimpse into a world that will both amaze and anger. The term itself *undocumented* puts emphasis on something lacking, something not done. An alternate perspective permits a fuller assessment of what *has* been done—what has transpired in the life of this person. It is from this richer understanding of the person's experience that insightful and effective care connections are developed. It is satisfying work and there is much work to be done. Estimates put the number of undocumented immigrants in the United States at 11 million. Zack Taylor, chairperson of the National Association of Former Border Patrol Officers, estimates that the number is actually more like 18 million (Dinan, 2013). Such a number has both social and political implications. Political implications are not the focus of this chapter. However, after reading this chapter it is anticipated that the reader will take these additional insights forward into such discussions.

The following cases are based upon real patients, but the names are pseudonyms. My role was as the psychiatric-mental health advanced practice nurse who saw them in a community-based clinic associated with a university.

Talia

This is all I knew about my 2:00 p.m. appointment: she is a 14 year old referred by a school counselor because she appears sad and is withdrawn. Talia was seated in a pillow-backed chair meant to be comfortable and homelike. Clearly, for Talia it was neither. She was tense and at the same time her eye contact was pleading. Her style of dress is what you would see on most any teenage girl: stylish jeans, fitted tee shirt, strappy sandals accented by bright purple toenails. There is nothing standard about undocumented immigrants—they come in all shapes and sizes. One year ago she was living with her father and two younger brothers in Ecuador. Her mother had immigrated to the United States a year earlier. Her father paid a "very large sum of money" to transporters who brought Talia and her 15-year-old cousin to the United States. At the border, both girls were sequestered and then taken by bus to a detention center. Several hundred children were housed at the center. They had medical examinations and were assigned a cot in a large dormitory. Talia was held at the detention center for 9 months. Her cousin was released a few months earlier. Talia remained at the center because she expressed suicidal ideation to one of the interviewers. Talia was very worried about her young brothers because her father drank heavily and often would beat the children. She had not wanted to leave her brothers. She felt helpless and hopeless. Talia's mother lived several thousand miles from the detention center. She didn't visit or call. Upon release from detention, Talia was transported to her mother's home. The mother had a new boyfriend and was not pleased to have her daughter added to the household; Talia was not pleased to be added. The mother proved to be both physically and psychologically abusive—and this abuse was not something new. When Talia was 8 years old she was walking home from school when a 17-year-old village boy raped her. She was crying so hard that the boy felt bad and gave her money. Her mother told her that meant she was now a whore and she beat her. Focusing on her story, that is, focusing on what she had done versus what she had been through allowed a connection that proved to be therapeutic. In a later session with her mother, this petite, beautiful, 14-year-old undocumented immigrant looked her mother directly in the eye and said "this is American you can't do these things to me ever again."

Roberto

In the 1980s Roberto was a 17 year old living in Cuba with his family. He was a typical teenage boy with perhaps one exception: he was academically gifted. Cuban President Fidel Castro arranged scholarships for promising students to attend university in Germany. Roberto had been in university for several months when he returned to Cuba "to visit." Much was going on in Cuba at the time. The United States and Cuba had negotiated the Mariel boatlift. Under this agreement a mass emigration of Cuban citizens occurred during April 15 through October 31, 1980. They were to be sent to the United States on a temporary basis. They would be given Social Security cards and I-94 papers. Roberto and a couple of his friends hid on one of the boats transporting criminals from Cuban jails and mental patients from institutions. It was an opportunity for freedom.

Upon arrival in the United States, Roberto and his friends were issued Social Security cards and I-94 papers just like all the other passengers. For almost a year, he made his way in a big city with the eagerness of youth. Unfortunately, he became involved in the sale of marijuana. When he was arrested, he had just enough marijuana on his person to send him to federal prison. He served his time as a model prisoner and was released a little more mature and a lot more motivated to build a good life for himself and a future family he so much wanted. That is exactly what he did. Roberto built a successful roofing company employing many workers and proudly paying his taxes as a business owner. He still had his Social Security card and I-94 paper (with no expiration date), which gave him refugee status, but he also had a criminal record from his stay in federal prison. He married and had children. In 2012, he was deported. It was a traumatic process. U.S. President Obama pulled all I-94s from the Mariel boatlift emigrants that could be located. Roberto's brief stay in federal prison made him easy to locate. He complied with the notification to go to the Immigration Customs Enforcement (ICE) office to register. Upon entering the office, he was stripped of his personal belongings and sent to a deportation camp for 90 days. From there he was sent to another camp in Key West, Florida, and then to prison in Cuba. His prison time was "hard time" due to the seriousness of his crime: he had "taken" a Cuban government scholarship and then fled the country. During his imprisonment in Cuba, he was forced to wear steel boots as punishment for running away. When he was finally released, he was 65 pounds lighter, physically ill, and depressed. When he walked into that ICE office, he walked in with 32 years (1980–2012) of contribution to society. Newly immigrated undocumented persons have heard these stories and live in fear that it could happen to them at any time. Roberto's child told me that immigrants fear the hospital because it can house an ICE processing center: "Entering a large building is always a risk. You never know if you will be allowed to walk out."

Maria/Hector

In some ways Maria was one of the lucky ones. She felt blessed to have been chosen by lottery to enter the United States. She joined a large group of family members and friends who had immigrated to United States years before. They were all undocumented. Maria was grateful to have family and friends in the United States because she had had to leave her children, aged 5 and 10 years, in Honduras. Her plan was to work hard, save money, and have her children join her. She wanted to provide a better life for her children in America. As the only documented person in the group, Maria was often called on to handle all matters of business for the others. It was Maria who convinced her uncle Hector to come to the clinic. He had become increasingly withdrawn. He rarely left the home. His sleep and appetite were poor. He felt emasculated, as he could not be a man to his full potential. In his view, he was a financial failure. He was "tired of sneaking around and looking over my shoulder ... I'm an empty, weak man with no rights." Maria warned me that Hector would be resistant to taking psychiatric medicine. That, to him, would confirm that he was indeed "loco." I prescribed a tea infusion of telio leaf—an herb Hector knew well for his "weakness." We discussed exercise: "Back home I was the dancer." I prescribed salsa dancing. Subsequently, Hector was comfortable taking S-Adenosylmethionine (SAM-e), which he could buy himself at a local store. I wish I could say Maria did as well. It would be years before she would also be challenged with depression. By the time she was able to bring her children to the United States, they wouldn't come. During the 10 years she struggled, her children had grown—the eldest was planning to marry. Maria then came to realize that she had given up years with her children that could never be recouped. She was angry that she, the only fully documented member, had "been so foolish with my time." She wasn't at all sure that she was one of the lucky ones.

Lester

Twenty-five years ago Lester, age 50, came to the United States. He is a talented woodworker who, despite his undocumented status, has been steadily employed throughout these years. He married, had a child, and later divorced. Two years ago Lester sustained a serious back injury at work. Even after more than 20 years in the United States, he was fearful of seeking medical care. Desperate for food, he went to a free pantry and met a social worker who was from Colombia, his native country. She convinced him to come to the clinic for reiki treatments. Reiki, an energy medicine technique, is frequently used in Colombia. This familiar practice served as entry to an otherwise intimidating environment.

Grace

Grace was not a patient. She worked at the clinic as a phlebotomist. One day she and I were talking about colleges because her daughter, a senior in high school, was working on applications. I mentioned that I did my undergrad at University of Arizona and I went on to say how much I loved Arizona. I asked her if she had ever been there. She said: "Oh yes, I will never forget Arizona." She then lifted her skirt to show me her legs. Angry looking scars covered her thighs, and her lower legs looked like the complex fine lines you'd see on a subway map. "The cactus in the desert was very difficult," she explained. At age 17, Grace came into the country alone, literally crawling across the desert and hiding among the tumbleweeds and, of course, the cactus. Exhausted and in pain, she fell asleep in the sandy soil. In the morning, she prayed—not a plea for help but a prayer of gratitude. She continued: "The desert in the spring has the most beautiful wild flowers. The cactus flower is a wonder to behold—I knew my life had just begun."

NURSING OPPORTUNITY

There is no group of healthcare professionals better positioned to significantly impact the health of undocumented immigrants than nurses. The core of nursing is and always has been the nurse–patient relationship. The challenge with undocumented persons is that they are essentially disconnected from the society in which they live. They move about the community in fear and distrust—always on guard. Stories of being apprehended, detained, and deported are circulated in the communities. Hearing these stories reinforces the distrust. Detention camps are real. The stories of deportation are real. ICE offices housed in various buildings are a reality. Skillfully building connections is the requisite first step in getting this population engaged in health care.

Nurses are rightfully concerned about immigrants being able to access health screenings and receiving care for chronic health conditions like hypertension, diabetes, and asthma. Community nurses are frustrated in their attempts to reach this population. One nurse who works on a mobile health van in a city heavily populated with undocumented immigrants put it this way: "We literally take the care to their doorstep yet they won't come—they wait until there is a health crisis and often then it is too late." Assessing the problem, I see a constant. That constant is fear and distrust. But what is it that allows the fear and distrust to persist? We cannot deny the reality of detention camps and deportation, but we can create another reality just as real. Nurses can create new stories—stories of safe interaction: stories of a nurse who asked: "What has it been like for you?" stories of a nurse who didn't interrogate to fill in blanks on a form but rather a nurse who listened. In homeopathy we see the Law of Similars. Simply put, the law posits that what caused the illness can cure the illness. When nurses listen to the stories of Talia, Roberto, Lester, and all of the other undocumented immigrants, we are establishing caring connections—we are creating new stories to flood the community. And as we listen, we see life through their lens, which gives us a richer understanding of their problems. Solutions are always most effective when we thoroughly understand the problem. I have found that using treatment approaches that are familiar to this population is very well received. Lester was comfortable with reiki and prayer, which set in motion a care connection that allowed additional healthcare interventions. Hector drank a telio tea infusion, which led to an agreement to take SAM-e (Papakostas, Mischoulon, Shyu, Alpert, & Fava, 2010).

Treatments

You cannot attend a nursing conference or pick up a journal without seeing emphasis on evidence-based practice. You may be concerned that immigrants from some less-developed countries will be more receptive to herbs or folk remedies than to FDA-approved pharmaceuticals. How will building care connections with immigrants mesh with an evidence-based standard of practice? The truth is that the timing couldn't be more perfect. American healthcare consumers have been demanding more complementary and alternative medicine (CAM) for several decades. The use of CAM is increasing yearly and research has responded to this trend. Changes in nursing education will play a major role in bringing CAM into everyday practice. As doctor of nursing practice (DNP) programs flourish, graduates will be positioned to translate research into practice. Nurse practice councils and committees in hospitals will update practice guidelines and nursing literature will bring evidence-based nutraceuticals and herbals to nurses practicing in a variety of settings. Already there is sufficient evidence to support the use of a wide range of natural modalities. As you listen to your patients from these "underdeveloped" countries you will learn about natural treatments. When you go to the literature, you may be surprised to find evidence to support the use of the herb or flower your patient cited (Blumenthal, Goldberg, & Brinckman, 2000; DeStefano, 2001; Lange, 1999; & Rotblatt & Ziment, 2002). Many undocumented immigrants, fearful of going to medical facilities, are purchasing herbs and medicines from sources that may or may not be safe. If the story gets into these communities that we are knowledgeable about these natural practices, it could encourage them to consult with us.

- *Epsom salts* are known in almost every country. Many people will tell of seeing their grandparents soaking their feet in a basin of water and Epsom salts. I keep a large container in my office and a supply of Ziploc bags. Epsom salts is magnesium sulfate and we know that magnesium is nature's tranquilizer. A soak in a bathtub is most effective but a foot basin will do. Its gentle chelating properties soothe sore muscles. Lavender-scented Epsom salts are useful for calming anxiety. Instruct that they are not to be taken orally.
- *Kava (Piper methysticum)* has been studied in numerous clinical trials (Pittler & Ernst, 2003; Stevinson, Huntley, & Ernst, 2002). Kava is an anodyne and an antianxiety

agent. It should not be used in conjunction with hepatotoxic medications (like acet-aminophen) or alcohol. Kava is less popular in the United States than in most countries, in large part due to a manufacturing contamination that was widely publicized in the 1990s in the United States. It is not intended for long-term use but can be very effective for acute stress episodes.

- *L-theanine* is very effective for anxiety and can be used long term (Kimura, Ozeki, Juneja, & Ohira, 2007). It is an amino acid that supports production of inhibitory neurotransmitters. The fact that it is inexpensive and can be purchased at many local stores makes it less intimidating than benzodiazepines. It increases alpha waves in the brain producing a state of *relaxed alertness*—a mode of action that is especially appealing to an undocumented immigrant.

- *CoQ10* (coenzyme Q10) can be an important adjunct for patients who have agreed to take a statin for hyperlipidemia. When patients experience muscle pain after taking a prescription, they can become fearful and distrustful. Statins deplete CoQ10 causing myalgia. There are two forms: ubiquinon and ubiquinol, which is the reduced form and therefore immediately bioavailable.

- *Reiki* is one type of energy healing. Many nurses are familiar with therapeutic touch, originally introduced to nursing by Dolores Krieger in the 1970s. Reiki is known and practiced worldwide. Reiki can be a power connector.

- *Pranic Healing* is familiar to many immigrants. I have a vibrantly colored poster of chakras hanging in my clinic office. While a clinic can offer a full range of primary health care, it is important to start with the patient's priority. I recall the first day Felix came to the clinic. In response to: "How can we help you?" Felix, with tears in his eyes, asked: "Can you, will you please clean my chakras?" A connection was made and a story begun.

REFERENCES

Blumenthal, M., Goldberg, A., & Brinckmann, J. (2000). *Herbal medicine: Expanded commission e monographs*. Newton, MA: Integrative Medicine Communications.

DeStefano, A. (2001). *Latino folk medicine*. New York: Ballantine Publishing Group.

Dinan, S. (2013). Nearly 20 million illegal immigrants in US former border patrol agents say. *The Washington Times*, September 09, 2013.

Kimura, K., Ozeki, M., Juneja, L., & Ohira, H. (2007). L-theanine reduces psychological and physiological stress responses. *Biological Psychology, 1*, 39–45.

Lange, A. (1999). Homeopathy. In J. Pizzorno & M. Murray (Eds.). *Textbook of natural medicine*. (pp. 335–343). London: Churchill Livingstone.

Papakostas, G., Mischoulon, D., Shyu, I., Alpert, J., & Fava, M. (2010). S-adenosyl methionine (SAMe) augmentation of serotonin reuptake inhibitors for antidepressant nonresponders with major depressive disorder: A double-blind, randomized clinical trial. *American Journal of Psychiatry, 167,* 942–948.

Pittler, M., & Ernst, E. (2003). Kava extract for treating anxiety. *The Cochrane Database of Systemic Reviews, 1,* CD003383. Retrieved from http://summaries.cochrane.org/CD003383/DEPRESSN_kava-extract-for-treating-anxiety

Rotblatt, M., & Ziment, I. (2002). *Evidence-based herbal medicine.* Philadelphia: Hanley & Belfus.

Stevinson, C., Huntley, A., & Ernst, E. (2002). A systematic review of the safety of kava extract in the treatment of anxiety. *Drug Safety, 25,* 251–261.

Chapter 22

Developing Population-Based Programs for the Vulnerable

Anne Watson Bongiorno and Mary de Chesnay

OBJECTIVES

At the end of this chapter, the reader will be able to

1. Describe the relationship between planning and success when designing new programs to serve the vulnerable.
2. Discuss the importance of stakeholders when proposing new programs.
3. Develop an idea for a new program that serves a vulnerable population.

INTRODUCTION

Population-based programs can strengthen communities by increasing the amount of resources available to promote social justice. This unit focuses on how nurses can structure programs to serve large numbers of vulnerable people. To maximize effectiveness, health professionals should serve populations by using efficient and cost effective methods to deliver programs that are based on best practices within the program domain. We discuss the importance of a common vision, the relationship between key planning elements and program success, and creating partnerships with major stakeholders. We discuss how to design programs to maximize their impact with scarce resources. This unit covers the multiple components needed for successful program planning.

BALANCING EFFICIENCY WITH NEED AND EFFECTIVENESS

In today's healthcare environment, well-conceived programs meet the needs of a population, and flow through a continuous quality cycle of improvement that is efficient and effective. It is important to establish a consistent program approach. An appropriate analysis of need and evaluation of effect of the program lead to improved efficiency and effectiveness of efforts. Concepts such as *Lean Six Sigma*, involve just such a process, where the lean concepts analyze need and effect, while minimizing excess steps to an outcome (Klefsjo, 2012). *Six Sigma* concepts complement lean by examining what the target audience needs, recommending specific approaches to care, and creating a workflow to maximize the effect of the efforts. Efforts to maximize efficiency and effectiveness should balance with the cultural and creative needs specific to the population of need.

FOCUS OF THE PROGRAM

Problem Statement

The *problem statement* captures the significance of a health issue in relationship to the focus of the program, clearly defines the purpose of the program, and identifies the population served by the program. It is vital to analyze the environment and determinants of health; this process leads to a problem statement and plan that better predicts program success. The problem statement should reflect what is important to both the target audience and major stakeholders, with all in agreement on the proposed program focus (Lewis, 2008).

Stakeholders

Programs targeting vulnerable populations implicitly seek to reduce health disparities. The program planner needs to learn who the stakeholders are and how to identify them. Stakeholders are representative of community engagement in the project and often function as the power brokers for the program. Stakeholders generally include nonprofit organizations or political entities that can help establish and sustain the program; they also encompass individuals who are the target of the program (Issel, 2014).

Stakeholder mix ought to demonstrate diversity in their perspectives. For example, the first author of this chapter (Bongiorno) consults with the Adirondack Tobacco Free Network, often designing service-learning practicums for nursing students. In one outreach, the collaborative goal was to improve outdoor smoke-free policies in the community. Students used a survey to measure effectiveness and acceptance of a county-level outdoor smoke-free policy. Surveys were distributed to a wide variety of stakeholders: community members, legislators, and self-identified smokers. Editorials were placed in the area newspaper. Focus group interviews were conducted to determine acceptability of the program. The coalition provided free consultation and materials to business leaders for development of tobacco-free worksite policies. Key stakeholders were honored at a recognition event that was well publicized; with a goal to share the benefits and success of implementing smoke-free policies in their workplaces.

Programs built with a broad stakeholder base clarify the sociopolitical and economic factors at play, and raise awareness of the scientific merit of interventions. A cohesive stakeholder group develops synergy through the influence of its members and empowers the group and its participants, a key tenant in *Lean Six Sigma* systems of care and a surefire indicator of potential success of the program. (Godin, Gagnon, Alery, Levy, & Oatis, 2007; Mader, 2007).

Gatekeepers

Closely related to stakeholders are *gatekeepers*—those people who have power and authority, usually by way of their positions within the setting. They can use this authority in one of two ways: to facilitate a project they support or to create barriers to programs they do not support. It does not matter whether the program is a service program or a study; gatekeepers need to be identified early in the process. At this juncture, the use of metrics from research and political and culturally competent acumen can be key strategies for engaging gatekeepers.

A positive example of gatekeepers was described in the first edition of this book, when the second author and colleagues (Colvin, de Chesnay, Mercado, & Benavides, 2005) designed a research project in a barrio of Managua, Nicaragua. Early in the process of beginning the study on mothers' access to health care in the barrio, the research team met with a key community leader. The woman who was the lead *brigadista* (community health worker) welcomed the team into her home, where we described the study and planned how to approach the community. She gave the researchers many helpful tips on the interview instrument, which women to invite first, best timing, and culturally appropriate incentives to participate in the study.

In contrast, a negative gatekeeper can effectively halt a program. Consider the doctoral student who planned a study in which she would access a rural African American sample through a local church. She obtained the permission of the pastor, who was enthusiastic in supporting her. When she arrived for data collection, however, the student was told by the deacon that he had not given his permission to collect data through the church and he would not allow her to enter. Inability to resolve the power struggle between the pastor and the deacon cost the student months of work, because she needed to revise her entire methodology.

Values

The values section is a list of the core values held by the designers of the program. For example, for those who work with vulnerable populations, a key value is social justice. The values section might include statements like the following examples:

- For a program to reduce violence against children: *Every child has the right to live free of abuse.*
- For a public education campaign to prevent HIV/AIDS: *The public has a right to know the risks of sharing needles.*

Mission

The *mission statement* is an opportunity for the program designers to clearly say what they plan to do and why they believe it is important. The following example is a mission statement from a prenatal program in Clinton County: *Every expectant woman should have access to prenatal care throughout her pregnancy.*

DESIGN PROCESS

Recruiting the Team

A useful place to start designing a program is to obtain help from like-minded people who share a concern about the issue and the population. It is very important to partner with members of the community who will be affected by the program.

For example, the first author of this chapter (Bongiorno) partnered with a group of key public health personnel, industry and nursing leaders, legislators, and community members to address high levels of obesity. The *Action for Health* committee addressed the built environment and access to quality health resources, such as grocery stores, pharmacies, and outdoor activities. The goal was to reduce obesity and increase physical activity from childhood through senescence. As part of the initiative, we assessed access to grocery stores among those with no private transportation. We conducted ridership surveys and key informant interviews on local buses to find out who rode them to obtain groceries. Findings showed that bus routes were incompatible with grocery store hours and that a bus policy of only carrying what can fit on your lap is incongruent with community need for access to weekly grocery shopping in large, inexpensive stores. Next steps include policy-level work to change bus route times and bag policies. As part of our strategy to increase physical activity we collaboratively developed free resources, such as a disc golf park and the Saranac river trail, a beautiful bike and walking trail. The success of these projects is directly related to broad community stakeholder representation that included recipients of the programs.

Feasibility Study

Proposed programs need to be realistic, cost-effective, and have the potential to achieve predetermined goals. A feasibility study will define the skills and resources needed to implement a program and offer alternative solutions. Needs and the proposed service are examined for practicality and usefulness. The feasibility study highlights strengths and weaknesses of the proposal, and its capacity to deliver and sustain the program (Stanhope & Lancaster, 2012).

The Saranac trail initiative is a positive example of how a feasibility study supports potential success of a program. An example where feasibility was not well considered was a local health department initiative designed to help increase healthy choices for children and their families. The target audience was children who were morbidly obese, but the program was open to any interested family. Although the program was well grounded in theory and evidence, the collaborative project was unable to recruit a sufficient number of families. Parents were not ready to label their children as obese. This example highlights how important it is to complete a feasibility study when planning a new program.

Capturing Data

Informal talks and formal interviews may yield important data about a particular need in a community and often serve as the catalyst for action. For example, in the upstate region, women of low socioeconomic status were not accessing the statewide Quit Line. Because the key to effective health communication is to understand the audience, we needed to determine message appeal, and how to strategically place the message so that it would attract the attention of women of low socioeconomic status. We recruited community members to participate in focus group discussions and conducted anonymous curbside surveys in places where the women congregated. Data showed that the print information was at a reading level beyond the capabilities of the target group and did not resonate with the audience. New, simplified outreach materials were then developed, tested, and placed in areas where the women congregated—thereby bridging a gap in previous outreach efforts.

Surveys and focus groups provide rich data about a population problem from the emic point of view. For example, Bongiorno worked with an upstate New York public health agency to determine need and effectiveness for use of electronic medical records (EMR) in home care. A mixed method of quantitative surveys and personal interviews provided rich data about acceptance among end users and transition to use. In the Caribbean, de Chesnay (second author) worked with a group of nurses to revise their mental health program. Her techniques included interviews with a variety of people and short surveys administered as a needs assessment.

Participant observation is an important data-gathering technique because data collected in this manner are nonlinear, contextual, and provide salient information about a problem whose dimensions cannot be gleaned from quantitative methods. In a study-abroad program for nursing students, interviews and observation of participants revealed rich insight into how the experience reframed participants' worldview regarding poverty and vulnerability of indigenous populations. Qualitative analysis revealed important information for program growth.

Good programs directed toward vulnerable populations are built upon a foundation of evidence that creates a compelling story of a need, a gap in service, and the ability to develop an effective strategy to improve the health of the population. Hence, program planners must also elucidate the scientific underpinnings for their proposal. The epidemiology of the health issue should be clearly and succinctly communicated. The cultural congruence of the program intervention needs to be addressed when gathering data, as well as the bicultural diversity of the program recipients.

A BUSINESS PLAN

Definition and Role in Seeking Funding

Experienced grant writers know all too well that funding will be awarded only for ideas that are feasible and sustainable. Funding agencies want to be assured that the grantee is functioning within the limits of his or her ability and experience. The business plan is the document that provides funding agencies with this kind of valuable information. A business plan is a vital tool in a grant proposal to identify and prioritize the resources needed to implement the program (Longest, 2004). It highlights both the strengths and the weaknesses of the proposal. In addition, it explains how the grantee will allocate resources to meet the current and future needs of the program.

At a minimum, the business plan should define the mission and goals of the program and outline how the grantee plans to conduct business to match the purpose of the program. Traditionally, the business plan describes the program, product, and purpose, and discusses the market for the program now and in the future. The plan provides a detailed financial analysis, management plan, and a personnel plan with dates and budget.

Business plans may range from simple to complex, depending on the scope of the program and request for funding. For example, the first author (Bongiorno) and a colleague wanted students to learn first-hand the role of advocacy for vulnerable populations. We developed a simple business plan for the proposed program. The mission of the program was to increase nursing students' awareness of advocacy as a nursing mandate. Two objectives of the program were to relate the importance of nursing's voice in the advocacy process and to apply knowledge of the legislative process to a vulnerable population. Our market analysis showed a complete lack of knowledge regarding the role of population-based advocacy among current students. Final steps in planning were to develop a specific strategy and implementation plan to meet the mission of the program.

In the program, students spent a semester investigating a vulnerable population and learning the legislative process, culminating with an advocacy presentation to their county legislator. The management team included faculty and administrators. The financial plan included a detailed budget of costs to the university and students and a projected cash flow from grants and other sources of funds.

Creating a business plan is an excellent exercise for students in a nurse practitioner program because they often take positions in physician practices that share profits. Nurse practitioners might at some point want to set up their own clinics such as the one described by Knestrick and Counts in this volume.

Costs and Budget

Anticipating costs is an important part of any business plan. Project financing should be identified, including accountability and communication regarding costs and current and projected revenues, surplus, and deficits. It is critical to the success of any program in staying within its budget to project the cash flow and create a balance sheet. Expenses, personnel costs, indirect costs, and issues such as inflation or market adjustments need to be factored into more complex program plans. The proposed budget must realistically match the amount of funds a grant agency is willing to award. The program developer's vision of the program and budget must be aligned for a funding agency to consider the proposal. Matching ideas to funding is a vital element in grantsmanship.

Sources of Funding

People who believe strongly in the programs they develop can be quite creative at seeking funding. *Grants* and *contracts* serve as an excellent way to seek funding, although writing and submitting the grant can sometimes take several months. Grants directories are valuable resources in this quest, as they detail the focus of the grant-sponsoring organization, contact information, guidelines for grant writing, and much other useful information. Because these folks are passionate about their causes, they can be quite persuasive at obtaining community support—either in the form or donations or support letters for grant proposals. Some students in the human trafficking course taught by the second author held a bake sale to raise money for a shelter that serves child sex trafficking victims. One student reported that her mother was so proud of her for participating that she donated an extra $100 to the student's project.

Public campaigns can generate large amounts of money targeted to the program of interest. Sometimes it is possible to designate a program as a new United Way agency. If not, creating a similar public campaign is not difficult if the team recruits the support of the local media. For example, the KSU Community Clinic Program was a nurse-managed clinic at Kennesaw State University under the WellStar College of Health and Human Services and staffed by a WellStar School of Nursing faculty member who is a nurse practitioner. After the clinic received favorable publicity in the local media during its new building dedication, KSU faculty and staff responded to requests for funding by asking that their Capital Campaign donations be designated for the clinic. Walk-a-thons are another popular way of raising funds. Student nurses' groups in many universities employ this method to raise money for their organizations or for health promotion awareness.

Grass roots fundraising should not be overlooked if relatively small amounts of funds are needed. Students often use bake sales and car washes to raise funds for airplane tickets to developing countries where they combine learning community health nursing with service. *Formal dinners* with highly visible speakers combined with *raffles* can earn thousands of dollars if the right community leaders are invited. For example, John Walsh (host of the *America's Most Wanted* television program) agreed to be the featured guest at a fundraiser for Prescott House, the Children's Advocacy Center of Jefferson County, Alabama.

Crowd funding is another way to support programs that are within the domain of nonprofit organizations. This method of fundraising has been very successful but is labor intensive. The key to successful crowd funding is to raise awareness of a fundraising effort for a few weeks prior to the funding period and to be realistic about the level of funds that can be raised. (Gore & DiGiammarino, 2014). Also needed is agreement from all partners, dedicated personnel for the fundraising event, and a clear picture of how the event will fund programs that support organizational goals.

EVALUATION

Process and outcome evaluation are a vital part of continuous quality improvement. Program evaluation can be accomplished through traditional research methods. Quantitative measures include tools designed to collect stakeholder demographic data and identify the satisfaction of participants, such as surveys and questionnaires. Qualitative measures for this purpose might include interviews and focus groups.

EXAMPLES

Native American Network for Health

The first author of this chapter (Bongiorno) and other faculty researchers with the State University of New York (SUNY) proposed a program for a Native American Health network in New York (NY). The network sought to reduce health disparity and improve health outcomes among Native Americans (AI) through a collaboration with AI tribes in NY. The AI population in NY hovers about 100,000 persons. Data shows that the AI group has some of the worst health of any ethnic group in the United States, with high post-neonatal mortality rates and a median age of 31 years, indicating low life expectancy rates. Adults suffer at disparate levels from heart disease, obesity, strokes, and substance abuse. Access to care is limited (Barnes, Adams, & Powell-Griner, 2010).

The goal of the network is to improve AI health. We would start with a planning period to gather individual AI communities together to build trusting relationships and culminate the planning work with a pan-NY state community health conference. Here, tribal leaders can determine priorities for care, with expertise from the SUNY faculty group. The second phase of the program included development of a collective database describing AI health and specific programs to tackle the most pressing health needs identified by the tribes.

Prescott House

In the mid-1980s, the second author of this chapter (de Chesnay) was involved in working with the district attorney to set up a children's advocacy center in Jefferson County, Alabama (de Chesnay & Petro, 1989). The intention of this program was to reduce further victimization of child sex abuse survivors through the criminal justice system and to improve prosecution rates of offenders. The team had been concerned about the extreme emotional distress experienced by children and their nonoffending family members as prosecution of the offenders proceeded through the slow-moving justice system. Grant funds became available for a project to model a new center after one that had been started by the district attorney in Huntsville, Alabama.

To assess the need for such a program in Jefferson County, the team conducted interviews with a variety of stakeholders. The most powerful finding from this research was that children were required to tell their stories over and over to many professionals in intimidating circumstances, such as in police stations and courthouses with big, adult furniture. The short-term goal was to require all individuals who needed to interview children to find a quiet, private place; the long-term goal was to create a new space with age-appropriate furniture and anatomically correct dolls.

On a short-term basis, the team designated a quiet space in the police station that was equipped with smaller furniture for children. Dolls and coloring materials were brought to the room to enhance the interviews. All interviewers came to the child. The effectiveness of this plan was limited, however, in that the child still needed to tell the story many times. With each subsequent telling of the story, many children become confused or numb and the story sounded false.

The long-term solution was to acquire a building that would be dedicated to interviewing the children. Funds were raised through private donations, and the house was named Prescott House in honor of the local citizen who donated the building. Prescott House is located away from the courthouse, in a residential neighborhood. The former residential space was renovated to accommodate a large conference room upstairs with age-appropriate interview rooms for young children and adolescents. The arrangement of rooms with closed-circuit television enables the child to be in the interview room with one interviewer who wears an earpiece. All other professionals are required to watch from the conference room and feed their questions to the interviewer.

CONCLUSION

This chapter has offered some basic ideas about program development with examples from the authors' experiences in developing programs that serve vulnerable populations. Nurses are in a unique position to provide such programs for vulnerable populations, and the following chapters offer examples of the fine work they do. We think program planning is an important role of Doctor of Nursing Practice (DNP) nurses and suggest fieldwork and exercises in those programs to develop the skills necessary for success. With appropriate planning and involvement by stakeholders, programs at the local level can make great contributions to their communities and nurses can play a major role in their development and implementation.

REFERENCES

Barnes, P. M., Adams, P. F., & Powell-Griner, E. (2010). Health characteristics of the American Indian or Alaska Native adult population: United States, 2004–2008. *National health statistics reports; No. 2*. Hyattsville, MD: National Center for Health Statistics.

Colvin, S., de Chesnay, M., Mercado, T., & Benavides, C. (2005). Child health in a barrio of Nicaragua. In M. de Chesnay (Ed.), *Caring for the vulnerable: Perspectives in nursing theory, practice and research* (pp. 161–170). Sudbury, MA: Jones and Bartlett.

de Chesnay, M., & Petro, L. (1989). The accountability of incest offenders. *Medicine and Law, 8*, 281–286.

Godin, G., Gagnon, H., Alery, M., Levy, J., & Oatis, J. (2007). The degree of planning: An indicator of the potential success of health education programs. *Promotion and Education, 14*(3), 138–182.

Gore, E. M., & DiGiammarino, B. (2014, May). Crowd funding for nonprofits [blog]. *Stanford Social Innovation Review*. Retrieved from http://www.ssireview.org/

Issel, L. M. (2014). *Health program planning and evaluation: A practical, systematic approach for community health* (3rd ed.). Sudbury, MA: Jones and Bartlett.

Klefsjo, B. (2012). Health. Quality function deployment and Lean Six Sigma applications in public health. *Quality Progress, 45*, 1–67.

Lewis, J. (2008). *Mastering project management* (2nd ed.). New York: McGraw-Hill.

Longest, B. (2004). *Managing health programs and projects*. San Francisco, CA: Jossey-Bass.

Mader, D. (2007). How to identify and select Lean Sigma Six projects. *Quality Progress, 40*(7), 58–60.

Stanhope, M., & Lancaster, J. (2012). *Public health nursing: Population-centered health care in the community* (8th ed.). St. Louis, MO: Mosby/Elsevier.

Chapter 23

Childhood Autism in a Rural Environment: Reaching Vulnerable Children and Their Families

Ellyn E. Cavanagh

OBJECTIVES

At the end of this chapter, the reader will be able to

1. Define autism spectrum disorder (ASD) in terms of key identifiers.
2. List the symptoms of ASD.
3. Describe the cultural components of ASD.
4. Describe how the practitioner engages the family in service delivery.
5. Understand the continuum of interventions in making evidence-based decisions.

INTRODUCTION

Autism spectrum disorder (ASD) is a lifelong neurodevelopmental medical condition associated with unique abnormalities in brain development. It is the second most common developmental disability following intellectual disability, more common than childhood cancer, cystic fibrosis, and multiple sclerosis combined. The Autism and Developmental Disabilities Monitoring (ADDM) network estimates overall incidence of ASD as 14.7 per 100 children or one in 68 children aged 8 years (Centers for Disease Control and Prevention [CDC], 2014). The overall incidence is the same around the globe, but it is five times more prevalent in boys than girls. ASD has no racial, ethnic, or social boundaries, and is not influenced by family income, lifestyle, or educational level. It is a lifelong disorder.

Autism exposes children to many risk factors, such as loss of important social relationships. Affected children do not experience typical human interaction with the outside world in a natural manner. Protective factors such as temperament, learned coping skills, consistent parenting, higher cognitive power, and supportive environment may all increase the child's ability to interpret and adapt to the stimuli from the external environment. However, these children and youth are easily overwhelmed and may become disabled by their behavioral disorder. Nurses have an impact from early diagnosis through childhood, adolescence, and young adulthood. The number of autistic children expected to need extensive adult services by 2023 is more than 380,000—roughly equal to the population of Minneapolis (Davis, 2009). These individuals will need caregivers and nursing case management.

This chapter covers inherent vulnerabilities, resilience, the central role of family, and implications for professional nursing practice, including how to access evidence-based practices for treatment of autism across the age span. The term *resilience* is most often used to describe the protective process that results in a more positive outcome for individuals who are at risk for either social or psychological factors (see **Table 23-1**). It is often thought of as the opposite of risk or vulnerability. The social confines of autism make affected individuals dependent on family support as they go from social isolation

---

Table 23-1   Five Points Every Provider Should Know About Autism Spectrum Disorder

1.   The medical home model is the ideal model for ASD service delivery. However, the care of an individual with autism is highly dependent upon the professional profile of the provider.

2.   Sometimes not all of the diagnostic features of ASD are present by age 3 years. Many children do not show clear repetitive behaviors at 2 years of age. Between 3 and 4 years of age, preschool children with autism exhibit the more classical picture.

3.   Early and continuous intervention in ASD is highly desirable and has measurable effects on later intellectual and communicative abilities.

4.   Parental stress is significantly greater for mothers of children with autism than for mothers of children with mental retardation or physical disabilities. Family life can end up revolving around the needs of the child with autism. Concerns may arise about taking the child into the community due to behavior challenges. ASD can be particularly challenging because the child appears "normal" physically, but may exhibit extreme behavior problems that are misunderstood by community members.

5.   There is the need for constant vigilance for children who have no understanding of danger. As the child grows bigger and stronger, some families struggle with addressing behavior challenges such as aggression.

to social perplexity. Resilience, as an outcome in autism, is a measure of the individual child's strengths, dependent upon the physical and social capital of the family and the larger community. The focus of this chapter is on nursing interventions to help the family understand the full range of potential resources and focused interventions to protect the child from risk and to support the human capital of family.

Individuals who have autism seem to manage well if they are identified early in childhood and if their families are taught to differentiate normal from abnormal behaviors, have specific strategies to enrich the child's early experiences and cognitive development (e.g., an intensive educational program). The needs of children with ASD straddle the education and healthcare systems from early identification until early adulthood, thus linking two major systems of care. The child cannot access educational services without a medical diagnosis, and the treatment for autism is largely educational. It is therefore critical for nurses to understand the educational team measurements and to be able to write prescriptive care plans that are realistic. Nursing priorities include recognition of autism as disordered development, an understanding of the autistic nervous system, and skill in facilitating family-focused care. The interplay between vulnerability and resilience is illustrated through case examples of ASD children attending school and living in rural New England communities.

THE AUTISTIC NERVOUS SYSTEM

The autistic nervous system is best understood according to symptoms. Common symptoms of ASD include delayed language, social unrelatedness, and unusual sensitivity to the environment. Behaviors include rigidity, necessitating highly structured routines, preoccupation with sameness, repetitive body movements, insensitivity to pain or temperature, and apparent deafness. Although commonly associated with intellectual disability, autism differs from other developmental disorders in that the behavioral features are distinctive and do not simply reflect developmental delay but rather a disordered development. Social and adaptive abilities, language level, and nonverbal intelligence are important predictors of independence and long-term prognosis. Most typically developing children will exhibit nonverbal communication and joint attention skills before the age of 1 year. Children with autism fail to develop social engagement and suffer impairments in social interaction and communication (Myers, Johnson, & American Academy of Pediatrics Council on Children with Disabilities, 2007).

Theoretically a congenital disorder, autism is often characterized by symptoms that appear during early infancy. There are four basic trajectories representing the potential outcomes for children who are diagnosed in early childhood:

• Recovery of language and development of compensatory social skills
• Failure to develop proficient language and persistent poor social interaction

- Progressive developmental gains and acquisition of maladaptive behaviors with variability in communicative skills
- Developmental regression and nonfunctional behaviors

These developmental pathways are established during childhood and operate across the lifespan. The goal is early screening and diagnosis within the first 2 years of life and initiation of a treatment program specific to autism. The American Academy of Pediatrics' Council on Children with disabilities states that the primary goals of treatment are to:

- Maximize the child's ultimate functional independence and quality of life by minimizing the core features
- Facilitate development and learning
- Promote socialization
- Reduce maladaptive behaviors
- Educate and support families (Myers et al., 2007)

Children with autism also face comorbidity that complicates the disorder and interferes with learning. Cognitive impairment or an intelligence quotient (IQ) equal to or less than 70 has been reported for 40% to 62% of children whose conditions were consistent with the case definition for ASD. Seizure disorders occur in 25%, central nervous system malformations occur in 20%, significant dysmorphology in 25%, microcephaly in 5–15% and macrocephaly in 30%. In addition, sleep problems are common in children and adolescents with ASDs at all levels of cognitive functioning (Myers et al., 2007).

VULNERABILITY AND RESILIENCE

The level of vulnerability is defined by the constellation of symptoms in the autism spectrum. Resilience includes the capacity of the family to navigate necessary resources and to sustain well-being in the face of this diagnosis. Parents are typically ill prepared for the challenges of having a child with autism, so they need resilience to deal with the unexpected diagnosis.

For example, one of the precursors of positive childhood development is attachment. Often parents' first clue is the social disconnect experienced by the child and their difficulty in establishing a reciprocal relationship with the child. The child never "connects" or connects and then quite unexpectedly disconnects. One mother explained: "He had been receiving early intervention services for 3 months and was improving, and then the light in his eyes began to go out. He stopped looking in my eyes, and when I caught his chin in my hands to look in his face, there was nothing there. He was irritable and spun in circles most of the time, and when he did sit down, he kept pushing the same button on a musical toy over and over and couldn't be engaged. My son was gone. There was no spark in his face, no sign of life, just dead eyes." (Leal, 2011, para. 13).

Social impairment is the central vulnerability, the defining feature of the disorder, and not explicable in terms of cognitive delay alone. The social dysfunction in autism is distinctive and disabling. Autism interferes with the ability of the child to recognize faces, use language, possess emotions, or develop self-awareness (Martinez-Pederast & Carter, 2009). In addition, children, adolescents, and adults with ASD often have comorbid psychiatric difficulties, with the most common being anxiety and depression (Howlin, 2005).

Resilient families facilitate and protect the child's core social skills. The child with social deficits relies on the primary social group—the family—to cope with the uncertainty of the outside world. The child may have difficulties with social reciprocity, appropriate conversational skills, and higher-order language ability. Behaviors may be perceived as bizarre or strange. Disordered social development in autistic children is characterized by deficits in affiliation skills such as eye contact, gesturing, pointing, or showing. Families often develop a system of knowledge as the child may not indicate needs and may have a low level of need for close physical contact. For example, the child uses people as objects, grabbing a hand and leading someone to the refrigerator door for food. The child attends poorly to social stimuli and may react with negative emotions and negative affect to social stimuli. The child fails to establish affective contact with others, driving the family to seek help.

Each family has a different level of resilience and each autistic child presents with strengths and weaknesses. Each family needs to recognize and exploit the child's strengths and create a relationship of mutual stimulation and elevation. The goal is for the family to tap into higher-order needs for affiliation, belonging, esteem, and efficacy, rather than mere survival or comfort. Families build daily interactions around their child and rely on professionals for expert opinion, anticipatory guidance, measurement, troubleshooting, and simple support. ASD has no cure, and there has been little examination of which factors might decrease parental perceptions of vulnerability after the diagnosis. The earlier the diagnosis is made, the more likely it is to affect the parents' developing view of their child. Thus, it is most important that practitioners recognize the disorder early and develop a long-term management plan.

Seltzer and colleagues (Seltzer, Kraus, Osmond, & Vestal, 2000; Seltzer, Shattuck, Abbeduto, & Greenberg, 2004) describe three ways in which families are affected by having a child with autism. First, compared with parents of children with other developmental disabilities, these families face greater stress, depression, anxiety, and other negative mental health outcomes. Second, the consequences of ASD are pervasive and lasting, changing from childhood through adolescence and adulthood. In earlier childhood years, families welcome intervention programs and extensive treatment regimens. As the child reaches adolescence, however, families recognize that the child's level of functioning or capacity for transition to independent living may not change dramatically. Third, social support and the use of specific coping strategies can buffer the magnitude and impact of stress among family members. The social ecology must provide the necessary resources, and resilience is measured by the ability of individuals, their families, and communities to negotiate culturally meaningful ways for resources to be shared. Resilience is a process of adaptation to environmental, social, psychological, and physiological processes (Cameron, Ungar, & Liebenberg, 2007).

ELEMENTS OF RESILIENCE

Environmental Components

One of the most insidious and insurmountable environmental vulnerabilities is resource insufficiency. The treatment plan for ASD involves intensive educational support and behavior therapy in all settings. Unfortunately, educational services are underfunded, sometimes grossly so. Without funds, it is difficult to build any kind of service system for autism treatment. Resource insufficiency inevitably leads to shortages in skilled staff and difficulties in training and recruiting appropriate personnel. Such shortages drive the search for treatment modalities that might be more cost-effective but are not as effective and, in some cases, are actually harmful.

The availability of educational services depends on local tax revenue, a key problem in rural poor and underserved communities. Services for children with ASD need to be delivered in the immediate, not years down the line. Poor rural areas are dependent on limited community resources and tax-based revenue. Environmental resources for local, early intervention are generally funded through the educational system. Jurisdictions make critical choices on the provision of these education resources.

Case 1: Thomas—Educational Support in the Preschool Environment

Thomas was diagnosed with autism at age 30 months, at which point early intervention services were started on a schedule of 1 hour per week. Thomas was eligible for preschool at 36 months and enrolled at the local elementary school. He was nonverbal, so he was assigned a one-on-one paraeducator who was well meaning but not skilled with autistic children. The role of the paraeducator is to support the child in a classroom, as a human attachment, but this role is typically a low-paying position with a minimal skill set expected.

Thomas' mother stepped in and asked the educational team and school board for financial support to receive training in applied behavioral analysis (ABA). ABA methods are used to teach social skills, enhance communication, and reduce interfering maladaptive behaviors. They agreed, and his mother became Thomas's paraeducator. The role evolved and today she is a leader within the small rural elementary school. For a year her son was the only child in the school system with autism. When a second child was diagnosed a year later, the school was ready for immediate intervention. Thomas's mother enlisted a certified ABA therapist to travel from the southern part of the state once a month to consult on both children. The cost was shared between the school and the two families. This intervention resulted in less disruption in the children's education and brought a collective gain in therapies for both children. In this way, the rural district provided ABA at the preschool level and effectively started a program for managing ASD.

Schools have the potential to support children with ASD at both policy and practice levels. The National Research Council, in *Educating Children with Autism* (Lord, McGee, & Commission on Educational Interventions for Children with Autism, 2001), recommends at least 25 hours per week of intensive early intervention as soon as a child is diagnosed. If diagnosis occurs prior to age 3, the Family, Infant and Toddler (FIT) program is responsible for coordinating services for the child and family. However, 25 hours per week of active engagement in intensive instructional programming is considerably more service than children in FIT generally receive in rural communities. Essential Early Education programs typically provide 3 to 5 half-days per week of a preschool program and some additional home visits for parent education or support. A preschool program may or may not be an intensive program and is frequently less than the recommended minimum of 25 hours per week (Lord et al., 2001).

Thomas was an autistic child living in a rural community school with 87 students in kindergarten through fifth grade. There was no therapist available to provide the recommended educational support. Such rural environments tend to have more single-parent families and young workers lacking a higher education and more vulnerable to income inequality. However, Thomas's mother—a single mother on a limited income—developed a cooperative agreement with the school board, negotiated a role for herself, and created an environment for justice and reduction of vulnerability.

Cultural Components

In New Hampshire, home of the famous "Live free or die" motto, the culture is inherently anti-tax. Local governments are lean and efficient. However, rural healthcare settings are challenged by limitations placed on providers. Vulnerability occurs when professionals are stretched beyond their comfort levels in caring for individuals with developmental disabilities. Rural families often have no choice in selecting a provider, and if the provider has a limited skill set, the family has no recourse. Further, it is a cultural expectation among these rural populations not to question the expertise or skill sets of their healthcare providers.

Case 2: The Reynolds Family—Cultural Factors and Delayed Diagnoses

The Reynolds family, living on a limited income, had three children under age 7. Two of the children had developmental delays. The family received primary care through a rural-based family practice group. When the children presented for well-child care, they were fearful and uncooperative, and saw a different provider each time. The providers within the group had limited experience with children who fall along the autism spectrum and did not refer the children to early intervention. At each provider visit, the children had tantrums, the exams were incomplete and developmental screens were never completed due to behavior problems.

When the children entered kindergarten and first grade, the educators identified their developmental problems. Both children had challenging behaviors and were not able to be taught in a group setting. The educational team requested a development evaluation, and the healthcare provider referred the children to a tertiary center. The parents had no money to travel to a tertiary center, the small health practice had no coordinator to help them fund the referral, and the family was left to negotiate with a tertiary health system on their own. After a conversation with the children's mother, an administrative assistant at the tertiary referral center recognized the dilemma and arranged a relatively simple intervention: a gas card and a 2-day stay at the tertiary center's family housing alternative. This action preserved the family's independence and did not require clinical expertise, just an empathetic approach using para-clinical skills. In this case, the para-clinical person who understood the challenge and made a decision to strengthen the system of care delivery laid the cornerstone for stability.

The cultural milieu can present challenges for families with an ASD child. Not only are special educators, therapists, and psychologists less available in small, rural communities, but teachers' expectations for education of the child can be lower. The follow-up on the Reynolds children illustrates a cultural synergy of both risk and protective factors. One of the Reynolds children received the diagnosis of ASD with the recommendation for an individualized educational program. The parents were not willing to have the child labeled with this diagnosis because teachers in the community had expressed the opinion that autistic behavior occurred secondary to poor parenting. Further, in this rural community, the parents were well known, and in the past both had experienced a rebellious relationship with local teachers. The parents were defensive, neither had completed high school, and they were not comfortable entering into a meeting with the teachers. The school district did not have a special education advocate.

The nurse practitioner at the tertiary referral center offered to be present at the meeting by teleconference. This intervention helped clarify expectations. The educational team was resourceful and made offers for accommodations. The parents expressed feelings of empowerment, and the child gained an individualized educational plan. The cost of this intervention was billed as a follow-up appointment and covered by the state health program.

A cultural risk in a small rural community is that the family is rarely anonymous when it seeks care. In this environment, individuals often arrive in the professional offices with a well-known past. It is important for practitioners to understand the subtle nuances that may derail a treatment plan. Mrs. Reynolds articulated the humiliation she felt about living on public assistance with an unemployed partner. She felt judged by the community and as a result, approached any gesture of help with suspicion. As a consequence, she was not able to take advantage of the local community resources.

The nurse practitioner recognized that resilience is not an individualized cultural phenomenon. The community must share resources to provide the opportunity for the child to flourish starting with the family. In this case, the gas card, housing, and a teleconference call buffered the risk in this child's life and built capacity for his parents. Later, a second nudge came from the nurse practitioner, who alerted the community mental health team about needed respite services. The system rallied around the family as community members offered services to repair their car and improve the living situation. This nurse created change and addressed vulnerability by working across disciplines and embedding culturally appropriate family-centered care into work settings, the home, and the classroom. Ultimately, the cultural strengths of the community contributed toward making necessary changes to foster attachment with their autistic child.

Social Components

Managing a child with ASD is extremely time-consuming for families. Thus, a key vulnerability associated with this diagnosis is parenting role stress. The types of parental stress experienced generally change over the child's life span, and families may have complications that challenge their ability to handle the additional stress. Initially, parents must deal with the emotional aspects of discovering that their child has a significant developmental disability (Beatson, 2008). As the child grows older, areas of weaknesses are likely to persist, even as areas of strength buffer vulnerabilities. Due to the high level of daily stress, crises can overwhelm the family and create dangerous situations. The child with autism has a very narrow range of attachment behaviors and, when threatened, often regresses developmentally, manifesting anxious behaviors. These behaviors may become too overwhelming for the family to manage. If the family is facing changing roles or housing or financial difficulties, the child's stability may be threatened. In a rural community, the availability of services outside of the educational system is often limited. Thus, when a family's social situation changes, crisis may develop rapidly.

Case 3: Phillip—Social Factors and Sleep Disorder

Phillip was a 9-year-old nonverbal youth with ASD and chronic sleep disturbance. He had difficulty getting to sleep at night and often awoke after a few hours. When awake, he screamed and required constant supervision. His parents took turns responding to this dilemma. They stayed awake in 4-hour shifts at night, and they slept during the day when Phillip was at school.

Then Phillip became physically aggressive during the wakeful periods and his behavior at school worsened. He bit his mother and she had difficulty controlling him alone, so his father was frequently called upon to intervene. There was no quality sleep for anyone. The sleep deprivation caused a decline in the well-being of the entire family. Phillip developed a pattern of falling asleep in the early morning. If awakened for school, he became combative. The parents often decided to let him sleep, keeping him home from school. Because the child was not attending school, he began to fail educationally.

The solution to this social dilemma involved an ecological approach. Foremost, the physical aggression was socially unacceptable. Parents who encounter this problem are usually not forthcoming in describing the situation until the risk of injury or actual harm occurs. In this case, the questions asked to parents were pivotal: "What is your threshold of calling for help?" and "Who would you call?" The threshold for alerting others was if Phillip bit his mother hard enough to draw blood, and the agency or person they would call was the police. When queried about why they did not consider the primary care provider, the mother said that the healthcare providers were uncomfortable with the behavior and were unable to come up with a solution, even on a short-term basis. When queried about using any health facility, such as an emergency room, the response was even more negative. The parents stated that this practice would create a larger problem. In small communities, public servants such as the police and fire personnel play a vital role in managing crises, because they make house calls, know how to assess risk, and possess skills to de-escalate a conflict situation.

The solution in this case involved the regional child development team. The child needed an assessment and a two-tiered approach to the problem. Having a child with autism imposes a higher level of social isolation on the family. Social isolation may reach a critical level rapidly as parents, working at maximum capacity, become helpless. In a rural setting, informal networks of support may not be in close proximity, or may be unavailable, overburdened, or unsuitable. It is important for practitioners to have a clear understanding of the social connectedness of the family.

The informal network of caregivers is a first line of defense, followed by alliances built with clergy, sheltered programs, skilled caregivers, and respite care. The formal network, defined as community health professionals, regional programs, and residential care, is another alternative. If a child's primary social network is failing, it is imperative to reduce the parenting stress and work toward stability. Phillip responded to sleep medication, but the treatment required almost 2 weeks to achieve a complete 6-hour sleep cycle. In the interim, the mother was hospitalized with chest pain and the father was left as sole care provider for a week.

Psychological Components

Psychosocial quality of life is predicted by autism severity. As a child with autism works to change behaviors or learn difficult skills, it is essential that the reward for this effort be substantial. Individuals with autism need a consistent approach in education and teaching/learning strategies. Some families do not show an interest in being interventionists on behalf of the child, some are already at their psychological limit and may also have other family responsibilities. Some parents expect the school to provide total care. Thus, some families do not accept a family-centered philosophy as an option. These cases are challenging for providers, and the practitioners need to accept the situation, using a positive tone laced with compassion. Such families may be in an evolutionary process, and they may become more supportive on a psychological level with time and patience.

Case 4: Sara—An Adolescent with Attention and Aggression Issues

Sara was an adolescent with autism. When educators noted a decrease in Sara's attention span and an increase in problem behaviors in school, the healthcare provider assessed the situation and prescribed central nervous system stimulants. Over the next few weeks, Sara had severe anxiety and became increasingly resistant to school. The medication used to increase her attention span was not effective and her behavior deteriorated. Her mother let Sara stay home because she believed the school was not providing her daughter with an appropriate education.

Treating a target symptom alone—rather than as a target symptom within a disorder, such as autism—often creates secondary problems. As demonstrated by this case, providers in rural areas have less training in handling mental health issues and the chronic needs of individuals with autism. The result for Sara was an exacerbation of her core symptoms of obsessive anxiety. Sara regressed and developed secondary problems related to her ASD. In general, individuals with autism have a higher degree of internal distractibility that can manifest as inattention. Although the medication prescribed for Sara was intended to make her more internally driven (i.e., hyperfocused), it actually caused her to develop heightened anxiety. This anxiety was manifested as refusal to participate in school. She was no longer willing to put forth the effort because the rewards were not great enough, and she reverted to self-stimulatory behavior. Once such behaviors overwhelm a rural educational system, few alternatives are typically available because there are few trained behavior specialists who can break down the problem in a systematic manner.

Sara was evaluated at the regional center, and started on medication to help reduce her aggression and school avoidance. The central nervous stimulants were discontinued and a low-dose selective serotonin reuptake inhibitor was started. While stimulant medications are prescribed to treat inattention and hyperactivity symptoms, they may exacerbate stereotypic behaviors, such as hand flapping, tic-like behaviors, and a paradoxical response, resulting in increased hyperactivity, obsessive behaviors, and mood liability (Di Martino, Melis, Cianchetti, & Zuddas, 2004; King & Bostic, 2006).

While autism is three to five times more common in boys, girls with autism are more likely to be severely intellectually impaired (Fombonne, 2005). When children with

ASD move beyond elementary school programs, it is necessary to focus on behavioral regulation. In adolescence, the term *transition* is used to describe movement from child-centered activities to adult-oriented activities. For some youth, the hormonal contribution of puberty makes this period even more challenging. Problematic emotional reactions and behaviors such as aggression and self-injury are common in older individuals with ASD. Recent surveys indicate approximately 45% of adolescents and as many as 75% of adults with ASD are treated with psychotropic medications. Increasing age, lower adaptive skills and social competence, and higher levels of maladaptive behaviors are associated with greater likelihood of medication use (Tsakanikos, Costello, & Holt, 2006).

The most common use of medications is for managing disruptive behaviors, such as self-injury, aggression, compulsions (repetitive behaviors), hyperactivity, mood lability, anxiety, and sleep disturbances (Kanne, Christ, & Reisersen, 2009). Such medications do not cure autism. The goal of treatment is to alleviate the most troublesome behavioral symptoms that impair or distress the child and/or interfere with therapeutic efforts, such as intensive education and socialization (Witwer & Lecavalier, 2005).

Social challenges occur with the onset of adolescence. The youth with autism is much more vulnerable, and at higher risk for regressive behaviors as a result of the physiology involved. Such behaviors may, in turn, overwhelm the family system. Teens with autism need individually focused care to minimize the anxiety and social disorganization that threaten their ability to achieve inclusion. At this point in development, the adolescent with autism needs to have a certain level of independence and any regression is problematic. A team approach during this critical period is necessary.

Physiological Components

The communication impairments characteristic of ASD may lead to an unusual presentation of atypical signs of common disorders; most prevalent are gastrointestinal and sleep disturbances. In a nationally representative sample, researchers found that children with ASD spent twice as much time with the physician per outpatient visit compared with children in control groups. A wide variety of physical illnesses and aberrant physiologic states in ASD can produce pain and discomfort that, in turn, generate high rates of problem behavior and impede psychosocial and educational development (Carr & Owen-DeSchryver, 2007).

Case 5: Camus—A Preschooler with Two Physiological Comorbidities: High Lead Level and a Seizure Disorder

Camus was a 3-year-old child diagnosed with autism. Prior to his third birthday, he was mouthing objects as one of his self-stimulatory behaviors. His blood level of lead, as measured at the child development center shortly after diagnosis, was 40 µg/dL. Camus lived in a 200-year-old farmhouse, and the source of lead poisoning was lead paint in the window frames. The home was owned by the family, who had lived there for many generations. However, the family was delinquent in its property taxes, so was not eligible for state funding for lead abatement until the balance was paid. The child remained in the house and received oral iron treatment, but his lead level remained toxic and his behavior worsened. This financial dilemma affected both the quality of his education and his ability to learn. Nurses were involved at the state and regional levels, but the interventions were ultimately determined by the ability of parents to complete their financial obligation. In consultation with the nurse practitioner at the tertiary level, the family was able to assess their situation and make the decision to tear down the house and live in a temporary house on the property. The cost of property taxes far exceeded the cost of a new modular home. This solution left them in the same situation of owing taxes, but the child was in a safer environment.

Camus continued to demonstrate behavioral regression as the lead was slowly absorbed into his system. He was diagnosed with a seizure disorder when his pica progressed to the self-injurious behavior of biting. He was excluded from his preschool program because his unpredictable biting injured the paraeducator. The nurses involved in his care collaborated across several agencies and coordinated efforts with parents as case managers. The family lived in rural isolation but had daily contact with a web of providers to improve their child's behavior to the point where he could safely be reintroduced to his school environment.

NURSING INTERVENTION

Development in children with ASD is not merely delayed, but also different and disordered. Autism affects development by interfering with socialization, communication, and learning. The goal of intervention is to potentiate human development through collaborative and responsive family partnerships with the educational and healthcare teams. Interventions should focus primarily on improving parenting practices, as they represent the most important factor in the adjustment of children. A focus on resilience calls for attention to be paid to building capacities in children through family-centered care by developing a flexible and responsive system in health care and education. At the level of clinical work, the focus is on well-child care and early identification of social impairment. Deficits in social interaction in autism change over the course of development but remain an area of great disability even for the highest-functioning adult with autism.

To manage patients with ASD, the nurse must be knowledgeable about normal and abnormal development, recognize developmental milestones, and be able to use a validated screening tool. General developmental screening at 9, 18, and 24 months of age will identify most children with autism. The early signs for an ASD diagnosis include the child's social skills, communication, and restricted or repetitive patterns of behavior, interests, and activities (American Psychiatric Association, 2000). A child should respond to his or her name by 1 year of age, and the lack of this pivotal social skill is concerning for ASD. An infant with a relative lack of social interest and an over-concern with environmental (nonsocial) change is considered to be at high risk. Various rating scales and checklists may aid in diagnosis but do not replace the need for thoughtful and careful assessment (Greenspan & Brazelton, 2008). It is important for the nurse to be cautious about terminology, such as high functioning and low functioning. "The difference between high functioning and low functioning is that high functioning means your deficits are being ignored, and low functioning means your assets are being ignored," stated one mother of an autistic child.

Developmental or behavioral regression describes a significant loss of previously acquired milestones or skills. Regression occurs in a minority of children with autism. The mean age at which parents report regression is 20 months. The most frequently reported aspect of regression is loss of language, followed by loss of social–emotional connectedness. Some groups of children are at risk for later diagnosis, especially those who have many primary care providers, those who live in a rural area, and those who live in poverty (Mandell, Maytali, & Zubritsky, 2005).

Resilience in ASD is a dynamic social process. To promote resilience, it is necessary to have resources available that provide a structure through which individual capacity may flourish. The healthcare provider working in rural areas needs additional training to understand how to implement and manage a family-centered plan of care. Healthcare providers need to partner with emergency responders, educators, and community activists to create a safety net for families (Carbine, Behl, Azor, & Murphy, 2010). It is critical to remain connected with families and willing to respond to their most pressing needs. A continuum of services across the lifespan is needed for individuals on the autism spectrum (Carbine et al., 2010; Elder & D'Alessandro, 2009). See **Table 23-2** for ASD resources.

Parenting an autistic child is an isolating experience, simply because of the nature of the disorder (Elder & D'Alessandro, 2009). A skilled and resourceful nurse can regulate the level of stress so that it becomes motivating rather than overwhelming. Home visits, teleconferences, and regularly scheduled clinic appointments create space and time to discuss hopes and aspirations as well as the daily reality. The nurse must establish a partnership with the educational team, building interdisciplinary care. Reliable partnerships help prevent distortion of information, focus on the child's strengths, and help the family to be realistic about the journey ahead. Families need a supportive, collaborative team to help their child reach his or her fullest potential. By putting these approaches into action, the nurse frees the family from the illusion that they could accomplish these goals in isolation or should carry the load alone.

Table 23-2 Autism Spectrum Disorder Resources for Nurses

Autism and Medication: Safe and Careful Use. A Guide for Families with Autism: www.autismspeaks.org

Autism: Caring for Children with Autism Spectrum Disorders: A Resource Toolkit for Clinicians—American Academy of Pediatrics: www.aap.org/healthtopics/autism.cfm

Autism Speaks, Family Services Department: www.autismspeaks.org/family-services

Center for Social Emotional Foundations for Early Learning: www.vanderbilt.edu/csefel

Developmental Screening Policy Statement: www.medicalhomeinfo.org/screening/indexx.html

Enhancing Developmentally Oriented Primary Care (EDOPC): www.illinoisaap.org/medicalhome.htm, www.illinoisaap.org/DevelopmentalScreening.htm

National Center of Medical Home Initiative for Children with Special Needs: www.medicalhomeinfo.org

Pathways to Independence Natural Supports Project: www.waisman.wisc.edu/naturalsupports

Pill swallowing: www.pillswallowing.com

Public Awareness Program on Early Childhood Development: www.cdc.gov/ncbddd/autism/actearly

Understanding Autism Spectrum Disorders—American Academy of Pediatrics: www.aap.org/heal;thtopics/autism.cfm

Zero to Three: www.zerotothree.org

Autism and Medication: Safe and Careful Use—A Guide for Families of Children with Autism http://www.autismspeaks.org/sites/default/files/docs/sciencedocs/atn/medication_safe_and_careful_use.pdf

By working closely with the family, the nurse supports their resilience. There is hope for the ASD child and family, as described in the book, *Born on a Blue Day*, written by an autistic adult diagnosed in infancy with both autism and a comorbid seizure disorder:

> I'm amazed to think how much my parents did for me even as they must have gotten so little back at the time. Hearing my parents' recollections of my earliest years has been a magical experience for me: to see for myself in hindsight the extent of their role in making me the person I am today. (Tammet, 2006, pp. 27–28)

REFERENCES

American Psychiatric Association. (2000). *Diagnostic and statistical manual for mental disorders* (4th ed.). Washington, DC: American Psychiatric Publishing.

Beatson, J. E. (2008). Walk a mile in their shoes: Implementing family-centered care in serving children and families affected by autism spectrum disorder. *Topics in Language Disorders*, 28(4), 309–322.

Cameron, C., Ungar, M., & Liebenberg, L. (2007). Cultural understandings of resilience: Roots for wings in the development of affective resources for resilience. *Child and Adolescent Psychiatric Clinics of North America, 16*, 285–301.

Carbine, P., Behl, D., Azor, V., & Murphy, N. (2010). The medical home for children with autism spectrum disorders: Parent and pediatric perspectives. *Journal of Autism and Developmental Disorders, 40*, 317–324.

Carr, E. G., & Owen-DeSchryver, R. (2007). Physical illness, pain, and problem behavior in minimally verbal people with developmental disabilities. *Journal of Autism and Developmental Disorders, 37*, 413–424.

Centers for Disease Control and Prevention. (2014). Prevalence of autism spectrum disorder among children aged 8 years—Autism and Developmental Disabilities Monitoring Network, 11 sites, United States, 2010. Surveillance summaries, March 28, 2014, 63 (SS02). Retrieved from http://www.cdc.gov/mmwr/pdf/ss/ss6302.pdf

Davis, L. H. (2009, April 4). Still overlooking autistic adults. *The Washington Post*. Retrieved from www.washingtonpost.com

Di Martino, A., Melis, G., Cianchetti, C., & Zuddas, A. (2004). Methylphenidate for pervasive developmental disorders: Safety and efficacy of acute single dose test and ongoing therapy. *Journal of Child and Adolescent Psychopharmacology, 14*(2), 201–218.

Elder, J., & D'Alessandro, T. (2009). Supporting families with autism spectrum disorders: Questions parents ask and what nurses need to know. *Pediatric Nursing, 35*(4), 240–253.

Fombonne, E. (2005). Epidemiological studies of pervasive developmental disorder. In F. R. Volkmar, A. Kiln, R. Paul, & D. Cohen (Eds.), *Handbook of autism and pervasive developmental disorders* (3rd ed., pp. 42–69). Hoboken, NJ: John Wiley & Sons.

Greenspan, S. L., & Brazelton, T. B. (2008). Guidelines for identification, screening, and clinical management of children with autism spectrum disorders. *Pediatrics, 121*, 828–830.

Howlin, P. (2005). Outcomes in autism spectrum disorders. In F. R. Volkmar, R. Paul, A. Klin, & D. Cohen (Eds.), *Handbook of autism and pervasive developmental disorders* (3rd ed., Vol. II, pp. 201–209). Hoboken, NJ: John Wiley & Sons.

Kanne, S., Christ, S., & Reisersen, A. (2009). Psychiatric symptoms and psychosocial difficulties in young adults with autistic traits. *Journal of Autism and Developmental Disorders, 39*, 827–833.

King, B., & Bostic, J. (2006). An update on pharmacologic treatments for autism spectrum disorders. *Child and Adolescent Psychiatric Clinics of North America, 12*(11), 161–175.

Leal, A. (2011) Little boy lost. *The Chronicle of Higher Education*. The Chronicle Review. Retrieved from http://chronicle.com/article/Little-Boy-Lost/129176/

Lord, C., McGee, J. (Eds.), & Commission on Educational Interventions for Children with Autism. (2001). *Educating children with autism*. Washington, DC: National Academies Press.

Mandell, D., Maytali, M., & Zubritsky, C. (2005). Factors associated with age of diagnosis among children with autism spectrum disorder. *Pediatrics, 116*(6), 1480–1486.

Martinez-Pederast, F., & Carter, A. (2009). Autism spectrum disorders in young children. *Child and Adolescent -Psychiatric Clinics of North America, 18*, 645–663.

Myers, S., Johnson, C., & American Academy of Pediatrics Council on Children with Disabilities (2007). Management of children with autism spectrum disorders. American Academy of Pediatrics. *Pediatrics, 120*(5), 1162–1182.

Seltzer, M., Kraus, M., Osmond, G., & Vestal, C. (2000). Families of adolescents and adults with autism: Uncharted territory. In L. Chidden (Ed.), *International review of research in mental retardation: Autism* (*Vol. 23*, pp. 267–294). San Diego, CA: Academy Press.

Seltzer, M., Shattuck, P, Abbeduto, L., & Greenberg, J. (2004). Trajectory of development in adolescents and adults with autism. *Mental Retardation and Developmental Disabilities Research Review*, *10*, 234–247.

Tammet, D. (2006). *Born on a blue day*. New York: Free Press.

Tsakanikos, E., Costello, H., & Holt, G. (2006). Psychopathology in adults with autism and intellectual disability. *Journal of Autism and Developmental Disorders*, *36*, 1123–1129.

Witwer, A., & Lecavalier, L., (2005). Treatment incidence and patterns in children with autism spectrum disorders. *Journal of Child and Adolescent Psychopharmacology*, *15*, 671–681.

Chapter 24

Developing a Nurse Practitioner–Run Center for Residents in Rural Appalachia

Joyce M. Knestrick and Mona M. Counts

OBJECTIVES

At the end of this chapter, the reader will be able to

1. Discuss the process of implementing and sustaining a nurse practitioner (NP)–run clinic in rural Appalachia.
2. Describe the attributes of Appalachian culture.
3. Transfer the information on this NP-run center to other vulnerable populations.

INTRODUCTION

In rural Appalachia, the population experiences barriers to primary care, a high risk of acute and chronic illness, inconsistency in healthcare services, and geographic separation from healthcare services. The barriers faced by this population impact their quality of life.

In a rural Appalachian area in Southwestern Pennsylvania, a need was identified to develop and maintain a NP-run primary care center to serve the primary health care needs of the community. Sustainability of the center and cultural competency were paramount in providing care to this population. The provision of evidence-based healthcare services by culturally sensitive providers is the mission of this NP-run primary care practice.

The purposes of this chapter are to describe a vulnerable population in the rural Appalachia region of Southwestern Pennsylvania and to discuss the planning, implementation, sustainability, and outcomes of a NP-run primary care practice.

DESCRIPTION OF THE POPULATION

Demographic Characteristics

In this Appalachian community, more than 13% of the patients are over the age of 65. This is consistent with the demographic profile of 15% elderly in the county and 15% state-wide in Pennsylvania (U.S. Census Bureau, 2010). These elders tend to be minimally educated, often unemployed, and frequently uninsured or underinsured (Counts, 1992; Russell, Gregory, Wotton, Mordoch, & Counts, 1996). The general population has limited economic resources and is also often uninsured or underinsured. They may leave the area to gain employment and then return to care for family. The average annual per capita income is $20,258, with 17.5% of residents living below the poverty level. The poverty level in the county is 13.5% versus the national average of 9.6 % (U.S. Census Bureau, 2010).

Core Values

Core values of this rural Appalachian population drive health behavior and health care seeking. The concepts of hardiness, family, acceptance, spirituality and neighboring are valued by the culture (Counts, 1992; Huttlinger & Purnell, 2008). This particular community exhibits many of the traits described in the literature on Appalachian populations (Huttlinger & Purnell, 2008). The authors of this chapter have the distinct advantage of being residents of rural Appalachia.

Being Hardy

Being *hardy* is a common cultural descriptor. The population has lived in this mountainous area for a long period of time and they have survived and carried on with their lives. They have sustained economic losses and have limited employment opportunities. *Health* is defined as the ability to function, regardless of circumstances, and encompasses physical, spiritual, and mental aspects of life (Counts, 1992; Huttlinger & Purnell, 2008).

For the population served by the center, health is "function." Members of the community will ignore health problems until they are not able to go to work, tend to their farm or household chores, or are completely incapacitated. For this population, as long as people are able to continue to work, they consider themselves healthy (Counts, 1992). Although health care is focused within the family, a sense of individual responsibility for self-care exists. As part of the self-care practices, the family may use folk medicines and treatments before they seek traditional healthcare services. The community generally accepts mental health problems as "fate."

Family

Family ties are important and strong in the community. Family is more than one's blood relatives. It includes individuals married into the family and individuals or families adopted into the family (formally or informally). Family is considered a stronger entity than an individual. A member of the community may reference the family when speaking (e.g., "We want a healthcare center that is going to stay here," or "We only want to see the nurse provider").

Families take pride in "doing for each other." Most people have extended families that live in close proximity. The entire extended family may become involved in an issue that other cultures would consider personal. For example, if a teenager is pregnant, the family may get together to offer advice and decide how to handle the teen and her pregnancy. Elders are respected and often live with family members. The elders often are the main providers of child care and also provide care for other less healthy elders in the extended family. The family ties are so strong that obligations to family may outweigh other obligations (e.g., school, work, or healthcare appointments).

Acceptance

Continuity of care and sustainability are essential for acceptance of healthcare programs in the community. The long-held distrust of outsiders is strengthened when services are started and are subsequently moved or closed. Previously, centers employing foreign medical graduates were started, but the language barriers created additional trust issues. The gathering of research data with no follow-up plan by faculty in universities and medical schools left a "bad taste" for outsiders querying about need for healthcare services.

Acceptance by the community is a slow process. The NPs must demonstrate respect for the individual and the family. When one of the authors first came to the center, a grandmother stated, "You can see my granddaughter but I will not see you, you are a Northerner." The NP, who lives less than 30 miles away in the same Appalachian region, acknowledged the grandmother and offered to make an appointment with the other NP. She turned around and the grandmother noticed the NP had Elvis on her shirt. The grandmother remarked: "You did a good job with my grandbaby, and you like Elvis, you are okay by me. I will see you now." This encounter is an example of acceptance of the provider.

Spirituality

Spirituality is defined as a deep-rooted belief in God and Christ. Many people have strong ties to their churches. The church often provides a means of social support and a mechanism for socialization. "Doing good deeds" and "living right on earth" are pathways to rewards in heaven. Because one cannot change the future, certain circumstances have to be endured on this earth. Health is intertwined with the mind, body, and spirit (Counts, 1992).

Neighboring

An essential concept in this community is *neighboring*, which is described as neighbors taking care of each other when needs arise. If a person is sick, the neighbors will do what they can to provide care. If the person is laid off from work, the neighbors will help with food and other services, such as babysitting while job searching. As a neighbor, the person receiving the services will help another neighbor in turn.

CASE STUDY

An Appalachian Farmer

Mr. Couch is a 56-year-old farmer who currently lives on a 20-acre farm with his wife, three children, and his mother. He has a positive history of one myocardial infarction, hypertension, and high cholesterol. He has a normal body weight and his record states that his blood pressure is controlled on lisinopril 20 mg with HCTZ 12.5 mg. The record also states he is on warfarin 5 mg and atorvastatin 20 mg daily. He presents to the center in November, complaining of excessive bleeding every time he gets a small cut. His wife and oldest son are in the room with him. His son notes that they have just finished tilling the garden for the winter fallow. His wife states they are stocked with food canned from their garden this past summer. She hands the NP jars of pickled beets and zucchini relish. As his last medication adjustments were done in July, the NP reviews the medication list with Mr. Couch and asks him if he taking any other medicines or any herbs. His wife volunteers that she is giving him gingko to help with his perceived memory loss.

Case Study Questions

1. What are the attributes of Appalachian culture evident in this case?
2. What are possible etiologies for the bleeding?
3. How does the understanding of the culture help guide the NP in appropriate teaching strategies?

DEVELOPMENT OF THE PRIMARY CARE CENTER

In the 1980s, healthcare services in this area of Appalachia were limited. Barriers to access to health care included lengthy travel to a tertiary care center in a neighboring state or to a tertiary care center 60 miles from the community. The establishment of foreign physicians' private practices provided an inconsistent supply of providers and limited access for individuals and families without health insurance. An NP living in the community was bombarded, on her porch, by community members seeking health care. The community asked her to start a center to provide healthcare services to the area.

In response, the NP did an ethnographic analysis of the community. The need for more data on the population emerged. A community assessment tool, the Appalachian Patterns General Ethnographic Nursing Evaluation Studies in the State III (Russell et al., 1996) was administered in the county. It further assessed healthcare concerns and needs. The study reinforced the need for culturally competent services, a sustainable commitment to the community, and integration of a primary care center within the community. Key cultural characteristics of this particular Appalachian community were defined.

The goal of the primary care center was not only to provide healthcare services but to partner with the community to make improvements in the lives of residents. Historically, the area has had several extraction industries. Coal mining continues to be an integral part of the area. Strip mining and gas drilling are becoming more prevalent. Workers often come from other areas to work in these industries. Recreational activities related to the beautiful mountains, lakes, and streams are owned or managed by outside agents. Therefore, to help the community economically, the goal has been to hire staff from within the community and to train the staff to become successful so that they can give back to their own community.

The Operational Plan

A plan was developed with the input of the community to establish a community-owned center, staffed by local residents and caring providers who are culturally sensitive. The primary care center was launched and staffed by a corporation of NPs. In order to increase community participation and to develop more intense community involvement, the structure was established as a 501(c)(3), nonprofit organization to enhance access to additional funding sources. The community residents became the owners of the practice and had a vested interest in the sustainability of the center. In addition to the community at large, stakeholders included the township supervisors, state representative, local businesses, churches, and senior organizations. From the group of concerned citizens, a board was established to oversee the operations and sustainability of the center.

The establishment of community ownership of the nonprofit organization led to becoming a Federally Qualified Health Center Look-Alike (FQHC-LA). To expand and optimize funds in the area, all FQHC-LAs combined under a Federally Qualified Health Center (FQHC), minimizing administrative costs and providing opportunity to expand services. Grants were written to fund the primary care center. Local state representatives were enlisted to help at the state level. In addition, the federal representative and a state senator were contacted to help fund the center. The granting of federal funds to build a new facility was obtained prior to the merger with the FQHC.

The center was established with four NPs (total of 1.2 full-time equivalents [FTEs]). Seven other personnel, including a registered nurse, a medical assistant, a receptionist, and a billing clerk were hired. As the center expanded, a merger with a local FQHC located in the same county was completed to ensure sustainability of services for the community. Over time, office staff went on for further education to become licensed practical nurses, registered nurses, and NPs.

Incorporation of Social Services

Early in the development of the primary care center, a need for social services became apparent. This area of Appalachia has high poverty levels and limited access to mental health services, leaving the community vulnerable for injuries related to violent acts and issues related to substance abuse. Mental health problems tend to be accepted by families and treatment is not sought unless the person is unable to function in the family.

The addition of a social worker to the primary care center was carefully assessed and initially funded by a grant from Staunton Farm Foundation. This person needed to be culturally competent, accepted by the community, and perceived by the community as providing services differently from a traditional social worker. Many of the residents expressed concerns related to prior bad experiences with social workers such as "they came and took my cousin's kids away" and "that social worker put my mother in a home." The role of this social worker was to provide mental health screenings and assessments, provide counseling services, and maintain a link with area mental health providers. In addition, the social worker would acquire services to keep the elderly and disabled patients in their homes. At this point, social services continue to be available at the FQHC.

Sources of Funding

The primary care center is funded by private insurers, Medicare, Medicaid and cash payments via a sliding scale, so some patients do not pay. Some private insurers recognize the NPs as primary care providers while others do not. A few private insurers do not recognize the NPs as primary care providers but rather list them as "specialists." The primary care center is also funded by donations, program grants, and contracts with companies for wellness and drug screening services.

Outcomes

The NP-managed center has been acknowledged by the state Medicaid managed-care insurer for providing excellent, highest quality standards of care. This designation noted accessibility, prevention of illness via immunizations, screening for potential illnesses, and efforts to minimize the impact of nonpreventable illness. The center has partnered with various agencies to provide preventive services such as cervical cancer screenings, breast exams, and mammogram services to women in the community.

Health Promotion

During the last 5 years, over 90% of adult patients had cholesterol screening with education on diet, lifestyle changes, and medications. In a sample of type 2 diabetes patients ($n = 40$), 84% with elevated glycohemoglobin A1C levels, has now decreased A1C levels to 6.5 or to the patient–provider goal. To decrease diabetic complications, a protocol change was implemented increasing diabetic education and promoting aggressive treatment strategies. In addition, smoking cessation programs were initiated.

Although the population acknowledges that eating healthy food can lead to better health, food choices are limited by cost. The sedentary lifestyle of the population coupled with the poor diet leads to an increasing prevalence of obesity. Programs for lifestyle changes, diet education, and exercise programs have been initiated with the use of community partners involved in recreational activities. These are examples of ways to work with the community to improve health and quality of life.

Access to Services

In 2008, a mobile unit was funded by the Pennsylvania Department of Health to provide county-wide health care, health promotion, and prevention services. In collaboration with a large university and smaller universities in the area, the mobile unit was staffed with NPs, volunteer registered nurses, nursing faculty, and students. The mobile unit visits senior centers, community centers, and schools throughout the county. Blood pressure, cholesterol, height, and weight screenings are provided. County residents who do not have a healthcare provider are offered appointments and follow-up care services. Funding was also received from the Pennsylvania Department of Health to retrofit the mobile unit to provide dental services. This mobile unit works in collaboration with the primary care center to extend services.

Barriers to Care

While the mobile van is an adjunct to care, access to services continues to be a complex problem. Money for food takes precedence over gasoline to drive to the primary care center for care. Severe weather conditions, such as extreme heat, rain, or snow influence access to care because many patients need to walk to the center.

Barriers to full scope practice for NPs continue to exist in the state. Although most local hospitals now accepted the NPs orders for diagnostic testing, some still do not. Problems with billing and reimbursement frequently occur. Although the community health center is accepted and listed on provider panels for multiple insurers, most patients have Medicaid (31%), Medicare (17%), other third-party payers (22%), or are self-pay (30%). Due to the FQHC-LA status, 48% of the visits are paid at base level. Funding is often dependent on payment from insurers who do not provide payment in a timely manner.

Growth Opportunities

Increase in patient numbers and continued stakeholder support provide opportunities for further growth of the primary care center. Healthcare reform legislation calls for more effective ways to deliver primary healthcare services. An opportunity exists to demonstrate how the NP model of primary care can effectively reduce healthcare costs while providing high quality and culturally sensitive services.

With changes in the healthcare system, the primary care center has become part of a larger health system in the county and it is now part of the FQHC that began operations in 1977. For several reasons, this partnership is a logical step to sustain culturally competent care to this vulnerable population. First, the evolution of this system and that of the primary care center are similar. Secondly, the types of populations are similar for both systems. Third, both were begun as NP-managed practices and have expanded to include services by other professionals.

CONCLUSION

This chapter describes the implementation of a NP-managed center to provide primary healthcare services to a low-income area of rural Appalachia. By living in this region, the NPs who started the center have a good understanding of the perceived needs of the community. NPs and other advanced practice nurses have the skills to provide high quality, cost-effective, culturally sensitive care to this vulnerable population. The NPs have worked to empower their patients to improve their quality of life and to limit the effects of chronic disease through primary care, screening, prevention, health education, and social services. Outcomes indicate that attention to community priorities and perceived needs can enable NPs to provide culturally competent primary health care to a vulnerable population.

REFERENCES

Counts, M. (1992). *GENESIS III: General ethnographic nursing evaluation studies in the state, 1985–2002.* Unpublished manuscript, Department of Nursing, West Virginia University, Morgantown, WV.

Huttlinger, K. W., & Purnell, L. D. (2008). People of Appalachian heritage. In L. D. Purnell & B. J. Paulanka (Eds.), *Transcultural health care: A culturally competent approach* (3rd ed., pp. 95–112). Philadelphia: F.A. Davis.

Russell, C., Gregory, D., Wotton, D., Mordoch, E., & Counts, M. (1996). ACTION: Application and extension of the GENESIS community analysis model. *Public Health Nursing, 13*(3), 187–194.

U.S. Census Bureau. (2010). Retrieved from http://factfinder.census.gov/servlet/ACSSAFFFacts?_event=ChangeGeoContext&geo_id=05000US42059&_geoContext=&_street=&_county=Greene+County&_cityTown=&_state=&_zip=&_lang=en&_sse=on&ActiveGeoDiv=&_useEV=&pctxt=fph&pgsl=010&_submenuId=factsheet_1&ds_name=ACS_2008_3YR_SAFF&_ci_nbr=null&qr_name=null&reg=null%3Anull&_keyword=&_industry=

Chapter 25

Negotiating the World: Nursing Interventions for a Vulnerable Prison Population Before and After Parole

Judi Daniels

OBJECTIVES

At the end of this chapter, the reader will be able to

1. Identify risk factors at pre-incarceration, incarceration, and post-incarceration.
2. Discuss the impact of the Affordable Care Act on the health of felons.
3. Describe nursing interventions to decrease risk at pre-incarceration, incarceration, and post-incarceration stages.

THE VULNERABILITY OF THE PRISON POPULATION

Over the past 30 years the expansion of the United States (U.S.) prisoner population has focused attention on the costs of housing inmates as well as searching for underlying variables that influence criminal behavior. Changes in mandatory sentencing laws have resulted in 1 out of every 35 adults being supervised in some manner (e.g., prison, jail, supervised probation, or halfway houses) (Glaze & Herberman, 2013). One common thread throughout the literature is the vulnerability of this population based upon their medical problems and lack of access to health care before, during, and after imprisonment. Using a progressive case scenario, this chapter focuses on these problems, along with potential interventions. Although this discussion focuses on men, women in the justice system are also vulnerable.

Healthcare costs incurred by prisoners have increased substantially over the past several years. In 2008, the latest figures recorded, healthcare expenditures had risen 52% in 42 of the 44 states surveyed (PEW Charitable Trusts, MacArthur Foundation, 2013). Costs are driven by an aging prison population, the complexity of chronic medical conditions, and the higher incidence of infectious diseases. Many of these conditions are both pre-existing and exacerbated by incarceration, placing a burden on the correctional system budget (Moore & Elkavich, 2008; PEW Charitable Trusts, MacArthur Foundation, 2013). The healthcare community is in a unique position to intervene at three distinct periods in the incarceration trajectory, reducing risk factors leading to incarceration, providing care within the prison system, and offering support post-incarceration. The progressive case study examines a typical scenario of one individual who moves through the prison system. Opportunities for intervention will be discussed at each point in the incarceration experience.

PRE-INCARCERATION

Robin, a 35-year-old African American single parent and her two sons, Quint, age 16, and Tobias, age 14, are patients at the Community Health Clinic (CHC). The boys have different fathers who are not active in their sons' lives. Robin thinks Quint's father is in prison on a drug charge. Robin does not work, lives in government housing, and attends a community college studying to be a medical assistant. She has had difficulties with her sons, especially Quint. As the oldest, he receives the least amount of her supervision and Robin says: "He is always in trouble."

At age 12, Quint was diagnosed with attention deficit disorder, oppositional defiant disorder, and bipolar disorder. He was prescribed Adderall, Risperdal, Clonidine, and Zoloft. Robin tries to make him take his medications but he often skips his mental health appointments, resulting in lapses in prescription refills. Recently, Quint was seen at the CHC for a sexually transmitted infection (STI). He reported having unprotected intercourse with his girlfriend who was later diagnosed with chlamydia. His mother accompanied him to the CHC and voiced concerns about anger episodes as well as truancy from school.

Quint smokes cigarettes and is experimenting with alcohol and street drugs with his friends. Robin does not like Quint's friends but feels she has no control over his social life. She lectures him that he will end up like his father. This approach does not change his behavior. Twice, he has been caught shoplifting and was scheduled to go to court. Quint was interviewed at court without his mother. He stated that the shoplifting charges were false, that he did not want to go to school, and he planned on taking online courses to obtain a GED certificate. He told the court he was unhappy at home and wanted to stay with his 16-year-old pregnant girlfriend. The court assigned a caseworker and Quint was instructed to stay in school. Robin stated: "These conditions will not make any difference, Quint will do what he wants, and someone will have to just lock him up."

Risk Factors at the Pre-incarceration Stage

This case is a typical scenario. Quint has several risk factors placing him on the path toward incarceration.

Ethnicity and Age

Quint's ethnicity and age are associated with higher risk for incarceration. Though he has no control over these demographics, it is worth noting that approximately 4–7% of all African American males between 20 to 49 years of age have been incarcerated at some point, serving an average sentence of 5 or less years (Carson & Golinelli, 2013). There are a number of contributing factors leading to disparity in the conviction and incarceration rates of African Americans. These factors include poverty, urban-centered crime, targeting of African Americans by the justice system, and lack of leniency in sentencing (National Association for the Advancement of Colored People [NAACP], 2014). Adult felonies subsequently occur among 30–60% of adolescents who engage in delinquent activities before the age of 18 (Ridgeway & Listenbee, 2014). Quint's criminal behavior in adolescence increases his risk.

Mental Illness

Quint's history of mental illness is also a risk factor increasing his chances of being incarcerated (Hawthorne et al., 2012; Schnittker & John, 2007; Schnittker, Massoglia & Uggen, 2012). Mental illness is one of the most well recognized variables associated with criminal behavior. In a study of 39,463 adults with known mental illness, 11% had been incarcerated in the past year and among those incarcerated, 26% were reincarcerated within 1 year (Hawthorne et al., 2012). Using data from the National Comorbidity Survey Replication ($n = 5,692$) Schnittker et al. (2012), reported a relationship between psychiatric disorders in childhood and adolescence and subsequent incarceration.

The most common mental disorders associated with incarceration are major depression, psychosis, schizophrenia, oppositional defiant disorder, and bipolar disorder (Schnittker et al., 2012). The lack of mental health treatment services is linked to incarceration as a means of institutionalization. Untreated mental illness is both cause and consequence, with incarceration compounding the problem. James and Glaze (2006) note that less than 22% of those diagnosed with mental illness prior to imprisonment had received mental health treatment. In Quint's case, it is the lack of consistency in mental health care. His refusal to go to appointments interfered with medication refills, and suboptimal management.

Substance Abuse

Equally important is the influence of drug and alcohol abuse, especially when paired with mental illness. Quint's use of both alcohol and street drugs is a red flag for potential incarceration. James and Glaze (2006) report that 74% of those incarcerated who have a history of mental illness also reported substance abuse. Hawthorne et al. (2012) note a fivefold increased risk of incarceration among individuals with both mental illness and a history of drug abuse. This relationship holds for reincarceration as well. The combination of mental illness and substance abuse is a red flag for providers of mental health services.

The complexity of drug abuse and imprisonment is difficult to untangle. Drug violations account for 50% of federal imprisonments and 26% of state incarcerations (Carson & Golinelli, 2013). The use of drugs is not only a direct cause of imprisonment but is frequently an indirect cause. Overall, 56% of those incarcerated used or were dependent upon illegal drugs prior to imprisonment (James & Glaze, 2006). The National Longitudinal Youth Database reports that persons with recent substance abuse (cocaine and crack) were twice as likely to be incarcerated compared to the general population (Schnittker & John, 2007). The use of drugs is a significant variable among imprisoned persons.

Socioeconomic Factors

Socioeconomic risk factors for potential incarceration include:

- Homelessness (Schnittker & John, 2007; Hawthorne et al., 2012; James & Glaze, 2006)
- Failure to complete high school (Davis, Bozick, Steele, Saunders, & Miles, 2013; Kulkarni, Baldwin, Lightsone, Gelberg, & Diamant, 2010; Schnittker & John, 2007)
- Childhood adversity (e.g., abuse, neglect, and abject poverty) (Schnittker et al., 2012; James & Glaze, 2006)
- One or more parents who have served time in a federal or state prison (James & Glaze, 2006)

This last factor brings full circle the problems that complicate the social fabric on causes, consequences, and influences that lead to incarceration. The children of parents who are or have been incarcerated experience multiple stresses. Parental incarceration may diminish household income, involve a move to a new home and school, and places the child at risk for a sense of shame. There is evidence that antisocial behavior is common in children after parental incarceration (Murray, Farrington, & Sekol, 2012). Quint had a number of risk factors that were out of his control but placed him at greater risk for gravitating toward deviant behavior: his father was incarcerated, the family was living below the poverty level, he was truant from school, and he was living with his pregnant girlfriend. This arrangement was tenuous at best and Quint was at risk of becoming homeless.

Intervention at the Pre-incarceration Stage

Adolescents crossing into a deviant lifestyle are a perplexing problem for families and communities. Early intervention may mitigate risky behaviors, directing the adolescent away from the criminal justice system. Some critical questions are raised. Does the answer lie in subjecting the adolescent to the adult world of harsh incarceration? Should the behavior be excused because of immaturity? What *has* been found to be most helpful is recognizing those adolescents at risk and intervening before an event occurs with a coordinated effort among schools, community action centers, and health clinics. Data compiled by The Future of Children (2008) identifies interventions found to be cost effective and successful in reducing youth violence. These interventions are as follows.

Parenting Education

The single best intervention is helping parents with specific child management skills. Information needs to be given proactively as well as when parents have a child with a problem. Parenting classes can be offered at clinics or schools. Providers must recognize the ongoing need by parents in high-risk situations.

Family Therapy

Families can benefit from learning to communicate better with each other. One of the most successful programs is Functional Family Therapy (Greenwood, 2008). This program is delivered in the home by trained therapists. Problem-solving skills, communications, and ways to set boundaries and provide structure are designed. Tobias, Quint, and Robin also needed the opportunity to grow and succeed. The approach must be coordinated and family centered in order to reduce adolescent criminal behavior and strengthen the family.

Coordination of Mental Health Services

Primary care providers need to be in contact with the child's mental healthcare provider. Prescriptions for ongoing medications must be coordinated to avoid a lag between prescriptions.

Community and School-Based Programs

Referral to Big Brothers or Big Sisters has been found to reduce youth violence, offer strong role models, and reduce youth crime. Nurses working in the community may be involved with school boards in helping to solve problems with truancy and dropouts. School programs with successful outcomes include adult mentors, peer mentors, and helping students who are struggling with coursework.

INCARCERATION

What does *not* work is to do nothing, to decide that Quint is destined to a life of imprisonment. By age 22, Quint had failed to obtain a high school diploma or a GED. He had spent the last few years wandering the streets. Homelessness introduced him to the drug subculture on the streets. His experimentation with crack cocaine led to addiction. Unemployed, without financial support, and needing money for drugs, he began stealing from his mother, who barred him from her government-subsidized home. At age 26, Quint was arrested for armed robbery, classified as a Class B felony with a deadly weapon. He was convicted and sentenced to 5 years in prison with a $15,000 fine. He was eligible for parole in 3 years.

The Experience of Incarceration

Quint was sent to a prison outside of his home state as the in-state facilities were over capacity. Upon admission to prison, he was evaluated for STIs, tuberculosis, hepatitis C, and HIV, screening negative for these diseases. He was also seen by the prison psychiatrist who diagnosed him with bipolar disorder, anger management problems, drug addiction, and depression. The psychiatrist prescribed an antidepressant, a mood stabilizer, and offered drug counseling. During his prison term, Quint withdrew from both crack cocaine and tobacco. He attended the drug rehabilitation meetings, avoided the gangs in the prison cell block, and enrolled in high school completion classes. He worked in the prison kitchen, earning spending money and points for early release. Participation in established prison programs provides evidence of good behavior, used in determining a shortened prison sentence.

Quint did not see his family during incarceration because of the distance they had to travel to see him. His mother wrote to him occasionally and in one letter she informed him that his grandmother, with whom he was very close and had lived with for a period, had died of cancer. His attempts to contact his girlfriend, the mother of his child, were unsuccessful, as she had broken off all contact with him. He kept this loneliness to himself but decided to get a couple of tattoos from a fellow inmate as a reminder of this time period.

While he was in prison, Quint was physically healthy and described himself as "OK," in spite of feeling depressed. He was seen by the psychiatrist periodically for his mood disorder and received the prescribed medications. He was anxious to return home and after 3 years, at the age 29, he was released to a halfway house 3 hours from his hometown. He was mandated to remain at the halfway house for 1 year, after which he would be allowed to move closer to home to finish his sentence on probation.

Social and Ethical Issues with Incarceration

Quint's incarceration history is not unusual. Prisoners often serve time away from their family, leaving them without an external support system. Families may not have the finances or transportation to visit and family ties become loosened. Ultimately this loss of family ties can affect reentry to the community (Moore & Elkavich, 2008).

Provision of Health Care

Health care in prison is mandated under the "equivalence of care" principle. Since 1976, the right to health care equal to those not imprisoned was acknowledged (Niveu, 2007). There are many issues in delivery of health care within a prison setting. Specialists are not readily available or may be limited, especially mental health providers. An unanswered question is whether a prisoner's rights outweigh the risk to others if he refuses medications for contagious diseases. For many prisoners, it is the first time they have ever had regular, direct access to health care and for those serving life sentences, there are issues of aging and chronic illness.

The cost of providing health care to inmates has increased exponentially, amounting to hundreds of millions of dollars annually (Schaenman, Davies, Jordan, & Chakraborty, 2013). With monies limited, prison health services have found ways to reduce cost by providing:

- Health education to target high-risk behavior while in prison
- Screening and treatment of contagious diseases (HIV, hepatitis, tuberculosis, and sexually transmitted infections)
- General preventive health care

Incorporating telemedicine, triaging medical conditions before transferring to an off-site facility, and instituting prisoner co-payment for nonemergency medical visits and medications are some ways to contain cost. Co-payment for services places a small barrier against unnecessary consumption of medical services. Yet, co-payment could pose a real barrier to care for some, especially those who are medically underserved (Schaenman et al., 2013).

Risk of Infectious Disease Transmission

Despite the mandate for screening, not all prisoners complete the required tests. Adding to the problem is the transfer of prisoners during screening periods and the subsequent effect on continuity of care. According to recent statistics 1.4% of male prisoners were living with either HIV or AIDS (Centers for Disease Control and Prevention [CDC], 2014). Treatment is often initiated upon diagnosis and has led to a decrease in overall mortality from AIDs in this population (American Foundation for AIDS Research [AFAR], 2008). However, 25% of long-term inmates have not been screened for HIV across the United States (Dumont, Gjelsvik, Redmond, & Rich, 2013) spreading the disease during unprotected sex, both consensual and nonconsensual, as well as sharing dirty needles. The latter can be from subversive drug use and/or tattooing (AFAR, 2008).

HIV is not the only disease spread among inmates. Hepatitis C infection is significantly higher among prison inmates as compared to the general population, most likely associated with the high-risk behaviors among incarcerated populations. Approximately 12–35% are chronically infected with hepatitis C compared to 1–1.5% of the free-living population. The infection is spread primarily through needles and tattoos. The outcome of untreated active hepatitis C is hepatic fibrosis, cirrhosis, and hepatocellular carcinoma cirrhosis of liver (CDC, 2013). Currently the cost of treatment ($84,000 dollars per person) prohibits most states from offering treatment unless the individual is symptomatic (Ollove, 2014). Because Quint obtained a couple of tattoos while in prison, he could have been exposed to both HIV and hepatitis C. Most likely he did not understand the risk to himself and to the community upon his release.

Management of Mental Health Disorders

Mental health disorders affect many prisoners. Approximately 10% have major depression and up to 50% are considered to have an antisocial personality disorder (Schnittker et al., 2012). Fortunately, most prisoners with mental disorders seem to be less dysfunctional while in prison because of constraints on their behavior. However, the experience of prison may have negative consequences on mental well-being. There is a heightened sense of vigilance, lack of privacy, loss of individuality, and erosion of social skills (Schnittker & John, 2007). Quint entered the system with a past history of suboptimal treatment of mental illness, which was screened and addressed upon admission to prison. This is not always the case as one out of three state prisoners and one out of six jail inmates receive no mental health treatment (James & Glaze, 2006).

Experiencing a family death while imprisoned is a complex problem. Prisoners cannot attend funerals and may not be able to express grief or work through the normal grieving process (Hendry, 2008). Bereavement in prison is often amplified by the constraints of confinement and the unwritten code of maintaining masculinity. Outwardly expressing emotion may be viewed as weak, leaving the inmate feeling vulnerable to physical abuse from other inmates. This stoicism has the unfortunate consequences of masking grief over loss of family members. Quint learned of his beloved grandmother's death in a letter. He was not able to process the death with other members of his family and he chose to deal with his grief by remaining quiet.

Issues of Aging and Chronic Illness

A problem surfacing in prisons is the growing health needs of older and chronically ill prisoners. As would be expected, this group brings unique challenges to the prison health delivery system (Williams et al., 2010). Prison systems struggle with deciding how to handle problems with inmates who have dementia, cancer, diabetes, and other debilitating illnesses.

Nursing Interventions with Prisoners

Nurses play an integral role within the prison system including:

- *Testing.* Nurses incorporate the CDC HIV Testing Implementation Guidance for Correctional Settings including "opt out" testing, measures to ensure retesting if the inmate is transferred during the testing period, measures to ensure confidentiality and treatment options.
- *Health screening.* Upon admission to or transfer within the prison system, nurses administer health screening. All transfers should include a health summary. Quality improvement reviews must be conducted routinely to ensure that all prisoners are screened for contagious diseases as well as other health conditions.
- *Advocating.* The Federal Bureau of Prisons has outlined standards of care for prisons. The standards for care for prisons can be accessed at http://www.justice.gov/oig/reports/BOP/a0808/final.pdf; nurses implement these standards. Nurses may need to advocate for completion of screenings and early intervention as ways to contain cost. Access to care must be reviewed and copayments, if instituted, evaluated for their effectiveness. If co-payments pose a barrier to care, nurses need to advocate for an alternate solution to insure care.

There is evidence that the prison population is in worse health than free-living counterparts of the same age (Schnittker & John, 2007). Several explanations are given for this health disparity. The majority of those imprisoned have not had access to regular health care in the past. For many, lack of consistent health care contributed to ongoing addiction and mental health disorders that ended with incarceration. Secondly, the mental stress of the prison environment compounds physical health problems (Dumont et al., 2013).

RELEASE FROM INCARCERATION

Upon release from prison, an inmate may be placed in a halfway house, given parole with supervision, or released to his community with no conditions. He may be given a nominal amount of money, a bus ticket to his community, a prison photo identification card, and medication for 7 to 17 days (Williams et al., 2010). From this point onward, he is expected to be self-sufficient.

After 3 years, at age 29, Quint was released from prison and sent to a halfway house located 3 hours from his hometown. He was instructed that he must follow the house rules, have negative drug screens, maintains curfews, find employment, and continues to attend Narcotic Anonymous meetings. If he complied, he would be able to leave the halfway house after 1 year. Any violation of the rules would result in return to prison to complete his full sentence. Upon discharge he was given a 2-week supply of his medications, his prison identification card, and transportation to the halfway house. Once he arrived, he received instruction on the rules and expectations. One of his primary concerns was where he could obtain his medications. He was given information about the Affordable Care Act (ACA) and told where to apply for a state card. While waiting for enrollment, he was instructed to go to one of the community's free clinic for medication refills. Quint needed to learn how to navigate the bus system, with tokens provided by the halfway house in order to get to his medical appointments and apply for a job.

Quint found life outside the prison more stressful than he had expected. He was unable to secure ready employment. He found the bus system difficult to navigate. His prison record was a deterrent in obtaining employment. He was uncomfortable with talking about his most recent past with potential employers. He found the halfway house rules confining, almost suffocating. He had not heard much from his mother. She talked to him once and told him that upon release he would not be able to live with her. He became overwhelmed and after 3 years without smoking cigarettes, he took up smoking again in order to relax. He began to feel the urge to escape into drugs. Yet, he knew that any lapse insured return to prison. As time passed, he felt that return to prison was most likely his destiny.

Adjustment Post-incarceration

Quint's experiences post-incarceration are not unusual. The challenges ex-prisoners face upon release can easily derail the individual. The rituals of prison life, now were no longer in place and providing a safety net with boundaries and basic necessities. Despite prisoners having overall worse health than the general population, Spaulding et al. (2011) report that ex-prisoners perceived that they were actually healthier during imprisonment than after release. They attributed better health to prison rules, substance-free facilities, and regular eating and sleeping patterns.

It is estimated that 40% of American ex-prisoners are reincarcerated within 3 years of release (Pew Center on States, 2011), inferring that prison is not a deterrent to post-discharge crime. The larger problems of prevention, incarceration, and re-entry into society have not been addressed sufficiently.

The transition period post-incarceration can be extremely risky. The first several weeks post-incarceration pose the greatest difficulty in remaining drug free. In a study conducted in the state of Washington, there was a 12.7 higher risk of death in the first 2 weeks post-incarceration compared to other state residents. The primary cause was drug overdoses, 129 times higher than other state residents (Binswanger et al., 2007). Beyond the first 2 weeks of release, mortality remained high. Causes of death were accidental drug overdose, homicide, cardiovascular disease, and suicide. (Spaulding et al., 2011).

Beyond the first month, health problems identified and treated within the prison system often continued. The burden of disease is costly among former prisoners (Rosen, Schoenbach, & Wohl, 2008). Prior to the passage of the ACA in 2012, inmates were given a limited supply of medication until they could find ongoing medical care. For many, this was challenging due to the cost of both medications and provider visits. These financial barriers force the ex-prisoner to seek free community-based clinics or emergency rooms or to discontinue treatment. None of these options are without consequences, putting the ex-prisoner at risk for reincarceration. Adding to this is the financial burden to hospitals, communities, and families. The advent of the ACA in 2012 has improved this situation.

Since passage of the ACA, an inmate can now be enrolled for medical benefits prior to release, facilitating continuity of a medical treatment plan. He is provided with both a medical discharge summary and an appointment with a medical provider who can see him within a few weeks after discharge (Bainbridge, 2012). The medical home model should ensure that providers coordinate community services, a key factor in reducing prison recidivism. Providing continuity in mental health treatment, coordinating medical services for the treatment of chronic diseases, and targeting services for addiction are key issues for healthcare providers working with ex-prisoners (Gaynes, 2005). Quint was fortunate to be in a halfway house where he received assistance in enrolling in the state's Medicaid program. The waiting period was bridged by a free clinic that provided his routine medications. The free clinic also rescreened him for hepatitis C and HIV because he had received tattoos in prison. His negative screening results were given to him to share with his new health provider.

Reintegration into society is far from easy and help is not always readily apparent. For the ex-prisoner to be successful in establishing a life outside the prison system, access to health care and the ability to meet personal needs must be met. Quint quickly encountered one of the most challenging aspects post-incarceration, the stigma of being a felon, a label that presents a number of overwhelming barriers for an individual trying to start a new life. There are legal barriers in seeking employment, housing, government assistance for food stamps, voting, obtaining student loans, and obtaining a driver's license. The ex-prisoners's criminal record is on the public internet domain (Samuels & Mukamal, 2004). These state and federal restrictions are designed to alert the community to potential criminal activity by ex-prisoners.

Navigation of the rules and conditions is not intuitive. Policies differ among states. A person with a felony record released in one state and then traveling to another may find the transition even more difficult. Each state has the authority to make independent decisions regarding post-prison restrictions. For example, housing agencies in 47 states make individual determinations for felons living in public housing. Three states, however, completely ban residence in public housing for those with a criminal record (Samuels & Mukamal, 2004). Such variance creates anxiety and confusion for the newly released inmate.

Housing is but one of the many stressors faced by ex-prisoners. There is a lifetime ban on food stamps in 17 states and 21 states limit access to food stamps. Employers in most states can deny jobs or fire anyone with a criminal record, regardless of individual history or business necessity (Samuels & Mukamal, 2004). There are 29 states with laws refusing an occupational license based upon criminal conviction (e.g., obtaining a barber's license). Obtaining a driver's license after incarceration can be difficult for anyone convicted of a drug or alcohol offense as many states revoke or suspend the license post-incarceration for a set period of time. Complicating rehabilitation for drug offenses is the federal law that prohibits anyone with a drug offense conviction from receiving student grants, loans, or work assistance (Samuels & Mukamal, 2004).

A social network is a critical variable in helping the ex-prisoners navigate the state and federal restrictions. In a study of 652 men, family support was a key factor in maintaining employment and avoiding substance abuse post-incarceration. The majority of men in this study, 84%, were still living with a relative 7 months after release and 92% were accepting financial help from relatives. The stability of their living arrangements was tenuous. Close to 50% were hopeful of living with relatives for a year or longer. Despite these potential issues, family relationships were key in providing for basic needs (Visher, Yahner, & La Vigne, 2010)

Not all ex-prisoners find family ready or able to accommodate them. Depending on how long the person was incarcerated, the family has had to make adjustments. They may have moved into public housing, which will not accept the ex-prisoners, or moved to housing that is too small for another person. The family may be expecting financial support, which may not happen, as the ex-prisoner finds employment a struggle. Nuclear families with children may be hesitant to reunite as emotional ties have changed. It is not unusual for an inmate to lose contact with significant others due to the length of the sentence and the location of the prison. Believing that one can simply pick up the relationship up where it was left upon incarceration is not realistic (Gaynes, 2005). In

Quint's case, his mother told him not to expect any help with lodging after discharge from the halfway house. This proved to be a challenge for him when he returned to his community, already feeling tenuous about his success with drug rehabilitation.

Another factor influencing successful transition to mainstream living is the rehabilitation services in which the inmate participated. In a study by Visher et al. (2010), 32% of participants expressed a desire to participate in rehabilitation programs within prison and 84% did participate in at least one in-prison program. Whether involved job training, learning work skills, or obtaining a GED, the percentage who were gainfully employed 1 year post-incarceration was higher among those who attended prison rehabilitation programs (Visher et al., 2010). In a meta-analysis of various studies by the RAND Corporation, educational programs within prison resulted reducing the odds of recidivism by 43% (Davis et al., 2010). Not all prisons offer such rehabilitation programs nor do all inmates agree to participate. Those who leave prison with the same skill and educational level they had upon entry are further hampered upon release, now carrying a felon designation. In Quint's case, he did complete his GED while in prison which helped him in his search for employment.

Nursing Interventions to Reduce Vulnerability Post-incarceration

The community must be involved in seeking solutions to reintegrating and rehabilitating ex-prisoners. Employment opportunities and housing are key areas of social concern. The need for continuous, coordinated, comprehensive, and accessible primary health care cannot be overly emphasized. Nurses providing primary health care, emergency care, in public health or in clinical leadership roles have a large sphere of influence. Some advocacy activities for ex-prisoners include:

- Contacting area prisons and jails to determine the discharge process for prisoners
- Making healthcare appointments available within 2 weeks of discharge
- Referring ex-prisoners to free clinics or providers who accept patients with ACA coverage
- Informing ex-prisoner clients of community resources (e.g., pharmacy assistance, free or reduced dental care, or mental health counseling)
- Coordinating services with churches, city action groups, schools, and free clinics

CONCLUSION

The problems facing ex-prisoners are daunting. For some, it may be easier to return to prison. Some deliberately do just that. There are no easy solutions. As noted in this progressive case study, the problems start early, often in childhood or adolescence. The nursing role is to provide an advocating response to actual or potential health problems and to help people who are at risk for prison, in prison, or facing the struggles of community reintegration to reach their highest state of health and well-being.

REFERENCES

American Foundation for AIDS Research (AFAR). (2008, March 1–12). HIV in correctional settings: Implications for prevention and treatment policy. *The Foundation for AIDs Research*, Issue Brief 5. Retrieved from http://www.amfar.org/uploadedFiles/Articles/Articles/On_The_Hill/summary%20of%20recs.pdf

Bainbridge, A. A. (2012). The affordable care act and criminal justice: Intersections and implications. Bureau of Justice Assistance, U.S. Department of Justice. Retrieved from https://www.bja.gov/publications/aca-cj_whitepaper.pdf

Binswanger, I. A., Stern, M. F., Deyo, R. A., Heagerty, P. J., Cheadle, A., Elmore, J. G., & Koepsell, T. D. (2007). Release from prison—A high risk of death for former inmates. *New England Journal of Medicine, 356*(2), 157–165.

Carson, E. A., & Golinelli, D. (2013). Prisoners in 2012: Trends in admissions and releases, 1991–2012. U.S. Department of Justice, Office of Justice Programs. Bureau of Justice Statistics. (Publication NCJ 243920). Retrieved from www.bjs.gov/content/pub/pdf/p12tar9112.pdf

Centers for Disease Control and Prevention (CDC). (2013). Hepatitis C. Centers for Disease Control and Prevention. Retrieved from http://www.cdc.gov/knowmorehepatitis/

Centers for Disease Control and Prevention (CDC). (2014). HIV in correctional settings. Retrieved from http://www.cdc.gov/hiv/risk/other/correctional.html

Davis, L. M., Bozick, R., Steele, J. L., Saunders, S., & Miles, J. N. V. (2013). Evaluating the effectiveness of correctional education. Bureau of Justice Assistance. Retrieved from http://www.rand.org/pubs/research_reports/RR266.html

Dumont, D. M., Gjelsvik, A., Redmond, N., & Rich, J. D. (2013). Jails as public health partners: Incarceration and disparities among medically underserved men. *International Journal of Men's Health, 12*(3), 213–227.

Gaynes, E. (2005). Reentry: Helping former prisoners return to communities. A guide to key ideas, effective approaches, and TA resources for making connections cities and site teams. Annie E. Casey Foundation. Retrieved from http://www.aecf.org/upload/publicationfiles/ir2980d32.pdf

Glaze, L. E., & Herberman, E. J. (2013). Correctional populations in the United States, 2012. U.S. Department of Justice, Office of Justice Programs, Bureaus of Justice Statistics. (NCJ 243936). Retrieved from http://www.bjs.gov/content/pub/pdf/cpus12.pdf

Greenwood, P. (2008). Prevention and intervention programs for juvenile offenders. *Juvenile Justice, 18*(2), 185–210. Retrieved from https://www.law.umich.edu/centersandprograms/pcl/ljjohnsonworkshop/Documents/Adolescent_Development.pdf

Hawthorne, W. B., Folsom, D. P., Sommerfeld, D. H., Lanouette, N. M., Lewis, M., Aarons, G. A., … Jeste, M. D. (2012). Incarceration among adults who are in the public mental health system: Rates, risk factors, and short-term outcomes. *Psychiatric Service, 63*(1), 26–32.

Hendry, C. (2008). Incarceration and the tasks of grief: a narrative review. *Journal of Advanced Nursing*, *65*(2), 270–278.

James, D. J., & Glaze, L. E. (2006). Mental health problems of prison and jail inmates. U.S. Department of Justice, Office of Justice Programs, Bureaus of Justice Statistics. Publication (NCJ 213600). Retrieved from http://www.bjs.gov/content/pub/pdf/mhppji.pdf

Kulkarni, S. P., Baldwin, S., Lightstone, A. S., Gelberg, L., & Diamant, A. L. (2010). Is incarceration a contributor to health disparities? Access to care of formerly incarcerated adults. *Journal of Community Health*, *35*, 268–274.

Moore, L. D., & Elkavich, A. (2008). Who's using and who's doing time. Incarceration, the war on drugs, and public health. *American Journal of Public Health*, *98*(5), 782–786.

Murray, J., Farrington, D. P., & Sekol, I. (2012). Children's antisocial behavior, mental health, drug use, and educational performance after parental incarceration: A systematic review and meta-analysis. *Psychological Bulletin*, *138*(2), 175–210.

National Association for the Advancement of Colored People. (2014). Criminal justice fact sheet. Retrieved from http://www.naacp.org/pages/criminal-justice-fact-sheet

Niveau, G. (2007). Relevance and limits of the principle of "equivalence of care" in prison medicine. *Journal of Medical Ethics*, *33*, 610–613.

Ollove, M. (2014, March 25). Should prisoners get expensive hepatitis C drugs? *Stateline: The Daily News Service of the Pew Charitable Trusts*. Retrieved from http://www.pewtrusts.org/en/research-and-analysis/blogs/stateline/2014/03/25/should-prisoners-get-expensive-hepatitis-c-drugs

Pew Center on the States. (2011). State of Recidivism: The Revolving Door of America's Prisons. The Pew Charitable Trusts, Washington, DC. Retrieved from http://www.pewcenteronthestates.org

PEW Charitable Trusts, MacArthur Foundation. (2013). Managing prison health care spending. Retrieved from http://www.pewstates.org/healthcarespending

Ridgeway, G., & Listenbee, R. L. (2014, May). Criminal career patterns: Justice research. National Institute of Justice, Office of Juvenile Justice and Delinquency Prevention. Retrieved from https://www.ncjrs.gov/pdffiles1/nij/242545.pdf

Rosen, D. L., Schoenbach, V. J., & Wohl, D. A. (2008). All-cause and cause-specific mortality among men released from state prison, 1980–2005. *American Journal of Public Health*, *98*(12), 2278–2284.

Samuels, P., & Mukamal, D. (2004). After prison: Roadblocks to reentry. A report on state legal barriers facing people with criminal records. Legal Action Center. Retrieved from http://www.lac.org/roadblocks-to-reentry/upload/lacreport/LAC_PrintReport.pdf#page=3&zoom=page-actual,0,-153

Schaenman, P., Davies, E., Jordan, R., & Chakraborty, R. (2013). Opportunities for cost savings in corrections without sacrificing service quality: Inmate health care. The Urban Institute. Retrieved from http://www.urban.org/UploadedPDF/412754-Inmate-Health-Care.pdf

Schnittker, J., & John, A. (2007). Enduring stigma: The long-term effects of incarceration on health. *Journal of Health and Social Behavior*, *48*(2), 115–130.

Schnittker, J., Massoglia, M, & Uggen, C. (2012). Out and down: Incarceration and psychiatric disorders. *Journal of Health and Social Behavior*, *53*(4), 448–464.

Spaulding, A. C., Seals, R. M., McCallum, V. A., Perez, S. D., Brzozowski, A. K., & Steenland, N. K. (2011). Prisoner survival inside and outside of the institution: Implications for healthcare planning. *American Journal of Epidemiology, 173*(5), 479–487.

The Future of Children. (2008). *Juvenile justice, 18*(2), Retrieved from https://www.law.umich.edu/centersandprograms/pcl/ljjohnsonworkshop/Documents/Adolescent_Development.pdf

Visher, C., Yahner, J., & La Vigne, N. (2010). Life after prison: Tracking the experiences of male prisoners returning to Chicago, Cleveland, and Houston. *Urban Institute Justice Policy Center.* Retrieved from http://www.urban.org/UploadedPDF/412100-life-after-prison.pdf

Williams, B. A., McGuire, J., Lindsay, R. G., Baillargeon, J., Cenzer, I. S., Lee, S. J., & Kushel, M. (2010). Coming home: Health status and homelessness risk of older pre-release prisoners. *Journal of General Internal Medicine, 25*(10), 1038–1044.

Chapter 26

Role Transition for Immigrant Women: Vulnerabilities and Strengths

Lisa R. Roberts

OBJECTIVES

At the end of this chapter, the reader will be able to

1. Identify important aspects of vulnerability among immigrant women seeking health care.
2. Describe how nurses can support resilience among immigrant women.
3. Analyze four case studies in terms of supporting resilience among immigrant women.

INTRODUCTION

There are many challenges facing new immigrants including leaving behind a familiar life to start anew, new languages, foods, expectations, health practices and beliefs, and navigating the healthcare system in their new home country. It takes tremendous strength to face all of this. Even resilient individuals may be made temporarily vulnerable by the situation (de Chesnay & Anderson, 2011). An immigrant's country of origin is an important determinant of post-migration health. The country of origin influences education, prior health care and income, exposure to discrimination, and attitude regarding traditional gender roles, which in turn influence health (Blau, Kahn, & Papps, 2011)

Immigrants are in transition, increasing their vulnerability. Another dimension is added when a newly immigrated woman is not only away from her country of origin but also assuming new roles (e.g., wife, mother), or working outside of the home for the first time (Hill, Lipson, & Meleis, 2003). Self-identity is inherently tied to one's roles in life. Poor self-confidence regarding the ability to fulfill new roles or internal conflict regarding different roles may produce psychological distress and negative effects on health (Thoits, 2013). Additionally, a young woman's self-efficacy during transitional periods in life is influenced by beliefs regarding traditional gender roles (Weiss, Freund, & Wiese, 2012). Social support is protective for women's psychological well-being during these transitional periods in life (Gjesfjeld, Weaver, & Schommer, 2012). Yet immigrants often lack social support. Nurses can play an important role in helping women in this situation in developing self-efficacy in new roles.

The nurse is in a good position to partner in care with immigrant women as they face these stresses. Being aware of one's own bias and being sensitive to cultural differences are the building blocks of developing an authentic relationship—the foundation for partnering in care. Care must be taken to avoid stereotypes and presumptions based on limited knowledge of another's culture. Likewise, the patient's concepts of health, how the healthcare system works, and the desired outcomes must be carefully explored. Respectfully proceeding with appropriate nursing actions within the framework of the patient's cultural context is cultural competency (de Chesnay & Anderson, 2011). It is a basic requirement for partnering in care with immigrant women. Such a partnership uses the nurse's clinical expertise in navigating the complex U.S. healthcare system. It is also guided by the patient's worldview, life history, and transition into the new country. Shared decision making is essential (Hain & Sandy, 2013; Matteliano & Street, 2012).

Shared information, leading to consensus regarding treatment choices, and mutual agreement regarding the treatment plan are the hallmarks of shared decision making. Shared decision making is a process that relies on information exchange, evidence-based practice tools, open communication, and patient participation. The process of shared decision making is guided by respect for patient autonomy. It requires that the patient is well informed, challenging the nurse to share knowledge at an appropriate level of health literacy (Hain & Sandy, 2013).

Nurses are distinctly poised to partner with immigrant women in shared decision making and to bridge the gap between patients' needs and the U.S. healthcare system. Innovative and capable of providing culturally competent care, nurses have a holistic framework of care and generally communicate well with other disciplines in the healthcare system (Matteliano & Street, 2012). These facets of nursing practice make nurses unique advocates for vulnerable immigrant women. The following vignettes illustrate the vulnerability of immigrant women who grew in resilience as result of nursing intervention.

AANJAY: A MAIL-ORDER BRIDE

In 1998, the "mail-order bride" industry was booming. Thousands of women or their families in other countries sought American husbands and American men sought brides from outside the United States. While Filipino and Russian women dominated the market, agencies listed women from around the world with 16% of the requests for Indonesian women. Among Indonesian requests, 63% resulted in mail-order marriages. Other Indonesian women immigrated as domestic workers (Scholes, 1999).

Aanjay, a 19-year-old Indonesian woman, signed on with a placement agency. She was looking for a way to leave her home where she had watched her alcoholic father beat her mother repeatedly. Her community was a place where she endured humiliation from the gossip about the many indiscretions of her father. She was sure she would end up with the same fate. She was already older than some of the girls listed with the agency and she worried that no one would pick her. She dreamed of an American husband, who would be gentle and faithful. The family nurse practitioner (FNP) met Aanjay for the first time when she presented at the clinic with a rash. The FNP described the first encounter with this client.

I entered the exam room to find Aanjay sitting anxiously on the exam table, her husband sitting on the only chair in the room. I introduced myself and began asking Aanjay about her complaint. She looked at her husband without saying a word and he spoke for her. Jim appeared to be about 20 years older than Aanjay and seemed irritable as he explained, without looking at Aanjay, that she had developed a rash all over her body. He wanted to know how she got it and if she could give it to him. Jim refused to leave the room for Aanjay's examination, reporting that she did not speak English well. However, when Jim stepped out to take a phone call, Aanjay quickly spoke up in thickly accented but understandable English: "He thinks I cheat on him and get rash. How I cheat? He home all the time except play golf." Jim re-entered the room as I was explaining that the rash was consistent with contact dermatitis caused by laundry detergent. Jim agreed to switch the detergent brand. This was Aanjay's first visit to a healthcare provider since immigration.

Over the next 6 months I saw Aanjay for a few minor ailments and trust was gradually developed. Jim stayed in the waiting room during her gynecological examination. During that visit, Aanjay confided that she was afraid there was something wrong with her because she consistently experienced dyspareunia. I discussed some explanations and solutions for dyspareunia.

Three weeks after this encounter, Aanjay appeared at the clinic without Jim. She had walked 4 miles from her home. She told the receptionist she was not sick but wanted to talk with the FNP about her last visit. The FNP instructed the scheduler to make time for Aanjay that day. The floodgates opened as Aanjay explained that she was completely isolated. In the 3 years she had been in the United States, she had made no friends because Jim did not want her to "become like American women." She was allowed to call her family in Indonesia once a month. She stated that Jim would not allow her to get a job, saying: "He says my job is clean the house every day and have sex with him." She wept bitterly as she recounted her lost dreams and aspirations. She indicated that while Jim was not cruel to her, she had hoped for so much more.

The mail-order bride industry continues to grow. While the divorce rate among mail-order marriages is lower than the general population, not all unions are pleasant and some are very dangerous. These women have three times the risk of being abused compared with other women in the United States (Wu, 2012) with increased risk for mortality due to intimate partner violence (Tran, 2012).

The FNP inwardly bristled, acknowledging that she had difficulty knowing how to respond to Aanjay's needs without imposing her own ideals. She realized that Aanjay lacked a support system to help her explain her needs to her husband. The FNP connected her with resources and Aanjay found inner strength and resilience. It was not a quick process, but 5 years later, she is happily volunteering 3 days a week at the local library, has made friends, and she and Jim delight in their 3-year-old daughter.

AZEEN: A PREGNANT IMMIGRANT WOMEN

Azeen, age 20, arrived in the United States with her 31-year-old husband, Taymur. Her husband had lived in the United States for 8 years and then returned to the Middle East for their arranged marriage. Azeen had graduated from secondary school prior to leaving her homeland and she looked forward to going to college in the United States once she became proficient in English.

Young Arab women are socialized to become wives and mothers. They are raised to be modest in order to ensure the reputation and honor of the family. As they grow into adolescence, their activity is progressively restricted by their parents and brothers, protecting them until they are married. Once a young woman is married and has at least one child, she transitions into adulthood (Hattar-Pollara, 2003). This socialization into marriage, motherhood, and a domestic role may be complicated by immigration with inherent language and cultural barriers.

The couple came to the clinic for confirmation of pregnancy after Taymur noted Azeen's absence of menstruation for 2 months. Azeen was embarrassed to talk about her menstrual cycle and conferred with her husband in Arabic before answering my questions. After confirming the pregnancy, the FNP returned to the exam room to discuss prenatal care. Azeen seemed to have limited knowledge of reproductive health, pregnancy, and prenatal care. I discussed these matters with the couple over several visits. When Azeen became comfortable with the idea of beginning prenatal care, I referred her to a female healthcare provider to manage her pregnancy and attend her birth.

Eight months later, Azeen and Taymur returned to the clinic with their infant son, requesting counseling on family planning. The FNP inquired about their beliefs and preferences. Although she now spoke English well, Azeen was still reticent to engage in discussion, letting him ask the questions. While they were most familiar with the rhythm method, they desired a more reliable method of birth control. The FNP discussed the options and provided language-appropriate written material. Then, she left them alone to consider their preferences. When she returned, Taymur stated they wished to proceed with an intrauterine device (IUD). The nurse asked Azeen what she wanted to do. She responded that it was her husband's decision.

The Arab patriarchal family structure may seem restrictive by U.S. cultural standards, but it is also protective. Including the husband in education and planning is essential to insure his cooperation and vital in providing holistic care for Arab women in traditional roles. When Azeen returned for IUD placement, her husband remained in the waiting room with their son. The FNP again reviewed the procedure with Azeen who appeared anxious but insisted that she was ready, stating: "It is best."

Over time, Azeen, Taymur, and the FNP grew increasingly comfortable in their cross-cultural relationship. Azeen's plans for higher education were delayed as she struggled with the demands of being a wife and mother without the close physical support of her extended family. She confided that she was glad that she did not have to worry about having another baby soon.

SANGITA: IMMIGRATION AND INTIMATE PARTNER VIOLENCE

Intimate partner violence (IPV) against women is pervasive. Conservative global estimates range from 37–45% of all women and the United Nation Population Fund reports as high as 70% of married women in India have suffered from IPV (Krishnan, 2008; Murray, 2008; Press Trust of India, 2005). Higher education is correlated with higher risk (Murray, 2008). According to the Asian and Pacific Islander American Health Forum, 66% of women from the Indian subcontinent who live in California hold a Bachelor's degree or above (Ethnic health Assessment for Asian Americans, Native Hawaiians, and Pacific Islanders in California, 2011). Further, among immigrant women from the Indian subcontinent living in the United States, 33% have experienced violence within the home (Puri, Adams, Ivey, & Nachtigall, 2011). The actual percentage may be higher due to underreporting in an effort to preserve family honor (Zachariah, 2003). For women who may already be marginalized as a result of immigrating to the United States, reporting IPV may be especially difficult.

Sangita's parents had arranged a good marriage. Her husband Ramesh had all the right qualifications: his family was of the right social standing; he was well educated; and he had a good job in the United States. Sangita joined her husband in the United States 1 year after their marriage to live in a joint-family home, which included her in-laws. Upon her arrival, her passport and visa were promptly put in the family safe. Her in-laws were aloof and she tried to please them by fulfilling her family duties. Her husband worked long hours and she was restless. She had a bachelor's degree in botany but at the age of 25, she had yet to hold a job outside the home. She suggested that perhaps it was time to use her education. The family agreed to her job search, but she was unable to find a job deemed suitable by her husband and his family. She grew despondent.

I saw Sangita for various complaints: headaches, dizziness, and indigestion. Then she came to the clinic asking about possible infertility. She had been in the United States for 14 months with her husband and had yet to become pregnant. She described her husband as quarrelsome. I recommended a complete history and physical with lab work before an infertility referral. The history form included a depression screen. I noted several red flags. When I questioned her about depression, her story unfolded. Her husband and in-laws accused her of secretly using birth control to prevent pregnancy. She was indignant and decided to plan a trip to visit her family in India. Her husband accused her of intending to leave him and refused to give her the locked-up passport. In the ensuing months he slapped and kicked her repeatedly. She had told no one about this abuse until this visit.

The FNP discussed reporting the abuse, but Sangita begged her not to, afraid that it would only make matters worse. She was also afraid no one would believe her, as she did not have any injuries at the time. She felt trapped without access to her passport and isolated without the support of her natal kin. The FNP told Sangita she was worried about her physical safety and her psychological welfare. She explained her responsibility to comply with reporting laws and to monitor for ongoing or escalating abuse.

Sangita and the FNP partnered to find a solution, and ultimately Sangita was able to contact her brother in India. He applied social pressure through his contacts within the community where Sangita lived. The community's leverage was enough to stop the abuse and her passport is now in her own safekeeping. Sangita had made movement toward resilience.

FAZIAH: MARRIAGE AND FEMALE GENITAL CUTTING

Female genital cutting (FGC) is common in 28 African countries and in a few Asian and Middle Eastern countries. It is increasingly encountered among immigrant women migrating to other nations (Sandy, 2011; World Health Organization, 2011). Many nations have national laws banning the practice although local practices may not comply. Likewise, local laws may prohibit the practice while there is no national consensus or legal protection. In Sudan, for instance, some of the states have banned FGC but there is no national law prohibiting the practice (Abbas, 2013).

FGC involves varying degrees of genital cutting and mutilation. It is usually a traditional rite of passage for purposes of preserving virginity, marriage eligibility, and perceived hygiene (Sandy, 2011). FGC can result in narrowing of the introitus due to infibulation and scar formation.

At the age of 17, Faizah immigrated to the United States with her parents on a humanitarian visa. She was glad her family was alive and free from the fear they had experienced in war-torn Sudan. However, it was difficult to adjust to life in America and to be identified as a refugee. She felt she had little in common with others adolescents of her age.

She attended a local community college and then a university studying dental hygiene. After graduation, she obtained a job in a dental office. There she became friends with a young man. They gradually fell in love and her family approved of their engagement. Faizah, however, was worried. Since arriving in the United States, Faizah had not seen a healthcare provider for anything except minor ailments. After much deliberation, she made an appointment with the FNP to discuss her approaching marriage. What would the FNP think? Would she know what to do? Faizah did not even know how to ask for what she needed nor did she know how to explain her condition.

At first I thought Faizah was trying to request birth control. With gentle probing as to why she came to the clinic, Faizah desperately blurted out that she did not think she would be able to have intercourse after her marriage. I wondered why this young woman thought she was incapable of having intercourse. I asked her about vaginal burning, discharge, or vaginal pain. Faizah denied all of these symptoms and then stated she had never had sexual relations. With further questioning, she told me the problem was that she was "too small." Then I realized she was talking about FGC. Faizah allowed me to do a brief, noninvasive examination of her external genitalia. Her introitus was significantly narrowed and she acknowledged that she had experienced FGC. She asked me again if she could have intercourse. I assured that she could and suggested she consider counseling and a surgical consultation for deinfibulation.

Appropriate referrals for surgical consultation and mental health counseling depend on the type of FGC, complications, cultural norms, and individual patient preferences. While looking relieved, Faizah stated she felt comfortable with the FNP and declined counseling. She did agree to a surgical consultation for deinfibulation, as long as the healthcare provider was a woman. The FNP partnered with Faizah in exploring the options compatible within her cultural framework. She praised Faizah for her courage in seeking care.

The FNP was able to locate a female surgeon who performed deinfibulation. This surgeon had worked in Sudan with the international organization Doctors Without Borders. She had cultural knowledge about the practice of FGC. The FNP accompanied Faizah to the consultation visit and was reassured that Faizah was in culturally competent hands. Faizah had the procedure and went on to plan her wedding. She never regretted the day she went to the clinic seeking help.

CONCLUSION

Each of the women in these case studies faced challenges, but also showed remarkable resilience. Women's needs are influenced by a variety of factors including their culture of origin, their living situation and support in the country of immigration, their level of education, and individual goals in life. By careful listening, advocacy, and appropriate cultural response, the nurse can partner with the immigrant woman presenting for care. Shared decision-making supports the woman's resilience. The nurse in these case studies developed trusting relationships and open communication, which promoted shared decision making and ultimately helped these women to become less vulnerable.

REFERENCES

Abbas, R. (2013). Female genital mutilation campaign in Sudan slammed for "not getting message across," *Huffington Post*. Retrieved from http://www.huffingtonpost.com/2013/08/19/female-genital-mutilation-sudan_n_3779524.html

Blau, F., Kahn, L., & Papps, K. (2011). Gender, source country characteristics, and labor market assimilation among immigrants. *The Review of Economics and Statistics, 93*(1), 43–58.

de Chesnay, M., & Anderson, B. (2011). *Caring for the vulnerable: Perspectives in nursing theory, practice and research* (3rd ed.). Burlington, MA: Jones & Bartlett Learning.

Ethnic health Assessment for Asian Americans, Native Hawaiians, and Pacific Islanders in California. (2011). Health Policy Fact Sheet, California Program on Access to Care, p. 66.

Gjesfjeld, C., Weaver, A., & Schommer, K. (2012). Rural women's transitions to motherhood: Understanding social support in a rural community. *Journal of Family Social Work, 15*(5), 435–448.

Hain, D., & Sandy, D. (2013). Partners in care: Patient empowerment through shared decision-making. *Nephrology Nursing Journal, 40*(2), 153–157.

Hattar-Pollara, M. (2003). Arab Americans. In P. Hill, J. Lipson, & A. Meleis (Eds.), *Caring for Women Cross-Culturally* (pp. 45–62). Philadelphia, PA: F.A. Davis.

Hill, P., Lipson, J., & Meleis, A. (2003). Caring for women cross-culturally. Philadelphia, PA: F.A. Davis.

Krishnan, S. (2008). Domestic violence. *The New India Express*. Retrieved from http://www.prajnya.in/16d08medianie.htm

Matteliano, M., & Street, D. (2012). Nurse practitioners' contributions to cultural competence in primary care settings. *Journal of the American Academy of Nurse Practitioners, 24*(7), 425–435.

Murray, A. (2008). *From outrage to courage*. Monroe, ME: Common Courage Press.

Press Trust of India. (2005). Two-third married Indian women victims of domestic violence: UN. *Express India*. Retrieved from http://www.expressindia.com/news/fullstory.php?newsid=56501

Puri, S., Adams, V., Ivey, S., & Nachtigall, R. (2011). There is such a thing as too many daughters, but not too many sons: A qualitative study of son preference and fetal sex selection among Indian immigrants in the United States. *Social Science & Medicine, 72*(7), 1169–1176.

Sandy, H. (2011). Female genital cutting: an overview. *American Journal for Nurse Practitioners, 15*(1–2), 53–59.

Scholes, R. (1999). The "mail-order bride" industry and its impact on US immigration. Paper presented at the International Matchmaking Organizations: A Report to Congress. AILA InfoNet Doc. No. 99030999, 1999.

Thoits, P. (2013). Self, identity, stress, and mental health. In C. S. Aneshensel & J. C. Phelam (Eds.), *Handbook of the sociology of mental health* (pp. 345–368). New York: Springer Publishers.

Tran, T. (2012). Mis-matched: Taking a state approach to enforcing the growing international matchmaking industry. *Family Court Review, 50*(1), 159–174.

Weiss, D., Freund, A., & Wiese, B. (2012). Mastering developmental transitions in young and middle adulthood: The interplay of openness to experience and traditional gender ideology on women's self-efficacy and subjective well-being. *Developmental Psychology, 48*(6), 1774–1784.

World Health Organization. (2011). An update on WHO's work on female genital mutilation (FGM). Retrieved from WHO/RHR/11.8 http://www.who.int/reproductivehealth/publications/fgm/rhr_11_18/en/

Wu, Y. (2012). They're the same as any woman: Professionals' awareness of the unique needs of mail order brides who experience domestic violence. Retrieved from http://conservancy.umn.edu/handle/11299/123436

Zachariah, R. (2003). South Asians. In P. Hill, J. Lipson, & A. Meleis (Eds.), *Caring for women cross-culturally* (pp. 263–285). Philadelphia, PA: F.A. Davis.

Chapter 27

Youthful Resilience: Programs That Promote Health in Adolescence

Victoria L. Baker and Wendy Steinkraus

OBJECTIVES

At the end of this chapter, the reader will be able to

1. Use risk factors and youthful resilience to promote the health of adolescents in clinical care.
2. Use the Theory of Reasoned Action to select appropriate health promotion recommendations to adolescent clients.
3. Assess clinical agency services in terms of appropriate components of a health promotion program for adolescents.

PREDICTORS OF VULNERABILITY IN ADOLESCENCE

Adolescents are a vulnerable group at risk for developing health problems. Three risk predictors identify vulnerability: social status, social capital, and human capital (Aday, 2001).

Social Status

Social status is the position that an individual or group occupies in society based on age, gender, race, or ethnicity (Aday, 2001). *Adolescence*, ages 11 to 21 years, is a period of transition between childhood and adulthood (American Academy of Pediatrics [AAP], 2013).

This time period is subdivided into three categories: early adolescence (11–14 years); middle adolescence (15–18 years), and late adolescence (19–21 years) (AAP, 2013). These periods differ substantially in terms of physical and neurocognitive development, including decision-making capacity (Dunn, 2009; Patia-Spear, 2013).

Neurocognitive capacity and executive function for rational, responsible decision making changes over time, beginning in early adolescence and continuing into the third decade of life (Patia-Spear, 2013). As they age, adolescents learn to process abstract concepts, begin futuristic thinking, and internalize the importance of health (Coleman & Rosoff, 2013; Dunn, 2009; Patia-Spear, 2013). This maturation includes increasing capacity to make decisions about their health, including sexual behavior, weight maintenance, and risky behaviors potentially damaging health (American College of Obstetricians and Gynecologists [ACOG], 2010; Patia-Spear, 2013). Parents, healthcare providers and educators aim to help adolescents develop sound decision-making skills, process abstract concepts and consider distant consequences in making decisions (Coleman & Rosoff, 2013; Patia-Spear, 2013). Concerned adults seek to protect adolescents from the long-term health consequences of risky behaviors, as adolescents take on increasing responsibility for behavior (AAP, 2013; Dunn, 2009).

In certain situations, the adolescent's social status, defined by age, creates legal limitations to accessing health care and impedes the mature adolescent's ability to make decisions about health care (Boonstra & Nash, 2000). Minor consent laws vary by state and often lack clarity. Healthcare providers need to determine if the adolescent is legally emancipated, thus capable of consenting for health services. An emancipated minor is defined in many states as an adolescent who is married, has joined the military, or is living independently of parents (Center for Adolescent Health and the Law [CAHL], 2010; Guttmacher Institute, 2014c). In 37 states, minors who are parents are considered emancipated, allowing the legal right to decide for their own and their child's healthcare needs. However, this right varies among states. For example, some states allow the adolescent parent to obtain contraceptives and accept care for sexually transmitted infections, but do not allow consent for routine preventive health care, such as a physical exams and immunizations (CAHL, 2010; Ford, English, Davenport, & Stinnett, 2009). Most states allow a minor to consent to mental health and substance abuse services, although this varies significantly among states and within a state, depending upon whether the healthcare facility falls under Title X Family Planning Program and/or Medicaid regulations or the adolescent's parent is present (CAHL, 2010; Ford et al., 2009).

Confidentiality of care is an age-related factor, complicating access to care by minors. Adolescents may be hesitant to seek care if health services are disclosed. In most states where minors are allowed to consent to a specific health service, privacy and protection from disclosure is assured. The U.S. Supreme Court has recognized a minor's right to privacy with regard to contraception, protected by the Constitution. It has struck down numerous attempts at establishing the need for parental consent for these services (CAHL, 2010). In all states, Title X Family Planning Programs and Medicaid programs provide confidential family planning services and contraceptive care to minors without parental consent, although they encourage parental participation (CAHL, 2010; Guttmacher Institute, 2014c).

Federal medical privacy regulations, through the Health Insurance Portability and Accountability Act of 1996 (HIPAA), generally support a minor's right to confidentiality of medical records accrued during legally consented healthcare services (CAHL, 2010). However, when a minor has the legal right to consent for services independently, third-party payers often report encounter information to parental/legal guardian policyholders. Adolescents desiring confidential care may need to pay for it out of pocket or find subsidized care. As high as 30% of adolescents avoid filing healthcare fees through insurance plans in order to insure confidentiality (Gold, 2013). Healthcare providers need to be aware of state laws as well as HIPAA requirements pertaining to minor's disclosure of health information (CAHL, 2010).

Social Capital

The second predictor of risk is social capital, defined as the quantity and quality of relationships experienced by an adolescent (Aday, 2001). Adolescents often benefit from supportive families, religious groups, youth clubs, and organized social structures. Marital status, employment, and peer relationships also influence risk. Highly influential in adolescence, peer relationships create the potential for decreased vulnerability or increased risk. Examples of unhealthy social capital include peer-influenced risky behaviors, electronic misinformation among peers, and personal and electronic bullying (AAP, 2010, 2013; Centers for Disease Control and Prevention [CDC], 2014a; Dunn, 2009; Guse et al., 2012).

Human Capital

Human capital is defined as the investment in skills and capabilities of an identified population and is the third predictor of risk, according to Aday (2001). Human capital investment includes education, employment opportunities, potential for income, and adequate housing (Aday, 2001). Educational levels, income, and insurance coverage are correlated to health status (Kaplan, Everson, & Lynch, 2000). Adolescents are frequently disadvantaged in the ability to access these investments.

Health literacy, linked to education level, is the ability to use baseline health information in making healthcare decisions (CDC, 2014a). Adolescents, with limited education and health literacy, may experience embarrassment and stress when discussing health issues, such as sexual behavior, substance abuse, or mental health (Ackard & Neumark-Sztainer, 2001). Low levels of health literacy are found among adolescent college students with advanced technological skills as well adolescents lacking a high school diploma. This indicates that formal education, by itself, is not necessarily a marker of health literacy (Institute of Medicine [IOM], 2004; Stellefson et al., 2011). Adolescents frequently lack quality information regarding access, cost, benefits of quality healthcare, and location of available services (Anderson & Lowen, 2010).

Many adolescents are students without an independent income, fully reliant on familial support. More than 20% of adolescents live in poverty (DeNavas-Walt, Proctor, & Smith, 2013). Employed adolescents typically occupy the lowest paying jobs, with15% of adolescents and young adults under 24 years of age earning at or below minimum wage. This income disparity is five times the rate for older workers (U.S. Census Bureau, 2012). Understandably, increasing age is directly correlated to the amount of formal education and skills an adolescent has achieved. In 2010, less than 10% of younger adolescents and up to 30% of 18- to 24-year-olds lacked access to insurance coverage (DeNavas-Walt et al., 2013; Moonsighe, Chang, & Truman, 2013). With the Patient Protection and Affordable Care Act (ACA) of 2010, more adolescents and young adults will be able to access needed health care (Department of Health and Human Services [HHS], 2014).

RISK AND RESILIENCE AMONG ADOLESCENTS

Adolescents frequently engage in riskier behaviors than other groups, resulting in poor health outcomes and the need for services focused on their needs. According to the Centers for Disease Control and Prevention Youth Risk Behavioral Surveillance Survey (CDC, 2014b), U.S. adolescents between 9th and 12th grade participate in many risky behaviors (see **Table 27-1**). Although support exists for specific interventions aimed at

Table 27-1 Self-Reported Participation in Risky Behaviors Among U.S. Adolescents (9th–12th Grade)

Safety
88% never worn a bicycle helmet
41% texting while driving
22% riding in a car with a driver who had been consuming alcohol
10% driving after consuming alcohol

Table 27-1 Self-Reported Participation in Risky Behaviors Among U.S. Adolescents (9th–12th Grade) *(Continued)*

Drugs

  41% Cigarettes

    9% before age 13 years

    16% regular cigarette use

  66% Alcohol

    19% before age 13 years

    21% binging

  41% Marijuana

    9% before age 13

    25% regular use

  Street drugs

    6% cocaine

    7% hallucinogenic drugs

    7% inhalants

    7% ecstasy

    3% methamphetamine

    2% heroin

Sex

  47% sexual intercourse

    6% before age 13 years

    With sexual initiation

      59% used a condom recently

      19% use birth control

      15% report 4 or more partners

Nutrition

  35% eat vegetables and 33% eat fruit 2 or more times daily

  19% do not drink milk

  17% skip breakfast every day

  17% report disordered eating behaviors

Exercise

  15% have less than 60 minutes of physical activity on at least 1 day weekly

  13% use tanning beds

  10% use sunscreen regularly

Sleep

  32% report sleeping at least 8 hours nightly

Source: Modified from: Centers for Disease Control and Prevention Youth Risk Behavioral Surveillance Survey (CDC, 2014b).

depression prevention in adolescents, additional research is needed to support those aimed at other health issues such as tobacco prevention (Merry et al., 2011; Stanton & Grimshaw, 2013).

Global morbidity and mortality trends in adolescent vulnerability and poor health status (see **Table 27-2**) have stimulated policy efforts toward adolescent health promotion (Spurr, Bally, Ogenchuk, & Walker, 2012; Toumbourou et al., 2000; HHS, 2012; Viner & Macfarlane, 2005). At the national level, adolescent health concerns have generated much discussion.

Promoting Resilience Among Adolescents

Communities can support long-term health and resilience among adolescents through the promotion of healthy lifestyles (Resnick, 2005; Watson-Thompson, Fawcett, & Schultz, 2008). The increased prevalence of chronic disease in adolescents may actually prompt

Table 27-2   Health Indicators Among American Adolescents

Health status

21% have asthma (CDC, 2014b)

18% report a currently chronic health condition (HHS, 2012)

14% are overweight (CDC, 2014b)

Injuries

About 50% adolescent mortality due to unintentional injuries

71% of this mortality is motor vehicle accidents (HHS, 2011)

3% injured in a physical fight (CDC, 2014b)

Mental health

19% report being bullied on school property (CDC, 2014b)

15% report being bullied electronically (CDC, 2014b)

8% report a major depressive episode (Substance Abuse and Mental Health Services Administration, 2012)

8% report having attempted suicide (CDC, 2014b)

Sexual health

7% report forced sexual intercourse (CDC, 2014b)

6% of female adolescents experience unintended pregnancy annually (Guttmacher Institute, 2014a)

Data from: Centers for Disease Control, USDHHS, Guttmacher Institute, Substance Abuse and Mental Health Services Administration.

system changes to support autonomous adolescent decision making. Participation in decision making may improve long-term health among adolescents (Chung, Burke, & Goodman, 2010).

Adolescent Strengths

While many adolescent characteristics produce vulnerability, they also contribute to resilience (Masten, 2001). Youth enthusiasm, eagerness to make decisions, desire to achieve adult status, and openness to mentoring relationships demonstrate resilience. Adolescents often accept respectful advice and assistance that adults might refuse. A healthcare provider can influence and support opportunities for youth to make important health decisions (Resnick, 2010). This mentoring may increase interest in healthy behaviors and skills in accessing care that may carry through a lifetime (Resnick, 2010; Taliaferro & Borowsky, 2012).

Adolescent Vulnerabilities

While positive health behaviors learned as an adolescent may continue into adulthood, the inverse can also occur (ACOG, 2010; Hensel & Fortenberry, 2013; Morrison-Beedy et al., 2013; Spurr et al., 2012; Toumbourou et al., 2000). The immediate, costly, and potentially life-threatening consequences of impulsive adolescent decisions have the potential to affect immediate and longer-term quality of life for the adolescent and the family (Hensel & Fortenberry, 2013; Spurr et al., 2013; Toumbourou et al., 2000; Viner & MacFarlane, 2005). Failure to guide adolescents in decision making increases their vulnerability and potentially delays development in autonomous healthcare decision making, resulting in negative health outcomes (Society for Adolescent Medicine, 2004).

Programs to Promote Resilience

Peer relationships have an enormous influence on adolescents. Adolescents often believe their peers are engaged in far more risky behaviors than is actually the case (Pape, 2011). Adolescents base many of their decisions on their perception of acceptance by those closest to them. A strong health promotion program may reduce misconceptions and restructure peer relationships as a source of quality information and healthy behavior. Central to acceptance of any health promotion program targeting teens is sensitive adult–adolescent communication. Essential talking points to facilitate communication and promote health with an adolescent include:

- Help the teen to understand adolescent changes
- Keep the message simple without information overload and at the appropriate literacy level

- Interact, don't talk down or be judgmental
- Show how to identify quality websites
- Explain the evidence, demonstrating what is happening "out there"
- Remember that developmentally, teens are egocentric and invincible
- Encourage the teen to talk to parents, adult role models, or mentors
- Respect the teen's desire for independence within reasonable options
- Use triggers, such as cellular notifications, to keep the teen focused
- Be authentic, demonstrating an approachable communication style (AAP, 2013; ACOG, 2010; National Campaign to Prevent Teen and Unplanned Pregnancy, 2012; WebMD, 2013).

The Theory of Reasoned Action is a strong framework for building health promotion programs targeting adolescents. This theory proposes that health behavior results primarily from an individual's intent to perform a specified behavior, influenced by personal beliefs and the perceived beliefs of others with a social network (Fishbein & Ajzen, 1975; Furneaux, 2005). Personal attitude about an intended behavior, as well as the perception of how others in a social network would decide or act in a similar circumstances, strongly influences adolescent decision making (Doswell, Braxter, Cha, & Kim, 2011; Fantasia, 2008; Fishbein & Ajzen, 1975; Furneaux, 2005; Guo et al., 2007; Wang et al., 2006). As a foundation for health promotion programming, the Theory of Reasoned Action can frame understanding of adolescent decision making across cultures. Some examples are:

- Sexual behaviors of African American adolescent girls (Doswell, Braxter, Cha, & Kim, 2011)
- Predicting reproductive health decisions in adolescent women with diabetes (Wang et al., 2006)
- Predicting smoking behaviors in Chinese adolescents (Guo et al., 2007)

Effective health promotion programs should include a defined population, health issues and concerns specific to the population, appropriate health education for the population, informed consent as indicated, and policies and procedures to support these activities (Fertman & Allensworth, 2010). The authors present their work on developing an evidence-based template for adolescent health promotion (see **Table 27-3**).

In any health promotion program, it is essential to have evidence-based materials available for both healthcare providers and for clients. The authors developed the following list of resources for adolescent health promotion, using a variety of media sources (see **Table 27-4**).

Table 27-3 An Evidence-Based Template for Adolescent Health Promotion

Focus	Considerations	Description of intervention
Population 13–21 years old	Developmental stage	Contraceptive interventions should vary for younger and older adolescents (AAP, 2013; Betz, Ruccione, Meeske, Smith, & Chang, 2008)
	Health literacy level	Assess health literacy using validated tools, such as those reviewed in Betz et al. (2008) or the REALM-Team (Davis et al., 2006).
	Access, cost of care, and confidentiality	Title X Family Planning Program may increase access for sexually transmitted infections, pregnancy, family planning services. Clinics should include funding outside of insurance, to avoid fear of disclosure to parents and for uninsured teens (Guttmacher Institute, 2014b, 2014d; Piepert, Madden, Allensworth, & Secura, 2012; Reese, Haydon, Herring, & Halpern, 2013).
		School-based clinics can be very effective (AAP, 2012; Keeton, Soleimanpour, & Brindis, 2012).
Health issues	General health maintenance	Provide annual wellness visits, including immunizations (Anderson & Lowen, 2010)
		Teen-focused program of self-management for those with chronic disease show early promise but lack overall support (Rees, Bakhshi, Surujlal-Harry, Stasinopoulus, & Baker, 2010; Wolf, Guevara, Grum, Clark, & Cates, 2002)
	Risky behaviors	Screen for risky behaviors, using the Rapid Assessment for Adolescent Preventive Services (Darling-Fisher, Salerno, Dahlem, & Martyn, 2014; Salerno, Marshall, & Picken, 2012; Salerno & Marshall, 2011).
		Counseling on risks associated with unprotected sexual activity may reduce such behaviors (Nettleman, Chung, Brewer, Ayoola, & Reed 2007; Shepherd, Frampton, & Harris, 2011).
		Brief interventions to reduce drug use are supported by initial studies (Carney, Myers, Louw, & Okwundu, 2014).
		Tobacco cessation interventions in youth need more study (Stanton & Grimshaw, 2013).
		Combined education/contraceptive services seem to reduce unplanned teen pregnancies (Oringanje et al., 2009; Stanton & Grimshaw, 2013; Morrison-Beedy et al., 2013).
		Screen for and counsel about sexually transmitted infections, skin cancer, and tobacco use (U.S. Preventive Services Task Force, n.d.).

(Continues)

Table 27-3 An Evidence-Based Template for Adolescent Health Promotion (*Continued*)

Focus	Considerations	Description of intervention
	Mental health issues	Psychological and educational interventions show promise of preventing depression in adolescents (Merry et al., 2011).
		Screen for depression and intimate partner violence (U.S. Preventive Services Task Force, n.d.).
Health education	Electronic media	Mobile phone apps and electronic websites are used by 93% teens to access health information (Guse et al., 2012).
		Early evidence supports mass media to discourage uptake of tobacco use among youth (Carson et al., 2012).
	Written, audiovisual media	Brochures, posters, and DVD complement face-to-face and electronic health education (Marks et al., 2006)
	Mentors	Mentoring seems a perfect fit with this population, but evidence lacking to date (Thomas, Lorenzetti, & Spragins, 2011).
	Peer-to-peer education	Peer education on medication adherence shows promise with adolescents, but additional evidence needed (M'Imunya, Kredo, & Volmink, 2012).
Informed consent	Minor consent for medical care differs state to state	Apply relevant state laws defining mature minor and ability to access various forms of medical care (Bruce, Berg, & McGuire, 2009; CAHL, 2010; Coleman & Rosoff, 2013).
		Teens age 12 years and up can access contraception, pregnancy, and STI testing without parental consent through federally funded Title X Clinics (CAHL, 2010; Guttmacher Institute, 2014d).
Policies and procedures	Support for clinicians	Provide electronic websites and EMR prompts such as Tips for Interacting with Teens (AAP, 2013; ACOG, 2010; Nemours Foundation, 2014)
		Prompt clinicians with
		· Teen-specific interventions
		· Tools for screening and assessment,
		· Sources of teen-friendly health information
		· Advice for communication with adolescents
		· Readability score website (Preston-Werner, Wanstrath, & Hyett, 2013)
	Handouts for Parents, Teens, Educators	Use evidence-based sources

Developed by Victoria Baker and Wendy Steinkraus, 2014.

Table 27-4 Resources for Adolescent Health Promotion

Source	Resources	Website
Written		
American College of Obstetricians and Gynecologists	Birth Control for Teens (pamphlet) You and Your Sexuality (pamphlet) Fact Sheet for Teens: Acquaintance and Date Rape (fact sheet)	www.acog.org
Get Yourself Tested	Talking Tips: Talking to Your Partner (booklet) It's Time to Know Thyself: Get Yourself Tested for Chlamydia Today (booklet)	www.gytnow.org
Planned Parenthood Federation of America	The Facts of Life: A Guide for Teens and Their Families (pamphlet) Is This Love? Evaluate Your Relationship (pamphlet) Is Abstinence Right for You Now? (pamphlet) Birth Control Choices for Teens (pamphlet) Sexually Transmitted Infections: The Facts (pamphlet)	ww.plannedparenthood.org
Centers for Disease Control and Prevention	Trichomoniasis: The Facts (pamphlet) Pelvic Inflammatory Disease: The Facts (pamphlet)	www.cdc.gov/std/
Electronic		
American Academy of Pediatrics	Ages and stages: link for all pediatric stages	www.healthychildren.org
Birth Control Support Network	Questions, answers, interactive	www.bedsider.org
Get Yourself Tested (extension of It's Your Sex Life with input from CDC)	Discussion with adolescents about sexual health and STI prevention	www.gytnow.org
It's Your (Sex) Life: Developed by Kaiser Foundation and MTV	Promotion of healthy sexual health, avoidance of unintended pregnancies, and STIs	www.itsyoursexlife.com
Nemours Foundation	Hundreds of topics for parents, kids, teens, and educators	www.kidshealth.org

(Continues)

Table 27-4 Resources for Adolescent Health Promotion *(Continued)*

Source	Resources	Website
Office of National Drug Control Policy	Adolescent substance abuse	www.abovetheinfluence.com
Planned Parenthood Federation of America	Information for teens, parents, and healthcare providers/educators	www.plannedparenthood.org
Audiovisual		
American Academy of Pediatrics	Ages and stages link	www.healthychildren.org
Planned Parenthood Federation of America	Short videos for teens, parents, and healthcare providers/educators	www.plannedparenthood.org
Centers for Disease Control and Prevention	Adolescent health link with electronic podcasts, videos, widgets and buttons	www.cdc.gov

Developed by Victoria Baker and Wendy Steinkraus, 2014

CASE STUDY: AN ADOLESCENT SEEKS HEALTH CARE

The following case study demonstrates multiple opportunities for health promotion. Trisha, an African American adolescent, age 16, walks into a Title X–funded Federally Qualified Health Center without an appointment or a parent. While this case study is set in Michigan, the legal considerations addressed in this case study may vary in other states.

The History

Chief concern: Possible sexually transmitted infection or unplanned pregnancy.

History of the present illness: Copious amount of thin gray vaginal discharge without a foul odor for last month. Extensive personal hygiene does not reduce the discharge or vaginal itch. Last menstrual period unknown, but "too long."

Medical history:

- Reports no surgeries or medical diagnoses
- Body mass index 94th percentile for past 4 years
- No known allergies
- State immunization record indicates she is due for her meningococcal and Tdap vaccines; she has not had the human papilloma virus vaccination series
- Last physical exam was 10 months ago, a sports physical for track and field scanned into electronic medical record

Ob/gyn history: G0 P0.
Family history:

- Father: alive and well
- Mother: morbidly obese with type 2 diabetes and hypertension
- Sister: obese

Social history:

- Limited financial resources to pay for her services, on Medicaid insurance system
- Not using contraception; uses condoms at times; reports three new sexual partners in the past year, six lifetime partners; last sexual intercourse 2 days ago
- Presenting without her single working mother; does not want her mother to know about her visit today
- Starts 11th grade next month; good student
- Denies tobacco use; avoids alcohol use; reports weekend cannabis; denies use of other drugs
- Participates in school track and soccer team; she swims in the summer

Considerations During the Healthcare Encounter

What developmental aspects should be considered?

- Assess developmental stage and health literacy level.

Can Trisha make an informed decision? What is her health literacy level? How can the healthcare provider best promote her health?

- Use a validated health literacy assessment tool. There is no legal requirement to perform these assessments, but it improves confidence in the patient's ability to comprehend healthcare materials and recommendations.
- Ask her how she gathers healthcare information Does she understand the risk with her sexual behaviors? Provide information through her preferred method of learning at an appropriate learning level. Health education materials via electronic, audiovisual, and written means support the information given during the encounter. Such resources have the potential to be shared with her peers, thus extending the healthcare provider's influence.
- Encourage Trisha to discuss her health issues with her mother or another adult mentor. Model this with her in your discussion at the office visit, by eliciting her ideas, and helping her to express them.

What access barriers to care does Trisha face?

- Informed consent: In Michigan, 18 years is the age of majority and for consent for medical services. However, federal law governs testing for sexually transmitted infection and pregnancy as well as contraception services under the Title X Family Planning Program. Trisha may give consent for services in this setting, but not in many other Michigan settings. Although the HPV series is strongly recommended in light of her high-risk sexual behavior, Trisha cannot initiate it because of the need for parental consent. Under Michigan Law (Michigan Department of Community Health, 2012), parental consent is required for wellness visits, identified as general medical care, including immunizations.
- Confidentiality: Reimbursement from Medicaid is not billed in a federally subsidized clinic. No explanation of services is sent to the parent, protecting Trisha's confidentiality. Trisha can legally consent for these services and her parents will not be able to access her health records for this encounter. Trisha should understand, however, about Michigan state mandatory reporting of specific infectious diseases.

What are her physical needs?

- Reproductive health: Trisha came for this health issue, so it should be addressed first. Start with a focused history and physical, including a report of her menstrual cycle pattern. Determine whether she understands the need for reliable contraception and help her determine which method would be most appropriate for her. The CDC Medical Eligibility Criteria Wheel for Contraceptive Use (CDC, 2014c) can guide providers in identifying an appropriate method. In Trisha's care, the copper intrauterine device would provide for emergency contraception and act as a highly effective long-acting reversible contraceptive method. Test for pregnancy and sexually transmitted and reproductive tract infections: gonorrhea, chlamydia, HIV, trichomoniasis, bacterial vaginosis, and vulvovaginal candidiasis. In spite of risk factors, she is asymptomatic and screenings are not recommended for hepatitis B, herpes simplex, or syphilis (U.S. Preventive Services Task Force, n.d.).
- General health maintenance: Given the limits of a problem-focused visit, Trisha should be encouraged to return to her school-based clinic for her next screening physical, where her borderline obesity and any other health concerns can be addressed. Because she participates in sports, she is likely to do this. The Michigan Community Immunization Record can be accessed electronically to review indicated immunizations. She should be asked to consent to record release of this visit to her primary care provider at the school-based clinic.

What screening should be done for risky behaviors?

- Trisha's chief concern offers an opportunity for screening and counseling about multiple areas of health: safer sexual behavior, tobacco use, exposure to sun, and intimate partner violence (U.S. Preventive Services Task Force, n.d.). Use the Rapid Assessment for Adolescent Preventative Services (RAAPS) (Darling-Fisher, Salerno, Dahlem, & Martyn, 2014; Salerno & Marshall, 2011) for screening teens with risky behaviors. Assess these issues within the context of her social history, explaining that the data helps to improve her care. Use a matter-of-fact approach in discussing these issues.

What screening should be done for assessing her mental health?

- Screening conveys that mental health issues are as appropriate to discuss as physical issues. It can normalize questions. Screening for depression is recommended for adolescents, providing referral to treatment is available. The usefulness of screening for suicide lacks evidence (U.S. Preventive Services Task Force, n.d.).

What follow up needs to be done?

- Follow-up visits should be scheduled to review test results, to evaluate her tolerance for the selected contraceptive method, to evaluate risk with sexual behavior, and to assess for further health promotion needs.

REFERENCES

Ackard, D. M., & Neumark-Sztainer, D. (2001). Health care information sources for adolescents: Age and gender differences on use, concerns, and needs. *Journal of Adolescent Health*, 29(3), 170–176.

Aday, L. A. (2001). *At risk in America: The health and health care needs of vulnerable populations in the United States* (2nd ed.). San Francisco: Jossey-Bass.

American Academy of Pediatrics (AAP). (2010). Sexuality, contraception, and the media. *Pediatrics*, 126(3), 576–582.

American Academy of Pediatrics (AAP). (2012). School-based health centers and pediatric patients. *Pediatrics*, 129(2), 387–393.

American Academy of Pediatrics (AAP). (2013). *Ages & stages: Stages of adolescence*. Retrieved from http://www.healthychildren.org/English/ages-stages/teen/Pages/Stages-of-Adolescence.aspx

American College of Obstetricians and Gynecologists (ACOG). (2010). *Primary and preventive health care for female adolescents: Tool kit for teen care* (2nd ed.). Retrieved from http://www.acog.org/~/media/Departments/Adolescent%20Health%20Care/Teen%20Care%20Tool%20Kit/ACOGPreventCare.pdf?dmc=1&ts=20130325T1200207968

Anderson, J. E., & Lowen, C. A. (2010). Connecting youth with health services: Systematic review. *Canadian Family Physician, 56*(9), 778–784.

Betz, C. L., Ruccione, K., Meeske, K., Smith, K., & Chang, N. (2008). Health literacy: A pediatric nursing concern. *Pediatric Nursing, 34*(3), 231–239.

Boonstra, H., & Nash, E. (2000). Minors and the right to consent to health care. Guttmacher Institute website. Retrieved from http://www.guttmacher.org/pubs/tgr/03/4/gr030404.html

Bruce, C. R., Berg, S. L., & McGuire, A. L. (2009). Please don't call my mom: Pediatric consent and confidentiality. *Clinical Pediatrics, 48*, 243–246.

Carney, T., Myers, B. J., Louw, J., & Okwundu, C. I. (2014). Brief school-based interventions and behavioural outcomes for substance-using adolescents. *Cochrane Database of Systematic Reviews, 2014*(2). Art. No.: CD008969.

Carson, K. V., Brinn, M. P., Labiszewski, N. A., Peters, M., Chang, A. B., Veale, A., ... Smith, B. J. (2012). Interventions for tobacco use prevention in indigenous youth. *Cochrane Database of Systematic Reviews, 2012*(8), Art. No.: CD009325.

Center for Adolescent Health and the Law (CAHL). (2010). *State minor consent laws: A summary* (3rd ed.). Retrieved from http://www.cahl.org/state-minor-consent-laws-a-summary-third-edition/

Centers for Disease Control and Prevention (CDC). (2014a). Health literacy: Accurate, accessible, and actionable health information for all. Retrieved from http://www.cdc.gov/healthliteracy

Centers for Disease Control and Prevention (CDC). (2014b). Youth risk behavioral surveillance: United States 2013. *Morbidity and Mortality Weekly Review, 6*(SS4), 160–168. Retrieved from http://www.cdc.gov/mmwr/pdf/ss/ss6304.pdf

Centers for Disease Control and Prevention (CDC). (2014c). United States medical eligibility criteria (US MEC) for contraceptive use, 2010. Retrieved from http://www.cdc.gov/reproductivehealth/UnintendedPregnancy/USMEC.htm

Chung, R. J., Burke, P. J., & Goodman, E. (2010). Firm foundations: Strength based approaches to adolescent chronic disease. *Current Opinion in Pediatrics, 22*, 389–397.

Coleman, D. L., & Rosoff, P. M. (2013). The legal authority of mature minors to consent to general medical treatment. *Pediatrics, 131*, 786-793.

Darling-Fisher, C. S., Salerno, J., Dahlem, C. H. Y., & Martyn, K. K. (2014). The Rapid Assessment for Adolescent Preventive Services (RAAPS): Providers assessment of its usefulness in their clinical practice settings. *Journal of Pediatric Health Care, 28*(3), 217–226.

Davis, T. C., Wolf, M. S., Arnold, C. L., Byrd, R. S., Long, S. W., Springer, T., ... Bocchini, J. A. (2006). Development and validation of the rapid estimate of adolescent literacy in medicine: A tool to screen adolescents for below-grade reading in health care settings. *Pediatrics, 118*(6), e1707–e1714.

DeNavas-Walt, C., Proctor, B. D., & Smith, J. C. (2013). Current population reports: Income, poverty, and health insurance coverage in the United States: 2012. Washington, DC: U.S. Census Bureau. Retrieved from http://www.census.gov/prod/2013pubs/p60-245.pdf

Department of Health and Human Services (HHS). (2011). Health Resources and Services Administration, Maternal and Child Health Bureau. *Child health USA 2011*. Rockville, MD: Author.

Department of Health and Human Services (HHS). (2012). Health Resources and Services Administration. Maternal and Child Health Bureau. *Child and Adolescent Health Measurement Initiative survey results*. Retrieved from http://childhealthdata.org/browse/survey/results?q=2473&r=1&g=448.

Department of Health and Human Services (HHS). (2014). The Affordable Care Act: Section by section. Retrieved from http://www.hhs.gov/healthcare

Doswell, W. M., Braxter, B. J., Cha, E., & Kim, K. H. (2011). Testing the theory of reasoned action in explaining sexual behavior among African American young teen girls. *Journal of Pediatric Nursing, 26*(6), e45-e54.

Dunn, A. M. (2009). Developmental management of adolescents. In C. E. Burns, A. M. Dunn, M. A. Brady, N. Barber-Starr, & C. G. Blosser (Eds.), *Pediatric primary care* (4th ed., pp. 132–149). St. Louis, MO: Saunders Elsevier.

Fantasia, H. C. (2008). Concept analysis: Sexual decision-making in adolescence. *Nursing Forum, 43*(2), 80–90.

Fertman, C. I., & Allensworth, D. D. (Eds.). (2010). *Health promotion program: From theory to practice*. San Francisco, CA: Jossey-Bass, Wiley.

Fishbein, M., & Ajzen, I. (1975). Formation of intentions. In M. Fishbein & I. Ajzen (Eds.), *Belief, attitude, intention, and behavior: An introduction to theory and research*. Reading, MA: Addison-Wesley.

Ford, C. A., English, A., Davenport, A. F., & Stinnett, A. J. (2009). Increasing adolescent vaccination: Barriers and strategies in the context of policy, legal, and financial issues. *Journal of Adolescent Health, 44*(6), 568–574.

Furneaux, B. (2005). *Theory of reasoned action*. Retrieved from http://istheory.byu.edu/wiki/Theory_of_reasoned_action

Gold, R. B. (2013). A new frontier in the era of health reform: Protecting confidentiality for individuals insured as dependents. *Guttmacher Policy Review, 16*(4). Retrieved from http://www.guttmacher.org/pubs/gpr/16/4/gpr160402.html

Guo, Q., Johnson, C. A., Unger, J. B., Lee, L., Xie, B., Chou, C. P., ... Pentz, M. (2007). Utility of the theory of reasoned action and theory of planned behavior for predicting Chinese adolescent smoking. *Addictive Behaviors, 32*(5), 1066–1081.

Guse, K., Levine, D., Martins, S., Lira, A., Gaarde, J., Westmorland, W., & Gilliam, M. (2012). Interventions using new digital media to improve adolescent sexual health: A systematic review. *Journal of Adolescent Health, 51*(6), 535–543.

Guttmacher Institute. (2014a). *Facts on American teens' sexual and reproductive health*. Retrieved from http://www.guttmacher.org/pubs/FB-ATSRH.pdf

Guttmacher Institute. (2014b). *Facts on publicly funded contraceptive services in the United States*. Retrieved from http://www.guttmacher.org/pubs/fb_contraceptive_serv.pdf

Guttmacher Institute. (2014c). *State policies in brief: An overview of minors' consent law*. Retrieved from http://www.guttmacher.org/statecenter/spibs/spib_OMCL.pdf

Guttmacher Institute. (2014d). *State policies in brief: Minors' access to contraceptive services*. Retrieved from http://www.guttmacher.org/statecenter/spibs/spib_MACS.pdf

Hensel, D. J., & Fortenberry, J. D. (2013). A multidimensional model of sexual health and sexual and prevention behavior among adolescent women. *Journal of Adolescent Health, 52*(2), 219–227.

Institute of Medicine (IOM). (2004). *Health literacy: A prescription to end confusion*. Retrieved from http://books.nap.edu/catalog/10883.html

Kaplan, G. A., Everson, S. A., & Lynch, J. W. (2000). The contribution of social and behavioral research to an understanding of the distribution of disease: A multilevel approach. In B. D. Smedley & S. L. Syme (Eds.), *Promoting health: Intervention strategies from social and behavioral research* (pp. 37–80). Washington, DC: National Academy Press. Retrieved from http://books.nap.edu/openbook.php?record_id=9939&page=37

Keeton, V., Soleimanpour, S., & Brindis, C. D. (2012). School-based health centers in an era of health care reform: Building on history. *Current Problems in Pediatric Adolescent Health Care, 42,* 132–156.

Marks, J. T., Campbell, M. K., Ward, D. S., Ribisl, K. M., Wildemuth, B. M., & Symons, M. J. (2006). A comparison of web and printed media for physical activity promotion among adolescent girls. *Journal of Adolescent Health, 39*(1), 96–104.

Masten, A. S. (2001). Ordinary magic: Resilient processes in development. *American Psychologist, 56*(3), 227–238.

Merry, S. N., Hetrick, S. E., Cox, G. R., Brudevold-Iversen, T., Bir, J. J., & McDowell, H. (2011). Psychological and educational interventions for preventing depression in children and adolescents. *Cochrane Database of Systematic Reviews, 2011*(12), Art. No.: CD003380.

Michigan Department of Community Health (MDCH). (2012). *Michigan laws related to right of minor to obtain health care without consent or knowledge of parents.* Retrieved from http://www.michigan.gov/documents/mdch/Michigan_Minor_Consent_Laws_for_Sexual_Health_292774_7.pdf

M'Imunya, J. M., Kredo, T., & Volmink, J. (2012). Patient education and counselling for promoting adherence to treatment for tuberculosis. *Cochrane Database of Systematic Reviews, 2012*(5), Art. No.: CD006591.

Moonsighe, R., Chang, M., & Truman, B. I. (2013). Health insurance coverage—United States 2008 & 2010. *Morbidity & Mortality Weekly Report, 62*(Suppl. 3), 61–64.

Morrison-Beedy, D., Jones, S. H., Xia, Y., Tu, X., Crean, H. F., & Carey, M. P. (2013). Reducing sexual risk behavior in adolescent girls: Results from a randomized controlled trial. *Journal of Adolescent Health, 52*(3), 314–321.

National Campaign to Prevent Teen and Unplanned Pregnancy. (2012). *With one voice 2007: America's adults and teens sound off about teen pregnancy.* Retrieved from https://thenationalcampaign.org/sites/default/files/resource-primary-download/wov2007_fulltext.pdf

Nemours Foundation. (2014). *Teen health from Nemours.* Retrieved from http://kidshealth.org/teen/

Nettleman, M., Chung, H., Brewer, J., Ayoola, A., & Reed, P. (2007). Reasons for unprotected intercourse: Analysis of the PRATRISHA survey. *Contraception, 75*(5), 361–366.

Oringanje, C., Meremikwu, M. M., Eko, H., Esu, E., Meremikwu, A., & Ehiri, J. E. (2009). Interventions for preventing unintended pregnancies among adolescents. *Cochrane Database of Systematic Reviews, 2009*(4), Art. No.: CD005215.

Pape, H. (2011). Young people's overestimation of peer substance use: An exaggerated phenomenon? *Addiction, 107,* 878–884.

Patia-Spear, L. (2013). Adolescent neurodevelopment. *Journal of Adolescent Health, 52*(2), S7–S13.

Piepert, J. F., Madden, T., Allensworth, J. E., & Secura, G. M. (2012). Preventing unintended pregnancies by providing no-cost contraception. *Obstetrics and Gynecology, 120*(6), 1291–1297.

Preston-Werner, T., Wanstrath, C., & Hyett, P. J. (2013). *Electronic code host: Reading ease, grade level, and text statistics.* Retrieved from http://www.readability-score.com/

Rees, G., Bakhshi, S., Surujlal-Harry, A., Stasinopoulos, M., & Baker, A. (2010). A computerized tailored intervention for increasing intakes of fruit, vegetables, brown bread and wholegrain cereals in adolescent girls. *Public Health Nutrition, 13*(8), 1271–1278.

Reese, B. M., Haydon, A. A., Herring, A. H., & Halpern, C. T. (2013). The association between sequences of sexual initiation and the likelihood of teenage pregnancy. *Journal of Adolescent Health, 52*(3), 228–233.

Resnick, M. D. (2005). Healthy youth development: Getting our priorities right. *Medical Journal of Australia, 183*(8), 398–400.

Resnick, M. D. (2010). The case for programs, policies, and practices that promote healthy youth development. *North Carolina Medical Journal, 71*(4), 352–354.

Salerno, J., Marshall, V., & Picken, E. (2012). Rapid assessment for adolescent preventive services: Validity and reliability of the RAAPS adolescent risk screening tool. *Journal of Adolescent Health, 50*(6), 595–599.

Salerno, J., & Marshall, V. (2011). Rapid assessment for adolescent preventive services: Validity and reliability of the RAAPS adolescent risk questionnaire. *Journal of Adolescent Health, 48*(2), S16–S16.

Shepherd, J. P., Frampton, G. K., & Harris, P. (2011). Interventions for encouraging sexual behaviours intended to prevent cervical cancer. *Cochrane Database of Systematic Reviews, 2011*(4), Art. No.: CD001035.

Society for Adolescent Medicine. (2004). Confidential health care for adolescents: Position statement of the society for adolescent medicine. *Journal of Adolescent Health, 35*(4), 160–167.

Spurr, S., Bally, J., Ogenchuk, M., & Walker, K. (2012). A framework for exploring adolescent wellness. *Pediatric Nursing, 38*(6), 320–326.

Stanton, A., & Grimshaw, G. (2013). Tobacco cessation interventions for young people. *Cochrane Database of Systematic Reviews, 2013*(8), Art. No.: CD003289.

Stellefson, M., Hanik, B., Chaney, B., Chaney, D., Tennant, B., & Chavarria, E. M. (2011). eHealth literacy among college students: A systematic review with implications for eHealth education. *Journal Of Medical Internet Research, 13*(4), e102.

Substance Abuse and Mental Health Services Administration. (2012). *Results from the 2011 National Survey on Drug Use and Health: Mental health findings,* NSDUH Series H-45, HHS Publication No. (SMA) 12-4725. Rockville, MD: Author. Retrieved from http://www.samhsa.gov/data/NSDUH/2k11MH_FindingsandDetTables/2K11MHFR/NSDUHmhfr2011.htm

Taliaferro, L. A., & Borowsky, I. W. (2012). Beyond prevention: Promoting healthy youth development in primary care. *American Journal of Preventive Medicine, 42*(6 Suppl 2), S117–S121.

Thomas, R. E., Lorenzetti, D., & Spragins, W. (2011). Mentoring adolescents to prevent drug and alcohol use. *Cochrane Database of Systematic Reviews, 2011*(11), Art. No.: CD007381.

Toumbourou, J., Patton, G., Sawyer, S., Olsson, C., Webb-Pullman, J., Catalano, R., & Godfrey, C. (2000). *Evidence-based health promotion: Resources for planning.* [No. 2 Adolescent Health]. Retrieved from http://www.rch.org.au/uploadedFiles/Main/Content/cah/HP-JT.pdf

United States Census Bureau. (2012). *State & county quick facts.* Retrieved from http://quickfacts.census.gov/qfd/states/26/26027.html

United States Preventive Services Task Force. (n.d.). *Recommendations.* Retrieved from http://www.uspreventiveservicestaskforce.org/recommendations.htm

Viner, R., & Macfarlane, A. (2005). ABC of adolescence: Health promotion. *British Medical Journal, 330*(7490), 527–529.

Wang, S. L., Charron-Prochownik, D., Serdika, S. M., Siminerio, L., & Kim, Y. (2006). Comparing three theories in predicting health behavioral intention in adolescent women with diabetes. *Pediatric Diabetes, 7*(2), 108–115.

Watson-Thompson, J., Fawcett, S. B., & Schultz, J. A. (2008). A framework for community mobilization to promote healthy youth development. *American Journal of Preventive Medicine, 34*(3 Suppl), S72–S81.

WebMD. (2013). *Talking with teens: Tips for better communication.* Retrieved from http://www.webmd.com/

Wolf, F., Guevara, J. P., Grum, C. M., Clark, N. M., & Cates, C. J. (2002). Educational interventions for asthma in children. *Cochrane Database of Systematic Reviews, 2002*(4), Art. No.: CD000326.

Chapter 28

Culture, Collaboration, and Community: Participatory Action Anthropology in Development of Senior ConNEXTions

Rosemarie Santora Lamm

OBJECTIVES

At the end of this chapter, the reader will be able to

1. Describe participatory action research as a strategy to build a community program for a vulnerable population of seniors.
2. Identify the key characteristics of a program to serve seniors in a community-based setting.
3. Explain the roles of healthcare providers in partnership with others to serve the population.

INTRODUCTION

In this chapter, a program to serve the senior citizens of a community is described. The program was designed through the use of *participatory action research* (PAR), a methodology suitable for organizational change. It is often applied to "create both action and change for social transformation to build community cohesiveness" (Breda, 2014, p. 9). *Action theory research* is closely related to PAR because the action process includes "community self-determination, scientific truth and, social organization" (van Willigen, 1986, p. 59). This chapter provides a window into the development of participatory action promoting cohesive community organization, in the creation of an integrated education and resource center for access by senior adults and their families.

IN THE BEGINNING

The Coalition on Aging Think Tank (CATT) began in 1997 as a vision of community collaboration and resourcefulness related to needs of the elderly. Mr. Alfred Rath formed a group representing education, medicine, politics, transportation, business, long-term care, home health care, the law, and consumers. This group identified the ongoing needs of an ever-growing senior population. Dr. Rosemarie S. Lamm, professor at the University of South Florida (USF) became the organizer for the CATT group and moved forward with the development of a gerontology program on the USF regional campus in Lakeland, Florida. She obtained several grants, which provided funding for the fledgling program that included PAR.

Grants were obtained from the West Central Florida Area Agency on Aging, the Retirement Research Foundation, the Bartow Community Healthcare Foundation, as well as the state of Florida. While the grants supported the ongoing research and development of the Rath Senior ConNEXTions and Education Center, the university assisted with the development of the gerontology cognate in interdisciplinary social science and aging studies. Dr. Lamm became the director of the Rath Center, integrating students with senior adults to promote intergenerational learning while providing assistance in PAR.

Partnerships were developed with community agencies that provide services for elders and their families, desks for each agency were provided at the Rath Center to enable easy access for clients when they visited the Rath Center. These agencies included: the West Central Florida Area Agency on Aging, Polk County Elderly Services, financial services, home healthcare agencies, Retired Senior Volunteer Program (RSVP), Alzheimer's Association, Volunteers in Service to the Elderly (VISTE), and individual volunteers.

THE RESEARCH ACTIVITY

Methods

Data were collected from intake information obtained by faculty and students. Information from persons age 50 and over was collected and analyzed using she Statistical Package for the Social Sciences (SPSS) software. Ethnographic information was collected using face-to-face interviewing. Ethnographies were obtained in special classes such as life writing and master class. Mixed methods were used to collect information applied in program development. During the tenure of the Rath Center's partnership with USF, between 2004 and 2012, 7,800 duplicated respondents provided information identifying and establishing the need for integrated services.

Results

This model was developed at the University of South Florida campus in Lakeland, Polk County, Florida. Polk County has a total population of 616,000 with 23% of which is over age 60 (U.S. Census Bureau, 2012). Data collected at the Rath Center identified the following:

- Age of respondents: 45–92
- Mean age: 72.8
- Illnesses reported: 90% reported illnesses (3.8 chronic illnesses each)
- Caring for another: 32% (Caring for another highest at age 72)
- Gender of respondents: 67% females and 33% male
- Marital status: Majority were married or widowed
- Living near family: 70%
- Social interaction: 32 % reported limited social interaction while caring for another
- Utilization of services greatest for persons with over $30,000 annual income
- Culture and access: white, 70%; African-American, 10%; Hispanic, 6%; Native American, 8% (Lamm, 2011, 2012, 2013, 2014)

The reasons reported for seeking services in order of the greatest number of participants are as follows:

1. Senior scholars
2. Information and referral
3. Socialization and group participation
4. Financial assistance
5. Health and mental health
6. Home assistance
7. Caregiver support, meetings, and training seminars
8. Other (Lamm, 2011, 2012, 2013).

The number of individuals accessing services was identified by participant action researchers embedded in the community. Students, faculty, and facilitators were actively involved in providing services while attending meetings, organizing programs, teaching Senior Scholar classes, and interacting with elder clients.

While data confirm the need to access services, Polk County, Florida is an underserved area that is now designated a Statistical Metropolitan Area. Demographics reveal that 18% of the population has an income below the poverty rate and 20% do not have a high school diploma. There persists a 6–9% unemployment rate, with 19% with no health insurance and 33% receiving Medicare. Another language is spoken by 18.5% of the population and 10.6% are foreign born. The elderly make up 23% of the population (U.S. Census Bureau, 2012). Lifeways have been identified in the population of Polk County: 55% have no physical activity and 33% are obese. The racial–cultural composition is: 80.4% Caucasian, 16.3% African American, 19.1% Hispanic-Latino, .03% Native American (U.S. Census Bureau, 2012). These demographics project a future with "a perfect storm" (Hyer, 2012, p. 1). Data (Lamm, 2012) from the Rath Senior ConNEXTions and Education Center provides a window into the lifeways and needs of seniors living in the community.

DEVELOPMENT STATEGY

Services developed at the Rath Center provide health intervention, educational information related to health and care giving, gerontological education, financial information and planning, insurance information and connection to providers, referral to community agencies serving seniors and their families, Senior Scholars classes for continuing education, and collaboration with community agencies providing services for elders and their families. An ongoing Parkinson's support group integrates medical information with interaction.

In a continuing effort to bring services to elders, the Rath Center represented by Dr. Lamm has been a member of the Polk Vision and Lakeland Vision organizations. These task force volunteers are studying elder needs and planning a vision for community action to support "aging in place." Information related to the PAR results confirms elder needs and the Rath Center has been identified as a hub for leadership and information related to seniors.

TRANSITIONS AND TECHNOLOGY

The Rath Center was an integral part of the aging studies and gerontology curriculum of the University of South Florida's interdisciplinary social science program. Students collected data from intake information and Senior Scholars classes. Classes included: health and wellness, computer education, Spanish, life writing, yoga, stretch and strength, painting, 100 years of Broadway, acting 101, chess, and photography. Lunch and Learn classes included: environmental lectures, home design, dementia education, and topics volunteers provided. These classes remain the most attended of all services provided.

With the recognition that a new, more tech savvy generation of elders was moving into the aging network, the integration of technology became a goal. Computer education included brain fitness, a program of computerized training to enhance memory. This program became a hallmark for further development of information related to technology that can assist seniors to remain living independently in their homes.

Kearns, Fozard, and Lamm (2011) present an integration of technology with an understanding of movement disorders related to age and disease. Sensor technologies can provide key information about an individual's general health. These concepts are integrated into Senior Scholars classes and the Parkinson's support group.

This educational information allows individuals to learn about modes of assistance in order to allow "aging in place."

JOURNEY THROUGH AGING

There is a persistent need for gerontological education to be presented to healthcare professionals. With the ever-growing population of seniors accessing health related services, geriatric and gerontologcal information remains scant. At the present time, geriatric nursing education has been integrated into adult health and in medical school geriatric education is a minor aspect of the curriculum even though elderly patients comprise over 50% of those needing care. In recognition of this plight, the Rath Center, in collaboration with USF, provided three geriatric continuing education programs in 2005, 2007, and 2010. Continuing education credits were provided for participants representing nursing, medicine, psychology, social work, mental health counseling, pharmacy, and physical therapy. The lecturers were researchers and providers of health care from the University of South Florida College of Medicine, the University of Florida College of Medicine, practitioners from Lakeland Regional Medical Center, the Polk County Health Department, and Watson Clinic.

Evaluations of these programs provided data supporting a need for specialized education for community practitioners and students. These programs also provided information from Medicare, Medicaid, and insurance issues related to elder care. Providers from community agencies presented their programs and networked with healthcare professionals, students, and elders.

PARTNERSHIPS FOR SUSTAINABILITY

Like a phoenix rising from the ashes, the Rath Senior ConNEXTions and Education Center emerged renewed! The Florida legislature voted to remove the University of South Florida-Polytechnic from the USF system. Ongoing development of USF-Polytechnic, which was administered by the USF system ceased, and a new legislative mandate created Florida Polytechnic University. With this change, the Rath Senior ConNEXTions and Education Center was closed as part of USF.

Given the reality of a challenge for sustainability, the CATT moved forward with the establishment of 501(c)(3) nonprofit status. This incorporation of the CATT-Rath center allowed ongoing facilitation of programs. The Rath Family Endowment Fund was transferred to the Foundation for Greater Lakeland. A new location was solicited under the direction of Dr. Lamm and the CATT board of directors.

The Lakeland Volunteers in Medicine (LVIM), a nonprofit medical clinic for working individuals without health care, provided an office. Family Fundamentals, a nonprofit facility for ongoing education for children and families allowed use of classrooms. Volunteers from the Rath Center continued to provide ongoing services with data collection of information from clients and Senior Scholars. Monthly meetings with providers of services, healthcare professionals, and stakeholders continued. Committees continued to meet and establish goals consistent with community needs. Established committees include: health and education, transportation, housing, legislative, memory disorders and chronic illnesses, programming, and the Rath Center. Chairpersons provided ongoing information that is the foundation for the development of educational programs provided by the Rath Center for the community.

Round table programs were developed and presented to community participants. A partnership with Florida Presbyterian Homes of Lakeland provided a location for the seminar. The first program presented representatives from government and agencies that provide services for elders. One hundred twenty persons attended and the interaction provided ongoing information related to identification of elder needs in the community. This information was collected and appropriate committees began goal development.

MODEL DEVELOPMENT

The CATT-Rath Center moved into a level of assessment derived from collected data with the integration of developed goals. Participant action anthropology allows the CATT-Rath Center to integrate data with "community self-determination, scientific truth, and social organization" as defined by van Willigen (1986, p. 59).

This CATT-Rath Center model integrates health services, social networks, and educational facilities, with a hub of services (Lamm, 2013). The community network process begins with contact through the Rath Center, moving forward with an intervention plan and culminating with referral to community partners. This collaborative process includes: the Rath Center, community partners and agencies, support groups, Lakeland Volunteers in Medicine, Family Fundamentals, and community residential facilities.

The ongoing educational program, Senior Scholars, provides classes of many and varied subjects. The classes are taught by volunteer educators with specialized skills. Classes are developed after assessing senior needs. These classes include: computer education, healthy living, strength and stretch, yoga, life writing, healthy cooking, life transitions, and brain training. Classes are held weekly for 6 weeks, three times yearly. Partnerships have been developed with the Women's Resource Center and the YMCA.

These partnerships are another example of community collaborations that enhance seniors' contact with ongoing educational experiences.

At the present time, advocacy continues with Lakeland Vision and Polk County Vision. "Before 2024, Polk County will have a quality of life that encourages persons with diverse backgrounds to live in harmony while developing physically, spiritually, mentally, and culturally within a healthy and safe environment" (Polk County Vision, 2013). With this statement as a goal, the visioning process provides collaboration with many senior services and organizations promoting integrated planning for clients.

The CATT-Rath Center has been recognized as a leader in connecting collaborative services for elders and their families. Dr. Rosemarie Lamm, executive director of the Rath Center, is the representative who serves on the Polk Vision and Lakeland Vision councils. Recently, the mayor of Lakeland appointed a Council on Seniors that comprises service providers, interested citizens, and government representatives. This council has the responsibility of bringing providers and citizens together collaboratively to plan a "hub."

This model provides a process that will begin at a point of entry with an assessment being facilitated by Rath Center–trained volunteers. Continuation of the process will occur when individuals are referred to partnership agencies and community resource providers. When needs are assessed and intervention is provided, continuity of care can be realized.

CONCLUSION

This narrative provides application of PAR in development of a community collaborative resource hub. The CATT-Rath Senior ConNEXTions and Education Center is a point of entry into a network continuum of services that support "aging in place."

REFERENCES

Breda, K. (2014). State of the art of nursing in participatory action research. In M. de Chesnay (Ed.) *Nursing research using participatory action research* (p. 9). New York: Springer.

Hyer, K. (2012). The opportunities and challenges from perfect storm. Presentation. Florida Policy Exchange Center on Aging.

Kearns, W. D., Fozard, J. L., & Lamm, R. S. (2011). How knowing who, where, and when can change health care delivery. In C. Rocker & M. Ziefle (Eds.), *E-health, assistive technologies and applications for assisted living* (pp. 139–160). NewYork: Medical Information Science Reference.

Lamm, R. S. (2011). Entrepreneurship in aging and community collaborative: Students and services. Proceedings of the 32nd Annual Meeting of the Southern Gerontological Society, p. 40.

Lamm, R. S. (2012). Concept to creation: A ten year retrospective of community needs for elders. [Summary]. Proceedings of 72nd Annual Meeting of the Society for Applied Anthropology, p. 121.

Lamm, R. S. (2013). Sustainability and action advocacy: Epic collateral damage. [Summary]. Proceedings of 73rd Annual Meeting of the Society for Applied Anthropology, p. 108.

Lamm, R. S. (2014). Community and planned living center: Partnership for sustainability. [Summary]. Proceedings of 74th Annual Meeting for Applied Anthropology, p. 164.

Polk County Vision. (2013). Building a healthier Polk initiative. Bartow, FL: Polk LEAD.

United States Census Bureau. (2012). Washington DC: United States Printing Office.

van Willigen, J. (1986). *Applied anthropology: An introduction.* New York: Bergin and Garvey.

Chapter 29

Adolescents and Low Glycemic Control in Type 1 Diabetes Mellitus

Mary Katherine White

OBJECTIVES

At the end of this chapter, the reader will be able to

1. Recognize the incidence and prevalence on type 1 diabetes and the effects of poor blood glucose management.
2. Understand the factors contributing to poor glycemic control in adolescents living with type 1 diabetes.
3. Learn about Camp Kudzu and their role to improve glycemic control in children and adolescents with type 1 diabetes.

INTRODUCTION

Type 1 diabetes mellitus (T1DM) is a worldwide problem that accounts for approximately 10% of all diabetes cases (Currie et al., 2013; Toussi et al., 2008). Approximately 1.04% of the national population and 1.35% of the total population of Georgia are living with T1DM (Novo Nordisk, n.d.). T1DM is usually diagnosed in people less than 40 years of age, of which a large percentage is diagnosed prior to adolescence. Nearly 480,000 children ages 0–14 are living with T1DM today, and the incidence is increasing (Soltesz, Patterson, & Dahlquist, n.d.). Seventy six thousand new cases are diagnosed yearly, equating to an annual increase of incidence at 3% per year (Soltesz et al., n.d.). The United States has the fifth highest incidence rate of T1DM worldwide of about 22%

of all children 0–14 years being diagnosed (Soltesz et al., n.d.) and from 2001–2009, the number of youth diagnosed with T1DM increased by 23% (Hino, n.d.). In the United States, from 2002–2005, 15,600 youth were diagnosed with T1DM (National Center for Chronic Disease Prevention and Health Promotion, 2011). Diabetes is widely prevalent in the world, the United States, and Georgia with an increasing incidence, especially in children and adolescents. Skocic, Marcinko, Razic, Stipcevic, and Rudan (2012) cite T1DM as the third most common chronic illness in children, trailing asthma and cerebral palsy. Although this disease is manageable, the treatment can be expensive with complex regimens that are difficult for patients to maintain. T1DM management requires juggling treatment regimens that include diet, physical activity, multiple daily finger pricks to monitor blood glucose levels, and insulin injections and adjustments to maintain glycemic control (Skocic et al., 2012; Anderson et al., 2009). Lack of proper T1DM management can lead to multiple complications that can be expensive to treat and accounting for about $14.9 billion in healthcare costs in the United States annually (JDRF, 2014). Unfortunately, complications from T1DM can lead to a decreased life expectancy of approximately 20 years less than the general population, although that number continues to improve (Currie et al., 2013). Complications can include but are not limited to cardiovascular disease, neuropathy, and premature death. T1DM is the second leading cause of death second only to asthma (Anderson et al., 2009; Borus & Laffel, 2010). The purpose of this paper is to examine the reasons that adolescents typically poorly manage their T1DM or have low adherence to treatment regimens and how Camp Kudzu addresses these issues.

Patient adherence to treatment protocols is important to achieve success with any medical treatment (Taddeo, Egedy, & Frappier, 2008). Adherence to the T1DM regimen is important as it predicts glycemic control and health outcomes (Markowitz et al., 2011). Patients adhering to their treatments have a 26% reduction in poor outcomes and the odds of a good outcome are three times as likely with treatment adherence (Taddeo et al., 2008). Low adherence to treatment regimens correlates with suboptimal glycemic control (Borus & Laffel, 2010), and thus increases in medical complications, which leads to a poorer quality of life and risk for premature mortality and morbidity (Borus & Laffell, 2010; Taddeo et al., 2008). Nonadherence and its impacts are well documented (Toussi et al., 2008), and are more common with adolescents than other age groups, despite the availability of effective therapies (Borus & Laffel, 2010). Strict insulin regimens and diet adherence are challenging (Haagen, 2011), and suboptimal glycemic control established during adolescence may be very difficult to overcome (Rausch et al., 2012). Lack of adherence may have many repercussions with consequences to patients, their families and the healthcare system.

Proper disease management can help to reduce and avoid complications and overuse of the healthcare system (Taddeo et al., 2008; Rausch et al., 2012). An improvement in glycemic control can significantly reduce the risk of future complications such as renal failure, cardiovascular disease, and neuropathy (Skocic et al., 2012; Carson, 2000), but suboptimal control can have major consequences on long-term health (Rausch et al., 2012). One may think that young people with diabetes would want to maintain control of their disease to enjoy a long and healthy life; however, the adolescent age group is subject to enormous pressures that influence their acceptance and maintenance of their disease (Carson, 2000). As a result, many teens do not adequately manage their diabetes regimen (Carson, 2000) and, during adolescence, there is a high prevalence of low adherence to T1DM treatment (Taddeo et al., 2008). It is necessary to understand the factors that contribute to poor glycemic control in T1DM adolescents.

The developmental stage of adolescence is a time of physical and cognitive maturation in addition to psychosocial changes and identity formation (Taddeo et al., 2008). This gradual process is full of turmoil and rebellion for most budding adolescents (Taddeo et al., 2008) and is made more challenging when living with a chronic illness like T1DM (Scholes et al., 2013). Teenagers want to move away from dependence and become more autonomous, and teens with T1DM are also expected to increase personal responsibility for their diabetes management (Taddeo et al., 2008). Typical neurodevelopment in the adolescent stage includes lack of concern for future implications of their current actions that show little to no impact of the threat of serious long-term complications (Haagen, 2011). When considering compliance with treatment regimens in adolescents, there are many areas of concern (Carson, 2000; Taddeo et al., 2008; Scholes et al., 2013).

Diabetes management is typically better when parents remain involved in care, because of the parents' overall knowledge of the teens' illness management (Osborn et al., 2012), yet parents' roles are to guide their children towards autonomous responsibility of their own diabetes management (Skocic et al., 2012). Parents with an overprotective parenting style can delay the teens' ability to take responsibility for their treatment, which can cause frustration for the adolescent (Taddeo et al., 2008). Negative or unsupportive parental behavior such as nagging, threats, or criticism, have been correlated with poor metabolic control and treatment adherence (Skocic et al., 2012). Low adherence and poor glycemic control is a way for adolescents to confront parents' authority (Taddeo et al., 2008). Teens will also keep secrets from parents about their diabetes management to avoid punishment and disapproval of negative behaviors, and this is associated with high levels of depression (Osborn, Berg, Hughes, Phum, & Wiebe, 2013).

The impact of self-management on lifestyle is another reason for treatment noncompliance in adolescents. Rausch et al. (2012) state that lower frequency of blood glucose monitoring (BGM) predicted a decline in glycemic control, especially among teens. They did a study and followed preadolescent and early teens age 10–14 for 2 years through the transition to adolescence and recorded BGM frequency (Rausch et al., 2012). The BGM average intercept was 4.9 (95% CI 4.7–5.2, $p < 0.0001$) and the average slope over time was –0.2 (–0.0 to –0.3; $p = 0.02$)(Rausch et al., 2012). Rausch et al. (2012) concluded that the decline in younger adolescents may be even greater than on older adolescents, thus setting a poor pattern of self-management even earlier. Practitioners often see a discrepancy in the BGM diaries that teens keep and their actual control when measuring their glycosylated hemoglobin (HbA1c), a 3-month snapshot of glycemic control (Carson, 2000; Haagen, 2011). Teens do not want to appear different from their peers, so often this leads to hiding their illness, including self-BGM, and denial of their diabetes (Taddeo et al., 2008).

Because T1DM regimens can be so complicated, teens may vary levels of adherence within their treatment regimens (Taddeo et al., 2008). As children with T1DM enter puberty, they become more insulin resistant, and significant declines in treatment adherence have been documented, although all the factors for changes in glycemic control are not well understood (Rausch et al., 2012). Taddeo et al. (2008) cite a study that found 25% of adolescents with T1DM were neglecting insulin injections, 81% were not following their diet, and 29% were not measuring their glucose levels and were falsifying daily diaries (Taddeo et al., 2008). Because of the complicated treatment regimen, teens often eliminate steps of the regimen out of denial of their necessity for optimal health outcomes.

Adolescents are particularly vulnerable in this life stage, and acceptance by their peers is the first step to make changes (Haagen, 2011). Teens want to be socially accepted by their peers and negative relationship with peers is related to poor outcomes (Taddeo et al., 2008). Currie et al. (2013) suggest that teens may be less compliant with insulin administration because of a fear of hypoglycemia and because of weight gain from insulin use. Both of these are embarrassing events in this identity-seeking life stage. Underuse of insulin is often a strategy teens use to avoid hypoglycemia, which is embarrassing if it occurs in front of peers (Carson, 2000). Deliberate restriction of insulin, also known as *diabulimia*, is a dangerous and prevalent practice with the highest rates among teen girls (Haagen, 2011). Hyperglycemia due to inadequate insulin results in the excretion of calories and weight loss (Haagen, 2011). If insulin is omitted, patients can eat as much as they want and still lose weigh (Carson, 2000). Studies have shown that teenage girls with T1DM have a higher body mass index, experience a greater dissatisfaction with weight, and use more unhealthy weight control methods than teen girls without diabetes (Haagen, 2011). A 5–38% prevalence rate of insulin omission has been documented among teenage women thus, leading to a threefold risk of premature death in 30% of women that have restricted insulin at some point in their lives (Haagen, 2011). Currie et al. (2013) also states that teen nonadherence is due to a lack of understanding of long-term complications such as a mean death age of 45 for insulin omission compared with 58 for women with appropriate insulin use (Haagen, 2011). The pathogenesis for devastating outcomes begins during adolescence with metabolic dysregulation that continues into adulthood (Haagen, 2011).

Psychological problems could also affect metabolic control indirectly through low adherence to treatment management in T1DM (Skocic et al., 2012). According to Taddeo et al. (2008), teens that experience social and emotional problems struggle more with adhering to treatment regimens. Skocic et al. (2012) found that externalized issues with teens such as aggressiveness and conduct problems may lead to poor glycemic control by interfering with the patient's ability to follow rules associated with the treatment regimen. Internalized problems like anxiety and depression can lead to a lack of interest or energy, feelings of hopelessness, helplessness, worry, and fear which can also negatively impact adherence (Skocic et al., 2012). Youth with diabetes experience increased rates of depression and these symptoms can undermine diabetes management (Osborn et al., 2013). Anxiety and depression can affect emotion-focused coping skills needed for living with a difficult chronic illness (Skocic et al., 2012). Emotion-focused coping and avoidance coping both significantly correlate with poor metabolic control, particularly in adolescent males (Skocic et al., 2012). Adolescent girls present more often with behavior problems and depression and thus have worse metabolic control than boys (Skocic et al., 2012). Low investment in treatment plans can be a sign of depression as well (Taddeo et al., 2008).

Camp Kudzu is a camp in Georgia that serves children ages 8–16 that live in the state and have T1DM. They offer three overnight sessions that each last 6 days, and one 5-day day camp for those less than 8 years of age. They serve just over 600 campers each summer and over 50% are adolescents. Their mission is to educate, inspire, and empower children with T1DM. The author is a former medical director for Camp Kudzu and has witnessed many experiences that exemplify the camp's mission. Campers receive informal education through discussions with medical clinicians, facts of the day that are posted around camp, carbohydrate counting is practiced at each meal, using the plate method for proportions and eating foods with lower glycemic index. Adolescent campers negotiate insulin management with their medical clinician based on their carbohydrate intake, physical activity, and blood glucose trends. Campers are inspired as they witness fellow campers win awards for learning and performing new skills and are encouraged to do the same. Many of the volunteers at the camp also live with T1DM. Campers feel empowered to live with and properly manage their diabetes when they see their camp role models living and thriving with T1DM. At the end of the camp week, all of the staff living with T1DM stand in a sequential line in front of the camp to announce how many years they have lived with diabetes. This range spans from months to 50 years. This lineup inspires campers and empowers them to properly manage their diabetes so they too can live long, healthy lives.

Through this camp experience, several factors related to poor glycemic control are addressed and discussed with both children and their families. Parents are not allowed to attend camp, and if they volunteer while their child is at camp, they are not allowed to interfere with the diabetes management or even look at the BG log for their child. In fact, these parents must sign a release to agree to this rule in order to volunteer. This is required so that parents cannot interfere with the campers, or be the overprotective parent, especially to adolescents. The teens are able to negotiate with their clinician on insulin dosing in regard to carbohydrate.intake, exercise, and BG trends during camp. This allows the teen to learn firsthand, in a supportive and safe environment, the effects of taking insulin while planning for diet and exercise based on their trending blood sugars. This negotiation and discussion aids the teenagers in learning some of the idiosyncrasies of diabetes management while becoming responsible and dependent for a complicated treatment regimen.

At camp, no one, especially adolescents, has to hide the fact that they have diabetes. In fact, they can't attend camp if they don't have T1DM; therefore, there is nothing for anyone to have to hide. Many campers have never met another person that has T1DM prior to coming to camp, so they are thrilled to not have to explain what diabetes is or hide doing finger pricks or giving shots. Because everyone is performing these diabetes requirements, this difficult lifestyle feels normal.

Many adolescents like to withhold insulin for a variety of reasons, but at camp that is not tolerated. Every insulin injection, via syringe or pump, is witnessed by an adult volunteer to avoid withholding or wasting of insulin. Because the teens are given the power to help calculate insulin doses, they are compliant in taking their medication. BG levels are closely monitored, as campers are checked 5 to 10 times each day. Fears of hypoglycemic episodes are relieved when campers know exactly how their BG is trending. The campers have all experienced some form of hypoglycemia, yet the camp has not had a severe hypoglycemic reaction in over 6 years. The adolescents see trends in how much less insulin is required due to the high level of activity during the week, and improved diets from the typical home protocol. Learning that simple lifestyle changes can decrease insulin intake is appealing, especially to the females, which can help with weight reduction.

The complexities of T1DM treatment regimens can be all consuming for anyone. The incessant monitoring and calculating of medications, diet regimens, and exercise, coupled with fear of severe hypoglycemia or hyperglycemia is anxiety producing and can lead to depression. Camp is fun and the campers are kept busy participating in a multitude of activities so that they don't have time to dwell on their disease. Campers want to manage their diabetes so they can partake in all that is offered. They are surrounded and supported by friends and volunteers that manage the same struggles every day, but are happily living their lives. This role modeling is essential for adolescents, as they too are maturing into adulthood and possibly prospective camp volunteers.

Various aspects of Camp Kudzu's effectiveness have been evaluated before. While at camp, campers receive awards for learning new skills while at camp. For example, they can be acknowledged for trying a new injection site or pump site or drawing up insulin for the first time alone or giving an injection by themselves for the first time. These are important skills that patients with T1DM must acquire. The camp also sends out a survey after the weeklong session to the parents of all campers that have attended. This survey tracks camper and parent satisfaction with the camping program as well as evaluating whether the camper has implemented any new skills learned at camp. Camp Kudzu feels they provide an ideal environment for their campers, specifically adolescents, to learn, be inspired, and empowered to properly manage their diabetes. Pediatric endocrinologists from the metro Atlanta area volunteer their time to be at the camp to oversee the medical management of the campers in attendance. Healthcare professionals monitor patients' long-term blood sugar control with a HbA1C test. They do not run any lab tests on the campers other than multiple daily blood glucose checks while at camp. Camp Kudzu wants to evaluate the effectiveness of their programing by comparing HbA1c values of adolescents that come to camp to those that do not.

CONCLUSION

Adolescents have been documented to maintain poor glycemic control of their diabetes. Many factors contribute to these issues including social pressure, emotional stability, and impact to lifestyle. Developmentally, adolescence is a challenging stage of development and T1DM is a difficult disease to manage. When these two are combined, poor glycemic control is typically noted. Camp Kudzu intervenes with children, adolescents, and their families in the state of Georgia in an effort to improve overall disease management. An evaluation of HbA1c values of Camp Kudzu campers and a comparative group of noncampers will take place to compare long-term glycemic control.

REFERENCES

Anderson, B. J., Holmbeck, G., Iannotti, R. J., McKay, S. V., Lochrie, A., Volkening, L. K., & Laffel, L. (2009). Dyadic measures of the parent-child relationship during the transition to adolescence and glycemic control in children with type 1 diabetes. *Family Systems Health*, 27(2), 141–152.

Borus, J. S., & Laffel, L. (2010). Adherence challenges in the management of type 1 diabetes in adolescents: Prevention and intervention. *Current Opinions in Pediatrics*, 22(4), 405–411.

Carson, C. (2000). Managing adolescents with type-1 diabetes. *NursingTimes.net*, 96(45), 36.

Currie, C. J., Petyrot, M., Morgan, C. L., Poole, C. D., Jenkins-Jones, S., Rubin, R. R., ... Evans, M. (2013). The impact of treatment non-compliance on mortality in people with type 1 diabetes. *Journal of Diabetes and Its Complications*, 27, 219–223.

Haagen, B. F. (Ed.). (2011). Insulin omission. *Journal of Pscyhosocial Nursing*, 49(2), 6–7.

Hino, S. (n.d.). Ongoing support: A critical component to strengthen peer support for adolescents in diabetes camps. The American Academy of Family Physicians Foundation. Retrieved from http://peersforprogress.org/pfp_idea_exchange/ongoing-support-a-critical-component-to-strengthen-peer-support-for-adolescents-in-diabetes-camps

JDRF. (2014). Type 1 diabetes facts. Retrieved from https://jdrf.org/about-jdrf/fact-sheets/type-1-diabetes-facts/

Markowitz, J. T., Laffell, L. M. B., Volkening, L. K., Anderson, B. J., Nanselt, T. R., Weissberg-Benchell, J., & Wysockis, T. (2011). Validation of an abbreviated adherence measure for young people with type 1 diabetes. *Diabetic Medicine, 28,* 1113–1117.

National Center for Chronic Disease Prevention and Health Promotion. (2011). Retrieved http://www.cdc.gov/chronicdisease/index.htmt

Novo Nordisk. (n.d.). Changing diabetes barometer: Measure, share, improve. Retrieved from http://www.changingdiabetesbarometer.com/diabetes-data/countries/usa.aspx?intmap=prev

Osborn, P., Berg, C. A., Hughes, A. E., Pham, P., & Wiebe, D. J. (2013). What mom and dad don't know can hurt you: Adolescent disclosure to and secrecy from parents about type 1 diabetes. *Journal of Pediatric Psychology, 38*(2), 141–150.

Rausch, J. R., Hood, K. K., Delamater, A., Pendley, J. S., Rohan, J. M., Reeves, G. R., … Drotar, D. (20012). Changes in treatment adherence and glycemic control during the transition to adolescence in type 1 diabetes. *Diabetes Care, 35,* 1219–1224.

Scholes, C., Mandleco, B., Roper, S., Dearing, K., Dyches, T., & Freeborn, D. (2013). Young people's experiences of living with type 1-diabetes. *Nursing Times, 109,* 23–25.

Skocic, M., Marcinko, D., Razic, A., Stipcevic, M., & Rudan, V. (2012). Relationship between psychopathological factors and metabolic control in children and adolescents with insulin-dependent diabetes mellitus. *Collegium Antropologicum, 36*(2), 467–472.

Soltesz, G., Patterson, C., & Dahlquist, G. (n.d.). Diabetes in the young: A global perspective. Retrieved from http://www.idf.org/sites/default/files/Diabetes_in_the_Young.pdf

Taddeo, D., Egedy, M., & Frappier, J-Y. (2008). Adherence to treatment in adolescents. *Paediatric Child Health, 13*(1), 19–24.

Toussi, M., Choleau, C., Reach, G., Cahane, M., Bar-Hen, A., & Venot, A. (2008). A novel method for measuring patients' adherence to insulin dosing guidelines: Introducing indicators of adherence. *BMC Medical Informatics and Decision Making, 8*(55), 1–9.

IV

Teaching–Learning

Chapter 30

Teaching Nurses About Vulnerable Populations

Mary de Chesnay

OBJECTIVES

At the end of this chapter, the reader will be able to

1. Discuss ways in which students can be helped to understand their own ethnocentrism.
2. Discuss specific things about other cultures that students need to learn.
3. For each model described, identify sources of commonality that can be used in other settings.

INTRODUCTION

The American Academy of Nursing (AAN) and the American Association of Colleges of Nursing (AACN) have devoted much attention to teaching students to be culturally competent. The AAN has an expert panel assigned to the topic (AAN, 2011; Giger et al., 2007), and the AACN has mandated cultural competence as an outcome of baccalaureate education. The *BSN Essentials* document lists five competencies that baccalaureate students are expected to demonstrate by graduation. A toolkit for graduate students is available on the website, along with competencies for graduate students (AACN, 2010). Much attention in the literature is devoted to teaching people how to be culturally competent; in fact, a book on this issue won a well-deserved *American Journal of Nursing* Book of the Year award (Jeffreys, 2010). Moreover, a cottage industry of cultural trainers has sprung up and consultants can easily be found who stand ready to teach courses on cultural sensitivity, competence, or awareness.

It would seem that cultural competence is a good thing to know and, therefore, must be taught. As with any bandwagon, however, it is essential to critically examine the nature of the concept and determine what it means to teach students to be culturally competent. Dreher and MacNaughton (2002) caution that we should pay attention to the fact that individuals and their cultures do not represent a settled, static relationship; in addition, culture evolves over time, making it difficult for clinicians to keep up. These authors assert that, in public health, which focuses on populations instead of individuals, it is useful to understand as many cultural factors as possible about the group, although such understanding might be difficult to achieve in acute care settings. They caution against the danger of attributing poor communication to cultural differences instead of to poor interpersonal skills on the part of the nurse. In short, their contention is that cultural competence is simply nursing competence.

Having said that, there still seems to be an important place in nursing education for teaching students to be competent communicators with people who are different from themselves. This chapter provides some ideas on this subject for faculty and students.

There are many ways to teach nursing students how to work with vulnerable people, and there are numerous activities students can undertake to gain practice in providing culturally competent care. This chapter presents some ideas for faculty with regard to the use of these strategies and seeks to inspire them to devise similar learning activities for their own students. For students who read this chapter, it is hoped that they find some of the experiences presented here inspirational with regard to their own fieldwork.

For any activity designed to prepare nurses to provide culturally competent care, it is critical to emphasize two key points: know yourself and show respect for others. First, the best way that nurses can prepare for working with vulnerable people is to know themselves. The more a person knows and acknowledges his or her own biases, the more easily the nurse can put these prejudices aside and concentrate on the patient as a person instead of a stereotype. *Ethnocentric bias* is a term derived from anthropology that refers to the notion that one's own cultural beliefs, practices, folkways, values, and norms are the right ones. Ethnocentric biases develop from our experience of living within our own cultures: growing up in families, attending educational institutions with certain emphases, and interacting with people we like or do not like. Ethnocentrism is neither good nor bad—it just is. To acknowledge that we all have biases simply indicates that we are human. People tend to get in trouble, however, when they act toward others as if their own way is the only right way or when they confuse bias with truth.

How do we learn to deal with ethnocentric bias? It is essential to recognize a particular feeling or attitude as bias and then to critically examine all of our own values and beliefs, particularly in terms of how we see others who are different from ourselves. This principle of self-examination relates to everyone, not just to members of majority groups. It might be helpful to apply the general system theory concept of *multifinality*, which holds that there are many ways to reach the same end. Appreciating that other ways of achieving the goal might be equally effective and valid is a key component of self-awareness.

The second way that nurses can prepare for working with vulnerable people is to learn to show respect. Novices tend to expend large amounts of time and energy trying to learn cultural material quickly so that they can interact "appropriately" in terms of superficial gestures, such as making eye contact or not, shaking hands or not, or touching arms. Yet, despite the best of intentions, these actions can sometimes be interpreted as mocking to the group. Being yourself, yet doing your best in terms of showing the most respect, according to your own cultural standards, is more likely to be understood by the patient as respectful than is adopting gestures or expressions that are obviously not your own. In this regard, cultural competence is a misleading concept because it implies that one is competent to practice another group's cultural behaviors. A more useful view of cultural competence is that it entails being comfortable while interacting with diverse people who behave in ways and hold values that are different from one's own without judging the other group by one's own standards.

Another key point in providing culturally competent care is to reframe compliance or adherence in light of the patient's or group's cultural norms, values, and folkways. For example, students might not understand food taboos and offer pork to a Muslim or Jewish patient, then wrongly interpret the patient's rejection of pork as loss of appetite. Many Arabs and Jews do not observe the dietary laws—but many do, so it is important to ask about this issue.

The patient and patient's family are always the best teachers of their culture. The salient point for the culturally competent provider is to ask and not to assume. Think of your patients and their families as your best teachers about their culture.

WHY TEACH NURSING STUDENTS ABOUT VULNERABLE POPULATIONS?

Global demographics are changing as populations evolve into ever more complex societies. Demographics of individual countries are also changing rapidly as people move within their countries or from one country to another to find food, jobs, or simply better lives for their families. As the costs of living and health care spiral higher, the most vulnerable members of the population become even more entrenched in the daily ordeal of living. The nursing profession cannot afford for its practitioners to be isolationistic in the way they treat patients and families, nor can it afford to ignore communities. Community-based care and focus on populations are aspects of nursing that students need to learn in order to provide cost-effective, culturally competent care.

The kinds of experiences students have in their basic educational programs can improve their confidence. This chapter presents three models from different universities. Although two of these universities happen to be private, the strategies and activities are universal and can be adapted by anyone interested in helping students develop or improve cross-cultural interpersonal relations. Many schools have implemented similar programs on behalf of the vulnerable populations of their own or international communities. Websites for the schools are a good source of information.

WHAT SHOULD STUDENTS LEARN?

Nurses need experiences that teach them to be comfortable with people who are different from themselves, which in turn, requires interaction with many kinds of people. It is not sufficient to simply review the literature and write papers on vulnerable populations. Although writing papers is useful, it can be an empty intellectual exercise if not combined with developing competence at talking with people. Fieldwork is an excellent way to develop interaction skills; immersion programs such as study-abroad programs in which students live with local families are even better.

Students need to develop an understanding of culture and become aware of their own ethnocentric biases. In doing so, they need a safe context for their own experimentation in which they will not be criticized by their faculty for attitudes they hold but rather coached to develop new ideas or views about the vulnerable. For example, it is not useful to berate students who believe that all homeless people should take menial jobs so they can get off the street. Instead, they should be guided to understand the complexities of homelessness and the reasons why even menial jobs are not an option for many people.

Even though statistical information on vulnerable populations often becomes obsolete before it is printed, due to health disparities that tend to increase with population increases, students still need to know who the vulnerable are and recognize the health disparities associated with vulnerable populations in their own communities. Students should be encouraged to review the literature critically for applicability to vulnerable populations and to formulate practices that better serve the vulnerable.

Finally, students should learn how to reverse vulnerability. Nursing means not only curing and preventing illness, but also strengthening the patient's resources so that the patient becomes less vulnerable. Once trendy, the term *empowerment* has fallen out of favor because it has a patriarchal connotation, yet the notion that people can be helped to attain autonomy is still useful in teaching students to care for the vulnerable. Perhaps a more appropriate intervention is helping patients develop or increase resilience. Everyone has strengths, and focusing on strength rather than weakness is a good therapeutic technique. Several chapters in this book, for instance, emphasize the nature of resilience.

MODELS OF EXPERIENTIAL LEARNING

Duquesne Model

Duquesne University is a small liberal arts institution founded in 1878 and operated by the Spiritans, an order of Catholic priests with strong service ties to developing countries in Africa and South America. Through its school of nursing, Duquesne confers under-graduate and graduate degrees, including a PhD, and it offers a variety of certificate and continuing education programs. During the author's tenure as dean of the school from 1994 to 2002, the faculty created a variety of programs and experiences for students and faculty in order to operationalize the service mission of the university. Two major outreach programs—local and international—are particularly relevant to the education of nursing students in caring for people from vulnerable populations, and these programs involve students at all levels: baccalaureate, master's, and doctoral.

Nurse-Managed Wellness Centers

The first outreach program was initially funded by the school of nursing and later by a grant from the U.S. Department of Housing and Urban Development (HUD). The faculty member who coordinated the gerontological clinical nurse specialist track in the master of science in nursing (MSN) program created a model for outreach into the community by starting a wellness clinic in a high-rise apartment building designated for senior citizens (Taylor, Resick, D'Antonio, & Carroll, 1997). Students and faculty conducted many health screening and health promotion activities. The model was evaluated as successful by residents, staff, faculty, and students, with the result that the clinic was replicated later in a federally funded project to expand services to African Americans in the poor neighborhoods near the university.

With the success of the prototype center, two additional centers were opened in the African American communities called the Hill District and East Liberty (Resick, Taylor, & Leonardo, 1999). Later, the Visiting Nurse Association in Butler County, Pennsylvania, adopted the model for a rural community north of the city. To prepare for the expansion of the clinic, the faculty used ethnographic methods to gain access to the community, to establish rapport with civic leaders and community residents, and to identify unmet needs that the school of nursing could fulfill (Resick, Taylor, Carroll, D'Antonio, & de Chesnay, 1997). The community members initially had reservations about the proposed clinic because they perceived previous experiences, when outsiders had come into the community for various research projects, as disrespectful to them. However, by using the principles of ethnographic research and the methods of participant observation and interviewing, the faculty found ways to involve the community in planning, so that when the second clinic opened, the community members reported that they felt a sense of ownership.

As of this writing, the original clinic and the Hill District clinic are thriving and provide a continuous educational experience for students and a practice setting for the nurse practitioner faculty. Faculty and students conduct health assessments, medication evaluations, teaching presentations, exercise classes in the form of dance therapy, and other health promotion activities. One of the projects at the clinics involved creating a chart audit system for measuring outcomes. This experience provided graduate students with the opportunity to apply theory to the practice of nursing in a functioning practice setting and allowed them to test the validity and reliability of the audit tool in an actual setting in a way that would be used by the staff (Resick, 1999).

When necessary, staff members refer residents to their primary care providers and, in some cases, directly to the emergency room. Students who rotate through the clinics obtain a sophisticated understanding of the healthcare issues of the elderly in the two independent-living high rises, one of which has a predominantly white population and the other a predominantly African American population. Through the clinics, students learn firsthand about the issues of the elderly as a vulnerable population.

Other activities in the local communities were initiated at the request of community leaders, who had identified problems. One highly successful program taught cardiopulmonary resuscitation (CPR) to residents of all ages. Faculty conducted a research project in order to examine community knowledge about CPR, and the results were helpful in developing the CPR programs (Winter, 2001). Certified faculty in the community centers conducted classes, and people of all ages completed the course.

Center for International Nursing

The Center for International Nursing was created in 1992 (Carty & White, 1993; White & Smith, 1997) to provide an administrative structure within which students and faculty could conduct educational programs, service projects, and research abroad. Initially, the center's focus was Nicaragua, but later the center expanded to South America, Africa, and Europe to complete specific initiatives. From 1994 to 2002, more than 130 students at all levels completed international projects, and each year 6 to 10 undergraduate students completed part of their community health nursing clinical requirement in a barrio in Managua in conjunction with Duquesne faculty and faculty in Duquesne's sister school, Universidad Politecnica de Nicaragua (UPOLI) (L. Cunningham & S. Colvin, personal communication, August 2000). The students conducted community assessments, performed health assessments, intervened in referrals to the community health clinics, and conducted health fairs to teach the community residents a variety of health promotion techniques. In another project, one of the critical-care faculty taught part of the trauma content to students in a hospital in Managua (C. Ross, personal communication, September 1999).

Due largely to the publicity about the activities of the center, the nursing school was approached by the Pittsburgh Rotary Club, whose members wanted to begin an international health project. They had built a clinic in partnership with the Rotary Clubs of Managua and Jinotega in a northern community of Nicaragua near the city of Jinotega. When the community residents were asked what they wanted to name their clinic, they indicated that they wanted it named for the late member of the Pittsburgh Pirates baseball team—La Clinica de Roberto Clemente. Clemente died in a plane crash while trying to deliver medical supplies after the Managua earthquake of 1972 and is still revered in Nicaragua. This clinic is used by nurse practitioner faculty as a clinical site for training graduate students, and the community was the site of an ethnographic study on men's health conducted as dissertation research by a doctoral student, as described in Chapter 34 of the first edition of this book (Ross, 2000).

A second international study was conducted as action research by a doctoral student who worked in Peru on the clean water project run by the Sisters of Mercy (Zolkoski, 2000). Other doctoral students have conducted independent studies in Nicaragua and served as teaching faculty for some of the programs offered to the local nurses and physicians.

Faculty made a commitment to UPOLI, and many other projects have been conducted among the poor of Nicaragua. The emphasis on the "train the trainer" approach meant that the faculty tried to work with local nurses as much as possible; many projects were accomplished with the support of UPOLI faculty. The study by Colvin, de Chesnay, Mercado, and Benavides (2005) described in Chapter 17 of the first edition of the book, "Child Health in a Barrio of Managua," was an outcome of the work conducted under the auspices of the *hermanamiento* (sister school relationship). Many other projects and programs have been conducted as well—too many to mention here.

Online Doctoral Program

Concurrent with the increasing international visibility of the Duquesne University School of Nursing, the faculty became aware of the desire of nurses in developing countries to improve nursing education for their people. Dr. John Murray, the university president, challenged the deans to experiment with distance learning strategies, and the faculty chose to meet his challenge by creating opportunities for nurses in developing countries to earn Duquesne's PhD in nursing through synchronous Web-based courses, coupled with residency on campus during the summers. The first course was taught by Dr. Jeri Milstead in the summer of 1997 (Milstead, 1998). Although some international nurses applied to the program, Duquesne's faculty were surprised at the popularity of the program among nurses who lived within driving distance of the university. Many lived in medically underserved areas where they needed to continue working because there was no one to replace them or because they had children at home; they were highly motivated, and the program became extremely competitive.

Seattle University Model

The Seattle University College of Nursing (SUCN) has a long tradition of furthering the mission of the university to promote social justice by serving the poor. In response to changes in health care during the 1980s, the faculty revised the master's degree program to teach advanced practice nurses to work with vulnerable populations (Vezeau, Peterson, Nakao, & Ersek, 1998). Originally developed as a clinical specialist program, the faculty recognized the need for a corresponding program for nurse practitioners and added a family nurse practitioner track. More recently, SUCN has developed an innovative second-degree immersion track for people with college degrees in other disciplines who wish to be nurses.

Many experiences in other courses (for example, the clinical courses and the thesis/scholarly project) enable students to develop comfort and skill in working with diverse patients, families, and communities. For their thesis or other scholarly project, students are expected to develop projects significant to their own future roles as advanced practice nurses and to vulnerable populations. Chapters 19, Grandmason; 23, Pasumansky; and 24, Cogen are reports of research that has implications for vulnerable populations in Africa and the United States.

In the BSN program, students work in the poor neighborhoods, called garden communities, located near the university. Garden communities are scattered around the city and students spend a good bit of clinical time there. Faculty members are assigned to each community and provide clinical supervision and support. The undergraduate course on vulnerable populations is a required two-credit course in which the students conduct fieldwork by interviewing people different from themselves in order to develop comfort with and competence at interacting with culturally diverse people and groups. Students discuss their fieldwork in a variety of settings in the United States and Belize.

Kennesaw State University Model

Located just north of Atlanta, Kennesaw State University (KSU) emphasizes global learning in a way that has moved the university onto the world stage in several disciplines, and its School of Nursing is a leader in this effort. For many years, the WellStar School of Nursing has sent students to Oaxaca, Mexico, to live with families, study Spanish, and learn in the local hospitals and community agencies. Students report that the experience is life-changing. Even though many may never travel abroad again, they express an appreciation for the Mexican culture of clients they serve in this country. A second

Mexican initiative for KSU graduate students in the nurse practitioner track is described in Chapter 35 in this book.

For a course on vulnerable populations, the author of this chapter assigned undergraduate students to conduct fieldwork with populations different from their own. The groups might be of different races or ethnicity or simply be members of a population that is medically underserved or disadvantaged, such as homeless people. Students interviewed a variety of service providers and group members and presented what they learned to the class. One group of students interviewed affluent adolescents for a life history research project conducted by the author; their work is reported in Chapter 18.

Finally, KSU's nurse-managed clinic serves as a primary teaching site for its students. Run by a nurse practitioner faculty member, Donna Chambers, the clinic staff have an average of 3,000 patient visits per year. Now that a formal agreement has placed the clinic under the auspices of KSU, plans are in place to rotate all nursing students (as well as social work and health promotion and sports management students) through the clinic at some point in their studies.

KEY COMPONENTS OF EDUCATIONAL EXPERIENCE

A plan for teaching nursing students how to care for vulnerable populations might include the following components:

- Identify the vulnerable populations within the community. If the school is interested in international nursing, then faculty might capitalize on their own international research or service experiences. Sister school relationships such as the Duquesne hermana-miento can provide wonderful opportunities for faculty and student exchanges, service learning projects, or collaborative research with nursing faculty in other countries.
- Develop a set of guidelines for students to follow for their fieldwork, with the expected outcomes clearly stated. (The *Instructor Guide* for this book contains sample syllabi and detailed guidelines.) Outcomes should include an expectation for improved self-awareness.
- Designate key faculty to coordinate or guide the process. Not every faculty member will want to be involved, but it is essential to have at least one faculty champion for each project.
- Establish the need for specific projects in concert with stakeholders who are key members of the population.
- Decide whether service learning projects will be part of the curriculum and conducted within specific courses or whether they will be free-standing efforts that are initiated as people express interest. One way to focus on vulnerable populations without undertaking major curriculum changes is to allow students to use independent study courses for fieldwork.

- Design and implement a small-scale project that can be funded through existing resources. Later, after individual faculty members have established a track record, more sophisticated projects can be funded through grants and contracts.
- Evaluate the projects not only in terms of student satisfaction and learning but also in terms of benefits to the population.
- Consider evaluation data carefully before designing subsequent projects.

CONCLUSION

The models presented here have several characteristics in common that contributed to their effectiveness in meeting the objectives of the courses and programs. Successful experiences for students include opportunities for developing self-awareness, fieldwork that enables them to develop communication skills and interact with people different from themselves, and review of available literature on the population of interest. Although these experiences are challenging, the students generally rate them as positive. In many cases in which students have traveled to other regions to become immersed in another culture, they indicate that their experiences were life changing. The success of these service learning programs demonstrates that providing such opportunities for undergraduate and graduate-level students is a crucial aspect of nursing education with regard to vulnerable populations.

REFERENCES

American Academy of Nursing (AAN). (2011). Cultural competence: Expert panel report. Retrieved from www.aannet.org/i4a/pages/Index.cfm?pageID=3555

American Association of Colleges of Nursing (AACN). (2010). Cultural competence in nursing education. Retrieved from www.aacn.nche.edu/Education/cultural.htm

Carty, R., & White J. (1993). *Nicaraguan–American nursing collaborating project*. Washington, DC: American Association of Colleges of Nursing, pp. 37–38.

Colvin, S., de Chesnay, M., Mercado, T., & Benavides, C. (2005). Child health in a barrio of Managua. In M. de Chesnay (Ed.), *Caring for the vulnerable: Perspectives in nursing practice, theory and research* (pp. 161–170). Sudbury, MA: Jones and Bartlett.

Dreher, M., & MacNaughton, N. (2002). Cultural competence in nursing: Foundation or fallacy? *Nursing Outlook, 50*, 181–186.

Giger, J., Davidhizer, R., Purnell, L., Harden, J. T., Phillips, J., & Strickland, O. (2007). American Academy of Nursing Expert Panel report: Developing cultural competence to eliminate health disparities in ethnic minorities and other vulnerable populations. *Journal of Transcultural Nursing, 18*(2), 95–102.

Jeffreys, M. (2010). *Teaching cultural competence in nursing and health care* (2nd ed.). New York: Springer.

Milstead, J. (1998). Preparation for an online asynchronous university doctoral course: Lessons learned. *Computers in Nursing, 16*(5), 247–258.

Resick, L. (1999). Challenges in measuring outcomes in two community-based nurse-managed wellness clinics: The development of a chart auditing tool. *Home Health Care Management and Practice, 11*(4), 52–59.

Resick, L., Taylor, C., Carroll, T., D'Antonio, J., & de Chesnay, M. (1997). Establishing a nurse-managed wellness clinic in a predominantly older African American inner-city high rise: An advanced practice nursing project. *Nursing Administration Quarterly, 21*(4), 47–54.

Resick, L., Taylor, C., & Leonardo, M. (1999). The Nurse-Managed Wellness Clinic Model developed by Duquesne University School of Nursing. *Home Health Care Management and Practice, 11*(6), 26–35.

Ross, C. (2000). *Caminando mas cerca con Dios [A closer walk with Thee]: An ethnography of health and well-being of rural Nicaraguan men.* Unpublished doctoral dissertation, Duquesne University, Pittsburgh, PA.

Taylor, C., Resick, L., D'Antonio, J., & Carroll, T. (1997). The advanced practice nurse role in implementing and evaluating two nurse-managed wellness clinics: Lessons learned about structure, process and outcomes. *Advanced Practice Nursing Quarterly, 3*(2), 36–45.

Vezeau, T., Peterson, J., Nakao, C., & Ersek, M. (1998). Education of advanced practice nurses serving vulnerable populations. *Nursing and Health Care Perspectives, 19*(1), 124–131.

White, J., & Smith, C. (1997). Developing an international nursing partnership with Nicaragua. *International Nursing Review, 44*(1), 13–18.

Winter, K. (2001). Bystander CPR in two Pittsburgh communities. *Cultura de los Cuidados, 5*(9), 82–89.

Zolkoski, R. (2000). *Clean water for Chimbote, Peru: Transcultural nursing in participatory action research.* Unpublished doctoral dissertation, Duquesne University, Pittsburgh, PA.

Chapter 31

Caring for Vulnerable Populations: The Role of the DNP-Prepared Nurse

Barbara A. Anderson

OBJECTIVES

At the end of this chapter, the reader will be able to

1. Describe the education and role of the DNP-prepared nurse in providing care to vulnerable populations.
2. Describe the eight essentials for DNP education and how they apply to caring for the vulnerable.
3. Discuss examples of DNP translational research that bring scientific evidence to the solution of problems that face vulnerable populations.

HEALTH STATUS IN AMERICA

Americans are sicker and die sooner than citizens in 16 other high resource nations. In comparison, the United States has worse outcomes with birth, injuries, homicide, adolescent pregnancy, sexually transmitted infections, HIV/AIDS, drug and alcohol mortality, obesity, diabetes, heart disease, chronic lung disease, and disability among older persons. These outcomes hold across age, ethnicity, and socioeconomic level. They are not only the problems of the poor. While the healthcare system in the United States is very expensive, health outcomes are suboptimal (National Research Council and Institute of Medicine [NRC & IOM], 2013). The health status of Americans makes them vulnerable.

Factors affecting vulnerability and resilience are: family and community support, religious systems, cultural norms, and individual characteristics (Greeff & Human, 2004). Limited or no access to health care and/or suboptimal treatment and follow-up can also increase vulnerability. Recent historical changes in the delivery of health care are addressing these vulnerabilities. Key policy documents discussed include:

- The Institute of Medicine (IOM) landmark document on the future of nursing (IOM, 2010)
- The Patient Protection and Affordable Care Act (ACA) (Department of Health and Human Services [HHS], 2010)
- The development of the DNP-prepared nurse (American Association of Colleges of Nursing [AACN], 2004)

The solutions outlined in these documents are not new; they have been discussed for many years. Annually, billions of dollars are invested in bench and foundational research, providing strong evidence on causes of healthcare problems and issues in healthcare delivery. Much of this research never reaches the clinical setting, or if it does, it takes years before innovation occurs. While primary research is essential, it does not solve clinical problems if it sits on the shelf (Melnyk, Fineout-Overholt, Gallagher-Ford, & Kaplan, 2012). This translation of research into practice is essential in improving the health of the nation. The profession of nursing has a responsibility to translate evidence-based research into clinical solutions. The profession of nursing has been hampered in the ability to bring forth changes.

UNDERUTILIZATION OF THE NURSING WORKFORCE

Vulnerable populations have the capacity to improve their health in partnership with strong healthcare providers (Anderson, 2012). The profession of nursing has demonstrated this kind of leadership in the past. Historical examples include the public health interventions of Lillian Ward among the urban poor in New York City, the development of the Frontier Nursing Service under the direction of Mary Breckinridge in Appalachia, and the courageous groundbreaking innovations of Margaret Sanger with Planned Parenthood International. Nursing has shown leadership but there is still much untapped potential.

Leaders from many disciplines across the nation have expressed concern about this untapped potential engendered in the practice restrictions placed before the nursing profession. Such barriers are exacerbated by the current and emerging global and national nursing workforce shortage (AACN, 2008, 2010; World Health Organization [WHO], 2010). The consolidation of health systems with greater delivery capacity and the ACA expectations for primary care have increased the healthcare workforce needs. Quality health care depends on a fully functional, team-based system with capacity to deliver primary and specialty care across the life span (Berkowitz, 2015).

The National Governors Association (NGA) recently released a report concluding that the ACA would increase demand for primary care services and demonstrate the significant shortage of primary care providers. The NGA supported nurse practitioners as being well prepared to deliver primary care. They called for the removal of restrictions on practice and the provision of adequate reimbursement (NGA, 2012). The looming national nursing shortage and the poor health status of Americans makes the underutilization of nursing skills, caused by regulatory and system-level barriers, an untenable situation.

In 2010, the IOM released *The Future of Nursing: Leading Change, Advancing Health*. This landmark document called for enabling nurses to practice to the full extent of knowledge and skills, consistent with academic preparation and without impediments from regulations or healthcare systems. It warned that failure to do so would exacerbate the critical shortage of primary care providers and adversely affect the health of the nation (IOM, 2010).

THE DEVELOPMENT OF THE DOCTOR OF NURSING PRACTICE DEGREE

In response to growing needs in health care, creative educational programs are being developed across the nation. Principles of health promotion, building resilience among vulnerable populations, and using evidence-based best practices are hallmarks of these programs. Healthcare delivery has not yet caught up, continuing to be based on tradition and the underutilization of evidence-based practices. These ways of practicing contribute to wasted healthcare dollars and many lost years for many Americans (Melnyk et al., 2012). The need to translate evidence-based research into the practice environment is urgent, beginning with educating providers pre- and post-service.

In 2004, AACN issued a position paper outlining the doctor of nursing practice (DNP) degree, a terminal professional practice degree for the nursing profession. The central premise was the translation of knowledge into clinical practice. This new degree was envisioned to be the entry point for advanced practice nurses (AACN, 2004). An adjunct to, but not replacing primary research degrees in nursing, the focus of this clinical doctorate is to prepare clinicians for leadership in translating research evidence into clinical care (AACN, 2006). PhD and doctor of nursing science (DNS) prepared individuals continue to be the primary generators of rigorous research evidence that guides translation into clinical practice (Melnyk, 2013). This team approach is consistent with the call to action from the IOM report (Anderson, Knestrick, & Barroso, 2015).

The DNP-prepared nurse needs in-depth knowledge and skills in understanding the evidence-based practice (EBP) paradigm, leadership in implementation, creating behavioral and cultural change, influencing policy, and evaluating outcomes (Melnyk, 2015). The components of this knowledge are built into the DNP essentials for DNP education and recognizable in DNP curricula across the nation. The DNP graduate needs to demonstrate competency and understanding of eight key areas:

- Scientific underpinnings for practice
- Organizational and systems leadership for quality improvement and systems thinking
- Clinical scholarship and analytical methods for evidence-based practice
- Information systems/technology and patient care technology for the improvement and transformation of health care
- Healthcare policy for advocacy in health care
- Interprofessional collaboration for improving patient and population health outcomes
- Clinical prevention and population health for improving the nation's health
- Advanced nursing practice (AACN, 2006).

Since inception of the clinical doctorate in 2004, there is a cadre of 2,443 graduated DNP-prepared practitioners serving in a variety of settings across the United States (AACN, 2014). At present, 243 universities offer the degree and 59 programs are in the planning stages (AACN, 2014). In 2004, 170 students were enrolled in DNP programs and by 2012, there were 11,575 students, demonstrating a strong and continued growth trend in the update of the clinical doctorate in nursing (AACN, 2013). Between 2012 and 2013, the number of enrolled students increased from 11,575 to 14,688 (AACN, 2014).

DNP TRANSLATIONAL RESEARCH REACHING VULNERABLE POPULATIONS

With a high rate of adverse health outcomes and poor health among many citizens, America has many vulnerable populations. These issues are recognized in the *Healthy People 2020* goals for the nation (*Healthy People 2020*, n.d.). With enormous wealth, yet a sick and frequently impoverished people, a fragmented healthcare system, and poor health outcomes, the U.S. population presents an unparalleled health paradox. The National Research Council and the Institute of Medicine define the key areas of vulnerability as adverse birth outcomes, injuries, homicide, adolescent pregnancy, sexually transmitted infections, HIV/AIDS, death from drugs and alcohol, obesity, diabetes, heart disease, chronic lung disease, and disability among the elderly (NRC & IOM, 2013).

With support from the IOM policy document, the DNP-prepared nurse has a growing opportunity to practice to the full scope of knowledge and skills, providing leadership in decreasing vulnerability from poor health. The ACA and the medical home concept further support the role of the DNP-prepared nurse (HHS, 2010). As a leader in translational research, close to and on the ground with primary care, the DNP-prepared nurse is an essential player in reaching vulnerable populations in the United States and contributing to the creation of healthy communities. **Table 31-1** provides some examples of completed translational research by DNP-prepared nurses who have addressed vulnerable population in America.

Table 31-1 Vulnerable Populations Reached by DNP Translational Research

Translational research topic	Specific vulnerable population(s) reached
Birth outcomes	
Preconception resilience	African American women
Preconception health: obesity, diabetes	Women in poverty
Pregnancy-related mood disorders	Women in rural and isolated areas; women with preexisting history of mental illness; women with deployed partners in the military
Physiological birth	Military women attended by CNMs
Place of birth	Birth center medical home model for rural, underserved women; Amish women attended for home birth
Early interaction with newborns	Skin-to-skin care for women delivering in military hospitals
Breastfeeding uptake	African American women; urban women in poverty
Violence	
Gun-related events in the emergency room	Rural emergency room nurses
Strangulation events in the emergency room	Women in violent relationships
Sexual violence	Young women in violent relationships
Child maltreatment	Native Alaskan children
Compassion fatigue	Emergency room nurses; veteran healthcare providers
Adolescence	
Poor nutrition and adolescent obesity	Alaska adolescents in rural settings
Human papilloma virus immunization	Adolescents in poverty, male adolescents; parents of adolescents
Depression	College students in Student Health Service settings
Prenatal smoking	Pregnant adolescent women
Sexual health and HIV/AIDS	
Sexually transmitted diseases	Women > age 50
HIV and hepatitis C	Men who have sex with men
Gender identity	Transgender male to female post-operatively; Transgender military personnel

(Continues)

Table 31-1 Vulnerable Populations Reached by DNP Translational Research (*Continued*)

Translational research topic	Specific vulnerable population(s) reached
Female genital cutting	Somali and Ethiopian immigrant and refugee women in primary care
Substance abuse	
Alcohol abuse	Native Americans in reservation setting
Opioid abuse	Urban homeless men; elders abusing opioids, alcohol
Methamphetamine	Long-distance truckers
Tobacco use	Coal miners; rural men in Southern states
Childhood asthma	Smoking parents
Prenatal substance abuse	Rural women; women in poverty
Prenatal smoking	Adolescent women; rural women
Chronic illness	
Childhood autism	Rural families without mental health services
Childhood obesity	Rural, underserved children; Hispanic children; Bottle-fed infants
Adult morbid obesity	Rural South African Americans
Diabetes	Rural Southwest Hispanics; Hopi Native Americans; Haitian immigrants; long-term incarcerated prisoners
Heart disease and hypertension	Middle age men with low social support
Lung disease	Coal miners; smokers in rural Southern states
Osteoporosis	Urban low income women > age 50
Colon cancer	Low-income rural Hispanics
Depression	Refugees with secondary relocation; low literacy refugees in healthcare system
New and emerging infectious diseases	Immigrants, refugees, international travelers
Disability among the elderly	
Medication reconciliation	Confused elderly
Pain management	Elders with chronic unremitting pain
Anxiety management	Elders with severe life stresses
Opioid abuse	Elders with chronic pain and anxiety
Advanced directives	Low literacy elders

Note: This table is an exemplar and in no way represents the full range of translational research addressing vulnerability by DNP-prepared nurses.

REFERENCES

American Association of Colleges of Nursing. (2004). *AACN position statement on the practice doctorate in nursing.* Washington, DC: Author. Retrieved from http://www.aacn.nche.edu/dnp/position-statement.pdf

American Association of Colleges of Nursing. (2006). *The essentials of doctoral education for advanced nursing practice.* Washington, DC: Author. Retrieved from http://www.aacn.nche.edu/publications/position/dnpessentials.pdf

American Association of Colleges of Nursing. (2008, September). *Ensuring access to safe, quality, and affordable health care through a robust nursing workforce.* Washington, DC: AACN Policy Brief.

American Association of Colleges of Nursing. (2010). Joint statement from the Tri-Council for Nursing on recent registered nurse supply and demand projects. Retrieved from http://www.aacn.nche.edu/Education/pdf/Tricouncilrnsupply.pdf

American Association of Colleges of Nursing. (2013, April). *DNP fact sheet.* Retrieved from http://www.aacn.nche.edu/media-relations/fact-sheets/dnp

American Association of Colleges of Nursing. (2014, August). *DNP fact sheet.* Retrieved from http://www.aacn.nche.edu/media-relations/fact-sheets/dnp

Anderson, B. (2012). Healthy communities and vulnerability: Enhancing curricula for teaching population-based nursing. In M. deChesnay & B. Anderson, (Eds.), *Caring for the vulnerable: Perspectives in nursing theory, research, and practice* (3rd ed., pp. 455–464). Burlington, MA: Jones and Bartlett Learning.

Anderson, B., Knestrick, J., & Barroso, R. (Eds.). (2015). *DNP capstone projects: Exemplars of excellence in practice.* New York, Springer Publishing (in press).

Berkowitz, B. (2015). The emergence and impact of the DNP degree on clinical practice. In B. Anderson, J. Knestrick, & R. Barroso (Eds.), *DNP capstone projects: Exemplars of excellence in practice.* New York, Springer Publishing (in press).

Department of Health and Human Services (HHS). (2010). *Affordable Care and Reconciliation Act.* Retrieved from http://www.hhs.gov/healthcare/rights/law/index.html

Greeff, A., & Human, B. (2004). Resilience in families in which a parent has died. *American Journal of Family Therapy 37*(1), 27–42.

Healthy People 2020—Improving the health of Americans. (n.d.) Retrieved from http://www.healthypeople.gov/2020/

Institute of Medicine. (2010). *The future of nursing: Leading change, advancing health.* Washington, DC: The National Academies Press. Retrieved from http://www.iom.edu/Reports/2010/The-future-of-nursing-leading-change-advancing-health.aspx

Melnyk, B. M. (2013). Distinguishing the preparation and roles of the PhD and DNP graduate: National implications for academic curricula and healthcare systems. *Journal of Nursing Education, 52*(8), 442–448.

Melnyk, B. M. (2015). Foreword. In B. Anderson, J. Knestrick, & R. Barroso (Eds.), *DNP capstone projects: Exemplars of excellence in practice.* New York, Springer Publishing (in press).

Melnyk, B. M., Fineout-Overholt, E., Gallagher-Ford, L., & Kaplan, L. (2012). The state of evidence-based practice in US nurses: Critical implications for nurse leaders and educators. *Journal of Nursing Administration 42*(9), 410–417.

National Governors Association. (2012). *The role of nurse practitioners in meeting increasing demand for primary care.* Retrieved from http://www.nga.org/cms/home/nga-center-for-best-practices/center-publications/page-health-publications/col2-content/main-content-list/the-role-of-nurse-practitioners.html

National Research Council and Institute of Medicine. (2013). *U.S. health in international perspective: Shorter lives, poorer health*, Washington, DC: The National Academies Press.

World Health Organization. (2010). 63rd World Health Assembly. International recruitment of health personnel: Global code of practice. Geneva, Switzerland: WHO Press. Retrieved from http://www.who.int/workforcealliance/media/news/2010/codestatementwha/en/index.html

Chapter 32

Community Action by Undergraduate Students on Behalf of Trafficked Children

Lady Collins, Kaitlin Chance, and Christine Meyers

OBJECTIVES

At the end of this chapter, the reader will be able to

1. Explain the interest of the three student authors in the topic of child sex trafficking.
2. Understand the power of undergraduate students in making change.
3. Describe possible interventions that undergraduate students can develop to influence health policy.

INTRODUCTION

This chapter describes the experience of three undergraduate nursing students who are active in their state and national student organizations and passionate about the problem of child sex exploitation. They turned their interest into community action by participating in a task force to address the problem in their state. The task force comprised professionals from social services, law enforcement, the criminal justice system, education, the business community, and interested citizens. Their stories are shared here to inspire other students to become involved in their communities—professional and personal communities.

LADY

After graduating from high school, I moved to downtown Atlanta to attend Georgia State University. I fell in love with the city and the culture. I considered myself a smart kid with a good head on my shoulders, but I was oblivious of the possibility that human trafficking was happening in my new neighborhood. I enjoyed taking on leadership roles and being involved on campus; therefore, I quickly became president of the Residence Hall Association (RHA) and a peer health educator. It was the first semester of my freshman year in 2008 when I was looking for an event to host in the residence halls. A resident assistant (RA) came to our RHA board meeting with the idea of hosting a Not For Sale campaign awareness event. It was the first time I had heard of Not For Sale and the first time I became aware of the issue of human trafficking. I was moved by the awareness campaign video and the survivor stories the RA shared. I became distraught and furious. These emotions became the fuel to my passion to help as many people as I could to become aware of this epidemic. I am not one to stand still and the best outlet I have is to lead projects that are effective in bringing about change. The RHA immediately jumped on board and we produced the largest event our residence hall had ever had to that day. We hosted several hundred students who pledged to raise awareness of human trafficking. From that day forward, I knew that even as a student, I could make a difference and collectively we created a movement.

A plethora of events stemmed from the Not For Sale campaign awareness program that I was involved in during my freshman year. Among the awareness events our organization hosted were: book, clothing, and food drives for human trafficking safe houses and local organizations. Additionally, any time I had to write a paper on a topic of my choice, I would find some way to focus on human trafficking. I would always point out that it was happening in our neighborhood and in our city.

My life was changed forever since my freshman year in college and when, a couple of years later, I attended the Passion Conference of 2010 hosted in Atlanta and was introduced to global and local organizations that are combating human trafficking. I partnered with Passion to increase awareness as part of what is known as the End It movement. In 2012, I began nursing school, and I continued my endeavors as a student leader. I became vice president of my school Student Nurses' Association chapter as well as Breakthrough to Nursing (BTN) director of the state chapter, the Georgia Association of Nursing Students (GANS). During my time as a nursing student, I began to seek out professional mentors in my community that were involved in projects to raise awareness and end human trafficking. During my search I came across Dr. Mary de Chesnay's textbook. Concurrently, my professionalism and ethics professor, Dr. Mareno, introduced me to Dr. de Chesnay. I was honored to be in the same school as Dr. de Chesnay and spent hours in her office discussing my interest and seeking guidance. Her passion to educate nursing students and nurses on human trafficking fueled my desire to become more involved as a nursing student. I obtained a copy of her textbook, *Sex Trafficking: A Clinical Guide for Nurses*, and learned more about her research (de Chesnay, 2013). I was happy to find a proposed policy and procedure within her textbook. I dove into the existing research, which proved to be primarily qualitative and anecdotal. I also continued to meet with Dr. de Chesnay over the next several months as we discussed ways to bring action to the nursing student body. I was shocked and could not believe that we, as members of a professional workforce devoted to the betterment of mankind, were so minutely involved in combating human trafficking through our practice. Further, I came across several stories of survivors who had gone in and out of the healthcare system unnoticed through emergency room visits or other encounters with healthcare professionals. This led me to speak up in my nursing organization and my community. I devoted my nursing career to human trafficking and became an emergency room nurse at a pediatric facility in hopes of being the one to notice patients who have been subjected to commercial or sexual exploitation. Through my role as BTN director, I became involved with the Governor's Office of Children and Families Statewide Commercial Sexual Exploitation of Children (GOCF-CSEC) task force and learned about ways that professionals were collaborating to decrease the incidence of trafficking in our state. My responsibilities as BTN director included but were not limited to: diversifying the professional nursing population, getting involved with reducing minority disparities, and seeking out vulnerable populations to serve. I used my leadership roles to network and voice my concern for our (nurses) involvement in being aware of and noticing human trafficking patients.

I presented my decision to join the task force to the GANS board of directors and my decision was welcomed. Our GANS Legislative Director at the time, Kaitlin Chance became particularly interested in my work and supported every effort I presented. She had also had an incredible encounter with local and global organizations combating human trafficking at the Passion Conference of 2013. I partnered with Kaitlin to present a resolution to GANS on setting policy and procedures for patients subjected to human trafficking. Our resolution was well received at the GANS annual convention.

Furthermore, I began to discuss our progress in the nursing associations with my classmates. My nursing school professors allowed me to share my experiences during lectures on vulnerable populations. I remember standing in front of my peers looking at some of the faces of shock, astonishment, and a fury of other emotions. Every time I speak in front of an audience about this issue, I am reminded of the same feelings I felt when I first heard that human sex trafficking still exists. During one of my open discussions, one of my fellow colleagues, Christine Meyers, approached me about getting involved with the statewide task force.

CHRISTINE

I have Lady to thank for my extreme interest in human trafficking and for my introduction to activism. When I first thought about becoming a nurse, I focused more on mental health issues, particularly those surrounding addiction, because the most difficult and horrific stories in my personal life related to mental health and the embarrassing lack of support that patients and their families receive when mental health problems are their main health concern. I noticed how few nurses and nursing students felt comfortable around these patients and how many disliked interacting with them. I really cared for and enjoyed working with individuals and families suffering from addiction; so, I thought I would fill a gap in this area once I officially started working as a nurse. However, after listening to Lady speak so passionately about human trafficking during one of my classes, I looked into myself and realized I was tired of waiting to find a special niche; I wanted to get heavily involved in something really big right now. I wanted to make a real immediate difference today. So, when Lady brought up the task force, I felt like I had to walk through the door. Somewhere within myself I just knew I had to grasp the opportunity. I could be a part of something today that other people could not. I could actually contribute in a way that would translate into better lives for these children and perhaps prevent other children from being victimized.

My first real step was coordinating with Lady to ride into downtown Atlanta for the quarterly meeting of the GOCF-CSEC task force. We went through security and signed into the meeting before entering an expanded conference room with tables and chairs set out into three different viewing areas. The room was full of professionals representing law enforcement, medical facilities, community outreach organizations, churches, and local businesses. Lady was able to point out a number of people such as the director of Street Grace and the woman behind Children's Healthcare of Atlanta's CSEC initiatives. Seeing so many people representing so many organization was intimidating, but it was also inspiring because surely such a collaboration could lead to positive results. The speaker that day was Jonathan Cloud. His empowered speaking about the reformatted task force and its revamped goals reinforced my own hopes and created a feeling of confidence within me. With prior agreement from the board, Lady signed GANS up as an affiliate member of the task force and applied for positions on three of the soon-to-be-formed work groups. I applied to represent GANS on work group 2: At-Risk Youth Identified. This work group focuses on identifying youth in our city that are at risk for being subjected to trafficking. The work group collaborates to create programs to decrease factors that put the youth at risk. Now, I am able to hold conversations with professionals and peers on the efforts that are effective in eliminating human trafficking.

Nonetheless, it always surprises me how much naïveté exists in our American culture. We persistently judge situations without understanding, and we tend to hold very impassioned positions on topics not because we know a lot about them, but merely because we think we have the right to do so. Some of the most pervasive and malicious ideas concern women who are outwardly sexually active, particularly those who "become" prostitutes. As I'm old enough to recognize that tendency within my own behavior, I make an effort not to do so. Strangely enough, what led me to work in support of stopping human trafficking was not any particular sad traumatic story. I learned that it was going on, and then I learned it was a global issue. When I realized the sheer immensity of the criminal system, which picks up a vulnerable girl or boy and binds them into a system of subjugation until death, it changed my mindset on a major scale. I never connected cases of child abuse and sexual assault that entered my awareness to the incidences of prostitution featured on the nightly news. I missed the impact of neglect and trauma that captures these unguarded children and breaks them down until they fit into the mold of the women you see for sale on corners or hear about in reference to backroom services at bars. The realization that no one would speak up for them, that people would look at them with disgust or contempt, called me to speak out on their behalf. It was something I could do, but more importantly, it was something I could do that others who are less in tune with the realities of a tragic childhood would not necessarily be able or willing to do.

LADY

I agree with Christine about our preconceived notions of people subjected to human trafficking. We, as a society, are so quick to judge others by their outward appearance or by what seems to be their choice. When in fact, the lives of people subjected to trafficking go much deeper than what we can see on the outside. Our work with this population must go further than an initial assessment. We must take the time to dig deeper, look at the historical trends in their lives, understand where they are coming from, and most importantly, let them know we are here to listen and notice them. Too often I read survivor stories of how they went unnoticed, and it is our goal and duty to change that. Our promise as nurses is to be committed to serve the welfare of those in our care.

As I transitioned into my professional nursing role, I entrusted the GANS directors to continue our student efforts. A great mentor once told me that being a great leader did not mean doing everything myself but entrusting a group of fellow leaders to carry on the work I have started. Knowing this from experience, I knew that GANS would do great things. Kaitlin and I have continued to collaborate on our GANS resolution and she has remained an advisor to the GANS board.

KAITLIN

The first survivor story I heard was from a girl who was 14 years old. We saw her in person, not on some Internet video. As she stood in front of me all I could focus on was her childlike features, and how unfair it was that this beautiful girl had her innocence and childhood taken away from her. Then it really clicked—she was the same age as my niece. My heart broke, the tears came, and I haven't been the same since. When I moved to Macon, Georgia in 2009 for college I started noticing "massage parlors" that were open 24 hours, and oddly enough, they were marketing their services to truck drivers. I distinctly remember a feeling of apprehension whenever I passed one of those businesses. Our culture had taught me that people went into businesses like these to buy sex from willing women. It was bizarre to me, surely people weren't paying for sex in these business that were in plain sight in Macon, Georgia. I thought I was alone in my uneasiness, but no one seemed to be trying to close down these parlors, so I convinced myself that there must not be anything wrong with what was happening. I mean the women were willing, right?

Regardless of whether I wanted to admit it to myself or not, I knew that what was happening inside that building with bars on the doors and blacked out windows was wrong. In February 2013, I learned that I was not alone in my feeling of angst toward one particular massage parlor. After a 4-year undercover investigation, the owners were indicted and the parlor was closed for good. It wasn't until then that the reality of what was happening in those massage parlors clicked for me—we like to call it our shock factor. For me, the shock factor came while I was attending a Passion Conference in Atlanta, Georgia. Passion Conference is a gathering of college students, ages 18 to 25, lead by Louie Giglio. These conferences challenge students to pursue a life that honors God. The bible verse, Isaiah 26:8, is on the banner over Passion Conferences. It states, "Yes, Lord, walking in the way of your laws, we wait for you; your name and renown are the desire of our hearts."

During the 2013 conference, a video sharing the story of a human trafficking survivor was shared. It was so horrific—for me it was the first time I had ever heard the harsh reality that these children are forced to live every day. When the video was over, a spotlight moved to illuminate the young girl whose story had just changed my world forever. As I looked at her, all I could see was her childlike features. She couldn't have been more than 13 years old, but she had already experience more pain than I ever would in my lifetime. The speaker, Bryson Vogeltanz, who currently serves as the Pastor of Growth and Spiritual Formation at Passion City Church in Atlanta, Georgia, began sharing statistics about the life expectancy of these children once they are brought into "the life." As stated by Vogeltanz, the entry age for a trafficked child averaged between ages 12 to 14. Once the child is trafficked, their life expectancy drops to a startling 7 years. Meaning that statistically, these victims are dead by the ages of 19 to 21. I was 21 in 2013, meaning that if this had been the path my life had taken, I would more than likely be dead. That realization changed me.

I read a quote once that stated, "It is both a blessing and a curse to feel everything so deeply." For me, this quote holds so much truth when it comes to the state of my heart regarding human trafficking and its victims. I am honored to have the opportunity to make a difference in these lives, to have a position in which I can fight this injustice, to play a part in the restoration of a beautiful life; but at the same time being involved in such a dark place allows for a heartache. It's the type of heartache that will wake you up at night, leaving you tossing and turning until the sun rises. When you become passionate about something it changes you, regardless of whether your passion is fighting against trafficking or something else. When you dedicate this much time and effort to anything there is a cost. What's the cost for me to stand in the fight against human trafficking? I bear a constant heartache caused by the deep awareness I have of the dark ways the world works. For me, that heartache is worth it.

After learning everything I could about human trafficking on my own, I decided that being able to define human trafficking was not enough to satisfy me. Many have said: "Indifference is not an opinion," and the realization that slavery still existed outraged me. An overwhelming desire to make a difference was ignited in me back in 2013, and it has only grown stronger as time has passed. At nursing school I did not have a ton of time to dedicate, so I was waiting patiently for that something to come along in which it made sense for me to get involved. Little did I know that Lady, who served as the BTN on the GANS Board of Directors, a state board of nursing students where I served as the legislative director, was just as outraged about this social injustice. As she mentioned, GANS joined the task force in the spring of 2013.

After a long conversation with Lady, I became educated on how little the healthcare profession knew about human trafficking. From there it became obvious to both of us that we were going to use our director positions on the GANS board to change that. It has been my experience that when a group of young people becomes outwardly passionate about something, when they use their voice to make positive noise, people pay attention. As passionate future healthcare professionals eager to see a change, we began brainstorming on how to be most effective with our time and resources.

As the legislative director, my responsibilities included keeping our members informed on current legislative action regarding health care, memorizing policies and bylaws, learning Robert's Rules of Order and how to chair the House of Delegates. Outside of those duties it was also my responsibility to pick the topic, research, and write a resolution that would ultimately be presented at the National Student Nurses Association (NSNA) annual convention the following year. Resolutions work kind of like a "call to action." Lady and I decided that calling all nursing students to take action is exactly what needed to happen. We started the education process by posting links to articles, videos, and anything that could be found useful on GANS social media outlets. The response was overwhelming; our fellow board members continually supported our efforts as they educated themselves. With a unanimous vote, the GANS Board of Directors decided the focus of our resolution would be human trafficking and it's relevance in today's healthcare profession.

Lady and I scheduled a meeting with Dr. Mary de Chesnay, and with her guidance, decided that our resolution could have a significant impact if we found a need to meet. Dr. de Chesnay pointed out to us that health care is often driven by policies and procedures, and it has been my personal experience that most healthcare professionals welcome step-by-step instruction. These sorts of directions leave little room for error, and they accurately guide us in providing the best care available for our patients. At the hospital where I currently work there are policies for everything, when questions arise. Unfortunately, there is nothing of the like for human trafficking patients, an extremely vulnerable, high-risk patient group. With this knowledge, the title of our resolution became: "In support of hospitals adopting established policy and procedures for patients who have been subjected to human trafficking."

We believe that establishing a policy and procedure specifically for the care of patients who have been subjected to human trafficking is essential in order to provide the most effective care for this vulnerable population. These patients present with complications of not only a sexual nature, but with severe physical trauma, communicable diseases, malnutrition, chronic pain, substance abuse, and a wide range of mental health issues. Having a protocol in place will guide healthcare professionals in recognizing victims' need for help. It will enable us to confidently move forward with treatment by knowing the resources needed are in one concise location, a policy and procedure protocol.

After researching and writing, our resolution was presented to the GANS House of Delegates in October of 2013, and the membership voted in an overwhelming majority to adopt our resolution. This meant that Georgia nursing students were behind our efforts to make this policy and procedure become a reality. At the conclusion of the convention, our terms ended as we elected new BTN and legislative directors for the 2013–2014 term. Thankfully, GANS decided to continue our efforts by allowing me to stay involved in the resolution process. It was now time to expand our Georgia-focused resolution to have a national focus. The results of these edits are included at the end of the chapter. That following April, I stood in front of the National Student Nurses' Association House of Delegates and presented my case for the proposed resolution. With an overwhelming majority vote, NSNA membership agreed to support us in our efforts to see this policy come to fruition.

At this point, we are still waiting to see what the next step will be. Lady and I have both joined the Emergency Nurses Association and spoken to them about the possibility of a resolution or position statement. All of the healthcare professionals with whom we meet, understand the need for this sort of policy and procedure to be created. I believe that with enough effort, we will see our resolution become a reality in the coming days.

The next step for me was taking my journey to a global level. I wanted to understand human trafficking as best as I could, by exploring it in all forms. Up until this point, the global impact of human trafficking was missing. It was not too long after this realization that I committed to a summer-long internship in Mumbai, India through an antitrafficking organization called Rahab's Rope. My time in India was very unique. I learned more in those 2 months than I could ever put into words, but I want to share a few lessons from India that further ignited my passion to see human trafficking ended.

During my internship, I lived among and worked for an orphanage of close to 80 children and that was growing larger every day. Along with caring for the children, this ministry cares for rescued women, widowed women and their families, and slum families who have approached the orphanage looking for a better life. During my time there, 8 of the children had been rescued directly from brothels, and the majority of the older women had past experiences filled with horror stories of how they were abused, manipulated, and forced to sell themselves. I spent every day for 8 weeks with these people, living life and loving them. Over time, the more I loved the more their stories became personal. The horrific stories were no longer stories, they were people with faces and names, people that I loved. Now that things are personal, I know that my decision to join in the fight to end human trafficking will be well worth it, even if it only helps one victim begin a new life.

When I have shared my experience with people, the common response I receive falls into the category of: I wish I could do something like that, but I'm too old/married/have kids/have a job. People are comfortable making excuses when, deep down they want to invest themselves into something that can make a difference. My team in India was made up of women from all walks of life, with at least 30-year age difference from the youngest to the oldest team member. Now is not the time to make excuses; it is the time to take action.

Moving to a foreign country is not for everyone, so I am not saying that is what everyone should do. What I want you, the reader, to realize is that no matter the stage of life you are in, you can do something to make a change. Tame your rage, ignite your passion, and take a step toward change. Even if your cause is not related to human trafficking, there are many worthy causes that serve vulnerable populations who need you to ignite your passion and get involved. Lady, Christine, and myself can all vouch for how rewarding this experience has been.

LADY

The best time to start getting involved in something you are passionate about is during your undergraduate school years. You have the opportunity to collaborate with colleagues in other departments and build up your network. Additionally, as a student you can get a glimpse into different areas that you are interested in before making an official commitment. I still get emails from people I have worked with in the past on combating human trafficking and I am thrilled to hear they are continuing the work in their professional careers that they started as a student. As for me, I am glad that I was able to use my leadership positions to carry out programs, events, and promote awareness among my student body population. Even if one person was touched enough to start their own movement or if one person realized they were being recruited to be trafficked, I am glad I put the effort into this cause. I believe there is no effort too small or too big in interceding this devastating occurrence.

KAITLIN

I agree with Lady in that the best time to get involved is during your undergraduate years. Once the passion is ignited in you, run with it. It will be worth it. For me, nursing school was one of the busiest times of my life. It felt like I was expected to be in three places at the same time and have read 300 pages of information before I ever got there. Just because I was in school, the responsibilities of being a daughter, friend, girlfriend, and employee did not disappear. My calendar was always full, but I made the decision to do something, anything, that would make an impact in helping to end this injustice. My time at Passion 2013 provided me with beginning resources; the End It Movement campaign had been launched during the conference and their website provided resources on how to get started. After reading about various organizations that were involved on local, national, and global levels, it was up to me to decide just how involved I wanted to be. With a simple Internet search, all of these resources presented themselves; there were countless options for involvement, with as little or as much of a time commitment as I wanted.

One key factor Kaitlin mentioned is how a simple Internet search will open the door to endless resources in terms of education and opportunities to directly intercede. All it takes is willpower and commitment. For me, I made a decision to walk through the door and do something that would help other people. I don't need to know these people. I just need to know that I did something to improve their life path at least a little bit. Hopefully, I opened a door for them. I feel like the best recommendation I can make to nursing students and people in general is to care about the issue. If you can find it within yourself to care, you can find the time or the resources to help. Maybe you can give a bit of money, maybe you can use your skills to volunteer at a clinic, or maybe you can just pay attention to your surroundings and call if you see something suspicious. My quote of choice for nursing students and people in general is by Edmund Burke: "All it takes for evil to succeed is for a few good men to do nothing .... "

OUR BIG DREAMS FOR THE FUTURE

LADY

My goal is to carry on the work of Dr. de Chesnay and continue to move policy and procedures on human trafficking patients forward so that my colleagues and I will be equipped to handle an encounter. I also plan to continue my work as a leader and use my leadership roles to stand up and advocate for the vulnerable population.

KAITLIN

Ultimately, my goal is to play a significant part in putting an end to human trafficking. To see it ended during my lifetime would be a true joy. While we are working to get there, it is my goal to continue carrying forward Dr. de Chesnay's work. Lady and I are very excited to move forward in the process of implementing a policy and procedure specifically for patients that have been trafficked. I believe that once our colleagues are educated and feel supported we will be able to intervene in the lives of these victims sooner, rather than later.

A personal dream of mine is to continue my work overseas as a nurse in places where trafficking is considered a normal part of life. I want to have a part in teaching this vulnerable population that they do not have to sell themselves. They deserve to know that they are worth more than what society tells them. What an honor it would be to be a part of the restoration process by providing medical care in the most sensitive of times.

CHRISTINE

It all seems overwhelming when you look at the big picture of global human trafficking, but any problem is manageable if approached one step at a time. You first have to see the problem as it is. Have empathy for the victims, but remember that the problem is one of finance and culture. In order for humans to be trafficked, a group of humans must view certain people as chattel rather than valuable persons; be willing to commit criminal acts for profit, for pleasure, or out of desperation; and be neglectful of the problem so trafficking continues to be a profitable industry. The various cultural and financial ramifications require that a multifaceted approach be used to seek its end.

Victims must be saved and the populations vulnerable to induction into Commercial Sexual Exploitation of Children (CSEC) must be protected. That means we must create an infrastructure to support those who are vulnerable due to their socioeconomic status or their psychosocial environment. We have to educate children who are vulnerable, but more importantly, we have to teach them of their own greater value and worthiness. We must help them see their own potential.

As sad as it is, the first step is always to investigate the issue thoroughly. You can't effectively combat criminal activities without information. It is even more difficult to combat cultural norms or false beliefs. To combat a mindset or belief system great amounts of data are necessary. Luckily, the growing awareness of global human trafficking is attracting people who not only care about the issue, but will also put their resources into finding its heart and ripping out the arteries that feed it.

COMMENTARY

Mary de Chesnay

From the beginning, what impressed me about these students was their sense of compassion for an extremely vulnerable yet highly invisible population. At this writing, there are more than 27 million victims of human trafficking, 80% of whom are women and children and most of these are in the sex trade (Bales, 2004, 2009). Human trafficking is at least a $32 billion a year business and is the fastest-growing criminal enterprise, second only to drugs (Kara, 2009; Polaris Project, n.d.; U.S. Department of State, 2014). What impressed me the most, as I got to know these students, was the incredible power of community engagement in shaping character that will last a lifetime. If these students accomplished so much as undergraduates, think what they will do as practitioners. Our profession is in very good hands.

REFERENCES

Bales, K. (2004). *Disposable people: New slavery in the global economy.* Berkeley, CA: University of California Press.

Bales, K. (2009). *The slave next door: Human trafficking and slavery in America today.* Berkeley, CA: University of California Press.

de Chesnay, M. (2013). *Sex trafficking: A clinical guide for nurses.* New York: Springer.

Kara, S. (2009). *Sex trafficking: Inside the business of modern slavery.* New York: Columbia University Press.

Polaris Project. (n.d.). Retrieved from http://www.polarisproject.org/index.php?gclid=CNKRk_T_s8ACFSMV7AodiRQAOg

U.S. Department of State. (2014). *Trafficking in persons report 2014.* Retrieved from http://www.state.gov/j/tip/rls/tiprpt/2014/index.htm

Chapter 33

The College-Bound Adolescent with a Mental Health Disorder

Cara C. Young and Susan J. Calloway

OBJECTIVES

At the end of this chapter, the reader will be able to

1. Identify personal factors that contribute to the vulnerability of the college-bound adolescent with a mental health disorder.
2. Identify environmental factors that contribute to the vulnerability of the college-bound adolescent with a mental health disorder.
3. Apply knowledge of vulnerabilities in developing strategies for anticipatory guidance for all college-bound adolescents.

BACKGROUND AND SIGNIFICANCE

In 2011, approximately 3 million students, or 68.2% of high school graduates, enrolled in postsecondary education (National Center for Education Statistics, 2014). While not traditionally considered a "vulnerable" population, college-bound freshmen find themselves in a pivotal transitional period. The novice college student must learn to be self-sufficient in navigating the educational, social, and physical environment of the university. While students look forward to this independence, many are at risk for engagement in high-risk behaviors, social isolation, and academic failure.

The freshman with an existing or latent mental health disorder is particularly vulnerable for academic failure secondary to potential destabilization of mental health. There is a high likelihood that the student who is predisposed to a mental health disorder will develop this disorder during the college years, as 75% of lifetime cases of mental health conditions begin by age 24 (National Institute of Mental Health [NIMH], 2005). The National College Health Assessment (NCHA) survey reported that within the past 12 months, 43.8% of college undergraduates reported feeling hopeless, 84.3% felt overwhelmed, 79.1% felt emotionally exhausted, and 60.5% felt very sad (American College Health Association [ACHA], 2013). In another survey of students at a large university, over 50% of students indicated that they had experienced depressive symptoms in the first few months of the academic year, while a majority (69%) reported symptoms of anxiety (Orzech, Salafsky, & Hamilton, 2011).

According to the National Alliance on Mental Illness (NAMI, 2012), 73% of students with a mental health condition experienced a mental health crisis on campus. The majority of these students (65.8%) stated the college was unaware of this crisis, suggesting that often students suffer in silence, failing to reach out when their mental health declines. This lack of help-seeking for psychological distress may shed light on the reason that suicide is a leading cause of death for college students (Centers for Disease Control and Prevention [CDC], 2013).

College life is fraught with threats to optimum mental health, and healthcare providers must provide anticipatory guidance to the college-bound adolescent with a mental health disorder. Mental health issues were cited by 64% of young adults as the reason for withdrawing from college or for not attending college (NAMI, 2012). The sections that follow address the personal and environmental factors impacting vulnerability to destabilization of mental health. They focus on giving specific considerations to the college-bound freshman with an active or latent mental health disorder. Each of the vulnerabilities can have independent adverse effects on the student's mental health and when combined may result not only in academic failure but also violence towards themselves or others.

PERSONAL FACTORS IMPACTING VULNERABIITY

Sleep Disruption

Sufficient sleep is essential for conserving energy, thermoregulation, homeostasis, and restoration (Saddock & Saddock, 2007). An 18 year old is estimated to need between 7 and 9 hours per night, yet almost 90% of students reported not feeling rested upon waking in the morning, and over 69% stated they felt tired, dragged out, and sleepy 3 to 7 days each week (ACHA, 2013). Late night study sessions and campus social events lead to a cycle of getting little sleep during the weekdays and subsequently spending significant time sleeping on weekends. Regular wake-sleep schedules are important to the overall quality of sleep, and irregular sleep schedules exacerbate poor sleep quality (Carney, Edinger, Meyer, Lindman, & Istre, 2006).

Inadequate sleep is associated with numerous adverse outcomes including reduced academic performance and productivity as well as negative mood (Curio, Ferrara, &

DeGennaro, 2006; National Sleep Foundation, 2000). Sleep deprivation was cited by students as a reason for missing class (54%) and receiving a lower grade on an exam (42%), while 29% reported receiving an overall lower grade in a course due to sleep deprivation (Orzech et al., 2011). Not only does lack of sleep result in daytime sleepiness, reduced academic performance, and negative mood (Lund, Reider, Whiting, & Prichard, 2010), but sleep deprivation also results in increased likelihood of stimulant (Calloway, Kelly, & Ward-Smith, 2012) and alcohol use (Lund et al., 2010).

Students struggling with mental health issues may have additional threats to maintaining effective sleep hygiene. For example, students with anxiety and/or depression reported poorer sleep quality than their peers (Orzech et al., 2011). This finding was supported by research that demonstrated individuals with insomnia were over 9.82 times as likely to have clinically significant depression and 17.35 times more likely to have anxiety (Taylor, Lichstein, Durrence, Reidel, & Bush, 2005). A vicious cycle can result with the insomnia worsening due to depression and anxiety and the subsequent increase in depression and anxiety worsening the insomnia.

A student with an existing or latent bipolar disorder is particularly vulnerable to the impact of poor sleep quality and quantity, as sleep disturbances can significantly worsen mood instability or trigger latent bipolar disorder. The chronobiological model of bipolar disorder proposes that individuals with bipolar disorder have a predisposition for circadian rhythm disturbances, which lead to the symptom expression of bipolar disorder (Frank, Swartz, & Kupfer, 2000). The social milieu of the college experience is in direct opposition to the establishment of regular sleep routines, which increases the vulnerability for symptom expression of bipolar disorder.

Poor Diet

"The freshman fifteen," "first year fatties," and "fresher spread," are expressions that allude to weight gain that often occurs among freshman college students. A combination of factors contribute to this widely acknowledged phenomenon: (1) parents are no longer available to encourage health dietary choices and provide nutritious meals, (2) on campus meal plans to the university cafeteria offer multiple buffets of highly processed foods and desserts, (3) late night study sessions with junk food, (4) lack of exercise, and (5) overindulgence in calorie-laden alcoholic beverages. Lloyd-Richardson, Bailey, Fava, and Wing (2009) examined weight changes in 904 students over their freshman and sophomore years and found that 77% of students gained weight during their freshman year. Rates of overweight/obesity in this same sample increased from 21.6% at college entrance to 36% by the end of their sophomore year (Lloyd-Richardson et al., 2009).

Research has identified associations between diet and mental health in adults (Nanri et al., 2010) and adolescents (Oddy et al., 2009). A large-scale prospective evaluation of over 3,000 Australian adolescents found that poor diets characterized by highly processed and sugary junk foods at baseline predicted poorer mental health (i.e., increases in anxiety and depressive symptoms) at follow-up (Jacka, Mykletun, Ber, Bjelland, & Tell, 2011). Several mechanisms underlying this association have been implicated including deficiencies of omega-3 fatty acids, vitamin D, folic acid, and B vitamins (Anglin, Samaan, Walter, & McDonald, 2013; Herbison et al., 2012; Papakostas, et al., 2013; Walsh, 2011). These findings highlight the direct effect of dietary patterns on mental health for all adolescents, thus college freshman with mental health disorders must be particularly cognizant of the impact of their dietary choices. Students with a history of eating disorders should receive special consideration. The highly restrictive eating patterns of anorexia nervosa or the cycle of binging and purging may resurface in an attempt to combat the anticipated weight gain of the freshman year or as a maladaptive coping strategy attempting to manage increasing stress levels.

Lack of Exercise

The high school student who was involved in team sports, physical education classes, or running clubs may become sedentary after arriving on campus if not involved in college athletics. The student may substitute exercise with video gaming, snacking, and drinking. These compounding factors can lead to significant weight gain as well as affect mental health. Exercise can reduce anxiety and depression, increase mental alertness, improve sleep, and reduce a sense of social isolation (Peluso & Andrade, 2005).

Numerous research studies have documented the inverse relationship between physical inactivity and mental health (Deslandes et al., 2009; Penedo & Dahn, 2005). Avoiding a sedentary lifestyle is particularly important for the college-bound adolescent with a mental health disorder. Not only will engaging in moderate physical activity several times each week maintain optimum bone and muscle health and reduce the risk of obesity and obesity related disorders, the positive effects on mood and general well-being cannot be overstated.

Alcohol, Tobacco, and Other Drug Use

Alcohol use on college campuses is often considered a rite of passage for students, as evidenced by fraternity and sorority initiations, rankings for "party schools," and deaths due to alcohol intoxication. Peer influence and the desire to be part of a lively social scene may influence individuals into drinking more heavily than anticipated. A survey of college students in 2012, revealed that the majority of college students (64.8%) reported alcohol use within the past 30 days, and 23.2% reported driving after drinking (ACHA, 2013). It is significant to note that for college students that reported drinking alcohol in the past 12 months, 35% indicated they had done something they later regretted, 29.9% forgot where they were or what they did, and 20% had unprotected sex (ACHA, 2013).

Tobacco use among college students has trended downward with 13.8% reporting they had smoked or chewed tobacco in the past 30 days. Marijuana use, however, has exceeded tobacco use with 16.7% of students using marijuana in the past 30 days (ACHA, 2013). One study found that one out of four college students used marijuana to cope with stress (Aselton, 2012). While marijuana is seen as a benign substance by many, it does have a permanent impact on brain development when smoking is initiated in the teens. A long-term study in New Zealand found that heavy marijuana use resulted in an IQ decline on average of 8 points (National Institute on Drug Abuse, 2014). Marijuana has also been implicated in the development of schizophrenia in individuals with a family history of this disorder (Parakh & Basu, 2013). Often youth with anxiety and/or depression use marijuana to self-medicate. The positive impact of using this drug, however, is lost once the effect wears off, resulting in increased depression and anxiety (Pacek, Martins, & Crum, 2013).

Self-management of Mental Health Disorders

Because they are solely responsible for managing their health while attending college, adolescents with chronic conditions are at higher risk in for worsening of their condition (Rosen, Blum, Britto, Sawyer, & Siegel, 2003). Often a parent has been the monitor and manager of the college-bound student's mental health through scheduling of appointments, arranging for medication refills, monitoring mood, providing structure for study and sleep, and making sure that medication is taken at the appropriate times.

Upon arrival on campus, the student becomes the manager of these variables, which can significantly impact mental health stability when neglected. The student may feel that a new start in a new location without parental oversight is the time to discard the old identity of someone with a mental health disorder and forego medication, therapy, or both. This sense of independence combined with the lack of preparation for managing one's health care and the stigma of a mental health diagnosis can result in a mental health crisis.

Adherence to medication regimens is difficult, even for adults. In a review of adherence issues in the general population, 45.9% of participants taking antidepressants reported not taking their medications as prescribed. The reason for nonadherence in the majority of respondents (74.5%) was due to forgetting (Bulloch & Patten, 2010). If less than 50% of adults take their medications due to forgetfulness, college students who are questioning whether medication is really necessary will most likely have even lower adherence rates.

In order to remain mentally healthy, the college-bound adolescent must effectively navigate and be proactive in mental health management strategies. In addition, the student must analyze the negative impact that engaging in particular activities may have on mental health. Although the student may have the knowledge and desire to make wise choices to maintain mental health, the desire to be one of the group may override healthy choices.

Development of Academic Competencies

Skill development in areas such as time management, note taking, and study habits is essential for success at the collegiate level. High marks as a high school student do not necessarily translate to academic excellence in college. The structure of college education is vastly different from secondary education, and students must adapt to the increased flexibility and need for personal accountability.

Numerous priorities compete for a college student's time and attention. Campus activities and clubs, intramural sports, new friends, and new experiences can easily be chosen over scholastic activities. As students adjust to the new structure and content of their education, developing effective time management is essential for ensuring success. Effective time management has been found to be associated with reduced academic stress (Krumrei, Newton, Kim, & Wilcox, 2013; Misra & McKean, 2000). Furthermore, Misra and McKean's (2000) findings with a sample of 249 undergraduate students indicated successful time management had a greater buffering effect on stress than participation in leisure activities. These findings highlight the importance of developing time management behaviors for scholastic success.

For the adolescent with an active or latent mental health disorder, developing the skills necessary for academic success may be particularly challenging. For example, an individual with social anxiety may avoid attending large classes, finding the experience too anxiety producing. Qualitative findings from a study with university students in Australia revealed that attending and participating in class was problematic for many students (Martin, 2010). One participant reported: "I don't want to attend class or lecture for fear of an anxiety attack and so my marks have suffered. I worry that people will find out about my condition" (Martin, 2010, p. 268).

Alterations in the Structure of Social Support

Social support is generally considered to be the perception or experience that one is loved and cared for by others, esteemed and valued, and part of a social network of mutual assistance and obligations (Wills, 1991). The transition to college exemplifies a major shift in the structure and context of a student's social support. In a high school setting, students are surrounded by teachers, administrators, mentors, and caregivers who keep close watch on student attendance, academic performance, and problem behaviors. Slipping grades or absenteeism is quickly identified in the hopes of preventing further decline. The same types of safeguards do not exist at a collegiate level. The college student may feel separated from previous support systems, and although surrounded by people, feel isolated and alone.

Research evidence clearly demonstrates the positive effects of perceived social support on both physical health (Uchino, 2006) and mental health (Hefner & Eisenberg, 2009; Lakey & Orehek, 2011). Hefner and Eisenberg (2009) found lower incidences of depression, suicidality, self-harm, anxiety, and eating disorders in college students who reported higher quality social support. Moreover, evidence also demonstrates that poor quality social support is associated with a six-fold increased risk of depressive symptoms in college students (Hunt & Eisenberg, 2010).

Stress Management

The ability to adaptively cope with stress underlies each of the personal and environmental factors discussed in this chapter. Lack of preparation for the transition to college places the adolescent at risk for high levels of stress, resulting in adverse outcomes (e.g., alcohol/substance use leading to legal problems, lack of effective study habits resulting in a failing exam grade, etc.). Adequate preparation is of paramount importance because stress has been hypothesized as a factor contributing to the etiology of several mental health disorders (Hankin & Abramson, 2001; Muris, Roelofs, Rassin, Franken, & Mayer, 2005; Nolen-Hoeksema, Wisco, & Lyubomirsky, 2008). Depression may occur after a stressor if an individual interprets the stressor through overly negative appraisals and rumination. An individual is more likely to develop an anxiety disorder when there is selective attention to a stressor (Ouimet, Gawronski, & Dozois, 2009). An example is a socially anxious individual who tends to interpret ambiguous facial expressions in an overly threatening manner (Yoon & Zinbarg, 2007).

College life brings a brand new set of stressors, and the mechanisms through which an adolescent coped during high school may need to be adapted. Perhaps a "stressed out" adolescent previously sought the advice of a trusted friend or a parent, but now, in college, the structure of social support has changed, and the friend or parent is not as accessible. Similarly, an adolescent who played high school sports may have found the participation and camaraderie with teammates as stress reducing. Now at college, if no longer a member of organized sports, the primary means of stress reduction is lost. Effective stress management is of vital importance for the college-bound adolescent with an active or latent mental health disorder. With stress playing a role in the development of a variety of mental health disorders, the more adaptively a college-bound adolescent is able to cope with stress, the less likely a mental health crisis will occur.

CASE STUDY

An Adolescent with Bipolar II Disorder

> Jacob, a healthy 18 year old with bipolar II disorder, has been managed effectively for the past 3 years with medication, psychotherapy, and healthy lifestyle habits. At the beginning of Jacob's fourth week as a university freshman, he is not doing well. While studying for his chemistry test, he was convinced by some guys in the dorm to go to a party. Although he

did not drink any alcohol, he stayed out until after midnight, overslept the next morning and missed his 10:00 a.m. chemistry test. He also forgot to complete the reading assignment for psychology 101 and failed the pop quiz given in class. Jacob headed back to the dorm worrying about his success in college. During high school he would erase the effects of a bad day by meeting his friends at the park for a game of pick-up basketball. Because he has no close friends at the university, he goes to the gym alone to shoot some hoops. However, after a short time, he leaves feeling dejected and lonely. He sees some acquaintances on campus who invite him to a local bar, showing him a fake ID he could use to get in. He has not eaten dinner, he has not taken his medication, and he will have another early class the next day, however he knows that drinking a couple of beers will pick up his mood and help him to relax, plus he will make some new friends. Jacob is at a crossroads.

1. What skills could enhance Jacob's ability to choose healthy options mentally and physically?
2. What types of anticipatory guidance and health promotion activities could minimize risks to the destabilization of his mental health and help to maximize his college experience?

ENVIRONMENTAL FACTORS IMPACTING VULNERABILITY

Accessibility and Quality of Counseling Services

Counseling centers at universities and small colleges are not required to be accredited, resulting in significant variation in the quality, accessibility, and availability of counseling services. While a large, urban university may have a counseling center with highly qualified therapists, other universities may have staff that are only prepared in educational counseling and advisement and may not be qualified to offer various types of psychotherapy. Not only is it essential that the counselors have qualifications for providing psychotherapy, services must also be accessible. Often the ratio of students to therapists is very high so that even when the student feels an urgent need to see someone the wait for an appointment may take several weeks.

Accessibility and Expertise of Health Center Providers

The size of the university, funding, and location may impact the services provided in a college health center. These can vary from a registered nurse being present daily for assessment and referral or treatment of minor issues to a multiprovider staff who are able to provide a full range of health services, including mental health screening and treatment. Many large, urban universities have a psychiatric-mental health nurse practitioner or psychiatrist who is available to students. However, cost and wait times for an appointment may be significant.

Another issue within the health center purview is the availability and accessibility of a pharmacy. If the student does not have reliable transportation and local pharmacies do not deliver to the campus, obtaining prescriptions may be challenging. There may also be restrictions by insurance companies on where medications may be purchased that create potential barriers to quick access to prescription medications.

University Policies Related to Accommodations for Mental Health Disorders

The Americans with Disabilities Act of 1990 defined a disability as "a physical or mental impairment that limits one or more major life activities." In 2009, the Americans with Disabilities Act Amendments Act (ADAAA) clarified and expanded the definition of a disability and major life activities to include learning, reading, concentrating, thinking, communicating, and working. Section 504 of the ADAAA is designed to provide students with disabilities the same opportunities, access, and benefits that are provided to those without disabilities. Section 504 states that in order to provide equal access and benefits, schools that receive federal funds are required to make reasonable modifications to policies, practices, and procedures in order to avoid discrimination on the basis of disability (ADAAA, 2009). Required services vary based on the educational level of the program. A postsecondary institution is required to make adjustments for students with disabilities as long as it does not cause significant changes in requirements for the student's program of study or create a burden for the university (Department of Health and Human Services Office [HHS], 2013).

Each university, in order to meet the standards of this law, must have policies that delineate access these services and reasonable accommodations. The willingness to provide accommodations (e.g., such as extra time for taking exams, a quiet testing environment, optional testing times, permission to turn in work after deadlines, and the ability to make up missed assignments) may vary from university to university.

A student with a mental health disorder should not be penalized for making a request for reasonable accommodations that would promote success. However there is often a concern by the student that the faculty member may view the student as less capable and therefore less likely to earn a high grade in the course. In a study by Martin (2010) only 30% of college students with a mental health disorder divulged their condition to university staff. Students may also fear that requests for accommodations may impact their ability to obtain entry into graduate school or other professional programs. One student stated: "When experiencing a particularly vulnerable episode ... [I] feel I will be judged or considered an inappropriate candidate for my chosen course/career" (Martin, 2010, p. 265). Therefore, while accommodations are made available to students with mental health disorders, the student, in order to avoid perceived discrimination, may choose not to divulge the disability.

University Housing

A significant number of college-bound adolescents will be moving out of their parents' home and into campus housing. This unique living situation provides numerous opportunities for socialization and recreation. However communal living has challenges. Policies governing university housing vary across institutions and are dependent on many factors such as size of the student body, public vs. private status, and institution traditions. The majority of colleges have a variety of on-campus housing options for students to consider. The choice of living accommodations while attending college should be given careful consideration, particularly by the student with a mental health disorder.

Where a student lives during college has a direct link with alcohol consumption. Rates of binge drinking are the highest for students living off campus (and not with parents) and those living in fraternity or sorority houses (Wechsler & Nelson, 2008). While exposure to excessive use of alcohol, tobacco, and illicit drugs is expected by many entering college freshmen, less obvious housing factors affecting mental health are bathing/showering facilities, policies regarding quiet hours, overnight guests, and the presence of residential hall advisors or other college staff.

Roommate Compatibility

An important component of a college student's living arrangement is the nature of the relationship with one's roommate. For many students, this is the first experience of sharing a living space with a peer, and discussions must occur regarding the responsibilities and contributions to the shared environment. Negotiating the roles and responsibilities of each roommate can be a difficult task. Conflictual roommate relationships predict increase in overall stress levels (Dusselier, Dunn, Wang, Shelley, & Whalen, 2005).

Depending on the nature and status of an adolescent's mental health disorder, establishing positive communication patterns with a roommate may present a challenge. Hanasono and Nadler (2012) identify three distinct roommate types based on their preferred patterns of communication. Their findings suggest that roommates who share communication styles have more satisfaction with the roommate relationship than those who do not share communication styles (Hanasono & Nadler, 2012). The feasibility of selecting or being assigned a roommate with a similar communication style may be limited, but understanding the importance of effective patterns of communication in a roommate relationship may serve to support the development of a positive roommate relationship.

Protocols for room selection and roommate assignment vary by institution. Some institutions follow the guidance of Lapidus, Green, and Baruh (1985) and match students according to living habits, such as study and sleeping habits, smoking, and cleanliness preferences (Lapidus et al., 1985). Additional research findings support the matching of roommates on cleanliness preferences. Ogletree, Turner, Vieira, and Brunotte (2005) found cleanliness preferences contributed substantially to roommate satisfaction. In their cross-sectional study with 457 college students, 48% had discussed housecleaning issues at least three times with their roommate, and 20% had changed living arrangements at least once in the previous 3 years because of cleanliness issues (Ogletree et al., 2005).

NURSING STRATEGIES TO REDUCE RISK

This chapter concludes with an action plan nurses can follow when working with a college-bound adolescent with a mental health disorder. The discussion demonstrates that an individual plan can emerge through collaboration between the nurse and the adolescent.

Shelby is a 19-year-old college freshman who was diagnosed with depression, anxiety, and an eating disorder when she was in middle school. With cognitive behavioral therapy, paroxetine (Paxil), and use of alprazolam (Xanax) as needed, her depression and anxiety is in remission, and her disordered eating behaviors are under control. What types of nursing interventions can be implemented in order to reduce her risk for mental health decline and promote academic and social success as she leaves for college?

Mental Health Self-management

Self-management of the adolescent's mental health disorder should be an evolving process where the adolescent assumes increased responsibility to become more independent. Ideally, Shelby would have been encouraged in early adolescence to spend private time with the healthcare practitioner at each healthcare visit. This confidential interaction provides opportunity to develop communication skills related to health, including a history of current health issues. Individualized patient-centered care focuses on the decision-making process between the healthcare team and the patient. The adolescent with a mental health disorder should be a full participant in this process. By being involved in all decisions with increasing responsibility in managing self-care, the risk of inappropriate management is reduced when the adolescent leaves home.

The primary responsibilities/tasks that should be mastered before the adolescent leaves for college are: (1) knows the name and purpose of each medication, (2) independently takes medications as prescribed, (3) anticipates need for and obtains refills as needed, and (4) schedules and attends follow-up healthcare appointments and adjunctive therapies (e.g., psychotherapy, Alcoholics Anonymous meetings).

As the adolescent applies for college, the parent and adolescent should be provided with a list of healthcare responsibilities to be assumed by the adolescent before leaving home. Decisions must be made regarding where the adolescent will receive mental health care, who will provide medication refills, and where refills will be obtained. The shift toward independent self-management should also include education regarding payment for healthcare services. Knowledge regarding co-pays and in-network provider agreements is essential in order to understand the financial impact of managing a health condition. Additionally, there should be a discussion regarding how healthcare costs will be paid.

Strategies to Identify and Stabilize Declining Mental Health

When Shelby was living at home, her mother reminded her about taking her medications and completing tasks. She could identify when Shelby was having visible depressive and anxiety symptoms. At the same time when these symptoms resurfaced, her eating behaviors would revert back to previous unhealthy patterns. It is important for the nurse to engage Shelby in self-reflection on triggers for these episodes. Additionally, asking her to identify the behavior changes that would serve as warning signs of declining mental health is essential. Unless Shelby is able to gain insight into the signs of a declining state of mental health, she will not be able to reverse a downward spiral.

One recommendation that the nurse can make to assist Shelby in identifying changes in mood and anxiety is using smart phone applications. These applications or "apps" provide visual displays that demonstrate trends in mood and can assist in identifying those factors that have a negative impact. For example, if Shelby noticed that she felt depressed and anxious on days when she had little sleep, she could increase the number of hours of sleep per night. These charts can then be sent to the student's healthcare provider or brought to the office visit. *Optimism*, *Expereal*, *Emotion Sense*, and *iMood Journal* are a few of the more popular apps for mood tracking.

If Shelby had bipolar disorder she would be particularly vulnerable for widely fluctuating emotions that are often distressing, intense, and lead to social isolation. In addition to mood, sleep, and medication tracking apps such as *Bipolar Disorder Uncovered* and *eMoods Bipolar Mood Tracker*, there is an app to connect with other individuals with the same disorder, *Bipolar Disorder Connect*. This is an app that serves the role of a support group for individuals with bipolar disorder. Individuals can follow discussions, ask questions and share experiences with others. This is particularly helpful if there are members of the group on the same campus who could meet for socialization and support.

A Plan of Action to Promote Optimum Mental Health

Discussion Point #1: Importance of Maintaining a Regular Schedule

Sufficient sleep and regular sleep-wake cycles are essential in reducing risk of mental health destabilization. Regular sleeping patterns support a regular exercise, eating, and studying schedule. Shelby should be guided through motivational interviewing to identify strategies that she can take to obtain sufficient sleep. The nurse could use websites such as the sleepfoundation.org to provide Shelby with additional practical sleep hygiene techniques.

Excessive caffeine consumption can exacerbate anxiety and insomnia. Shelby should be counseled on the effects of excessive caffeine consumption and cautioned against the use of popular "energy drinks" that cause an initial increase in energy followed by a significant decrease (or "crash") in energy and, at times, mood. Additionally, because the FDA does not require manufactures to provide caffeine content on nutrition labels, hidden sources of caffeine should be discussed including decaffeinated coffee, noncola sodas, chocolate (particularly dark chocolate), coffee ice cream, weight loss pills, energy waters, and certain types of teas.

Maintaining a regular schedule also includes developing an exercise routine. The nurse can assess the types of exercises Shelby enjoys and her current fitness level. Shelby should be encouraged to consider joining an intramural sport team or find a group fitness classes. Participation in these types of activities is a wonderful way of getting physical activity while promoting peer connectedness and developing new means of social support. If Shelby is not comfortable with the social aspect of intramural sports or is not interested in team sports, she could be encouraged to go to the college fitness center.

Another threat to maintaining a regular schedule is inconsistent study habits. "Pulling an all-nighter" may be considered a rite of passage for many college freshman, but Shelby should be cautioned that this practice is not good for knowledge retention or her physical and mental health. Some ideas to discuss with Shelby include scheduling dedicated study times between weekday classes, hiring a tutor to ensure regular study sessions, and joining a study group. Shelby will need to develop a schedule that works best for her, but consistency is key.

Discussion Point #2: Alcohol and Drug Awareness

Shelby should be asked in an open, nonjudgmental manner her views toward alcohol and other drugs. Even if Shelby reports a plan to abstain from substance use, she should be instructed that the maximum recommended amount of alcohol for a female is two drinks in one day and only two days per week. She should also know the definition of binge drinking for a female is four or more drinks in a 2-hour time span. If she were to consume this level of alcohol, her blood alcohol level would be above the legal limit, her judgment would be impaired, and it would be illegal for her to operate a motor vehicle. Additionally, alcohol can worsen symptoms of depression despite feeling an initial short-term improvement in mood. Substances such as marijuana and cocaine are illegal in most states, and regular use of these substances would certainly impact her ability to maintain a regular schedule and increase risk for destabilization of her mental health.

Shelby also needs to be given information on the interaction between her medications and alcohol. Simply telling a patient to avoid alcohol without providing a rationale may have little impact on behavior change. Knowing the potential effects of combining alcohol with a benzodiazepine, in particular, is essential information to share. Because alcohol and most drugs are metabolized in the liver, alcohol can reduce the metabolism of benzodiazepines and paroxetine resulting in increased serum levels, increased side effects, and potential toxicity. Conversely the benzodiazepines and paroxetine also reduce the metabolism of alcohol causing an additive effect that increases sedation, drowsiness, and impaired motor skills.

Discussion Point #3: Stress and Coping Strategies

As previously discussed, minimizing stress is the foundation of many of the strategies suggested for promoting optimum mental health. Stress is an unavoidable reality for most college freshman. Stressors within various domains will inevitably arise (e.g., challenging assignments, romantic relationship conflict, homesickness), and the nurse should address these with Shelby. The focus of this discussion should be on identifying primary sources of stress (i.e., "What tends to stress you out?") and coping mechanisms she typically utilizes. In the past Shelby reverted back to restrictive eating patterns in times of high stress, but her mother was available to intervene when this was identified. Now on her own, she will need to be aware of this tendency and have an action plan in place.

General stress reduction techniques would also be helpful for Shelby. Research supports the use of cognitive behavioral therapy techniques to reduce stress in both adolescents (David-Ferdon & Kaslow, 2008; Rew, Johnson, & Young, in press) and adult populations (Goldin & Gross, 2010). Transcendental meditation and mindfulness-based stress reduction are two popular techniques that have been systematically studied and found to contribute to decreases in anthropometric measurements (i.e., blood pressure, heart rate, cardiac reactivity) as well as anxiety and stress levels (Barnes, Treiber, & Johnson, 2004; White, 2012).

Additional stress reduction techniques that have less research support may also be utilized. Perhaps she enjoys calming essential oils or watching a favorite movie for relaxation. The nurse could introduce Shelby to stress reduction mobile apps such as *Breathe2Relax* or the Canadian application *Self-hypnosis for Complete Relaxation* that is purported to achieve relaxation in 15 minutes. YouTube is another technology medium that provides instant access on the practices of yoga, tai chi, qigong, etc. Identifying the stress reduction techniques should remain secondary to Shelby's ability to recognize when she is experiencing increased levels of stress and her proficiency at reducing that stress in healthy and adaptive ways. Shelby and the nurse can discuss current practices and proactively develop a repertoire of strategies that can be turned to in times of high stress.

REFERENCES

American College Health Association (ACHA). (2013). *National college health assessment II: Reference group undergraduates executive summary spring, 2013.* Hanover, MD: American College Health Association.

Americans with Disabilities Act Amendments Act (ADAAA). (2009). 42 USCA § 12101. (Note: approved Sept. 25, 2008; effective date, Jan. 1, 2009). Retrieved from http://www.eeoc.gov/laws/statutes/adaaa.cfm

Anglin, R. E., Samaan, Z., Walter, S. D., & McDonald, S. D. (2013). Vitamin D deficiency and depression in adults: Systematic review and meta-analysis. *British Journal of Psychiatry, 202,* 100–107.

Aselton, P. (2012). Sources of stress and coping in American college students who have been diagnosed with depression. *Journal of Child and Adolescent Psychiatric Nursing*, 25(3), 119–123.

Barnes, V. A., Treiber, F. A., & Johnson, M. H. (2004). Impact of transcendental meditation on ambulatory blood pressure in African-American adolescents. *American Journal of Hypertension*, 17, 366–369.

Bulloch, A., & Patten, S. (2010). Non-adherence with psychotropic medications in the general population. *Social Psychiatry and Psychiatric Epidemiology*, 45(1), 47–56.

Calloway, S., Kelly, P. J., & Ward-Smith, P. (2012). Barriers to help-seeking for psychological distress among rural college students. *The Journal of Rural Mental Health*, 36(1), 3–10.

Carney, C. E., Edinger, J. D., Meyer, B., Lindman, L., & Istre, T. (2006). Daily activities and sleep quality in college students. *Chronobiology International*, 23, 623–637.

Centers for Disease Control and Prevention (CDC). (2013). College health and safety in a nutshell. Retrieved from http://www.cdc.gov/features/collegehealth/

Curio, G., Ferrara, M., & DeGennaro, L. (2006). Sleep loss, learning capacity and academic performance. *Sleep Medicine Reviews*, 10(5), 323–337.

David-Ferdon, C., & Kaslow, N. J. (2008). Evidence-based psychosocial treatments for child and adolescent depression. *Journal of Clinical Child and Adolescent Psychology*, 37(1), 62–104.

Department of Health and Human Services (HHS). (2013). *Know the rights that protect individuals with disabilities from discrimination*. Office for Civil Rights. Retrieved from http://www.hhs.gov/ocr/civilrights/resources/factsheets/504ada.pdf

Deslandes, A., Moraes, H., Ferreira, C., Veiga, H., Silveira, H., Mouta, R., … Laks, J. (2009). Exercise and mental health: Many reasons to move. *Neuropsychobiology*, 59, 191–198.

Dusselier, L., Dunn, B., Wang, Y., Shelley II, M. C., & Whalen, D. F. (2005). Personal, health, academic, and environmental predictors of stress for residence hall students. *Journal of American College Health*, 54, 15–24.

Frank, E., Swartz, H., & Kupfer, D. (2000). Interpersonal and social rhythm therapy: Managing the chaos of bipolar disorder. *Biological Psychiatry*, 48, 593–604.

Goldin, P. R., & Gross, J. J. (2010). Effects of mindfulness-based stress reduction (MBSR) on emotion regulation in social anxiety disorder. *Emotion*, 10, 83–91.

Hanasono, L. K., & Nadler, L. B. (2012). A dialectical approach to rethinking roommate relationships. *Journal of College Student Development*, 53, 623–635.

Hankin, B. L., & Abramson, L. Y. (2001). Development of gender differences in depression: An elaborated cognitive vulnerability-transactional stress theory. *Psychological Bulletin*, 127, 773–796.

Hefner, J., & Eisenberg, D. (2009). Social support and mental health among college students. *American Journal of Orthopsychiatry*, 79, 491–499.

Herbison, C. E., Hickling, S., Allen, K. L., O'Sullivan, T. A., Robinson, M., Bremner, A. P., … Oddy, W. H. (2012). Low intake of B-vitamins is associated with poor adolescent mental health and behaviour. *Preventive Medicine*, 55, 634–638.

Hunt, J., & Eisenberg, D. (2010). Mental health problems and help-seeking behavior among college students. *Journal of Adolescent Health*, 46, 3–10.

Jacka, F. N., Mykletun, A., Ber, M., Bjelland, I., & Tell, G. S. (2011). The association between habitual diet quality and the common mental disorders in community-dwelling adults: The Hordaland Health study. *Psychosomatic Medicine, 73*(6), 483–490.

Krumrei, E. J., Newton, F. B., Kim, E., & Wilcox, D. (2013). Psychosocial factors predicting first-year college student success. *Journal of College Student Development, 54*(3), 247–266.

Lakey, B., & Orehek, E. (2011). Relational regulation theory: A new approach to explain the link between perceived social support and mental health. *Psychological Review, 118*(3), 482–495.

Lapidus, J., Green, S. K., & Baruh, E. (1985). Factors related to roommate compatibility in the residence hall: A review. *Journal of College Student Personnel, 26*(5), 420–434.

Lloyd-Richardson, E. E., Bailey, S., Fava, J. L., & Wing, R. (2009). A prospective study of weight gain during the college freshman and sophomore years. *Preventive Medicine, 48*(3), 256–261.

Lund, H. G., Reider, B. D., Whiting A. B., & Prichard, J. R. (2010). Sleep patterns and predictors of disturbed sleep in a large population of college students. *Journal of Adolescent Health, 46*, 124–132.

Martin, J. M. (2010). Stigma and student mental health in higher education. *Higher Education Research & Development, 29*(3), 259–274.

Misra, R., & McKean, M. (2000). College students' academic stress and its relations to their anxiety, time management, and leisure satisfaction. *American Journal of Health Studies, 16*(1), 41–51.

Muris, P., Roelofs, J., Rassin, E., Franken, I., & Mayer, B. (2005). Mediating effects of rumination and worry on the links between neuroticism, anxiety and depression. *Personality and Individual Differences, 39*, 1105–1111.

Nanri, A., Kimura, Y., Matsushita, Y., Ohta, M., Sato, M., Mishima N., … Mizoue, T. (2010). Dietary patterns and depressive symptoms among Japanese men and women. *European Journal of Clinical Nutrition, 64*(8), 832–839.

National Alliance on Mental Illness (NAMI). (2012). *College students speak: A survey report on mental health*. Retrieved from www.nami.org/collegereport

National Center for Education Statistics. (2014). Postsecondary education. *Digest of Education Statistics: 2012*. Retrieved from http://nces.ed.gov/programs/digest/d12/ch_3.asp

National Institute of Mental Health (NIMH). (2005). *Mental illness exacts heavy toll, beginning in youth*. Retrieved from http://www.nimh.nih.gov/science-news/2005/mental-illness-exacts-heavy-toll-beginning-in-youth.shtml

National Institute on Drug Abuse. (2014, January). Department of Health and Human Services, *NIDA InfoFacts: Marijuana*. Retrieved from http://www.drugabuse.gov/publications/drugfacts/marijuana

National Sleep Foundation. (2000). *Adolescent sleep needs and patterns: Research report and resource guide*. Washington, DC: National Sleep Foundation.

Nolen-Hoeksema, S., Wisco, B. E., & Lyubomirsky, S. (2008). Rethinking rumination. *Perspectives on Psychological Science, 3*(5), 400–424.

Oddy, W. H., Robinson, M., Ambrosini, G. L., O'Sullivan, T. A., de Klerk, N. H., Beilin, L. J., … Stanley, F. J. (2009). The association between dietary patterns and mental health in early adolescence. *Preventive Medicine, 49*, 39–44.

Ogletree, S. M., Turner, G. M., Vieira, A., & Brunotte, J. (2005). College living: Issues related to housecleaning attitudes. *College Student Journal*, *39*(4), 729–733.

Orzech, K. M., Salafsky, D. B., & Hamilton, L. A. (2011). The state of sleep among college students at a large public university. *Journal of American College Health*, *59*(7), 612–619.

Ouimet, A. J., Gawronski, B., & Dozois, D. J. A. (2009). Cognitive vulnerability to anxiety: A review and an integrative model. *Clinical Psychology Review*, *29*, 459–470.

Pacek, L. R., Martins, S. S., & Crum, R. M. (2013). The bidirectional relationships between alcohol, cannabis, co-occurring alcohol and cannabis use disorders with major depressive disorder: Results from a national sample. *Journal of Affective Disorders*, *148*(2–3), 188–195.

Parakh, P., & Basu, D. (2013). Cannabis and psychosis: Have we found the missing links? *Asian Journal of Psychiatry*, *6*, 281–287.

Papakostas, G., Shelton, R., Zajecka, J., Etemad, B., Rickels, K., Clain, A., ... Basu, J. (2013). L-methylfolate as adjunctive therapy for SSRI-resistant major depression: Results of two random-ized, double-blind, parallel-sequential trials. *American Journal of Psychiatry*, *169*(12), 1267–1274.

Peluso, M. A., & Andrade, L. H. (2005). Physical activity and mental health: The association between exercise and mood. *Clinics*, *60*, 61–70.

Penedo, F. J., & Dahn, J. R. (2005). Exercise and well-being: A review of mental and physical health benefits associated with physical activity. *Current Opinion in Psychiatry*, *18*(2), 189–193.

Rew, L., Johnson, K., & Young, C. C. (2014). A systematic review of interventions to reduce stress in adolescence. *Issues in Mental Health Nursing*, *35*(11), 851–863.

Rosen, D. S., Blum, R. W., Britto, M., Sawyer, S. M., & Siegel, D. M. (2003). Transition to adult health care for adolescents and young adults with chronic conditions. A position paper of the Society for Adolescent Medicine. *Journal of Adolescent Health*, *33*, 309–311.

Saddock, B. J., & Saddock, V. A. (2007). *Kaplan & Sadock's synopsis of psychiatry* (10th ed.). Philadelphia: Lippincott Williams & Wilkins.

Taylor, D., Lichstein, K., Durrence, H., Reidel, B., & Bush, A. (2005). Epidemiology of insomnia, depression, and anxiety. *Sleep*, *28*(11), 1457–1464.

Uchino, B. N. (2006). Social support and health: A review of physiological processes potentially underlying links to disease outcomes. *Journal of Behavioral Medicine*, *29*, 377–387.

Walsh, R. (2011). Lifestyle and mental health. *American Psychologist*, *66*, 579–592.

Wechsler, H., & Nelson, T. F. (2008). What we have learned from the Harvard School of Public Health college alcohol study: Focusing attention on college student alcohol consumption and the environmental conditions that promote it. *Journal of Studies on Alcohol and Drugs*, *69*, 481–490.

White, L. S. (2012). Reducing stress in school-age girls through mindful yoga. *Journal of Pediatric Health Care*, *26*, 45–56.

Wills, T. A. (1991). Social support and interpersonal relationships. In M. S. Clark (Ed.), *Prosocial Behavior. Review of Personality and Social Psychology* (Vol. 12, pp. 265–289). Thousand Oaks, CA: Sage Publications.

Yoon, K. L., & Zinbarg, R. E. (2007). Threat is in the eye of the beholder: Social anxiety and the interpretation of ambiguous facial expressions. *Behaviour Research and Therapy*, *45*, 839–847.

Chapter 34

Homeless College Students

Jennifer A. Minick, Jennifer Emmons, Buffie Cole, Marcia A. Stidum,
Joshua Gunn, and Mary de Chesnay

OBJECTIVES

At the end of this chapter, the reader will be able to

1. Describe the extent of the problem of homelessness among college students.
2. Develop strategies nurses can use to facilitate success programs for this population.
3. Describe a model program that addresses the needs of homeless college students.

INTRODUCTION

The purpose of this chapter is to describe a fieldwork assignment for an undergraduate elective nursing course. A small group of students investigated the problem of homelessness among college students for their fieldwork assignment in the nursing course elective on caring for vulnerable populations. In so doing, they learned that their own university has one of the few programs in the country designed to address the needs of this vulnerable and somewhat invisible population. Organized under the Counseling Center, the program was created to identify students who are homeless and devise ways the university could assist them to be successful. The students were inspired by the commitment of their less fortunate fellow students to dedicate whatever funds they had to completing their college programs, even at the expense of living in cars, under bridges, or on their friends' sofas.

THE PROJECT

Project Requirements

The seminar requirement was worth 30% of the final course grade and was structured as a group project in which students selected a population (of which no one in the group was a member.) Groups comprised 3–5 members and were given release time during the course to review the literature, identify community resources for the population, visit appropriate agencies, and prepare a 20-minute presentation for the class about their topic. Although it was not necessary to interview individuals in the group, one of the students knew several homeless college students at another university and did conduct informal interviews with them. The group presented their project and subsequently decided to develop a publication. This chapter represents a collaborative effort of the students in the program with the coordinators and professor.

The Issue of Homeless College Students

We completed this project for our vulnerable populations nursing course. The assignment was to review the nursing literature on a vulnerable population and prepare a presentation that describes the population and addresses the health risks, conditions, and cultural aspects of the chosen population. Minick and Emmons had other classes together, and Cole was sitting near us when the class broke into groups. With the addition of another student nearby, Konneh, we formed a group and deliberated about a vulnerable population to choose for our topic. We considered the population of homeless people in the United States, but rejected it because we already had a firm knowledge on the subject and wanted to explore something different. I suggested we investigate homeless college students because I learned in a course on homelessness that we actually have a number of homeless students at our own university. Cole chimed in that she knew two students at other universities nearby who were also homeless. We were all surprised that this phenomenon was actually occurring so close to home, and we naturally wanted to learn more about this vulnerable population with whom we had so much in common.

Cole volunteered to conduct interviews with homeless college students with whom she was acquainted; they became our case studies. The rest of the group searched the literature to discover the extent of the problem and the risk factors for this vulnerable population. When we did not find much in the literature regarding homeless college students, I visited the student resource centers on campus to discover the staff's knowledge on this issue and what resources they offered for homeless students. I was surprised to find that some of the staff were unaware of the presence of homeless students on campus, but eventually someone referred me to Marcia Stidum—the "powerhouse" behind the university's developing program for homeless students.

EXTENT OF THE PROBLEM

About 58,158 students identified themselves as homeless in the 2013–2014 version of the Free Application for Federal Student Aid (FAFSA; Ellis, 2013). This number had increased by about 75% since the 2010–2011 FAFSA when about 33,000 students claimed they were homeless (Young, 2013). These numbers may underrepresent the actual population of homeless on college campuses as some students may be deterred from reporting due to stigma or lack of awareness of available aid (Young, 2013).

According to the U.S. Department of Housing and Urban Development (HUD), the total number of homeless in the general U.S. population is estimated to be 610,000, and of these 32.7% are children and youth (HUD, 2013). The National Alliance to End Homelessness (NAEH) reports point-in-time estimates in January 2013 that include 40,727 unaccompanied 18 to 24 year olds in the United States, which is the typical age range of traditional college students (NAEH, 2014). While the homeless population on college campuses comprises various age groups, the numbers are likely to increase as the population of homeless youth increases and students seek education as a means to personal betterment and an escape from homelessness.

We found the existing literature to be lacking on homelessness within the population of college students. However, more research was available when we considered the broader topic of homelessness in the general population, with specific stratifications for youth, individuals, and families. HUD (2013) considers a person homeless if they lack permanent housing or live in a place not meant for human dwelling such as an emergency shelter, transitional housing, out of a car, doubled up with friends or family, or on the streets (HUD, 2013). For the purpose of our project, we applied what the existing literature said about the general homeless population to college students experiencing homelessness.

Contributing Factors

The term *homeless* is a broad category that covers a wide variety of cases of individuals with different needs. While it is true that a small percentage of homeless Americans choose homelessness as a lifestyle, most find themselves in tough circumstances that render them homeless. There are some common contributors to the homelessness of our nation's students and youth. Societal trends, such as the downturn in the economy or the rising costs of housing, are major contributing factors to homelessness in America. However, individual issues including illnesses, disasters, and the breakdown of family often send individuals into the downward spiral of homelessness as well. In some cases, a combination of both factors contributes to an individual student's homelessness (McBride, 2012).

Lowe and Gibson (2011) and McBride (2012) found that lack of employment opportunities often leads to homelessness (Lowe & Gibson, 2011; McBride 2012). Although the economy is picking up, Americans in poverty are still weighed down by the effects of the Great Recession of 2007 to 2009, and there are still many without jobs as evidenced by the unemployment rate of 8.1% (NAEH, 2014). The narrow job market has pushed many people back to school in hopes of making themselves more marketable, including those that cannot afford stable housing. Some students who become unemployed and find themselves homeless make sacrifices in other areas in order to continue pursuit of their education, as they see it as the only route to a better life (Young, 2013).

Lowe & Gibson (2011), McBride (2012), and Shinn (2007) all agree that lack of affordable housing is the overarching contributor to homelessness (Lowe & Gibson, 2011; McBride, 2012; Shinn, 2007). In 2012, the U.S. poverty rate was 15.9% and over 6.5 million Americans were burdened by severe housing costs, spending over half their income on housing (NAEH, 2014). With such a limited budget, individuals and families are forced to choose between housing and other necessities such as food, clothing, or health care. Financial aid and scholarships are available for students with limited income or means to acquire housing. However, many colleges and universities shut down their dorms during school breaks, forcing students who have nowhere else to go to sleep on the streets or on the couches of charitable friends (Ross, 2012).

McBride (2012) listed availability of quality education as a societal factor that, if lacking, may lead to homelessness. Shinn (2007), in consideration of international homelessness, found that lack of education is a risk factor for becoming homeless. The average in-state tuition at a public 4-year university in the United States is $8,893, making education unattainable for the poor without financial aid (College Board, 2014). Still, some diligent students, like those whose stories are told by Allec (2014), Ross (2012), and Young (2013), are willing to make sacrifices, such as housing, in order to earn their education (Allec, 2014; Ross, 2012; Young, 2013).

The price of health care is on the rise, and many low-income students cannot afford coverage. While the literature does not support cost of health care as a major contributor to homelessness, Shinn (2007) describes health problems as barriers toward securing employment (Shinn, 2007). Health care is a need that often goes unmet for many homeless persons (McBride, 2012). Those who cannot afford health care may be unable to work, but without a steady income they cannot pay medical bills, thereby creating a vicious cycle that hinders the homeless from breaking free of their situation. While the issue of unaffordable health care in the United States is a societal factor, specific health problems can contribute to homelessness on an individual level.

The literature commonly refers to individual's struggles as contributing factors to homelessness, separate from societal problems. These micro-level causes of homelessness include disabilities and/or mental illness, addictions, domestic violence, breakdown of family structure, and natural disasters (Lowe & Gibson 2011; McBride, 2012).

Disabilities, mental illness, and addictions are highly associated with homelessness, but it is difficult to determine which is the cause and which is the effect (Lowe

& Gibson, 2011). Nearly a quarter of the nation's homeless people have some type of mental illness and they are more likely to suffer from depression than those with homes (McBride, 2012). Disabilities and mental illness can make it difficult to secure employment and create fundamental needs that rival the need for housing. Manea, Fletcher, and Beck (2014) identified one homeless veteran pursuing higher education whose depression hindered him from maintaining employment (Manea, Fletcher, & Beck, 2014).

Addiction and substance abuse, considered a mental illness by some, affects about 30% of homeless individuals (Lowe & Gibson, 2011). Substance abuse goes hand in hand with homelessness, sharing similar contributing factors and risks. The isolation, shame, depression, and lack of self-worth experienced by homeless persons often lead to substance abuse, and, in turn, substance abuse fuels the cycle of homelessness by taxing resources and decreasing potential for employment (Lowe & Gibson, 2011). Domestic violence and breakdown of family structure also contribute to homelessness on a micro-level (McBride, 2011). Many victims of domestic violence become homeless when they are forced to flee their homes for safety (NAEH, 2014). Child abuse and neglect are also factors that put an individual at a higher risk of becoming homeless (Lowe & Gibson, 2012). Shinn (2007) suggests that breakdowns of family structure, including divorce and single parenting, are primary contributors to homelessness in the United States (Shinn, 2007). Lastly, McBride (2011) cited natural disasters as an individual issue that contributes to homelessness (McBride, 2011). However, one could also argue that a disaster is merely a circumstance that provokes homelessness among those already impoverished. Shinn (2007) suggests that those who come from poor backgrounds have fewer resources to retain housing when disaster strikes (Shinn, 2007). Therefore, poverty may be the actual cause masked by the disaster, as those with ample financial resources are often prepared to weather such storms.

Culture

As mentioned above, scant literature exists on the culture of homeless college students, so we gathered information from reports found on the Web, our case studies, and personal communication with Marci Stidum and compared this to the experiences of the general homeless population. We found several common themes and attitudes associated with the lifestyle of homeless college students, which may serve as the basis for future research development of a potential framework.

Homeless students spend the night in their cars, unsheltered locations on and off campus, homeless shelters, and on other students' couches (Ross, 2012). Some students are fortunate enough to achieve housing on campus through financial aid, but during school breaks they are forced to sleep elsewhere (Ross, 2012). Others who do not receive aid for housing face the problem of homelessness throughout their semesters. HUD updated their official definition of homelessness in 2011 to include places not meant for human accommodation, such as cars and campus buildings, as well as *doubling up* (NAEH, 2014). This term refers to individuals and families who are temporarily living with friends or relatives and would otherwise be homeless (Hoback, 2007). One form of doubling up commonly practiced by homeless college students is *couch surfing*, which refers to staying the night on friends' couches, moving from dorm to dorm or apartment (Hoback, 2007).

Along with the lack of permanent housing, comes a lack of privacy. Students who live out of their cars or in unsheltered locations do not have private locations to perform their usual hygiene routine, so they must be resourceful and make do with convenience store or campus bathrooms. The inconvenience and possible embarrassment of such practices can hinder students from adequately caring for their hygiene needs (M. Stidum, personal communication, May 20, 2013).

Shinn (2007) points out that some homeless people are isolated from their families because of the shame that accompanies their lifestyle or circumstances (Shinn, 2007), however in some of the accounts we found that homeless college students admitted that they had severed ties with their families before becoming homeless (Ross, 2012; Gross, 2013). In Lowe & Gibson's study of homeless individuals (not homeless college students) in Florida, 80% of the 75 participants identified with feelings of isolation (Lowe & Gibson, 2011). The stories we found of homeless college students reflect the trend of isolation among the general homeless population. One college student does not like to refer to himself as homeless because of the stigma the name carries, and he relates the way people perceive the homeless population as similar to how they would relate to an "alien" (Allec, 2014).

In addition to feeling isolated, homeless college students experience a great deal of stress from living without permanent housing. It is no secret that college students face many stressors that come along with the journey toward higher education, but a student facing those struggles without a place to go that they can call home experiences a much deeper level of stress. Jennifer Martin with the National Association of Student Financial Aid Administrators described homeless college students as having additional obstacles that other students do not have to deal with, such as attaining the necessary supplies and books that they need (as cited in Ross, 2012). One homeless college student said that she had difficulty completing coursework because she was plagued by fears related to finding food and performing hygiene and other needs that ordinary students take for granted (Allec, 2014).

Marci Stidum describes the homeless student population she works with as being bright students with good grade point averages and determination (M. Stidum, personal communication, May 20, 2013). Ross (2012) also describes one student who graduated from high school with a 4.2 GPA and plans to enroll at a university despite being homeless (Ross, 2012). The policy director for the National Association for the Education of Homeless Children and Youth, Barbara Duffield, respectfully admonished these students as defying society's expectations for them, by choosing to pursue an education, despite their circumstances, in order to improve their lives (as cited in Ross, 2012).

RISKS

Homeless college students encounter several risks, both social and health related. Their poverty and lack of housing make them vulnerable to exploitation and poses health risks, which in turn may lead to serious health issues. For example, risk for malnutrition can lead to the risk of being overweight and obese, which can lead to developing type 2 diabetes and/or hypertension. Furthermore, homeless college students are at high risk for certain mental illnesses. Substance abuse and various other mental illnesses are common.

Homeless individuals are at risk of many kinds of exploitation, whether in college or not. As mentioned above, persons who are homeless are at a high risk for substance abuse, which often makes them vulnerable to exploitation such as robbery, rape, and other injuries. Those living on the streets, eager for work, are often driven to sell sex in order to survive, or to feed their addictions (Lowe & Gibson, 2011). This form of exploitation is called sex trafficking, and it often coincides with other forms of human trafficking such as slave labor, a fate more likely to befall those who are impoverished and homeless (Wheaton, Schauer, & Galli, 2010). McBride (2012) also suggests that the homeless population is exploited by being unfairly treated by police officers and criminalized for their situation (McBride, 2012). In addition to exploitation, homeless college students are also at risk for various health problems.

Malnourishment presents a large problem in the homeless college student population. A common myth is that the homeless population in America is underweight due to malnourishment. However, more homeless are actually overweight or obese as a result of malnourishment because they must eat whatever they can find. A study by Tsai and Rosenheck (2013) of 436 homeless persons showed that 7.6% were underweight while 57.3% were overweight or obese. Their diet does not contain all of the nutrients they need because a healthy balanced diet is often unaffordable and inaccessible (Dorsen, 2010). The food this population eats is insufficient to accurately nourish their bodies and maintain a healthy weight.

In addition to causing body weights to be higher than the healthy weight, malnourishment may lead to type 2 diabetes. A combination of factors puts this population at risk for diabetes. Dorsen (2010) suggests that lack of access to healthy foods, cost and unavailability of diabetic medications and testing supplies, and lack of healthcare provider compassion toward this population are the factors that put the homeless at risk for type 2 diabetes. One homeless diabetic stated his fears of his sugar deviating from the normal range. He said: "I try to eat right, I am diabetic, but I eat what I can get." (Nickash & Marnocha, 2009). The homeless man's statement confirms that food conducive to a proper diabetic diet is hard to find for the homeless population.

Similarly, the homeless population is at risk for hypertension. Kinchen and Wright (1991) state that hypertension is the second most common chronic physical health problem in the homeless population. Along with inability to maintain a healthy diet, they state that the population's high rate of alcohol abuse; inaccessible and unaffordable hypertension medications, the high stress environment in which they live in as a result of an unstable environment, shelter, or home; and the lack of motivation they have to treat the beginning stages of the disease contribute to hypertension in the homeless population. Therefore, because of alcohol abuse, stress, unattainable medications, and lack of incentive to treat the illness, the homeless population is at risk for both hypertension and uncontrolled hypertension.

Another health risk of the homeless population is the risk of mental illnesses such as substance abuse, depression, anxiety, and other psychiatric issues. McBride (2012) states that about 30% of the homeless abuse substances, 23% are labeled mentally ill, and they have a higher rate of depression and anxiety symptoms than the general population. In addition, Lowe and Gibson (2011) conducted a study of 75 homeless individuals to determine percentages of the homeless population with certain characteristics and emotional issues caused by mental illnesses. There is some debate about whether substance abuse or homelessness comes first, because they share similar risk factors and often coexist. These studies show the prevalence of mental illness in the homeless population and demonstrate how the illness may contribute to homelessness or how homelessness may cause the occurrence of mental illness.

In seems clear from these studies that nurses can play an important role in identifying and treating homeless college students. College health centers employ nurse practitioners that see enrolled students, but they may not recognize patients as homeless unless the student discloses this information. Routine intake assessments should include an item to determine whether or not the student has a safe home environment.

CASE STUDIES

Interviews were conducted with three homeless college students. The interviews were summarized and assessed in an effort to understand how a college student becomes homeless as well as to explain the vulnerability of the population through examples. The case studies reflect some of the risk factors of the homeless population discussed previously. These three individuals are personal contacts who have been assigned pseudonyms.

Case 1: Anna

Anna is a 46-year-old woman who decided to attend college "to better [her] life." She was unaware of the amount of money she would end up spending on classes and books in order to attend. Because of the cost of school, lack of a job, a small savings account, and medical bills accumulated from diabetes and hypertension treatments, she was evicted from her house. Additionally, she lost a fair amount of her belongings during the eviction because her belongings were left outside of her house and were claimed by others because she was not home at the time. With homelessness, she noted a loss of self-esteem and depression. Because of this situation, she has forced to delay her education to find work and shelter. The student noted: If there could have been a program for these kinds of things for the first 6 months, I could possibly have got on my feet and graduated. Because she lost her home, she began spending the night on a different couch in a different friend's house every couple of nights, otherwise known as couch surfing, so that she could obtain shelter. She did not have enough money to treat her diabetes and hypertension so she signed up for a diabetic medication clinical trial to provide income as well as diabetic treatment. She was able to find a full-time job. However, the side effects of the medication from the clinical trial resulted in her inability to work and the loss of her job. Soon after, a friend allowed her to move in indefinitely without paying rent.

However, living in her friend's home without paying rent did not last long. The student developed diverticulitis, and a ruptured sigmoid colon put her in the hospital for a week. When she returned from the hospital, she found herself in a form of debt bondage. Her friend told her that she must pay $300 per month for rent and that she could earn that money by cleaning her house along with taking her daughter to school and various other places. Because she did not have another place to live and no money to pay the rent, she took the offer. Shortly, the rent increased to $500 month and the homeowner became verbally abusive. For this reason, Anna decided to take a job as a nanny and save enough money to move out. At the same time, however, her daughter coincidentally lost her home in another state due to a natural disaster, so she sent much of the money she had earned to her daughter, prolonging the time she had to spend at the house before she could move out.

Once Anna finally saved enough money to move out, she began renting a home. She was not able to stay there long because the owner decided to sell the home. She quickly found another place to live, but the family she worked for as a nanny began to increase her hours without extra pay. Regardless, she continued to work at that position so that she could continue to make money to pay her rent. All the while, she suffered from depression and post-traumatic stress disorder (PTSD) as a result of her circumstances.

Case 2: Heather

The student in this case study is a 19-year-old New York resident and the daughter of the student in the first study. Heather was living in New York when Hurricane Sandy hit and devastated the area in which she lived. All of the student's belongings were lost in the storm and she was left with no place to live. As a result she noted depression and stated: "All I could do was cry." Because she lost her books and place to live, she was forced to drop her classes and retake them during the next semester. She borrowed money from a friend to fly to another state to live temporarily with her mother. Her mother was living with a woman who required her to complete chores in return for rent. Once the daughter arrived at the house, the owner had her clean the house as payment for rent as well. In addition, the landlord made her give some of the few clothes she had to her daughter in exchange for rent. Therefore, she left the place her mother lived and began to couch surf. After 3 months, she was able to return to her apartment and restart classes. She suggested that she may now be suffering from PTSD as a result of her situation.

Case 3: Lisa

Lisa, the student in this case study, is a 20-year-old member of a wealthy, controlling family. Once the student began college, she started consuming alcohol and various illegal substances. Because her family did not agree with these choices, they told her to move out of their house and stopped supporting her financially. She dropped her classes and began living out of her car and washing her hair in public sinks. She noted that she often went without food and therefore suffered from malnutrition. The student heard about a house (mentioned in Case 1) where tenants were allowed to live free of rent, so she went to the house. The landlord allowed her to live there free of charge. She re-enrolled in classes. After a semester living rent free, the landlord started requiring her to complete housework to earn rent. Consequently, the student moved into a friend's house. The friend asked her to drive her wherever she needed to go in return for a free place to live. Because of the amount of time the student had to spend driving her friend, she had to drop her classes again. She decided to move out and live in her car. She lived in her car for about a month until she found a job. She began to couch surf as she saved up money to rent a studio apartment. The student noted severe depression and PTSD during this time of her life as a result of homelessness.

Analysis of Case Studies

The case studies demonstrate that homeless college students are at risk of increasingly serious mental and physical illnesses, such as complications of chronic diseases (diabetes) and stress-related disorders (depression, PTSD, anxiety, low self-esteem). Although the women interviewed by the student did not discuss their risk for sexual assault and other forms of violence, their efforts to find safe houses (couch-surfing) rather than living on the street reduced this risk for them. However, in Dr. de Chesney's clinical practice as a psychotherapist, she had several clients who had experienced rape and beatings while living on the street.

The case studies also provided examples of health problems resulting from malnourishment and unavailable medications. They also showed the population's vulnerability to human trafficking through a form of debt bondage along with abuse and mistreatment. It is not unreasonable to view the people who allowed the students to live in their homes as human traffickers when they changed the rules about the rent and responsibilities after promising no or low rent with minimal responsibilities. If there were college programs in place for the students to use as resources once they became homeless, some of these circumstances may have been prevented. The following section describes one such program.

THE KENNESAW STATE UNIVERSITY PROGRAM

In 2006, Kennesaw State University (KSU) Student Health Services, in conjunction with Staff Senate, began the Feed the Future Program. This program is a box-style pantry that maintains a small stock of food for any KSU student with ongoing financial need. The pantry serves on average 10–20 students per month.

On October 13, 2008, KSU provided an opportunity for students to learn more about homelessness via the annual Homelessness Awareness Week (HAW) event. The activities typically include a 1-day conference and an on-campus sleep-out, which increases knowledge and understanding of living without reliable shelter and food, and sometimes living without hope. HAW is the result of the passion and dedication of Professor Emeritus Dr. Lana Wachniak in collaboration with community organizations and campus departments. HAW has been recognized nationally and locally. In July 2012, U.S. Senator Johnny Isakson, (R-GA) read a proclamation into the Congressional Record praising the efforts to raise awareness about the problem. In September 2012, the program received proclamations from the state of Georgia, Cobb County, and the city of Kennesaw.

After students continued to be identified and the number of referrals began to increase, KSU's Counseling and Psychological Services of Student Success Services officially established the Campus Awareness, Resource and Empowerment (CARE) center in May 2013. The CARE Center is dedicated to empowering and supporting students faced with issues surrounding homelessness while operating purely on the generosity of sponsors through donations, both tangible and monetary. In June 2014, the CARE Center was designated by the University System of Georgia as KSU's Campus Point of Contact for Homeless and Foster Care Youth. Both Feed the Future and annual HAW events were consolidated under the direction of the CARE Center by August 2014.

The CARE Center addresses homelessness by focusing on providing six key service needs: case management, emergency linens/clothing, urgent food resources, housing referral assistance, transportation, and finances. Within the CARE Center, the Owl's Closet serves as a donation-based collection program providing emergency linens such as towels and blankets, toiletries, immediate food assistance and winter coats and hats for students dealing with homelessness issues.

Through both on- and off-campus collaborations, the center affords it students many opportunities. For example, via reciprocal relationships with community consignment shops, the CARE Center provides clothing and/or shoes. When clothing items are collected by the CARE Center they are given to the consignment shops; the shops provide store credit to fulfill the clothing and footwear needs of students referred by the center. Additionally, the center has created a network of housing referral options for students, both on and off campus. It has worked with campus parking and transportation staff to secure the availability of drop-off locations near the local Wal-Mart to improve accessibility to nutritional food resources. The CARE Center assists students with meeting their financial needs by helping them locate on- and off-campus job opportunities, connecting them with the campus Financial Aid Office to ensure students have access to all available funding resources, assisting them in applying for scholarships and/or grants, and locating/connecting them with other community groups that offer services that students cannot afford. Lastly, the center is linked to two need-based scholarships, the Dr. Bruce

Thomason Memorial and Homelessness Awareness 20/4/1 Endowed Scholarships. These scholarships are available to any student in need at KSU and meet scholarship application requirements.

Homelessness on a college campus is not exclusive to KSU, the state of Georgia or the Southeast; it is affecting college students across the nation. Nationally over 58,000 students reported on their 2012–2013 FAFSA they were struggling with homelessness issues; yet it remains an underserved and/or unrecognized population. KSU aspires to be a leader for social justice and change by eradicating homelessness on its campus, hoping other campuses will follow suit.

OTHER UNIVERSITY-BASED PROGRAMS

City College of San Francisco

The Homeless At-Risk Transitional Students Programs (HARTS) of City College of San Francisco provides various services for students, including referrals for financial aid assistance to receive a monthly MUNI Fast Pass (San Francisco's public transportation system), assistance food vouchers, and shelter resources. Additionally, their outreach program presents at community agencies, collaborates with on-campus departments and programs, and promotes awareness and education for students, faculty, and staff.

Oregon State University

Oregon State University's Human Services Resource Center provides services for OSU students to help alleviate issues surrounding hunger and poverty. The center provides a food pantry for students and nonstudents on a bimonthly schedule as well as assisting students in applying for government food assistance. Through the MealBux program, students are able to apply for financial assistance for on-campus dining. The center also serves as an intermediary agency to connect students to agencies that provide rental and utility assistance, childcare, food boxes, and health insurance. Additionally, they provide workshops and seminars regarding internships and employment and connect students to those opportunities. They also help students maintain university health insurance through a student health insurance subsidy. Finally, the HSRC partners with the Center for Civic Engagement to host a Hunger and Homelessness Awareness Week annually.

Florida College System

The Florida College System, formerly known as the Florida Community College System, provides financial assistance for students who are homeless, among others. Through an exemption and waiver program, students who are designated as homeless are "exempt from the payment of tuition and fees, including lab fees."

CONCLUSION

In this chapter, undergraduate students electing a nursing course in working with vulnerable populations described their project to learn about homeless college students. They collaborated with program coordinators at their university to convey not just the seriousness of the problem for a largely invisible population, but to describe what other universities are doing to address the problem.

REFERENCES

Allec, R. (2014, March 18). Homelessness on rise for college students. *The Cabrillo Voice*. Retrieved from http://www.cabvoice.com/2014/03/18/homelessness-rise-college-students/

College Board. (2014). *Average published undergraduate charges by sector, 2013–2014*. Retrieved from http://trends.collegeboard.org/college-pricing/figures-tables/average-published-undergraduate-charges-sector-2013-14

Dorsen, C. (2010). Vulnerability in homeless adolescents: concept analysis. *Journal of Advanced Nursing*, 66(12), 2819–2827.

Ellis, B. (2013, October 24). Student homelessness hits record high. *Cable News Network*. Retrieved from http://money.cnn.com/2013/10/24/pf/homeless-students/

Gross, L. (2013, October 21). College campuses see rise in homeless students. *USA Today*. Retrieved from http://www.usatoday.com/story/news/nation/2013/10/21/homeless-students-american-colleges/3144383/

Hoback, A. (2007, March 18). National Coalition for the Homeless. Retrieved from http://www.nationalhomeless.org/publications/precariouslyhoused/index.html

Kinchen, K., & Wright, J. (1991). Hypertension management in health care for the homeless clinics: Results from a survey. *American Journal of Public Health*, 81(9), 1163–1165.

Lowe, J., & Gibson, S. (2011). Reflections of a homeless population's lived experience with substance abuse. *Journal of Community Health Nursing*, 28(2), 92–104.

Manea, E., Fletcher, E., & Beck, C. (2014, March 12). Student homelessness on the rise. *Independent: Clark College's student news publication*. Retrieved from http://www.clarkcollegeindependent.com/featured/student-homelessness-on-the-rise/

McBride, R. G. (2012). Survival on the streets: Experiences of the homeless population and constructive suggestions. *Journal of Multicultural Counseling & Development*, 40(1), 49–61.

National Alliance to End Homelessness (NAEH). (2014). *The state of homelessness in America 2014*. Washington, DC. Retrieved from http://b.3cdn.net/naeh/d1b106237807ab260f_qam6ydz02.pdf

Nickasch, B., & Marnocha, S. (2009). Healthcare experiences of the homeless. *Journal of the American Academy of Nurse Practitioners*, 21(1), 39–46.

Ross, A. (2012, December 17). More attention, resources focusing on homeless college students as numbers rise. *The Palm Beach Post*. Retrieved from http://www.campuscircle.com/review.cfm?r=16763

Shinn, M. (2007). International homelessness: Policy, socio-cultural, and individual perspectives. *Journal of Social Issues*, 63(3), 657–677.

Tsai, J., & Rosenheck, R. (2013). Obesity among chronically homeless adults: Is it a problem? Public Health Reports (Washington, DC: 1974), *128*(1), 29–36.

U.S. Department of Housing and Urban Development (HUD). (2013). *The 2013 annual homeless assessment report (AHAR) to congress part 1: Point-in-time estimates of homelessness.* Washington, DC: Office of Community Planning and Development. Retrieved from https://www.onecpd .info/resources/documents/ahar-2013-part1.pdf

Wheaton, E. M., Schauer, E. J., & Galli, T. V. (2010). Economics of human trafficking. *International Migration, 48*(4), 114–141.

Young, E. (2013). No shelter: Community colleges grapple with ways to help students without housing. *Diverse Issues In Higher Education, 23*, 32.

Chapter 35

Teaching Nurse Practitioners About Sex Trafficking: An Honors Capstone Project

Emily Peoples

OBJECTIVES

At the end of this chapter, the reader will be able to

1. Describe a capstone honors proposal in human trafficking.
2. Explain the need for nurse practitioner students to recognize sex trafficking survivors.
3. Develop a lecture on sex trafficking for nurse practitioners.

INTRODUCTION

The issue of human trafficking first came to my attention in the spring of 2012 when I enrolled in an honors course on the topic given by Dr. Mary de Chesnay. Before this course, I possessed little to no knowledge on the topic, but I quickly developed a passion for this subject and the persons affected by human trafficking. When the opportunity arose for me to conduct a service learning project, I knew immediately that human trafficking was the topic I wanted to pursue. My only question was how to incorporate it with nursing, my field of study. With the assistance of Dr. de Chesnay (2013) and her vast knowledge and experience in this area, I decided to create a lecture for nurses and nursing students on identification and treatment of human trafficking victims, specifically those trafficked for sex, in settings where nurses might possibly encounter these individuals. There is a tremendous lack of education among nurses and nursing students on this topic, a fact that was first brought to my attention by Dr. de Chesnay and later verified through my own research and literature review. Because nurses are in a prime position to help these individuals, it became clear this was an area of need and would be a perfect topic for my service learning project. In addition to the lecture, I wanted to include a research component to the project. I decided to develop and administer pre- and post-tests to students receiving the lecture to determine the level of prior knowledge on the topic and the effectiveness of the teaching.

THE PROJECT

Preparation

I began by reviewing the current literature on the topic. I read several books on human trafficking in general and sex trafficking specifically as well as relevant scholarly articles and publications found on Galileo and through Internet searches. The literature review continued for several months although I was able to begin working on the rest of the project after a short time.

Dr. de Chesnay put me in touch with a teacher from the nurse practitioner graduate student program at Kennesaw State University. This teacher agreed to let me present my lecture to her class. Having identified the audience, I began working on the pre- and post-tests that would be administered to the class. Each questionnaire comprised eight true or false questions related to some aspect of sex trafficking included general knowledge, identification of potential victims, and treatment of victims. Care was taken to ensure post-test questions matched the specific concepts covered by the pre-test in order to evaluate student learning on those specific concepts. The questionnaires were reviewed and critiqued by Dr. de Chesnay, whose feedback was incorporated to produce final versions of the pre- and post-tests.

Because I was conducting research in addition to preparing the lecture, I developed a consent form for student/participants to sign, detailing the nature of the research and all relevant information. Dr. de Chesnay, who has extensive research experience, also reviewed the draft consent form. With her approval, I finalized the consent form.

As soon as my pre- and post-tests and consent forms were finalized, I submitted my project to the Kennesaw State University (KSU) Institutional Review Board (IRB) for approval. This project fell under the IRB category of "exempt review" which involves initial review by the IRB but no further review of the project. The IRB responded to my application and required that I complete a designated online research ethics training module prior to their approval of my project. Upon receipt of my certificate of completion, the IRB approved my project.

I had originally planned to prepare handouts for the class in the form of pocket-sized reference cards with relevant facts to remember when identifying potential victims and how to proceed. The intention was for nurses to carry the cards on their person at work to have an easy reference on hand in case they ran across an individual whom they suspected might be a sex trafficking victim. However, during my research, I came across the website of the United States Department of Health and Human Services' Rescue and Restore Victims of Human Trafficking campaign (U.S. Department of Health and Human Services, n.d.). They offered a multitude of free resources, including pocket reference cards exactly like what I had intended to make. These reference cards, as well as other materials from the website, were distributed to the students after the lecture.

At this point in my project, I had everything assembled except the lecture itself. I began the process of reformulating all the relevant information I had gained into a cohesive presentation. Keeping my lecture audience in mind, I tailored my presentation to what information would best suit graduate nursing students. For example, I avoided explanations of medical conditions that would be common knowledge and therefore a waste of time to define. Instead, I was able to focus on explaining the ties between these medical conditions and sex trafficking victims. Additionally, practice scenarios within the presentation were written to coincide with settings and roles in which this audience will likely practice, such as nurse practitioners working in outpatient clinics within the community. I compiled all of the relevant information into a Power Point presentation that followed a logical sequence of events from identification to how to respond and initially treat sex trafficking victims. Both Dr. de Chesnay and the graduate student class' teacher reviewed the presentation and approved it.

Delivery

On the day of the presentation, I handed out packets to each student. Each packet contained a pre-test, a post-test, and two copies of the consent form, one for them to keep and one to give back to me. I allowed the students about 10 minutes to read and sign the consent form and complete the pre-test. The consent forms were collected and I asked the students to place the completed pre-tests back in their envelopes. When all of the students had completed the pre-test, I began the lecture. The following is a transcript of the lecture content that was delivered to the nurse practitioner students.

Lecture Content

In recent years, there have been many awareness campaigns bringing this issue to the public's attention, which is wonderful; however, we need to take it a step further and start focusing on how to make a positive impact on this population. Just knowing about it is not enough. As nurses, we are in a special position to be able to positively impact trafficked individuals. However, most healthcare professionals do not have the knowledge needed to identify and appropriately treat this group. Today, I am going to teach you how to identify potential victims of sex trafficking and what you can do about it.

I want to start by sharing with you some statistics on how often healthcare providers come in contact with this population and current education levels regarding trafficking victims.

One study showed that 56% of trafficking victims in the United States were brought to the emergency department for treatment at some point during their captivity and 25% of victims came to the emergency department more than once during their captivity yet were not identified as victims of trafficking (Raymond & Hughes, 2001). Another study reported that 28% of the victims interviewed had visited a healthcare provider outside the emergency department during their captivity, yet again, were not identified as victims of trafficking (Family Violence Prevention Fund, 2005). Clearly, we see these individuals in the healthcare setting more than we realize.

Unfortunately, it is rare anything that gets done about to help these individuals when they present because there is a significant lack of education on identifying and treating victims of human trafficking. An article I reviewed reported a survey of emergency department healthcare providers regarding this population. Only 13% responded that they felt they could identify a human trafficking victim and only 3% reported having had training on human trafficking (Chisolm-Straker & Richardson, 2007). Another article reported on a study of medical school students: 94% reported having no knowledge or only a little knowledge about human trafficking victims, 89% said they did not know the signs and symptoms of human trafficking victims, and 94% believed it was unlikely that they would encounter a victim of human trafficking in the clinical setting (Wong, Hong, Leung, & Steward, 2011). But, as displayed by the first set of statistics, that is not the case.

So, how do we fix this? The first step in identifying a potential victim of sex trafficking is to know what to look for. I have put together a fairly extensive list of red flags. These are things you should be on the lookout for and that should stand out to you as being "off." Victims may display several of these red flags, only one, or none at all. This is a particularly difficult vulnerable population to identify and there is no one profile of a sex trafficking victim. I will go through this list of red flags one by one and explain how you might see them present with a sex trafficking victim.

Signs of physical abuse is an obvious one. You want to look for bruising, especially in the more central, proximal areas. Distal bruising, on lower legs and arms, is more likely to be accidental while bruising on the more central areas of the body are potential indicators of physical abuse. Keep an eye out for burns. There may be large, obvious burns, or smaller, circular burns from cigarettes. Another sign of physical abuse to look for is marks on the wrists or ankles from being tied up.

Look for evidence of old injuries, especially injuries that do not seem to have healed properly which would have resulted from the individual being denied medical attention at the time of the injury. Look for multiple injuries that are in various stages of healing. This would indicate multiple instances of abuse or chronic abuse versus a single incident or an accident where an individual incurred several injuries simultaneously such as in a car crash or a fall.

If the individual has come in for treatment of a particular injury, ask how they got it. If the story is vague, inconsistent, or does not add up with the injury, this is a red flag. You can also ask about any old or partially healed injuries you notice, even if that is not what they came in for.

Note any tattoos on your patient. Of course, having a tattoo does not mean an individual is being trafficked. In this case, what you are looking for is a tattoo of a name or a sort of brand. Many pimps brand their girls with their name or a specific symbol as a sign of ownership. If you see a patient with a tattoo like this, ask about it and evaluate their response and their attitude when you mention it.

Poor eye contact is another red flag. This results from low self-esteem and/or fear. Both of these are bred by the situation they are in and encouraged by their traffickers as a control mechanism.

The attitudes of sex trafficking victims will vary. Some individuals will appear very frightened, timid, nervous, depressed, or detached. On the other hand, some will come off as quite hostile and exhibit a tough attitude. It is important to keep in mind that just because they do not seem like victims, it does not mean they are not victims. When you consider what these people have been through, it is not surprising they may treat others with hostility. Additionally, victims may seem confused and unaware of their surroundings, the time of day, etc.

If an individual is seeing you for late maternity care, that is also considered a red flag. You should investigate the reason for the delay in seeking maternity care. Sex trafficking victims are not allowed to receive maternity care until very late, when it is absolutely necessary, or often not at all throughout the pregnancy.

Another person almost always accompanies the potential victim: the trafficker or pimp. This person may be male or female, so do not dismiss it just because the accompanying individual is a woman. Pimps sometimes use one of their girls that they trust to keep the other girls in line. This woman is entrusted to accompany and to keep an eye on the girl receiving treatment and make sure she returns to the pimp. Male or female, this accompanying person is often overbearing, answering questions and filling out paperwork for the patient. They often claim to be needed as an interpreter, which may or may not be true. Even if interpretation is needed, a third-party hospital interpreter should be used as with all patients. The accompanying person will stick very close to the patient and will often refuse to leave them alone with healthcare providers. They may claim to be a relative even though they look nothing like or may not even be the same race as the potential victim.

When the potential victim is a child, the accompanying individual may claim to be a parent or guardian or they may simply say they are a friend or neighbor. While these claims could be legitimate, it is important to evaluate them on an individual basis in the light of other contextual factors. Another thing to look for with younger girls is if the accompanying man is supposedly her boyfriend or husband yet appears too old for her. Even if she agrees that the man is her boyfriend or husband, it is still very possibly a trafficking situation. Similarly to domestic violence situations, emotional manipulation is often involved and depending on the individual situation, the girl may honestly believe this man is in love with her or cares for her despite circumstances that may seem obviously contradictory to you or me.

A major red flag is when the individual is unable to provide information such as what city, state, or even country they are in. Not knowing this information, as well as being unable to provide an address, is very indicative of being trafficked. An individual trafficked across borders would have no idea where they are or know the address where they "live." Additionally, they may give very vague or inconsistent information about where they live, where they work, or where they go to school. This point is a really good one to keep in mind because most people, even children, are able to provide pretty detailed information about their homes, jobs, and schools. Also, these are things that are easy to bring up conversationally. You can ask about these things casually without seeming unusually inquisitive.

Paying for services in cash is another red flag. The trafficker will want to leave as little of a paper trail as possible with as little identifying information as possible. Therefore, paying in cash is common with this group.

Finally, an individual with a history of delayed care and/or who comes in repeatedly for treatment of STIs or abortions merits further investigation. This is unusual and an indicator of a potential sex trafficking victim. As we will discuss a bit later, this group has high risk for STIs and pregnancy and is rarely allowed to seek care unless the medical problem has escalated to a point where it interferes with their work.

I also want to include one non–red flag. Some people would think to use dress as a red flag. For example, if you had a provocatively dressed patient, you might think that would be a red flag as a stereotypical prostitute. However, trafficking victims are more likely to be dressed conservatively to avoid drawing extra attention. So don't dismiss anything that seems off just because your patient does not fit the look you might be expecting.

So you have a patient, you have noted some red flags, and you suspect they might be a victim of sex trafficking. What do you do next? Your first step is to separate the individual from whoever is accompanying them. As I mentioned before, the accompanying person will be very reluctant and may refuse to leave the individual. One strategy for dealing with this includes citing hospital policy. Say the rules state that the patient has to be examined in private. Another very simple method for separating victim from trafficker comes from Dr. de Chesnay. Say you need a urine sample and take the patient down the hall to the bathroom. Not many people want to be involved in collecting a urine sample. Even if they still try to go, say the bathroom is only big enough for the two of you. This should buy you some time alone with the individual to further investigate the situation. Again, if an interpreter is needed, you absolutely must use a third-party approved interpreter, never the accompanying individual.

The next step is to establish trust and an intent to help. Of course, establishing trust is much more easily said than done, especially with this population who has no reason to trust anyone. In the interests of establishing trust, you should assure the patient that you are on their side, that "this is a safe place and I am a safe person," and that anything they share with you is confidential, will not be shared with the accompanying individual, and will only be shared with other trusted people who need to know. Some examples of trust-building messages include:

- We are here to help you.
- Our first priority is your safety.
- We can find you a safe place to stay and get assistance for you.
- If you have been held against your will (trafficked) and cooperate, you will not be deported and can receive help to stay safely in this country.

After doing your best to assure the individual you are trustworthy and want to help them, you should ask questions to confirm whether or not this is a trafficking situation. One of the articles that I reviewed in preparation for this lecture presented interviews between the authors and sex trafficking victims. These victims had all come in contact with healthcare providers at some point during their captivity and none of them had ever been asked about their situation (Baldwin, Chuang, Eisenman, Ryan, & Sayles, 2011). So please remember to question it if you notice any of the red flags we talked about or even if something just seems a little off. Another thing to remember about asking questions is that you cannot just ask "are you being trafficked?" because these individuals most likely will not have any idea what "being trafficked" means. Another point to keep in mind is that victims may have been kidnapped or have gone willingly. This does not mean they chose to be trafficked, but many victims are lied to and tricked into their situation although they did actually make the initial choice to go with their trafficker. Thus, if you ask a person if she was forced or kidnapped, she may say no even though she was ultimately the victim of trafficking.

The Polaris Project suggests asking assessment questions that can help you determine whether or not an individual is being trafficked:

- Are you free to come and go from your work or living area as you please?
- Are you being controlled?

- Can you leave your job if you want to? Are you or your family threatened when you try to leave?
- Do you owe your employer money?
- What type of work do you do?
- Are you getting paid? Is anything taken out of your pay?
- What are your working and living conditions like? Are there locks on your doors or windows so you cannot get out?
- How are you treated? Do you have to ask permission to eat, sleep, or go to the bathroom?
- Has your identification or documentation been taken from you (passport, birth certificate, etc.)?
- Where are you from? What brings you to the United States? How did you get here?
- Is anyone forcing you to do anything that you do not want to do? (de Chesnay, 2013).

At this point, you have asked enough questions of your patient to determine that they are being trafficked. If there is immediate danger, call 911 and/or hospital security. If there is no immediate danger, your better option is calling the human trafficking hotline. This number connects you to the National Human Trafficking Resource Center sponsored by the Polaris Project. This hotline is toll-free, operates nationwide, and is available every day of the year, 24/7. They provide interpretation for 170 languages and can put you in touch with human trafficking resources in your area. Something to consider is that because victims are often labeled and treated like criminals by the judiciary system, contacting the police often is not the best option although it may be your first instinct. Advocacy groups like the hotline sponsors are your best first contact. Now, what we need to do for our patient is to provide them with resources and options. It is important to inform the patient that she is a victim of a crime and that it is not her fault. Inform her that there are resources available to help her and you will gladly get her in touch with those resources at any time. I am briefly going to touch on a point that we are going to discuss in more depth later on. That point is that, probably more often than you expect, you will encounter individuals that are resistant to your efforts to help them. We will to talk about why, that is later on, but what you need to know for now is that if they do not want immediate assistance, it is important to communicate that this is a safe place and they are welcome to come back any time they are able to or want to for help. If you can discreetly give them the hotline number, try and do that as well.

One of the most important things to keep in mind throughout is your own attitude and reactions. A friendly, nonjudgmental, accepting attitude is critical. One victim in an article I reviewed reported that she never said anything because she was ashamed and afraid the healthcare provider would laugh at her, call her stupid, or be angry she did not say anything sooner (Baldwin, Chuang, Eisenman, Ryan, & Sayles, 2011). It is important to remain calm and collected because expressing shock or surprise at what a patients reveals to you can be interpreted as disbelief. If they think you do not believe them, they tend to shut down and quit talking. Additionally, appearing shocked or surprised by their story may cause victims to stop sharing for fear of traumatizing the listener. On the flip side, while being kind and nonjudgmental is important, you want to avoid appearing overly sympathetic because this can distress the individual and reinforce feelings of shame and embarrassment about their situation.

Remember, it is not important to get the full, detailed story right off the bat. That can be handled later. You just need to know enough to identify that there is a problem and to put them in touch with the right resources. It is not your job to prove that an individual has been trafficked, but it is your job to offer them help if you suspect trafficking.

Some victims of sex trafficking may not view themselves as victims. They often do not know what trafficking is and, as I mentioned earlier, are often deceived by the trafficker and may have gone willingly, believing they were going to do honest work with a real chance of making a better life for themselves and their families. In some countries, situations we would define as trafficking are viewed as an unfortunate yet normal part of life. These countries tend to be places where trafficking is common and where they do not share the same beliefs about human rights. Along the same lines, some victims may not understand that what the trafficker is doing is wrong. They may not be aware that it is against the law or abnormal for people to be treated this way. They do not know that there is anything anyone can do about it. Individuals who do not think anything can be done or who believe their situation is normal are not going to be out seeking rescue or expecting help from anyone.

Another barrier to rescuing victims is fear of authority figures. Victims tend to be distrustful due to the trauma they have endured. Additionally, many victims are commonly conditioned to be distrustful of authority figures, including healthcare providers, by their traffickers as a method of ensuring they do not try to escape. Sex trafficked individuals are taught that if they tell anyone their situation they will be sent to jail, abused by law enforcement, or deported—which unfortunately is sometimes true.

Traffickers use fear as a control tactic. From day one they do their best to ensure that their victims are terrified of them and they generally succeed. Victims live in fear of injury to themselves and their families. As an example, I heard one story about a girl who was trafficked and the trafficker had a picture of the girl's little sister. He would show her the picture and tell her what he would do to her sister if she did not cooperate. Traffickers commonly use similar threats to family and loved ones to control their victims.

Victims suffer psychological abuse as well as physical abuse. The situations these women are in breed shame and embarrassment. These feelings are reinforced by their traffickers, again, as a method of control. Many of these women experience self-esteem so low they do not value themselves at all. They internalize the messages they are fed that they are "dirty" and "worthless." Many feel guilt as well as shame, as if they somehow brought this on themselves and deserve what is happening to them. These sorts of feelings contribute to why victims do not try to escape. Many victims are trafficked internationally—brought into the United States from other countries. They often do not speak any English. If they have no way to communicate with anyone around them, they are less likely to attempt an escape.

Some pimps deliberately impregnate their victims as a method of control. They use the child to bind the woman to them. For some women, escaping this life would mean abandoning her child.

Another method of control commonly used by pimps and traffickers is substance use. An estimated 85% of sex workers in the United States have addictions to some kind of substance. Drugs are sometimes forced on victims initially to addict them to the substance. If the victim leaves, access to the substance will be cut off. Some victims initiate drug or alcohol use themselves as a coping mechanism to deal with the horrors of their everyday lives.

Understanding what keeps the women from seeking rescue or accepting aid is an important aspect of treating this population. It can be very easy to be judgmental in a situation in which a woman refuses, help but you have to try and view the situation through her eyes. You cannot force an adult to leave unsafe conditions. Rescuing an adult against their will is counterproductive as well as an infringement on their right to autonomy. If they are not ready to leave, they will likely end up back in a similar situation. What you can do is be sure they know "this is a safe place and I am a safe person" and that if they ever need help or want to leave, "we are here and available at any time." You can also provide information and a course of action for her if she decides that she wants help later.

Now we will move on to a discussion of common health problems seen in this group. One of the commonly encountered health issues with victims of sex trafficking is sexually transmitted infections [STIs]. STIs are prolific among this group because they are forced into a lifestyle that puts them at increased risk for contracting an STI. These individuals do not have the option to practice abstinence or safe sex, our usual methods for prevention. In addition, they may have multiple sex partners, which further increases their risk for contracting an STI. Having an STI also increases the individual's risk of contracting another STI due to inflammation of the genitals. You will most likely see these patients only when the infection has become severe because they are typically not allowed to seek medical care until the problem interferes with their ability to work. These patients may present with multiple, simultaneous infections and these infections can be vaginal, oral, or rectal. STIs can lead to issues like pelvic inflammatory disease (PID), which is another issue I've listed here as common in this group due to a variety of causes. PID increases risk for infertility and ectopic pregnancies as well as chronic pelvic pain. These are all issues this group often experiences due to the multiple and various risk factors to which they are exposed.

Another major problem for this group is HIV and AIDS. Again, victims of sex trafficking are forced into many behaviors that increase their risk for HIV infection, such as inability to use condoms and having multiple sex partners. These individuals routinely experience forced and violent or "rough" sex, which is more likely to cause tearing of genital tissue, increasing the chances of HIV transmission.

This genital trauma is itself a problem commonly experienced by sex trafficking victims. It may take the form of hematomas, lacerations, perforation, abrasions, hemorrhage, abdominal and pelvic pain, and fistulas. Fistulas are an abnormal connection between the vaginal wall and the bladder, urethra, or rectum as a result of physical trauma such as rape or childbirth, especially in young girls. Complications of fistulas include urinary and fecal incontinence, shame, and self-consciousness due to incontinence. Genital trauma may be internal and not appear externally. Rectal trauma is another health issue you are likely to encounter with this group.

Victims of sex trafficking often can be faced with unintended pregnancy. They are usually not given any sort of birth control and are not allowed to use condoms. The decision to keep or terminate the pregnancy is not theirs. As I mentioned earlier, the pimp sometimes decides to keep the child for a variety of reasons. If the woman carries the child to term, she is rarely allowed prenatal care. Her risk of pregnancy complications is very high due to lack of prenatal care and lifestyle factors. She is not going to be given maternity leave, she is likely malnourished, she may be using substances, and she often experiences physical trauma. The woman may or may not be allowed time off to give birth and amount of time off varies. I read about one woman's experience in which one of the other women delivered her child, she cleaned herself up, and was back on the street the following day. If the pimp decides to terminate the pregnancy, the chance of the girl receiving a safe abortion is basically nonexistent. Some of the abortion methods used by traffickers and pimps that I have encountered in my research include: blunt force trauma to the abdomen, sharp foreign objects like a broken glass bottle inserted vaginally, and instilling chemicals such as bleach into the vagina. As you can imagine, these women are at risk for severe complications from unsafe abortions including: hemorrhage, fistulas, poor wound healing, infertility, internal organ damage, and sepsis. Post-abortion sepsis is a major problem faced by this population and is significant cause of death for this group.

Other problems commonly experienced by victims of sex trafficking include urinary difficulties, urinary tract infections, menstrual irregularities, and cervical cancer. Many of these problems are not something they would come in for specifically since they are not allowed to seek treatment for anything unless it gets in the way of their ability to work. If you have a patient that you have identified as a victim of sex trafficking, these are things you want to ask about specifically or assess because they are common in this population and may need to be treated.

All of these common health issues are important to keep in mind not just so you know what to look for if you have already identified your patient as a victim of sex trafficking, but also because you can use these issues as red flags, too. We touched on some of these conditions specifically when we were discussing red flags but if you are examining a patient who has many of the issues described here, yet did not display any other red flags, you will still want to investigate further in order to determine whether the patient is a potential trafficking victim.

These patients suffer a lot of physical trauma. They receive beatings, get hit by cars, thrown out of moving cars, thrown down flights of stairs, etc. You will likely to see the results of beatings on these patients. They will often have abrasions, bruises, broken bones, and burns. Cigarette burns and acid burns are common. These injuries may be current or you may just notice the scars. Pimps tend to inflict damage in places that will not impact the girl's appearance in order not to "devalue" what they consider their property. For this reason, you will often see scars in areas such as the lower back.

Victims may present with stab or gunshot wounds. These are mandatory to report to law enforcement. It is important to obtain detailed and precise documentation of these wounds for use by law enforcement. Document the size, shape, and appearance of the wound and take photos if you are able. As I mentioned earlier, sex trafficking victims often end up getting labeled as criminals by the judicial system, so be sure and contact the hotline to get in touch with local resources who can ensure the victim is treated appropriately and given the help she deserves.

Victims of sex trafficking may also suffer ill effects from untreated chronic diseases. Under normal conditions, an individual with a chronic disease such as diabetes, asthma, or some cardiovascular conditions would have routine doctor's visits and be on medications. These resources are not available to individuals living in captivity and their conditions can cause any number of problems if left untreated.

Due to poor living conditions and overcrowding, these individuals are at risk for lice or scabies infestations as well as any number of contagious diseases. Some of the more common diseases include hepatitis, pneumonia, and tuberculosis. Some more common health issues include rashes; skin sores; itching; back, jaw, and neck pain; malnutrition; sleep deprivation; dental problems; abdominal pain; vomiting; and diarrhea.

Sex trafficking victims experience psychological trauma as well as physical trauma. While mental health issues are not going to be the reason for their visit, nor will they be the focus of immediate treatment, they still play a vital role in the overall health and recovery process of these individuals and it is important to be aware of common mental health issues faced by this population. An author of one of the articles I reviewed stated that the majority of women they had worked with felt the physical issues they faced were much easier to manage and overcome during recovery than the psychological issues, which many victims of sex trafficking struggle with for their entire lives, even many years after their captivity if they have been rescued (Sabella, 2013). Anything beyond immediate, emergency treatment should include psychological interventions as well as physical treatment.

I will identify some common psychological issues faced by this group but we will not spend much time on them, because the focus of this presentation is on initial, emergency treatment and response. I mentioned substance abuse earlier and here it is again. Some traffickers deliberately addict their victims to substances as a control method and some victims turn to drugs on their own as a means of coping with the horror of their everyday lives. It is hard enough to quit for persons with access to care and treatment but this population does not have access to any substance abuse resources if they wish to quit. This group commonly experiences post-traumatic stress disorder (PTSD). One study reported that 67% of victims of sex trafficking met the diagnostic criteria for PTSD (Farley et al., 2003). Other mental health issues faced by this population include depression, anxiety, insomnia, irritability, suicidal ideation, self-destructive behaviors, mood disorders, disassociation, panic attacks, agoraphobia, poor self-esteem, OCD, eating disorders, self-blame, self-loathing, shame, and guilt.

At this point in my presentation, I had finished with the delivery of content and moved to a case study, with the intention of tying the information together and allowing the students to practice applying what they had learned. The following case was presented to the students:

You are a nurse practitioner working in a community clinic. Your client is a young woman with a broken ulna. Her companion is another young woman who greets you politely when you enter the room. When you ask your client how she broke her arm, her companion says the client does not speak English, but that she fell and broke it. While examining your client, you notice several healing bruises on her arms and neck. Your client avoids eye contact and appears sullen. She has remained very quiet the whole time. What red flags did you notice? What should you do? What questions would you ask?

The class was very responsive to the case study and came up with several answers for each question. Their answers demonstrated a good grasp of the information that I had presented. I continued with the second part of the case study that read as follows:

Through screening questions, you have determined your client is a victim of sex trafficking. She has become agitated during your questioning. Your client has stated she was kidnapped from her home, does not know where she is, and is forced to have sex for money. Her companion is sitting calmly in the waiting room. What should you say to your patient? What should you do?

Again, the students appropriately answered the questions using the material they had learned. After the case study, I provided the class with several resources for further information and relevant phone numbers to keep on hand in case they encountered a potential sex trafficking victim. I conducted a brief question-and-answer segment and then the class completed their post-tests.

The pre- and post-tests had no personal identifiers on them in order to maintain anonymity. To match each individual's pre-test with their post-test, I instead used a numbering system on the test papers. I collected all the pre- and post-tests and had handouts available at the front for the students. These handouts were very well received.

DISCUSSION

Research Results

Following the lecture presentation, I took all completed pre- and post-tests and graded them. A total of 29 students filled out and returned the pre- and post-tests. Pre-test scores averaged 64.2% with a median score of 62.5%. The average of the post-test scores was 86.2% with the median falling at 87.5%. I was pleased with these results because they showed an average score improvement of 22% following the lecture. Twenty-eight of the 29 test takers showed improvement from the pre-test to the post-test. Many of the students approached me after the lecture and said they found the presentation very informative and that they learned a good deal. Overall, I feel this project was successful in increasing education levels of nursing students regarding human trafficking, specifically how to identify a potential sex trafficking victim and what they should do in that situation.

Plans for the Future

The results of my research showed an improvement in knowledge levels of nursing students who received the lecture. Therefore, I intend to pursue delivering this simple 45-minute lecture to nurses and nursing students in as many settings as possible. I am currently working on scheduling a presentation that will be available to all undergraduate nursing students at KSU through the Student Nurses Association. I am also pursuing offering the presentation at the annual convention of the Georgia Association of Nursing Students. In the near future, I plan to look into offering this lecture to nurses working in local hospitals, specifically nurses in the emergency department, as well as local urgent care centers and clinics. Additionally, I would love to have the opportunity to present the program at other nursing schools and hospitals within Georgia. I would happily go and present this lecture anywhere that invited me.

I would like to continue the research portion of this project as well. In intend to make the consent forms and pre- and post-tests available to any nurses or nursing students who are willing to participate at future presentations. This will allow me to build a larger body of data regarding the effectiveness of the teaching. Also, this will provide a greater variety in the types of students and the settings in which the teaching is provided. In the future, I would also like to add a control group of nurses and/or nursing students who could take the pre- and post-tests without receiving the lecture to strengthen the quality of data gathered.

Conclusion

I have enjoyed my time working on this service learning project and I hope to continue presenting it to provide needed education to others. I gained a significant amount of experience performing a variety of tasks I would otherwise not have had the opportunity to do. Research projects and presentations that I have completed for other classes have not approached the level of magnitude and could not have hoped to provide the same level of real life experience.

Lecturing to a group of graduate students as an undergraduate student is an experience like no other. I was nervous leading up to the presentation but ended up enjoying myself while delivering it. I had spent several months immersed in the material, expanding my own personal body of knowledge, and was prepared to share it with others. I became quite confident in my knowledge on the topic while still realizing the vastness of what was still available to learn. I have never had a great fear of public speaking but have always experienced being nervous before and during presentations. Since this project however, I have found a level of confidence in my abilities to present that I have never experienced before. Now, I find that I simply enjoy sharing information and presenting.

Working on this capstone project has been a unique and wonderful experience that stands out on my resume. It is beneficial for me to have accomplished this. It has opened up other doors for me as well. Dr. de Chesnay has given me the opportunity to publish an account of my project in her upcoming textbook, *Caring for the Vulnerable*, another unique experience I can proudly include in my résumé. Additionally, I have the opportunity to continue presenting my project in a variety of settings and to a variety of audiences. These benefits are experiences I would be much less likely to encounter without having done this service learning project.

The benefits of this project extend to more than myself. The students I have already lectured benefitted by gaining knowledge that few other nurses or nursing students possess. The opportunity to have a lecture on this important topic is not widely available and not commonly given in nursing school. These students have been provided with important knowledge and a special skill set that sets them apart from their peers. My hope is that this project can continue to benefit nurses and nursing students in the same way, as I continue to offer this presentation in different venues. My belief is that all nurses and nursing students should be provided education on this topic.

Finally, this project stands to positively impact victims of sex trafficking. As presented in the lecture content, the statistics show that a fair number of sex trafficking victims come in contact with medical professionals but are not offered assistance due to lack of education on the part of the medical professionals. After receiving the information provided through my project, a nurse would be equipped with the knowledge to identify potential trafficking victims and the appropriate course of action to take. As more and more nurses and nursing students receive education such as that which my lecture provides, victims that present to healthcare settings will be noticed and offered appropriate assistance more frequently.

REFERENCES

Baldwin, S., Chuang, K., Eisenman, D., Ryan, G., & Sayles, J. (2011). Identification of human trafficking victims in healthcare settings. *Health and Human Rights*, *13*(1), 1–14.

Chisolm-Straker, M., & Richardson, L. (2007). Assessment of emergency provider knowledge about human trafficking victims in the ED. *Academic Emerging Medicine*, *14*(5), Supp. 134.

de Chesnay, M. (2013). Sex trafficking: A clinical guide for nurses. New York: Springer.

Family Violence Prevention Fund. (2005). Turning pain into power: Trafficking survivors' perspectives on early intervention strategies. Family Violence Prevention Fund. Retrieved from http://www.futureswithoutviolence.org/userfiles/file/ImmigrantWomen/Turning%20Pain%20intoPower.pdf

Farley, M., Cotton, A., Lynne, J., Zumbeck, S., Spiwak, F., Reyes, M. et al. (2003). Prostitution and trafficking in nine countries: An update on violence and posttraumatic stress disorder. *Journal of Trauma Practice*, *2*(3/4), 33–74.

Raymond, J. & Hughes, D. (2001). Sex trafficking of women in the United States: International and domestic trends. Coalition against trafficking in women. Retrieved from http://www.uri.edu/artsci/wms/hughes/sex_traff_us.pdf

Sabella, D. (2013). Health issues and interactions with adult survivors. In M. de Chesnay (Ed.), Sex trafficking: A clinical guide for nurses (pp. 151–166). New York: Springer.

United States Department of Health and Human Services. (n.d.). Retrieved from http://www.acf.hhs.gov/programs/orr/programs/anti-trafficking

Wong, J., Hong, J., Leung, P., & Steward, D. (2011). Human trafficking: An evaluation of Canadian medical students' awareness and attitudes. *Education for Health*, *24*(1). Retrieved from http://www.educationforhealth.net/

Chapter 36

Family Nursing Clinical Immersion in Lac du Flambeau

Cheryl Ann Lapp

OBJECTIVES

At the end of this chapter, the reader will be able to

1. Describe how a domestic intercultural clinical experience conducted on a Native American reservation might compare to an international immersion experience.
2. Reflect on the cultural characteristics of the Ojibwa population described in the chapter.
3. Explore how a similar project might be implemented in other settings.

INTRODUCTION

This chapter describes a clinical immersion project that was piloted and implemented on an Indian reservation in northern Wisconsin. Initially designed for graduate students of nursing, the clinical immersion was developed with the assistance of Family Nurse Practitioner Dana Irmick, Nursing Manager of the Peter Christensen Health Center in Lac du Flambeau, Wisconsin.

In the evolution of modern nursing, we have seen a shift in ethics from unqualified loyalty to the physician, often recited in the classic Nightingale Pledge, to a newer nursing ethic of patient advocacy (Nauright & Wilson, 2012). Patient advocacy is a core nursing value, just as population advocacy is a core value for public health (Thomas, Sage, Dillenberg, & Guillory, 2002). The question for educators is: How then might we prepare students to use empathy to care about advocacy and incorporate social responsibility into their practice? This question becomes critical when nurses are charged with preparing students for leadership roles in advanced practice with vulnerable populations. By virtue of their vulnerability for various reasons, these populations may be at greater than average risk for developing health problems. The nurse must be prepared for advocacy by being able to assess patients within their operating social context. Simply stated, this means breaking the mold of the individual unit of service in clinical settings, in favor of considering the many influences of family and community, as well as the socioeconomic and cultural features of everyday life. This degree of awareness is characterized as practicing holistically. What matters most is achieving optimal health outcomes by applying best practices.

As a nursing educator, it has been surprising to me how many experienced nurses are bypassing the assessment of their patients beyond the individual level. This happens when nurses consider the assessment to be complete when it primarily involves the classic review of physical systems along with a few brief questions with fixed-response answers to "cover" any socioemotional problems. As a consequence, nurse practitioner students are themselves at risk for embracing the constraints of their physician counterparts—being time bound and focused almost exclusively on maximum efficiency in treatment, diagnosis, and medication disbursement. The danger for the nurse, of course, is in losing one's way within the medical model through abandoning the nursing identity of loyalty as it translates into advocacy for patients. For example, several of my graduate students—typically those from emergency departments or intensive care units—have disclosed in our family nursing seminars that they often view the family as an inconvenience. They identify examples where family members "get in the way of getting my work done" and they would rather not think about routinely incorporating the family into the overall healthcare process. As startling as this perspective may sound, it is not inconsistent with nursing literature (Benzein, Johansson, Arestedt, & Saveman, 2008).

As an educator, it is important to examine with students the structure and climate of their healthcare settings and to generate some strategies to work with patients within the context of their families and community supports. It is instructive and important to identify with students how work settings they have experienced can support, or not support, their role as family and population-based advocates. One teaching strategy I selected for exploring what best practice may mean in family nursing was to work together within a culture where family and social context cannot be ignored.

At our university, our mission statement for excellence includes diversity, empathy, cultural awareness, and high-impact educational practices. In my clinical supervision with the Human Development Center, an interdisciplinary assessment clinic, I had been regularly visiting the Lac du Flambeau Indian Reservation in connection with the HDC's interdisciplinary activities in the Head Start program and connecting with the Lac du Flambeau Indian School's nursing office. Upon touring the community's new tribal health center and discovering that one of my former nursing graduate students was now employed there as an advanced practice nurse, I recognized the possibility for a comprehensive and challenging practice experience for my current students. At our university, the educational initiatives for cultural exchange, diversity projects, and other "high-impact" experiences are typically located within a funding domain exclusive to undergraduate students because of differential tuition. However, my personal connection with Dana Irmick, Family Nurse Practitioner and Nursing Manager, motivated me to negotiate a clinical contract and to pilot this opportunity with the Peter Christensen Health Center Clinic and the associated Community Health Department services as our anchor.

BACKGROUND: A DOMESTIC INTERCULTURAL IMMERSION PROJECT

A funding opportunity revealed itself coincidentally, when our campus Associate Chancellor's office invited proposals for development of a "domestic intercultural immersion project." After consultation with this office, I was enthusiastically encouraged to submit my proposal to benefit graduate students. It did not qualify for differential tuition funding (reserved for undergraduates), but it was supported and subsequently funded by an internal university grant. The pilot project's budget request was funded to cover six students' shared travel mileage, lodging in a nearby hotel, admission to two cultural heritage centers on the reservation (The George W. Brown Jr. Ojibwe Museum & Cultural Center, and the Waswagoning Indian village), and miscellaneous educational supplies. Although food expenses were not funded for the students, an additional sum of several hundred dollars was allocated by the funders with the instruction that this money be allocated to provide gifts and meals for Ojibwa community leaders who contributed as cultural guides to our clinical learning experience.

The pilot was funded on a one-time basis, with projected sustainability possible with private donors through the foundation office. In the absence of ongoing funding, this experience has since been repeated several times, in response to student requests. As news of the pilot opportunity spread to subsequent cohorts of graduate students, they offered to absorb all of their personal and travel expenses for the chance to have this immersion clinical placement before they graduated. For these graduate students, individual costs may have been less problematic due to their already established nursing positions. However, the logistics of planning for interruption in personal life, involving family, children, and work schedules remained a reality and a responsibility that they readily met without complaint. From my planning perspective in our nursing college, ongoing community access to this setting was greatly enhanced by the university Human Development Center's 10-year history of sponsoring the Lac du Flambeau Service Learning Project. This long-standing relationship paved the way for new collaborative possibilities for exploring credit-bearing opportunities for MSN candidates. Our university's essential course content in family nursing (theory and clinical) was designed to develop confidence and beginning expertise in the family specialization. As reflected in our course objectives, students are being prepared to plan nursing interventions together with families, as appropriate within the social and cultural context of their communities. Special attention is paid to learning about vulnerable populations, with a focus on health promotion, risk reduction, and clinical decision making that uses population data and evidence-based research. In addition to integrating healthcare ethics, cultural influences, and social awareness in providing holistic care for families in the advanced practice role, learning outcomes for students include demonstration of an ability to collaborate with families and with other members of an interdisciplinary healthcare team of providers.

On the Lac du Flambeau Reservation, students rotate through the clinical setting at the Peter Christensen Health Center; the Community Wellness Center, where they participate in public health programs such as diabetic education, family home visits; and finally, the nursing office of the Lac du Flambeau Indian School. In the words of Dr. Mike Axelrod, Director of the Human Development Center at University of Wisconsin–Eau Claire: "An immersion experience is perhaps the most practical way to help family nursing graduate students begin to develop culturally competent clinical skills."

COMMUNITY HISTORY AND HEALTH IMPLICATIONS FOR IMMERSION PLANNING

The Lac du Flambeau Reservation in north central Wisconsin is home to the Lake Superior Band of Chippewa Indians, historically known as the Ojibwa. The year-round population, which expands considerably in the summer months, is estimated at 3,000, with at least two-thirds of the population being Native American. The reservation was established in 1854, although the area had been a permanent settlement of the Chippewa Indians for more than a century. The Lac du Flambeau ("Lake of the Torches") area acquired its name from French traders and trappers, who harvested fish at night by torchlight. The geographic area is beautiful, characterized by lakes, rivers, and woodlands with abundant wildlife. All contribute to play a major role in the economy, as this is one of Wisconsin's popular recreational centers. The Lac du Flambeau Chippewa operate LDF Industries (pallet manufacturing), the Ojibwa Mall, campground, fish hatchery, gas station, smoke shop, and Lake of the Torches Hotel and Casino.

In planning for this immersion, population data from the Wisconsin Department of Health and Family Services were examined, and indicators of vulnerability for health risks were detected. For example, it was noted that the percentage of Wisconsin's Native American population that lives in poverty is more than double the rate for the entire state of Wisconsin. The median age of Native Americans in Wisconsin was 27 years, which suggests that this population does not share the longevity of other residents in Wisconsin.

According to Irmick's experience in Lac du Flambeau, local culture designates that an individual becomes an elder at age 50. On a national level, the Department of Health has reported that the pattern of life expectancy for Native American men was 6 years less than the life expectancy of Caucasian men (Ho, 2009).

In Wisconsin, at the time of the immersion experience, vital statistics indicated the existence of other disparities related to health. The age-adjusted death rate showed American Indians having more deaths (1031.5 per 100,000) than the state as a whole (769.4 per 100,000). The leading causes of death among this population were heart disease, cancer, unintentional injury, and diabetes. American Indians were three times more likely to die from diabetes than whites, twice as likely to die from unintentional injury as whites, and almost four times more likely to die from homicide than whites (Wisconsin Department of Health and Family Services, 2008).

Other health disparities observed by the school nurse and by the director of the reservation's Family Resource Center and Indian Child Welfare Program include higher rates of drug and alcohol use. Historically, we know that fur traders and trappers often used alcohol as part of the barter process with Native Americans, but today's challenges are multilayered. It was noted by the school nurse that more aggressive gang recruitment activity is encroaching on the reservation to target elementary and middle school–age youth. The proliferation of these influences, in addition to poverty, has a great impact on the lives and health of community members.

Some features of diet affect the health of today's Native American community. Dana Irmick points out that the traditional diet of wild rice, game, berries, and nuts was relatively low in fat. Along with government assistance to these groups, however, came "commodities"—that is, food subsidies items that are inexpensive and high in fat and carbohydrates. The introduction of a Western diet can be correlated to many of the comorbidities seen in this community. Prevalent health problems among this population today include diabetes, hypertension, cardiac disease, hyperlipidemia, and obesity.

For health providers trying to gain understanding of any diverse community, Irmick reminds nurses that they need to attend not only to cultural similarities, but also to individual variations within a group. Nurses need to take time to learn about the history of a culture, the socioeconomic realities of an area, verbal and nonverbal communication styles and practices, spirituality, rituals, dietary practices, and family relationships and dynamics of power and respect within the community. Irmick recalls: "One of the first things I needed to examine prior to starting my clinical rotation were my own beliefs and prejudices. I think in order to understand another culture you must understand your own culture as well." Irmick goes on to recommend self-reflection as a necessary strategy to identify what prejudices exist, and to discover what their basis. She explains, "It is harder to imagine the lifestyle or decisions of others, if you already accept that your beliefs and practices are better." This ability to confront preconceived notions and challenge our internal barriers in order to gain new understanding is critical to the development of empathy and our ability to care about and for others. It has been known for some time that empathy is declining among nursing and medical students (Ward Cody, Schaal, & Hojat, 2012; Spencer, 2004; Shapiro, 2008), immersing ourselves in life experiences different from our own is a worthwhile endeavor, and it could be argued, the role of responsible educators of health professionals.

Irmick recommends that students read about a culture beforehand, keeping in mind that there is diversity between and within tribes. She explains that she went to the reservation's museum, cultural center, and to the Waswagoning Indian village to learn as much as she could about the area, culture, and people of Lac du Flambeau. Once she was employed by the tribe, her learning continued as she attended traditional ceremonies, funerals, memorials, and feasts. She emphasizes that this activity was not merely a show of respect on her part, but it became an avenue to begin to actively build trusting relationships and was essential to her acceptance into the community.

Before arriving in the Lac du Flambeau community, Irmick had earlier exposures to other community members through the emergency department (ED) and urgent care settings of an area hospital. She recalls that she was influenced at the time by her lack of knowledge and her own ideas of the concept of *noncompliance* in relation to patients' and family members' lack of follow-through for appointments, instructions, or medications. She explains:

Since working within this community, both as a student and a nurse practitioner, I have learned to forgo these prejudices and to work with patients and their family members to understand their view of health and work proactively to maintain or improve it. I no longer think of noncompliance, but rather I see the apparent inability to follow through resulting from a need for better rapport and further trust building. [As a provider,] I need to understand what each patient wants to know, and how I can be a part of their health care ... it is also vital to understand how a lack of resources (education, money, knowledge) can affect health care and the management of any illnesses that occur.

Her message is this: "As nurses we offer compassion, understanding, and education, while continually reassessing readiness for intervention. This shows respect. Lecturing about noncompliance does not work."

Clearly, this advanced practice nurse is operating within the nursing framework of intentionality, where a heightened awareness enhances the practitioner's ability to look beyond the surface and join families as they are (Hartrick Doane & Varcoe, 2005). Nurses who are intentionally engaged with others in relational moments of practice are actively shaping the health and healing process.

Wright and Leahey (2013), experts on family nursing practice who are embraced internationally, have their own way of driving this point home for seasoned and novice nurses alike. In the sixth edition of their guide to family assessment and intervention, they have devoted an entire chapter to discussing the three errors that they believe occur most frequently in relational family nursing practice: (1) failing to create a context for change, (2) taking sides, and (3) giving too much advice prematurely. Identification of these errors is instructive for nurses in any family practice setting, but is especially applicable when working with families whose culture and worldview differ from our own.

While it is important to identify how a particular population may be vulnerable to health risks, it is equally important for providers to absorb what the community or culture can teach them. When providers are open to learning, the use of alert and keen listening skills can help them reach a therapeutic level of consciousness that can only enrich their knowledge and enhance their own best practice.

THE IMMERSION EXPERIENCE

Although nursing students at the advanced practice level were participating fully in providing health services, this immersion was very much a service–education exchange. In other words, in return for providing health services, students gain an education culturally and contextually, from community members. In the Native American culture specifically, they learned new norms for verbal communication, such as the skill of astute listening to find an answer within a story, while resisting any urge to interrupt or interject. They also encountered new norms for nonverbal communication, such as respecting the importance of silences and pauses in discussion, allowing for a few feet of personal space, and accepting the avoidance of prolonged eye contact (a practice regarded as a sign of respect in Native American culture). In addition, students learned about combining herbal remedies, spiritual practices, and ritual health practices with modern medicine and pharmacology. Moreover, there is much to be learned about family relationships, the parameters of which are very likely to include extended family and close friends. Native American youth are taught to respect elders; likewise, healthcare providers can learn a great deal from elders through their stories. This reciprocity of service–education exchange is rare and precious. It is also one sure way of building a necessary foundation for advocacy.

The course objective when planning this immersion was to critically examine social, cultural, and community influences that affect advanced nursing practice with families. At our university, the planned activities that met this objective also directly satisfied liberal education learning goals of understanding human culture and developing respect for diversity among people. The major participants in the immersion included six graduate students; the faculty clinical instructor; the designated on-site preceptor with advanced nursing practice skills in family health nursing; the clinic staff, which included several Native American physicians and nurses; a physician's assistant; the school nurse at the Lac du Flambeau public school; the public health nurses and dieticians at the Community

Wellness Center; and the individuals and families who agreed to meet or work with us in the clinic, in their homes, and at community gatherings.

In the Peter Christensen Health Center, each student rotated between two designated providers, for both chronic and acute care, and these providers sometimes served as cultural guides. Students participated directly with the seasoned providers in completing assessment updates, and collaborated directly with staff and family members on each plan of care. At the Community Wellness Center, students worked with public health nurses to facilitate group discussion on smoking cessation programs, sexually transmitted infection (STI) awareness, and other topics in funded clinics for Women, Infants, and Children (WIC). Students also accompanied the public health nurses on scheduled home visits to families with newborns or to see adults for chronic disease management. The school nurse's busy routine provided opportunity for interaction with family members when children were sick or injured and needed to be taken home. There was much to be learned from the school about life on the reservation, including how cultural heritage is visibly promoted and honored in the school, yet is complicated by negative forces such as drug involvement and gang recruitment that affect the children outside of school.

The immersion activities for graduate students were designed to be participatory rather than observational. The goals were to encourage students to use appropriate assessment skills, actively promote targeted health teaching, and give direct care when needed, such as dressing changes, to individuals and families using the health services on the reservation. Additionally, students interacted with cultural guides at the reservation's cultural centers, with community and tribal leaders, and they attended informal community gatherings when possible. The reservation was a 4-hour drive from the university, and the on-site lodging for the 7-day duration of the immersion was a nearby hotel, located 12 miles from the reservation.

Cultural Immersion

The cultural opportunities of this immersion were rich. Students worked directly with Native American individuals and families, and the experience was designed to enrich student learning about Native American perspectives on health, which could best be described as a journey as opposed to a labeled health status. Students were directed to expand their parameters of health assessment beyond the individual, progressing to family (clan) and community. Through preparatory reading, students were encouraged to develop an awareness of the Native American core connectedness to the Earth, and to a greater power that teaches reverence for all life forms. The role of family is omnipresent and it typically extends intergenerationally. The students were able to pick up on the ease of collective responsibility for parenting young children within what we would call a closely knit community. Families who observe traditional ways were occasionally observed deferring to their elders in the clinic appointments, at least in matters of decision making regarding health issues.

The providers who worked in this community graciously shared with the students their own knowledge and wisdom gained through years of service. This kind of immersion as a "lived experience" was a privilege for the students and one that could not have been duplicated in its intensity through classroom content or video presentations. Each student created his or her own experience and gave meaning to it in proportion to the student's depth of personal preparation. In turn, this attention to assigned reading and focused orientation activities opened the environment to purposeful reflection, cultural self-examination, and at times, a committed passion.

Immersion Design

A pre-immersion seminar was held on campus prior to travel. A student handbook was prepared for the experience, which included immersion expectations, objectives, and historical and demographic population data to provide initial community background. The handbook documented scheduled events, activities, assignment guidelines, instructions regarding clinic dress code, driving directions, and of course, restaurant information. The "critical guidance plan" seminar, encompassing 6 to 8 hours of discussion, focused on course expectations, clinical activities, and invited speakers. Speakers were guests from surrounding agencies and the historic Indian village, to teach about Ojibwa heritage and cultural traditions, both present and past. Because this was a clinical experience, the usual protocols for healthcare confidentiality were observed as well as review of expectations for individual conduct in etiquette, courtesy, and professionalism. As a group, the students were asked to complete exercises that included an assessment of personal background with socioeconomic survival skills, awareness of individual communication styles, and personal assessment of listening ability.

The on-site immersion experience consisted of an introductory orientation day; 5 consecutive working days, and a post-immersion, on-site debriefing.

EVALUATION OF THE IMMERSION EXPERIENCE

One choice for the on-site debriefing and evaluation was a focus-group format to provide students with an immediate opportunity for verbal feedback, both in the assessment of formal learning content and in the self-appraisal of personal growth toward cultural awareness. In addition to quantitative post-surveys, examples of qualitative post-immersion survey questions were as follows:

- Describe one learning experience from this opportunity that stands out for you.
- Were your expectations met? Explain.

- What did you contribute to your own learning to make it a more valuable experience for you?
- Considered both professionally *and* personally, how did this experience change/influence you?

Post-immersion activities were designed to enhance shared reflection and evaluation of the experience. Although this area cannot necessarily be reflected in the grading process, achieving a greater consciousness is most assuredly transformative. Nursing participants who are able to articulate the personal meaning of the experience will improve their likelihood of becoming more consciously effective and intentional in serving future diverse populations.

The immersion experience yielded many benefits for students. Many times classroom dialogue and the discussion of reading assignments are valuable, but not sufficient to achieve a full understanding of a vulnerable population's perceived needs and challenges. As an enhancement, a focused experience in a contextual environment can be highly effective for high-impact learning. Another benefit of an on-site immersion is the fact that students can be physically transported and "immersed" into a new setting. With some thoughtful planning and concentrated effort in the pre-immersion preparation, students can be coached to instill their own "buffers" to maintain some separation from the distractions of familiar "life as usual."

The immersion experience is based on the premise that meaningful engagement with persons whose shared meanings are different from our own helps us to reflect on the assumptions underlying our own culture, and gives us a way to see the other persons as if for the first time. By becoming more aware of multiple perspectives, we may accomplish the transformative experience of getting to know ourselves in a new way. Guided clinical reflection can be life altering for students who are able to reflect on questions of the human experience, including how experience is created and how it gives meaning to life. With increased understanding of others comes increased understanding of self. Such meaningful engagement can yield greater tolerance, appreciation, and empathic compassion for the well-being of others.

As discussed earlier, the skill of engaged practice is appropriately described as "relational practice" (Hartrick Doane & Varcoe, 2005). My goal for these immersion students was to have them experience the best that education could offer. A cultural immersion can open and enrich one's world in ways that cannot be anticipated.

Students were asked to keep a journal of all of their activities, whether their role was as a participant, observer, or some combination of both. This journal was meant to serve as a basis for guided reflection of each student's journey of exploration and learning and was shared (to a degree) in the post-immersion group session. In addition, a family assessment paper was completed, following guidelines that included a number of socioeconomic, environmental, and cultural factors affecting the health of one family. Finally, a presentation, poster representation, or artistic interpretation of a selected aspect of the immersion experience was developed by each student and shared with a larger peer group on campus. One student organized a display case for the enjoyment ctorsof the college, depicting cultural artifacts and photographs to illustrate her learning about traditional and modern healthcare practices in the immersion community.

In evaluation comments prepared by Dana Irmick, the students revealed to her that they were surprised at the welcoming and friendly nature of both staff and patients. This experience was their first clinical rotation as a nurse practitioner student, and some stated it helped them determine which practice specialization they would seek after graduation. Some participants also mentioned that "working with a whole family seems to be ideal." Irmick characterized the students' response to the experience as "eye opening" and "enjoyable." She reported that the patients and family members also enjoyed meeting the students and sharing their stories with them. All preceptors were given the opportunity to fill out feedback forms for the students who worked with them, and I later shared this information with students individually.

Pre- and post-immersion surveys were administered to the students to document their expectations and to what extent they were met. Students were also asked provide written answers to qualitative questions describing memorable learning experiences and to reflect upon and explain any actions taken or contributions they had made before or during the immersion, to contribute to the value of their own learning.

Students reported that the cultural guides on the tours were very helpful. As one student stated: "Our guide welcomed our questions and appreciated the opportunity to talk about his tribe and their culture." Another student elaborated: "I felt that the guided tour at the village and the museum helped me understand how the tribe portrays itself. The two guides explained what the tribe enjoys, how they live now compared to the past, what they have held onto … what is important in their lives. The history shaped what and how I saw things." She went on to make an important connection:

> With this understanding, I had a better perspective when observing and working with the healthcare providers and community health staff. It explained why they interacted with their patients the way they did. I also had more respect for the providers themselves, if they did not address certain issues I felt were important. They often did this since they are aware that the tribe's culture did not accept certain things.

In response to the question of whether expectations were met, a student replied: "My week of cultural immersion at Lac du Flambeau will be ever present in my life as I share my experiences with others. I will be reflecting on my own experiences but also use these opportunities to educate others about the Ojibwa culture. I believe this experience will continue to affect my personal life and professional career in ways I am only beginning to comprehend and it will continue to have a profound effect on me."

Under "other comments," a student wrote the following:

Most Americans know very little about the governments of indigenous people and even less about their diverse cultures, values, and lifeways ... Instead, they receive information through popular culture, mass communication outlets, and not through personal contact. Academic programs and teachers need to influence students to learn as much as they can about the history and partner with tribal people to help eliminate negative stereotypes about Native Americans and address unconscious racism that may be involved. I will be forever grateful to UW–Eau Claire for initiating this cultural immersion experience for graduate students and that I was able to participate.

Another student remarked:

I would highly recommend continuing this experience with future classes; it provided an opportunity I don't believe can necessarily be offered in a traditional once- or twice-a-week clinical experience. I'm very thankful I was able to participate.

Another student wrote of an immersion highlight:

The home visit with a new mom with breastfeeding concerns was an excellent experience. The nurse provided great teaching for the family while providing positive reinforcements. Being welcomed into an Indian home was a humbling experience. I was able to witness their current culture first hand. Were my expectations met? Yes. My expectations were exceeded daily.

CONCLUSION

The goal of the immersion was to combine required family nursing skills for advanced practice nursing with self-growth in areas of cultural sensitivity and awareness. Whether this immersion can fully achieve cultural competence depends on how one defines cultural competence. However, if this term is taken to mean sensitivity to differences and respect for client values and traditions as an integral part of our nursing care, then we are surely moving closer to the goal. This immersion sought to give students confidence in approaching new situations with increased wisdom and curiosity. With the emphasis on listening skills in cultural immersion experiences, future nurses will be equipped to approach diverse patients and vulnerable populations with greater empathy, more open minds, and greater generosity of spirit in the goal of creating an environment for health and healing.

REFERENCES

Benzein, E., Johansson, P., Arestedt, K. F., & Saveman, B. I. (2008). Nurses' attitudes about the importance of families in nursing care: A survey of Swedish nurses. *Journal of Family Nursing*, *14*(2), 162–180.

Hartrick Doane, G., & Varcoe, C. (2005). *Family nursing as relational inquiry: Developing health-promoting practice*. Philadelphia, PA: Lippincott Williams & Wilkins.

Ho, V. (2009). Native American death rates soar as most people are living longer. Retrieved from http://www.seattlepi.com/local/403196_tribes12.html

Nauright, L., & Wilson, A. (2012). Preparing nursing professionals to be advocates: Service learning. In M. de Chesnay & B. Anderson (Eds.), *Caring for the vulnerable* (3rd ed., pp. 465–474). Burlington, MA: Jones & Bartlett Learning.

Shapiro, J. F. (2008). Walking a mile in their patients' shoes: Empathy and othering in medical students' education. *Philosophy, Ethics, and Humanities in Medicine, 3*, 1–11.

Spencer, J. (2004). Decline in empathy in medical education: How can we stop the rot? [Editorial]. *Medical Education, 38*, 916–920.

Thomas, J., Sage, M., Dillenberg, J., & Guillory, V. J. (2002). A code of ethics for public health. *American Journal of Public Health, 92*(7), 1057–1059.

Ward, J., Cody, J., Schaal, M., & Hojat, M. (2012). The empathy enigma: An empirical study of decline in empathy among undergraduate nursing students. *Journal of Professional Nursing, 28*(1), 34–40.

Wisconsin Department of Health and Family Services. (2008). *Minority health report, 2001–2005*. Retrieved from http://www.dhs.wisconsin.gov/publications/P4/P45716.pdf

Wright, L., & Leahey, M. (2013). *How to avoid the three most common errors in family nursing*. In L. Wright & M. Leahey (Eds.), *Nurses and families: A guide to family assessment and intervention* (6th ed., pp. 309–319). Philadelphia, PA: F.A. Davis.

Chapter 37

Teaching Psychiatric and Community Health Simulations for Vulnerable Populations

Mary de Chesnay, Dori Cole, Johnathan Steppe, and Jennifer Bartlett

OBJECTIVES

At the end of this chapter, the reader will be able to

1. Explain the role of the nurse educator graduate student.
2. Explain how developing nursing simulation experiences can provide a meaningful preceptorship for nurse educator graduate students.
3. Describe simulation experiences in community health nursing and psychiatric-mental health nursing.

INTRODUCTION

In this chapter, the role of the nurse educator graduate student is explained with special attention to how the student might use a precepted course to develop simulations for undergraduate courses in community health nursing and psychiatric-mental health nursing. Precepted courses are those in which students identify a faculty member with whom they would like to work, assist with the teaching load of that faculty member, and often engage in scholarly activities with the faculty member. The second author is a current graduate student writing this chapter as part of her precepted experience. The third author is a new graduate who conducted his preceptorship with the coordinator of community health nursing and who has experience with developing psychiatric simulations. The fourth author is a simulation coordinator at a state university.

Previous editions of this book have highlighted how some creative graduate faculty members prepare their students to work with vulnerable populations. In the first edition, Phillips and Peterson (2005) described projects their students completed for a master's-level course on vulnerable populations. In the second edition, Peterson and colleagues (2008) discussed the process of mentoring master's degree students as they sought to develop innovative practice models for vulnerable populations. These projects generated a vulnerability assessment model, a way to help students understand the complexity of vulnerability by using a game (Jenga) and a form of play with visual symbols as a way of modeling (a bicycle and barbells). The third edition described international fieldwork in Mexico by nurse practitioner students (de Chesnay, Dorman, & Bennett, 2012). The current edition presents ideas from nurses who integrated individualized experiences throughout their master's education that were specifically designed to support their professional development as nurse educators.

SIMULATION

In the current climate of competition for traditional clinical placements, nurse educators have had to develop innovative strategies to prepare students for the clinical agencies. Although nursing, a practice-based profession, has traditionally incorporated basic forms of simulation throughout nursing curricula, recent technologies provide the opportunity for enhanced teaching and learning. For example, it is now possible to teach basic concepts such as aseptic technique by using manikins that not only provide body parts, but also talk and respond to students' actions, thereby increasing the level of interaction and fostering critical thinking and clinical reasoning. Because this chapter focuses on community health and mental health nursing, a brief review of the literature on simulation in those specialties is presented here.

Psychiatric-Mental Health Nursing Simulation

There is emerging literature regarding use of simulation in psychiatric-mental health nursing, with an emphasis on developing communication skills. Experienced practicing nurses were likely trained under live supervision, in which clinical supervisors and peers observed interaction with real clients in mirrored rooms. They did not have the benefit of access to simulations prior to interactions with real patients or clients. Presently, virtual patients and computerized scenarios are being used that enable students to practice in a safe environment in which mistakes cause no harm (Becker, Rose, Berg, Park, & Schatzer, 2006; Brown, 2008; Dearing & Steadman, 2008; Guise, Chambers, & Valimaki, 2012; McGarry, Kashin, & Fowler, 2012). These virtual environments, similar to those depicted in the video game *Second Life*, provide the opportunity to create a customized scenario that simulates specific environments, patients, and details, thus providing the opportunity to depict vulnerable patients in a myriad of situations designed to drive student learning. Although many ready-made virtual simulations focus on the medical-surgical client, including a National League for Nursing (NLN) collaboration with Laerdal Medical (Laerdal Medical, 2014), not many of these virtual simulations depict vulnerable populations. There is certainly room for expansion into the specialty of psychiatric-mental health nursing.

Although the use of standardized patients (SPs) provides the opportunity to introduce nuanced behaviors and facilitates the development of interpersonal relationships, high-fidelity simulation is a model that can be used to teach core principles of psychiatric-mental health nursing. Gasper and Dillon (2012) recently introduced structured, evolving simulation scenarios on the topics of: (1) narcotic overdose/bipolar disorder, (2) paranoid schizophrenia, and (3) lithium overdose. The simulations were designed to be used with high-fidelity manikins and/or with simulated patients. In a study comparing traditional format with high-fidelity simulation, self-efficacy was significantly improved in the simulation group and students rated the experience positively (Kameg, Mitchell, Clochesy, & Suresky, 2009; Sleeper & Thompson, 2008). Similarly, simulation can be useful in teaching mental health students to recognize and intervene appropriately when psychiatric patients experience physical illnesses. In a United Kingdom study, nurse faculty devised three videotaped scenarios for senior undergraduate students and found improved recognition of and response to alcohol intoxication, drug-induced psychosis, and chest infection in patients with Alzheimer's disease (Unsworth, McKeever, & Kelleher, 2012). In a phenomenological study with 52 senior-level nursing students, the researchers found that simulation training helped participants to improve intervention in patients hearing voices (Dearing & Steadman, 2009).

Community Health Nursing Simulation

Many of the techniques of therapeutic communication, family interviewing, and group process in psychiatric nursing are appropriate to community health nursing, but because community health nursing encompasses such a diversity of settings and strategies, simulation techniques need to be refined. Two studies were found in which specific strategies for using simulation for community health patients were used. An older study conducted in the UK used simulation and post-simulation interviews to examine students' knowledge base for community health nursing. While the researcher found considerable strength in simulation, they argue that the post-simulation interview is crucial to establish that learning did indeed take place (Bryans & McIntosh, 2000). In a recent study, Smith and Barry (2013) examined the outcomes of a simulation study with 56 senior community health nursing students. The experimental group participated in a home care visit and high-fidelity simulation experience with an elderly client with diabetes. While no differences were found between groups on performance, the simulation students reported significantly higher satisfaction and confidence.

In a book dedicated to promoting the creation, implementation, and evaluation of quality simulations for nursing students, Jeffries (2012) and her contributing authors prepare examples and templates that incorporate caring for vulnerable populations. For example, a simulation template designed to incorporate the tenets of the Quality and Safety Education for Nurses (QSEN) competencies highlights the nursing role when interacting with a patient for whom English is a second language (Durham & Alden, 2012). Aschenbrenner, Milgrom, and Settles (2012) provide a template that uses several different home visits with the student as the home care RN. In 2010, the NLN released unfolding cases as part of their Advancing Care Excellence for Seniors (ACES) initiative; three of these cases are specifically related to the care of patients with Alzheimer's disease. These toolkits include pre-work that introduces the patient simulation scenario templates that move the story forward, and post-work that encourages students to "finish the story" (NLN, 2013). All of these resources provide concrete ideas for nursing educators as to how to incorporate simulation into nursing education that addresses diverse populations in varied healthcare settings.

COMMUNITY HEALTH NURSING SIMULATION CASE STUDY

Case 1: Cole

One of the requirements for obtaining my online MSN with a concentration in nursing education was to precept with a college faculty professor in an academic setting for one semester. At first, I was very concerned I would not be able to find a professor willing to serve as my preceptor. However, I reached out to several universities and professors and was very fortunate to receive an opportunity to precept under Dr. de Chesnay at Kennesaw State University, WellStar School of Nursing and participate in an undergraduate community health nursing class. As part of the preceptorship experience, I developed two alternative simulations, visited undergraduate students at clinical sites throughout the greater Atlanta area, attended faculty meetings, gave two lectures, and assisted in grading journals and papers. The preceptorship activities and close interaction with my preceptor and other faculty members was a very positive teaching/learning experience and provided this graduate student with a glimpse of what it might be like to work in a university environment as a nurse educator.

Faculty and students have both expressed concern about the difficulty students may have in fulfilling their clinical hour requirements in the community health nursing course because of the limited number of clinical sites available for students to attend and limitations on the hours of operation at these sites. For example, one student was assigned to an elementary school and the combination of school hours, holiday breaks, and the student's own class schedule made it difficult for the student to complete all her hours. Alternative simulations can be designed for students to take at their leisure and allow the students to fulfill any unmet clinical hours.

Developing the simulations was a significant component of my preceptorship. Dr. de Chesnay selected two topic areas for which I developed alternative simulations for vulnerable populations. The first simulation I created was designed to provide the baccalaureate nursing student with an opportunity to assess health status, living conditions, and potential home hazards involving elderly and children living together and to identify ways to eliminate or mitigate those hazards. The first step involved creating a case study for the assignment that introduced unique family traits, cultural background, and circumstances that the student nurse would need to take into account when developing a patient family–centered care plan. Developing a case study generally has no bounds and is only limited by one's knowledge, experience, and imagination.

The family that I created for this case study included six people living together who recently immigrated to the United States with ages ranging from 15 months to 72 years. The baby had acid reflux and the grandmother was a recently diagnosed type 1 diabetic. For this simulation, I walked around Dr. de Chesnay's home and assessed it for potential hazards for children and elderly populations. I assessed the home for hazards that are specific to children (e.g., outlet covers) and for elderly people (e.g., throw rugs). I then made a list of the potential hazards, developed a checklist against which the observations of the students could be measured, and prepared a plan for how the simulation would be run.

By participating in the assignment, I was a co-learner and able to share my experience and background with the nursing students and appreciate their learning experience and be able to improve the simulation based on my experience. The assignment demonstrated that there are many home hazards that are often overlooked and the simulation allowed me to make my own home safer and eliminate potential hazards to elderly visitors and children. The simulation also emphasized the importance of how nurses need to communicate with families and build a trusting relationship so that the family members will act on the nurse's recommendations to mitigate home health hazards. The simulation could be improved by having students visit multiple homes, thereby exposing students to a larger number of potential home hazards; however, this would require greater student time commitment and coordination. Students were also requested to suggest ways to improve the simulation. This student feedback can be useful for helping to identify ways to improve the teaching/ learning experience. Unfortunately, no nursing students participated in this simulation because the simulation was not ready until the end of the semester and students did not need additional hours.

The second simulation was designed to provide nursing students with an opportunity to understand, through role playing, how a person with a disability functions in society and to assess the barriers that they face in performing activities of daily living. This activity and the first alternative assignment helped me to meet the course objectives in my graduate class: (1) to define self as a co-learner with students, (2) analyze the dynamics of the teaching/learning process in the clinical setting, and (3) evaluate teaching strategies and methods for education effectiveness.

In this simulation, students were assigned to go to a local grocery store that has a motorized wheelchair on their own time with a partner (could be a classmate or friend.) Students were instructed to inform the store manager that they are nursing students and ask for permission to use the motorized wheelchair. The assignment was to shop for a healthy yet affordable meal in the motorized wheelchair, assess the conditions for shopping (availability and maneuverability of motorized wheelchair, aisle width, shelf height, crowding, etc.), and observe people's behavior in treating someone with this disability. Based on the experience, students described what changes, if any, should be made to accommodate persons with disabilities in the store.

Students were also asked about who should be contacted to make these changes because future nurses need to become change agents and must be able to work with public and private policy makers to facilitate changes on behalf of the vulnerable populations they serve.

I participated in the assignment and found it to be a very humbling experience. Wheelchair-bound people should be able to go anywhere in the community and certainly be able to shop for food. I found the motorized wheelchair to be very difficult to maneuver in the grocery store aisles. It was also extremely difficult to reach for and take items off the shelves. The grocery store that I visited does however offer to do the shopping for shoppers who are disabled. I was not aware of this service, as it is something that is not well advertised due to the demand and number of workers available to provide this service. Nurses need to learn about the different services and support networks that are available for people with disabilities so that they can teach patients about different available strategies to meet their individual needs.

PSYCHIATRIC-MENTAL HEALTH NURSING CASE STUDY

Case 2: Steppe

Before my nursing career, I worked as an actor and received a bachelor of arts from a state university. While there, I participated in a standardized patient program that the university's medical school had developed to assist their students with therapeutic communication techniques for mentally ill patients. The program was designed as an interdisciplinary partnership between the school's medical and theatre departments, with all actors recruited from students who were enrolled in the college of fine arts. I became eligible to participate in the program during my junior year, and I continued my participation until graduation. In addition to providing experience with improvisational acting, the program paid a small stipend. During the experience, I portrayed patients with a wide range of psychiatric illness, including bipolar disorder, schizoaffective disorder, borderline personality disorder, and major depressive disorder. Although the program's main objectives were to facilitate development of communication techniques in medical students, it also had a lasting impact on many of the actors. My participation broadened my understanding of the challenges faced by those living with mental illness, giving me a new level of empathy for this population.

Accurately portraying a person with mental illness can be challenging. Therefore, theatre faculty selected potential participants enrolled in junior- or senior-level acting classes. They provided interested students with contact information for the coordinating faculty, who then set up interviews with potential participants. Once accepted, participants received packets that contained the information and resources necessary to accurately construct their characters. The packets included selected readings that detailed each patient's diagnosis. Often, they provided transcripts from interviews with persons living with the selected illness. When available, the packet offered lists of resources such as movies, novels, or works of nonfiction that actors could use to supplement their character study. Sometimes, specific objectives for the scenario were identified. For example, I once played a patient who was at risk for suicide, and one of the major objectives of the simulation was for the interviewing students to identify that risk.

Generally, we had 4 to 6 weeks to prepare for a simulation. After receiving our packets, we studied them for a week, and then met with coordinating medical faculty who discussed the case with us and offered guidance for our character building. We then spent several more weeks preparing for our role. During this time, we might delve into some of the additional resources provided, or rehearse with fellow theatre students. If necessary, medical faculty were available to further discuss the case. As we rehearsed, we also constructed our characters physical appearance, deciding on whatever clothes or props we felt would enhance our performance. We developed movements, mannerisms, patterns of speech. The theatre department's costume shop loaned any materials that we could not ourselves provide. As the simulation grew closer, we participated in a rehearsal with supervising medical and theatre faculty who provided recommendations to strengthen our performance. For the actor, this preparatory phase was crucial. Without adequate preparation and guidance, our performances would not have been authentic, and the verisimilitude of our portrayals directly impacted the quality of the simulation experience.

The simulation was held several times throughout the semester. Each simulation day lasted 6 to 8 hours, with a break for lunch halfway through the sessions. The sessions involved pairs of students who, in the role of healthcare provider, engaged the actors in conversation using therapeutic communication techniques learned earlier in the semester. The interviewing students directed the course of the session, while we reacted to their performance. Although the sessions were not scripted, the actors had been taught to recognize predetermined triggers that would signal them to advance the scenario in certain directions. These triggers included helpful, therapeutic techniques as well as those that were considered counterproductive. Based on the situation, the actors rewarded students who used appropriate communication; for example, the actor might decrease their level of hostility or begin sharing their feelings with the interviewer. Conversely, the actors escalated the situation when confronted with inappropriate techniques or behavior. The interviewers then had a chance to modify their strategies based on the actor's responses. Each simulation ran between 15 and 20 minutes, followed immediately by a short debriefing session.

Overall, students responded positively to the experience. Many commented how the use of actors kept them focused in the simulated scenario. Some found the actors' portrayals so convincing that they became uncomfortable during the process, and afterward stated that they felt they were interviewing a real patient. However, there were always some students who initially struggled with suspending their disbelief. These students found it challenging to remain "in the scene;" they might laugh or make comments that broke out of the simulated encounter. In these cases, the actors were instructed to remain in character and to treat such comments as unhelpful communication. This might mean they escalated the situation in response to the break in simulation protocol. Interviewing students quickly learned to remain in the situation to avoid unnecessary escalations.

At the end of each session, supervising faculty conducted a debriefing session during which they provided feedback on students' performances. The students in turn discussed what worked well for them, as well as how they could improve future interviews. They described any particular challenges they faced. The faculty then offered suggestions for overcoming these difficulties. Debriefing sessions also included the actors, who discussed their perceptions of the students' performances. The actors described the rationale behind their reactions, identifying for students the triggers that led to a particular change in behavior. Debriefings were relaxed and nonjudgmental; participants were never berated for taking a particular course of action.

Upon completing the simulation, participants were given the opportunity to evaluate the process. Faculty distributed evaluation forms not only to the interviewing students, but also to the actors, who provided feedback from their perspective. Faculty then modified the experience as needed. The program quickly became popular among theatre students who recognized an opportunity to hone improvisational skills (while earning their first paychecks as actors). Overall, the program was a success on several levels: it gave medical students practice using therapeutic techniques with mentally ill patients in a safe environment, it provided theatre students a chance to perform professionally, and it forged an interdisciplinary alliance between the university's medical school and the theatre department.

CONCLUSION

In this chapter the authors provided examples of how simulation can be used to enhance graduate education and preparation for undergraduate teaching using simulation in community health and psychiatric-mental health nursing. These examples are a beginning attempt to show cost-effective strategies for expanding undergraduate clinical experiences in a safe environment as well as to facilitate interdisciplinary collaboration among students in the humanities and healthcare fields. The highly technological simulations used in the adult health, pediatric, and obstetric arenas clearly have their place, but community health and mental health lend themselves to low-cost simulations that can be accomplished without expensive equipment.

REFERENCES

Aschenbrenner, D. S., Milgrom, L. B., & Settles, J. (2012). Designing simulation scenarios to promote learning. In P. Jeffries (Ed.), *Simulation in nursing education: From conception to evaluation* (2nd ed., pp. 217–230). New York: National League for Nursing.

Becker, K., Rose, L., Berg, J., Park, H., & Schatzer, J. (2006). The teaching effectiveness of standardized patients. *Journal of Nursing Education, 45*(4), 103–111.

Brown, J. (2008). Applications of simulation technology in psychiatric-mental health nursing education. *Journal of Psychiatric and Mental Health Nursing, 15,* 638–644.

Bryans, A., & McIntosh, J. (2000). The use of simulation and post-simulation interview to examine the knowledge involved in community health assessment practice. *Journal of Advanced Nursing, 31*(5), 1244–1251.

de Chesnay, M., Dorman, G., & Bennett, D. (2012). Working with graduate students to develop cultural competence. In M. de Chesnay & B. Anderson (Eds.), *Caring for the vulnerable* (pp. 475–482). Sudbury, MA: Jones and Bartlett.

Dearing, K., & Steadman, S. (2008). Challenging stereotyping and bias: A voice simulation study. *Journal of Nursing Education, 47*(2), 59–65.

Dearing, K., & Steadman, S. (2009). Enhancing intellectual empathy: The lived experience of voice simulation. *Perspectives in Psychiatric Care, 45*(3), 173–182.

Durham, C. F., & Alden, K. R. (2014). Integrating the QSEN competencies into simulation. In P. Jeffries (Ed.), *Simulation in nursing education: From conception to evaluation* (2nd ed., pp. 217–230). New York: National League for Nursing.

Gasper, M. & Dillon, P. (2012). Clinical simulations for nursing education. Philadelphia: FA Davis.

Guise, V., Chambers, M., & Valimaki, M. (2012). What can virtual patient simulation offer mental health nursing education? *Journal of Psychiatric and Mental Health Nursing, 19,* 410–418.

Jeffries, P. R. (Ed.). (2012). *Simulation in nursing education: From conception to evaluation* (2nd ed.). New York: National League for Nursing.

Kameg, K., Mitchell, A., Clochesy, V., & Suresky, J. (2009). Communication and human patient simulation in psychiatric nursing. *Issues in Mental Health Nursing, 30,* 503–508.

Laerdal Medical. (2014, February 12). *NLN content featured in virtual simulation product from Laerdal Medical and Wolters Kluwer Health: vSim for nursing/medical-surgical based on curricular content developed by the National League for Nursing.* Retrieved from http://www.laerdal.com/us/News/49212597/NLN-Content-Featured-in-Virtual-Simulation-Product-from-Laerdal-Medical-and-Wolters

McGarry, D., Kashin, A., & Fowler, C. (2012). Child and adolescent psychiatric nursing and the "plastic man": Reflections on the implementation of change drawing insights from Lewin's theory of planned change. *Contemporary Nurse, 41*(2), 263–270.

National League for Nursing (NLN). (2013). *Faculty program and resources: Advancing care excellence for seniors–Unfolding cases.* Retrieved from http://www.nln.org/facultyprograms/ facultyresources/aces/unfolding_cases.htm

Peterson, J., Anderson, H., Mercado, J., Shellhorn, J., Speyer, J., & Thiagarag, L. (2008). Designing a model for predicting or working with vulnerable populations based on graduate fieldwork. In M. de Chesnay & B. Anderson (Eds.), *Caring for the vulnerable* (pp. 483–496). Sudbury, MA: Jones and Bartlett.

Phillips, D., & Peterson, J. (2005). Graduate studies' approach to vulnerability. In M. de Chesnay & B. Anderson (Eds.), *Caring for the vulnerable* (pp. 385–394). Sudbury, MA: Jones and Bartlett.

Sleeper, J., & Thompson, C. (2008). The use of hi-fidelity simulation to enhance nursing students' therapeutic communication skills. *International Journal of Nursing Scholarship, 5*(1), 1–12.

Smith, S., & Barry, D. (2013). An innovative approach in preparing students for care of the elderly in the home. *Geriatric Nursing, 34*(1), 30–34.

Unsworth, J., McKeever, M., & Kelleher, M. (2012). Recognition of physical deterioration in patients with mental health problems: The role of simulation in knowledge and skill development. *Journal of Psychiatric and Mental Health Nursing, 19*, 536–545.

V

Policy Implications

Chapter 38

Public Policy and Vulnerable Populations

Jeri A. Milstead

OBJECTIVES

At the end of this chapter, the reader will be able to

1. Identify key concepts of vulnerability that are terms used by policy makers.
2. Describe how agendas are set, implemented, and evaluated by policy makers.
3. Discuss the ways in which nurses can influence legislation.

INTRODUCTION

Government policies that target vulnerable populations may seem like an oxymoron (if we can use that word to explain a phrase). On the one hand, vulnerable populations may be difficult to define. On the other hand, vulnerable populations may not have much of a voice to articulate their plight. How and to whom in government do "populations" direct their pleas—agencies? programs? This chapter seeks to define vulnerable populations, examine the policy process, and consider issues inherent in linking the two. Examples are provided of how nurses can work within the policy process for the benefit of vulnerable populations.

DEFINITIONS

The term *vulnerable populations* is a latecomer to nursing literature; "special populations" first appeared in 1995 as a descriptor in *The Cumulative Index to Nursing and Allied Health Literature* (CINAHL) in 1995, but "vulnerability" did not appear until 1997.

Users of the term vulnerable populations often mean to refer to groups of low socioeconomic status (the poor and those out of work), the underserved (i.e., those who lack health insurance or lack access to healthcare delivery), persons with diagnoses in certain disease categories (e.g., diabetes, congestive heart failure), persons with chronic illness (arthritis, AIDS), or those at risk for developing disease or illness. These terms are not really interchangeable, however. For example, all diabetics are not poor, and low socioeconomic status may not indicate the presence of chronic disease. Thus, these terms may not accurately reflect either vulnerability or populations.

CINAHL (2002) includes a category of vulnerability that is defined as "the state of being at risk or more susceptible physically, mentally, or socially" (p. 405). Flaskerud et al. (2002) define vulnerable populations as "social groups who experience health disparities as a result of a lack of resources and/or increased exposure to risk" (p. 75). The two major concepts incorporated in these definitions appear to be the degree of risk and the experience of health problems without access to resources. However, a full understanding of vulnerable populations requires a deeper look.

Flaskerud et al. (2002) addressed the evolution of knowledge about vulnerable populations from the 1950s to the early 2000s through a study of articles published in *Nursing Research*. Although the study was not comprehensive, in that writings from other journals or other sources were excluded, the researchers chronicled terms that were used in investigating groups or aggregates. Only one study was published in the 1950s, which focused on chronically ill aged adults. Group identity was based in the 1960s on socioeconomic status, education, occupation, gender, or race. The literature of the 1970s noted "race, ethnicity, and gender" (p. 76), with research at this time focusing on high-risk parents, infants, women, and immigrants. The concept of culture and its effect on the delivery of health care came into the literature in the 1980s (Leininger & McFarland, 2002). Reported as an "influence" in outcomes of social groups, culture became the context for studying a variety of societal problems that were not limited to either health or health care.

The concept of health disparities did not surface until late in the 1990s, when this term was introduced to reflect differences in health care and outcomes among many groups, such as adolescents and the elderly, women and infants, and low- and middle-income families. Ethnic groups also were studied as groups, often with a focus on the quality (or lack thereof) of health and health care. Quality was approached through professional accountability (vis-a-vis ethics and standards), marketing accountability (as evidenced in informed choices), and regulatory accountability (as reflected in government action) (Taub, 2002). Although the marketing method seemed prominent at that time, the regulatory scheme used the Health Plan Employer Data and Information Set (HEDIS), hospital discharge data from the now-defunct Health Care Financing Administration (HCFA), and information on the quality of managed care organizations from the National

Committee for Quality Assurance. Since 1991, the Medicare Current Beneficiary Survey collects "data on the utilization of health services, health and functional status, healthcare expenditures, and health insurance and beneficiary information (such as income, living arrangement, family assistance, and quality of life" (Office of Disease Prevention and Health Promotion, n.d.).

In the early years of the 21st century, many terms surfaced that referred to vulnerable populations. *Uninsured* became a blanket term for poor and low-income people, regardless of their gender, ethnicity, or employment status. Researchers discovered that the uninsured, which included the working poor, had more health problems than persons who carried insurance. The homeless, as a group, were uninsured (often because they were also unemployed) and exhibited many physical and mental health problems. The range of health disparities was great. Migrant workers were considered *disadvantaged* (Ward, 2003), and often less attention was paid to their health concerns than the health issues of established workers. African Americans (Plowden & Thompson, 2002; Richards, 2000) and Latinos (Campinha-Bacote, 2002) experienced much inequity related to health care. The disabled were identified as having social and physical barriers to health (Harrison, 2002). Those who lived near hazardous waste sites were considered at increased risk for serious health problems (Gilden, 2003). Finally, the term *vulnerable populations* evolved to include whole populations, not just aggregates of individuals, as identifiable groups.

On an international scale, migration is occurring from rural areas to urban areas. Nurses often are the key care providers in rural areas. Resettlement of individuals and populations from farm to city, although providing greater opportunities for jobs and higher salaries, often results in a serious lack of healthcare services for the rural underserved population (Buchan, 2006).

POLICY PROCESS

When they hear the term *policy*, many people think of legislation or laws. Although legislation may be its most recognizable component, the policy process includes many other components. When discussing public policy (as opposed to private-sector policy), the author of this chapter means the process of taking problems to the administration that can or should be addressed by government and obtaining a governmental response. (The author notes her opinion that not all social problems warrant governmental action.) Within this broad approach, four major aspects are evident: agenda setting, government response, program and policy implementation, and program and policy evaluation.

The policy process is not always linear or sequential. That is, one does not always start with agenda setting and move immediately to government response. A nurse, for example, may initially become involved during program implementation after a law has been signed. A garbage can model of organizations (Cohen, March, & Olsen, 1982) provides a foundation for considering the process of making public policy as the inter-weaving of streams of problems, policies, and politics. These streams mingle in government circles, often joining and breaking apart as ideas and solutions are considered, rejected, or reconsidered (Kingdon, 1995). At times, a solution hooks up with a problem, and a window of opportunity opens that results in creation of a program that addresses the difficulty. The following brief discussion of each component of the policy process reveals opportunities for becoming involved in these activities.

AGENDA SETTING

The national agenda is a list of items to which the president and his advisors (known as the administration) attend. Agenda setting is the activity in which problems are brought to the attention of the administration. If the president is not interested in a problem, it has little chance of being addressed. The issue is how to get the president's attention (Furlong, 2015). Crises can propel an issue onto the national agenda. For example, the attacks of September 11, 2001, brought immediate attention to the issue of terrorism, and funding was made available for projects and programs such as the establishment of the Department of Homeland Security.

One of the issues in agenda setting is defining a problem so that it is palatable to the administration and to the public. When HIV/AIDS was first discovered, for example, it was defined as a problem of intravenous drug users and homosexuals. The Reagan administration believed that the public would not support funding for research into the cause or treatment of the disease, so little funding was forthcoming. When children like Ryan White and heterosexual non-drug users began to get the disease (most often from infected blood products), the disease was redefined as a community health problem, and funding was made available.

Nurses are experts at choosing words and scenarios to describe problems. Creative use of language may not be necessary in alerting an administration to a problem, but one should know how to use key words to advantage. The point in defining a problem is to pique the interest of the administration so that a solution can be found. Knowing that the public will scrutinize funding options is part of the context of defining the difficulty.

GOVERNMENT RESPONSE

The government may respond to a problem in several ways. The three most common responses are enactment of a law, a regulation, or a program. Policy experts develop these activities in policy communities. Policy communities are loosely knit groups of people who can provide expertise about an issue and who, for the most part, work in government agencies. Policy experts often know one another through professional associations, the literature or other media exposure, or prior experience. In many situations, legislative aides, who serve as staff in the offices of legislators, are good contacts for nurses who want to connect with "insiders." Experts discuss problems, suggest solutions, and exercise their opinions about the relative political worth of issues. Legislative aides in one legislator's office often talk informally with legislative aides in other legislators' offices and with staff in government agencies, faculty in university settings, and members of special-interest groups to establish a priority list and to consider alternative solutions. Nurses who have cultivated relationships with government policy staff have a golden opportunity to be recognized as experts who are sought out to consider problems (Wakefield, 2008).

Laws are made in legislative sessions that last 2 years. Bills (potential laws) are introduced throughout the session, but bills introduced early have a better chance of action. The "how a bill becomes a law" page that can be found in nearly every basic government or political science textbook provides a simplified overview of the steps for moving a bill from introduction to signature by the president. Neither legislators nor their aides are expected to know everything about the myriad issues brought to their attention, as these issues range from health to transportation to the economy to defense and beyond. Nurses have a wonderful opportunity to serve as experts on many health issues. A nurse can provide a one-page overview of a problem, a summary of relevant research in ordinary language, and phone or email information to pave the way for a serious contact.

Seasoned nurses understand the importance of informal processes—political processes. Many nurses shun the idea of politics, thinking it to be a tainted process that skews judgment and biases legislators. On the contrary, the political process is merely the exercise of persuasion and education to one's perspective. What nurse has not spoken informally to others before a decision was made in an effort to gather support, challenge a conclusion, or talk out a problem? The same communication techniques are used with legislators and their staffs or anyone in the policy community. Reflection, active listening, and clarification are therapeutic communication skills that are integral to how nurses approach others. The art of using talents in this way should be natural for nurses.

The legislative process must be followed carefully, and nurses must be vigilant for amendments that may either help or hurt their causes. Developing strong, positive relationships with legislators, staff, and other interested parties' results in a network that leads to "inside" information. Working at the subcommittee level is a more efficient use of time than letting a bill get to the committee level, but it is important to stay with a bill through its passage by both houses of Congress and, in many instances, a conference committee where final negotiations are completed. Nurses may recommend language for inclusion in drafting a bill or an amendment and must be cognizant of amendments that could derail or inhibit passage of the legislation.

Once a bill becomes a law that establishes a program, the program is assigned to a government agency for implementation. The choice of which agency is designated as the controller of the program is very political. Not all health programs go to agencies in the Department of Health and Human Services. Some, for example, go to the Department of Defense (for piloting by the military), the Department of Education (school health programs), the Department of the Treasury (drug enforcement programs), or other departments and agencies. The choice may be based on past experience with similar programs, the chance for an infusion of new funding needed by an agency, rejection of a program due to lack of time or expertise, or many other reasons.

The regulatory process is similar to the legislative process in that legislative action is required. However, the regulatory process is governed by the Administrative Procedures Act, which dictates a specific format and course. All proposed rules require notification of the public, an established period of time for public comment, and public announcement of the final rule. The *Federal Register* is the vehicle for publication of information on federal issues.

Public comment can take the form of letters, email messages, phone calls, or in-person visits to the appropriate agency. All comments must be considered before the final rule is adopted. The comment stage is a particularly easy way for nurses to involve themselves in expressing their opinions about potential rules. Communication should be brief, focused, and identifiable (i.e., specific to the rule on which you are commenting). Arguments should be stated clearly and prefaced by whether you are for or against the issue or section of the rule. Solutions are welcomed.

IMPLEMENTATION

Implementation is a fluid process that involves getting a program up and running. Agency staff may need assistance in determining eligibility. That is, who is entitled to participate? Who is excluded from participation? What are the criteria, and who monitors participation? Nurses can suggest policy tools, such as incentives (waivers, coupons), educational brochures, posters advertising a program, or learning tools (training sessions), to assist staff in operating a program (Smart, 2015).

Nurses should confer with agency personnel, known as street-level bureaucrats, who are putting the programs into operation. These street-level bureaucrats often use ideas from program participants or program staff about how to streamline programs or make them more efficient or user-friendly. Nurses may provide tips about the population being served or thoughts about how a program could be conducted. Sometimes programs can be expanded to include broader involvement or shrunk to remain within the legislative intent and purpose. Nurses can provide concrete assistance and guidance by recommending ideas about how to alter the provision of a program.

In his classic work on implementation, Bardach (1977) identified games that are played by agency personnel during the implementation phase of a program. Many of the games have to do with budget, policy goals, and administrative control. For government agencies, spending funds early and requesting additional funding later is one way to increase a budget. Encouragement of overspending, known as boondoggling, can be seen when consultant fees exceed the budget. Inflation of the estimated cost of a program is a way of padding a budget so that some of the funds can be used later (e.g., as discretionary funds) or in ways different from the original intent.

Nurses study implementation to determine to what extent programs meet the original policy goals (Wilken, 2015). They investigate any modifications that were made and seek explanations for changes. Researchers examine the level of difficulty or "tractability" of the initial problem and whether technology was accessible to address the problem. On one hand, the range of services provided by a program may produce variation in program performance such that many services might dilute operations negatively. On the other hand, successful programs can become a target for piling on additional objectives. The idea is to be part of a thriving program, but to avoid the inclusion of too many extra activities that may result in program failure.

EVALUATION

Evaluation is rarely conducted and usually is not part of an original program plan, despite the vast body of literature that recommends appraisal as part of monitoring program success. Such an evaluation should be both formative and summative.

Formative data can help bureaucrats determine progress during implementation, informing decisions about whether the program should continue to function as usual or whether a change in direction should be sought. Formative data can also indicate whether resources are adequate and are being distributed appropriately.

Summative data can be useful for evaluating public programs for effectiveness or outcomes, not just efficiency or outputs. That is, what difference does it make to the public good if thousands of poor women are offered free mammograms? Has this screening method resulted in significant prevention or early treatment of breast cancer? This is not to say that efficiency is not worth assessing, because a poorly run program will waste tax dollars.

Evaluative reports should be provided to agency personnel, legislators, and the public. Charts and other visual media can be used to present aggregate data, identify trends, and track progress. Reports may contain recommendations for adjusting goals and objectives or implementation strategies.

LINKING THE POLICY PROCESS AND VULNERABLE POPULATIONS

Agenda Setting

Nurses can propel issues of vulnerable populations onto the national agenda by defining needy groups, serving as a voice for vulnerable populations, and alerting legislators to problems that affect the public health. For example, the homeless usually are not organized in any formal way and have little voice as a group. Their worries about health care may go unheard unless someone, known as a policy entrepreneur, makes available his or her reputation, money, or other resources on their behalf. A nurse can serve as an entrepreneur or can mobilize the media to take up a cause.

Issues of social justice are political issues. Discrimination against marginalized populations and against people based on health status, income, employment status, or type of disease or disability is unethical and unjust and may be illegal in the United States. The distribution and allocation of resources is also a political process. The choice of which problems get on the national agenda is very political, and nurses are skilled in political interaction because of their expert ability to communicate and think critically. Nurses must take up the mantle of social problems, especially health problems, for those who cannot or do not speak for themselves. In the truest sense of the term *advocacy*, nurses also must educate vulnerable populations about how to advocate for themselves. Self-advocacy is empowering for every population.

Nurses can help bureaucrats define problems in ways that help the public understand and value them. Drug users, for example, are often unemployed or financially poor, and may be disenfranchised in the public eye because of related crimes. (In contrast, employed drug users often go undetected by the general public and escape bias [Milstead, 1993].) Legislators ignore or shun known drug users as a group, often because officials perceive that the "druggies" create violence, do not vote, and are not organized politically.

In the 1980s, social activists (including nurses) formed groups such as the Association for Drug Abuse Prevention and Treatment (ADAPT) and the AIDS Coalition to Unleash Power (ACT UP) as vehicles to address drug use and health. Members recognized the link between gay men, intravenous drug users, and HIV/AIDS, and a few created needle exchange programs and served as policy entrepreneurs. These volunteers changed the terminology used from drug "addict" to drug "user," recognizing this transformation as one way to change the public's perception of a vulnerable group. Notably, volunteers in Tacoma, Washington, and New York City educated legislators, bureaucrats, and public health officials about HIV transmission and the need for research on diagnosis and treatment (Milstead, 1993). Communications techniques such as consciousness raising and the use of sound bites were developed to a high level.

Policy entrepreneurs may take years to attain their goals. Indeed, some of the first groups of volunteers related to drug use and health are still staffing needle exchange programs on the streets and working with state legislatures to obtain legitimacy for their programs. Most needle exchange programs in the United States are still operating.

Government Response

Laws are composites of language that reflect the wishes and priorities of those who craft them. Laws often are the result of negotiation and compromise among many people with disparate philosophies and values. Nurses can help shape laws by means of their expertise in health care and healthcare delivery. Congressional representatives usually do not know much about diseases such as diabetes or tuberculosis. A nurse who has nurtured relationships with elected officials by becoming a contact for health issues and providing understandable explanations of medical terminology has a great opening to contribute to language as a bill is being constructed. A nurse's knowledge of current issues can be a tremendous help to legislators or their staff. Nurses also bring anecdotes to the policy community that put a personal face on an issue.

The elderly, for example, are often considered a vulnerable population. This designation may be confusing because the term does not necessarily refer to low socioeconomic status, the underserved, or disease categories for older persons. Instead, "elderly" cuts across all types of categories. As a vulnerable population, there is inference of risk and lack of resources for health care for the elderly, specifically in relation to an increased danger of suffering disease or disability and a lack of resources because of fixed incomes. The elderly have a strong, organized lobby through AARP. During the early years of the 21st century, AARP waged a campaign in the U.S. Congress to create protection for members (aged 50 years or older) in the form of a program for funding prescription drugs.

The Medicare Prescription Drug, Improvement, and Modernization Act of 2003 (MMA) amended Title XVIII (Medicare) of the Social Security Act to add a new Part D (Voluntary Prescription Drug Benefit Program), under which each individual who is entitled to benefits under Medicare Part A (hospital insurance) or Medicare Part B (supplemental medical insurance) is entitled to obtain qualified prescription drug coverage. The law was passed by both the House of Representatives and the Senate and became public law 108-173 on December 8, 2003 (MMA, 2003). Many people found that prescription costs soared under this law and vulnerable populations who were supposed to have been helped actually suffered when they could not afford needed medications. Nurses, physicians, and other healthcare providers participated in a focused assault on legislators in an effort to influence the form of the bill before it became law. Senators and representatives held hearings, met with lobbyists and AARP members, talked with constituents, and discussed issues within the policy community. The issue evolved into a hotly debated partisan battle, but compromise language created a bill that was acceptable enough to pass the Republican-dominated House and Senate. Herein lies a caveat: Although the bill has been signed into law, many changes must be made as the program continues to be implemented.

The Medicare prescription plan is an example of how the streams of agenda setting, government response, and implementation interconnect. During efforts to move the issue of prescription costs onto the national agenda, work already was in process to determine alternative solutions, and the basic rudiments of a program were already being conceived.

Implementation

An example of a purely symbolic policy action is the Stewart B. McKinney Act of 1987. Vladeck (1990) studied the homeless, including their characteristics, causes of homelessness, and health status of homeless persons. He chronicled the evolution of a joint initiative between the Robert Wood Johnson Foundation and the Pew Charitable Trusts that became a model for a program that would provide federal support for the homeless. Even though there was agreement among policy makers that homelessness was a problem worthy of government intervention, authorization of funding did not eliminate the problem or even address most of the social, economic, health care, and other issues. The McKinney Act was symbolic in that legislators could document an attempt to address the issue of homelessness, even if the issue had little probability of being resolved.

A brief search for initiatives about the homeless in the 111th Congress shows a plethora of attempts in which bills were introduced but stalled in committee or subcommittee (www.loc.gov). (Note that relief for vulnerable populations can be addressed within a variety of committees and through a variety of topics.) House of Representatives (H.R.) 4484 Strengthening Healthcare Options for Vulnerable Populations was referred to the subcommittee on Health, a subset of the House Ways and Means, Energy, and Commerce Committee. H.R. 834 Improving Access to Child Care for Homeless Families Act of 2013 was referred to the House Health, Education, Labor, and Pensions Committee. S. 2646 Runaway and Homeless Youth and Trafficking Prevention Act was referred to the Senate Committee Judiciary. Two companion bills, H.R. 3120 and S. 1522, Comprehensive Dental Reform Acts, would have amended titles XVIII (Medicare) and XIX (Medicaid) laws by authorizing dental care for low income, underserved, prisoners, and Indian tribes. These two bills were referred to the House subcommittee on Military Personnel and the Senate committee on Finance, respectively. None of the bills were voted out of committee.

Evaluation

Evaluation of health policy that affects vulnerable groups does not occur often at the program level. Rather, policy itself is more typically evaluated through research. Nurse-led studies in the 1990s and the early 2000s reported in *Nursing Research* (Flaskerud et al., 2002), for example, evaluated resources available for Hispanics, Cubans, African Americans, Filipinos, lesbians and other women, men, low-income families and age-related groups, and the homeless. Disease categories included mental illness (including depression), chronic illness, addictive disease, pregnancy, injuries, and specific populations with asthma, hypertension, HIV/AIDS, lung and heart disease, sexually transmitted diseases, and tuberculosis. The discovery of health disparities between vulnerable groups and the general population indicated that the former have higher levels of risk and less access to healthcare providers and resources.

Research has also uncovered problems in defining vulnerable populations, specifically in relation to issues of race and ethnicity. The Institute of Medicine, for instance, challenged the National Institutes of Health (NIH) to replace the term *race* with *ethnic group* (Oppenheimer, 2001). The Office of Management and Budget (OMB) sets policy about which racial and ethnic classes are to be referenced by any federal agency, although OMB recognizes that these terms are based on ill-defined social or political types, not scientific categories. The American Anthropological Association adopted the concept of race/ethnicity as an interim combined term, but the category of race was eliminated in the 2010 national census. Thus researchers must take care to define race or ethnicity clearly as they study various groups. Issues related to vulnerable groups will be subject to increased scrutiny in the future, and federal agencies that authorize programs, initiate policies, and appropriate funds must take into consideration the legal, governmental, cultural, and historic implications of terms.

Sudduth (2015) asserts that nurses "are not strangers to evaluation" (p. 194). She urges advanced practice nurses to transfer the skills they use to determine outcomes in a healthcare setting to evaluation of government programs. "Social programs are public policy made visible" (p. 197), and nurses are well equipped to determine the worth, efficacy, and efficiency of many programs.

CONCLUSION

Nurses work with vulnerable populations in the provision, administration, and evaluation of health care. Public officials design policies in response to problems that rise to the agenda-setting attention of the president and his advisors. The policy community is involved in defining problems, prioritizing their value, and seeking and considering alternative solutions. Legislators, their staff, special-interest groups, and others in the community of interest draft government responses to the problems, often in the form of laws, regulations, and programs.

Nurses must integrate their political knowledge and skill into their professional lives. Nurses can identify problems, bring them to the attention of lawmakers, keep them from fading from public view, suggest redefinitions, and propose alternative solutions. Nurses must persevere throughout this process by using their expertise to help legislators choose policy tools and implement and evaluate programs and policies. Public officials are not used to nurses participating actively in the process of policy making; therefore, nurses must initiate the contacts, provide information that a layperson can understand, and acknowledge those legislators or bureaucrats who respond positively and move government to action.

Nurses are experts in the provision of health care, especially for the vulnerable. Not only do nurses have an ethical obligation to inform policy makers on issues for which at-risk populations have little or no voice, but as professionals they must recognize that they will cede their societal accountability if they do not.

REFERENCES

Bardach, E. (1977). *The implementation game: What happens after a bill becomes a law.* Cambridge, MA: MIT Press.

Buchan, J. (2006). The impact of global nursing migration on health services delivery. *Policy, Politics, & Nursing Practice, 7*(3), 16S–25S.

Campinha-Bacote, J. (2002). The process of cultural competence in the delivery of healthcare services: A model of care. *Journal of Transcultural Nursing, 13*(3), 181–184.

Cohen, M., March, J., & Olsen, J. (1982). A garbage can model of organizational choice. *Administrative Science Quarterly, 17*, 1–25.

Cumulative index to nursing and allied health literature (CINAHL). (2002). Glendale, CA: EBSCO Publishing. Retrieved from www.ebscohost.com/cinahl

Flaskerud, J. H., Lesser, J., Dixon, E., Anderson, N., Conde, F., Kim, S., … Verzemnieks, I. (2002). Health disparities among vulnerable populations. *Nursing Research, 51*(2), 74–85.

Furlong, E. A. (2015). Agenda setting. In J. A. Milstead (Ed.), *Health policy and politics: A nurse's guide* (5th ed., pp. 45–68). Burlington, MA: Jones & Bartlett Learning.

Gilden, R. C. (2003). Community involvement at hazardous waste sites: A review of policies from a nursing perspective. *Policy, Politics, & Nursing Practice, 4*(1), 29–35.

Harrison, T. C. (2002). Has the Americans with Disabilities Act made a difference? A policy analysis of quality of life in the post–Americans with Disabilities Act era. *Policy, Politics, & Nursing Practice, 3*(4), 333–347.

Kingdon, J. W. (1995). *Agendas, alternatives, and public policies* (2nd ed.). New York, NY: Harper Collins.

Leininger, M., & McFarland, M. R. (2002). *Transcultural nursing: Concepts, theories, research and practice* (3rd ed.). New York, NY: McGraw-Hill.

Medicare Prescription Drug, Improvement, and Modernization Act of 2003 (MMA). (2003). Retrieved from http://www.gpo.gov/fdsys/pkg/BILLS-108hr1enr/pdf/BILLS-108hr1enr.pdf

Milstead, J. A. B. (1993). *The advancement of policy implementation theory: An analysis of three needle exchange programs.* PhD dissertation, University of Georgia, Atlanta, GA. Retrieved from Dissertations and Theses A&I (Publication Number AAT 9329821).

Office of Disease Prevention and Health Promotion, (n.d.). Retrieved from http://www.healthypeople.gov/2020/Leading-Health-IndicatorsHealthy People.

Oppenheimer, G. M. (2001). Paradigm lost: Race, ethnicity, and the search for a new population taxonomy. *American Journal of Public Health, 91*(7), 1049–1054.

Plowden, K. O., & Thompson, L. S. (2002). Sociological perspectives of black American health disparity: Implications for social policy. *Policy, Politics, & Nursing Practice, 3*(4), 325–332.

Richards, H. (2000). And miles to go before we sleep: Rising to meet the challenges of ending health care disparities among African-Americans. *Journal of National Black Nurses Association, 11*(2), 2.

Smart, P. (2015). Policy design. In J. A. Milstead (Ed.), *Health policy and politics: A nurse's guide* (5th ed., pp. 151–169). Burlington, MA: Jones & Bartlett Learning.

Sudduth, A. L. (2015). Policy evaluation. In J. A. Milstead (Ed.), *Health policy and politics: A nurse's guide* (5th ed., pp. 189–217). Burlington, MA: Jones & Bartlett Learning.

Taub, L.-F. M. (2002). A policy analysis of access to health care inclusive of cost, quality, and scope of services. *Policy, Politics, & Nursing Practice*, 3(2), 167–176.

Vladeck, B. (1990). Health care and the homeless: A political parable for our time. *Journal of Health Politics, Policy and Law*, 15(2), 305–317.

Wakefield, M. (2008). Government response: Legislation. In J. A. Milstead (Ed.), *Health policy and politics: A nurse's guide* (3rd ed., pp. 65–88). Sudbury, MA: Jones & Bartlett.

Ward, L. S. (2003). Migrant health policy: History, analysis, and challenge. *Policy, Politics, & Nursing Practice*, 4(1), 45–52.

Wilken, M. (2015). Policy implementation. In J. A. Milstead (Ed.), *Health policy and politics: A nurse's guide* (5th ed., pp. 171–188). Burlington, MA: Jones & Bartlett Learning.

Chapter 39

The Samfie Man Revisited: Sex Tourism and Trafficking

Mary de Chesnay

OBJECTIVES

At the end of this chapter, the reader will be able to

1. Differentiate between sex tourism and sex trafficking.
2. Discuss the health implications of the sex tourism and trafficking industries.
3. Describe the roles of specialty nurses (psychiatric-mental health, community health, and nurse practitioners) in helping people who have been trafficked.
4. Explain the kinds of policy changes that need to occur in order to eliminate human trafficking.

INTRODUCTION

This chapter calls attention to some key issues related to the growing problem of modern-day slavery—in particular, sex slavery. Sex tourism and sex trafficking are described herein and clinical reports presented that illustrate some of the health issues encountered by the vulnerable women and children who are the major victims of sex traffickers and tourists.

It is important to distinguish between prostitution and the majority subset of prostitutes who are slaves (Butcher, 2003). Some confusion persists in the literature and media about the two, and Cusick, Kinnell, Brooks-Gordon, and Campbell (2009) warn that prostitution is not always a result of trafficking. Some would argue that there is a population of prostitutes who are consenting adults and that they should not be viewed as criminals, but this is a discussion for another place and detracts from the major problem of women and children enslaved in the sex trade.

This chapter focuses on those sex workers who are the victims of traffickers and those who are in the business of providing sex to tourists. The term *samfie man* is used to capture the essence of those who prey on people around the issues of sex. Samfie man is a Jamaican word meaning con man, often one who pretends to use witchcraft to trick people. This chapter was inspired by meeting one of these individuals who happened to come from Jamaica, but the term can easily be used to describe any scam artist. In this chapter, it may be difficult to tell the difference between the samfie man and his prey, as some of the victims eventually become the exploiters.

Sex tourism refers to travel for the express purpose of engaging in sexual encounters with people of different races, with individuals of different ethnicities, or, frequently, with underage partners. Sex trafficking is modern slavery functioning as a global business that promotes exploitation of men, women, and children primarily for sex but also as a source of cheap labor. For the purposes of this chapter, the samfie man is the villain in each of the case studies—the man or woman who introduced the person to a life of exploitation and abuse.

SEX OFFENDERS

There would be no market for sex tourism and trafficking if there were not a huge number of sex offenders worldwide. Whether they are pedophiles, rapists, wife beaters, or just sociopaths who indulge their own needs at the expense of others, consumers of sex trafficking and sex tourism create both victims and opportunities for the criminal organizations that make money by selling sex. In a bizarre twist of logic, however, victims of child sex trafficking are often treated as criminals because they are trained to be seducers and the "johns" are simply seen as customers instead of child sex predators (Jayasree, 2004; Raymond, 2004; Williamson & Prior, 2009). Thus prostituted children are placed in juvenile detention facilities, while their customers go free.

One argument made in the literature is that legalizing prostitution might provide an answer to decriminalizing the victims. Similar to those who advocate legalizing certain drugs (marijuana, for instance), proponents of this view suggest that legalization of prostitution would not only decriminalize "consensual" prostitution but also remove the need for involvement of criminal organizations in the sex industry and decrease the level of violence associated with prostitution. This argument seems to assume that prostitutes engage in selling sex for money because they prefer to earn a living this way. While sex between consenting adults is one thing, it is difficult to view women engaged in prostitution as choosing prostitution as a career, when the stories they tell about how they entered the life so obviously focus on coercion—that is, coercion by family or friends who destroy their sexual innocence, cons by people they meet who take advantage of their gullibility to pretend to help them find their dream of modeling or acting, and kidnapping by organized rings of traffickers.

SEX TOURISM

Sex tourism refers to vacations to destinations where the primary purpose of the trip is to have sex with people far away from home—that is, away from the home-based rules of conduct and social controls. In some cases, the prostitutes are "consenting adults"; often, however, they are current or former victims of predators who have coerced or finessed them into a life of selling sex for the profit of their handlers.

The Caribbean has experienced shifts in mobility of locals from agricultural jobs in isolated rural areas to cities and resort areas that support a growing tourism industry. The shift has accounted for some residents' increased vulnerability to foreigners looking for sex. These rural people come to the city looking for work, which is often unavailable, so they sell their bodies to survive. They are transformed from what they grew up believing they were (traditionally heterosexual) to what the market demands (homosexual or bisexual). In one study in the Dominican Republic, interviews with 72 Dominican male sex workers with male clients revealed how they maintain their own sense of masculinity in what the researchers called "staged authenticity" to counteract the negative stereotypes of homosexuals and increased risk of HIV/AIDS (Padilla, 2008).

In Peru, tourists come not just to look at Machu Pichu (Bauer, 2008), but also to engage in sex with locals who are different from themselves. The phenomenon of "bricherismo," which is practiced in Cuzco, exploits the Incan culture for the purpose of sex with foreigners who favor men with long hair who speak Quechua and claim to be descended from the Inca. This practice creates new disease trends in isolated areas and a need for public health education for hospitality employees.

The people whom the tourists seek for sex are often minors. This demand for minors, in turn, creates a market for trafficking in children both in the United States and abroad (Kotrla, 2010; Williamson & Prior, 2009). The preference of customers for young victims feeds the virginal fantasies of the johns (Dickson, 2004).

SEX TRAFFICKING

Bales (2009) estimated that 27 million people are victims of human trafficking at any one time and that 80% of these are women and children trafficked for sex. However, women and children trafficked for forced labor are likely to be sexually abused as well. A conservative estimate is that approximately 50,000 women and children are trafficked into the United States each year for the purposes of sex slavery (Miller, Decker, Silverman, & Raj, 2007). Others are trafficked for labor but will not be discussed here, as this chapter focuses on the sex trade. Although governments increasingly recognize trafficking as a serious problem, few have found ways to help the victims (Svrivankova, 2006).

ORIGINAL FIELDWORK

The clinical cases presented in this chapter resulted from fieldwork in Jamaica to examine family structure (de Chesnay, 1986a, 1986b). At that time, the author was conducting doctoral research on family variables as part of a cognate in anthropology. In the course of field trips and subsequent visits to Jamaica and later Central America, she came across individuals who were involved in sex work. As a nurse, she found that people felt comfortable talking to her about the most intimate details of their lives. They often shared problems and issues spontaneously, similar to what nurses and physicians experience at social gatherings when people tell them about their ailments.

THE CLINICAL REPORTS

The cases reported here were inspired by real people but have been substantially disguised to protect their privacy, to the extent that the clinical reports are essentially fictional and represent the stories of hundreds of people who have been victimized by traffickers and tourists. It is important to stress that these people were telling their stories openly but not within the context of research. The institutional review board (IRB) permission covered the family structure study; the clinical cases were outside that context. However, over the years, the author has had interactions in other parts of the world that have focused her attention on the extent of the problems of sex workers and victims of the traffickers. As a nurse, the author wants to call attention to the health issues of people, but the wider social context is social justice health policy.

Ideally, presenting these stories will call attention to the necessity for governments to do more to protect their citizens. The implications for nurses include the critical need to take thorough histories for people who present with any indications they might have been sex workers at some point.

The dangers of the sex trade inhibit people from calling the authorities. People who are sold are commonly told that they or their families will be killed if they tell, resist, or try to escape. Therefore, it is imperative that nurses and other health professionals who treat these patients do so within a climate of safety and security, protecting not only their confidentiality under privacy laws, but also shielding them from further abuse at the hands of the predators.

Magda

Magda is a 25-year-old woman from Russia who entered a contest at the age of 13 in Moscow to fulfill her dream of becoming a high-paying fashion model. From a poor family, she had three younger siblings and yearned to help her parents provide a better life for them. Her family was happy and hard working but poor, and she wanted to ease the financial burden on her parents. Magda was told that she had made the contest finals and would be flown to Paris, where she would be photographed by a famous fashion photographer whose name she recognized from the magazines she and her friends read at the library. She was escorted onto an airplane by a "husband and wife," who told her that they had her parents' permission for the trip, but that she could not see them to say goodbye because they had to make the next flight in order to meet with the busy photographer. The couple also said that she must pretend to be their daughter because she did not have her own passport. If she refused to play along, they said, her parents "would get in a lot of trouble with the police." Magda was told how pretty she was and how much money she would make as a model, and the couple promised to help her set up a bank account to send the money back to her parents.

Once she arrived in Paris, Magda was placed in a warehouse with a dozen other women of many nationalities. The woman who escorted her learned she was a virgin and let slip that she would earn much money but she had to be "prettied up." She had her hair styled and cosmetics applied, and she was given beautiful clothes to wear for the photoshoot by a man who said he was an assistant to the famous photographer. Then she was placed in a locked room separate from the other women. By the time she realized she had been sold to traffickers, she had no way to communicate and no one to ask for help.

Magda was sold to a wealthy man who treated her well at first but tired of her when she reached her 15th birthday. At that point, he gave her to his friend, who preferred teenagers. She was passed around until she became so sick from sexually transmitted diseases (STDs) and malnutrition that she was sold to a pimp who turned her out on the street. Repeated beatings and threats to kill her if she tried to escape or return home were successful at intimidating her, to the point that Magda lost the will to resist. She was told that her parents and younger siblings would be killed if she did not cooperate. Eventually rescued by an aid organization, Magda was malnourished, diseased, and broken in spirit. Her prognosis for recovery is minimal without help beyond what the organization can provide.

Rita

Rita and David prey on affluent men and women from the United States and Europe who go to the Caribbean as sex tourists looking for partners of a different race. They specialize in heterosexual activities but are not averse to homosexual encounters if the price is right. As attractive people, they command a high price. They save their money with the idea of retiring early and leaving the business—they dream of a life in Europe, living among the jet set.

Rita is David's partner both in life and in crime. She is a beautiful, light-skinned black woman who keeps fit and wears expensive clothes and jewelry that she can well afford or that are given to her as gifts by her regular clients. Her story begins at the age of 20, when her parents disowned her after they discovered she was servicing the wealthy American and European men who came to the Caribbean. Rita was making enough money to support herself and then became involved with David, who rescued her from a pimp. The two became business partners and backed each other up as well as designing their cons for the tourists.

Rita is not retired. She states that she is young and beautiful enough to attract the wealthiest clients and that she can afford the luxury of accepting only men (or women) she can tolerate in bed. Her body is fit, and she maintains her sexual health. She becomes angry at any thought that she is vulnerable, preferring to view herself as completely in control of her life.

David

David is a handsome man in his mid-30s with dark hair, soft brown eyes, and extremely polite manners that mask his contempt for most people. He describes himself as a sex worker who specializes in affluent white American women who come to the Caribbean as sex tourists to have sex with black men. He is independent but works with a partner (Rita). David emphatically refuses to work with pimps—individuals whom he sees as the lowest form of humanity. He is very protective of Rita and backs her up when she is with a client. At the same time, he reports that he has no difficulty taking advantage of the wealthy women he services since "they get what they deserve and I give them their money's worth."

David takes good care of himself and sees a doctor regularly for STD check-ups. His presenting problem to the nurse is gastrointestinal pain and frequent diarrhea for which he takes Imodium and ibuprofen, but he is beginning to think there is something more seriously wrong than indigestion. When he learns that his diagnosis of Crohn's disease could seriously affect his business, he begins a series of doctors' visits in an attempt to find someone who can "make this go away" without surgery. During the period of doctor shopping, he becomes severely depressed and considers suicide. David's income and lifestyle depend on his clients seeing him as desirable sexually, and he is terrified of living with Crohn's disease with its unpredictable and embarrassing flare-ups.

Luisa

Luisa is a young woman in her late teens from Guatemala who was sold to sex traffickers at the age of 5 by her parents, who were desperate for money to feed their 10 other children. The contrast between the poverty of her family's life and her own lifestyle as a sex worker often makes her wonder whether she would have been better off at home with her parents, yet she does not blame them for selling her. She views the sale of their oldest daughter as her parents' desperate attempt to save the family, and she has convinced herself that she is tough enough to handle the 20 to 25 men she is expected to service daily. If she falls short, she is beaten and deprived of what little food the handler gives her.

Luisa was 5 years old when she was first sent to a brothel, where she was brutally raped by a man whose job was to prepare her for her new life. She was hurt, confused, and terrified not only at the brutality but at the whole of her world crumbling. She had been starved for lack of food at home, but her family treated her with kindness to the extent that they were able. She held onto the idea that she is saving her family, which allowed her to tolerate her unbearable life.

At the age of 12, Luisa was swept up in an undercover sting operation. A police officer posing as a john was able to arrest her current handler, but the handler was part of a ring with major financial backing and the ringleaders went free. Luisa was placed in a juvenile detention facility because her family could not be found. Even if they could be found, authorities would not have released her to the people who sold her to traffickers. In a misguided attempt to convince her that her lifestyle was her parents' fault for selling her, the "therapist" assigned to her by the aid organization paradoxically took away the only comforting thought that had maintained Luisa during her years of abuse—that she was helping her deserving family. Immediately after this session with her therapist, Luisa succeeded in killing herself with an overdose of aspirin.

HEALTH ISSUES

HIV/AIDS and STDS

Perhaps not surprisingly, trafficking is largely responsible for the AIDS pandemic. In China, for example, commercial sex workers and injection drug users have introduced HIV into the population of Yunnan province, which has a higher rate of HIV than other provinces (Xiao, Kristensen, Sun, Lu, & Vermund, 2007). It seems clear that there is a relationship between trafficking and HIV/AIDS due to the increased rates of infection that trafficked individuals face in destination countries (Vijeyarasa & Stein, 2010). The authors Dharmadhikari, Gupta, Decker, Raj, and Silverman (2009) focused on the trafficking of Nepalese women and girls to India and found lower but significant rates of infection, with 15 of 287 trafficked individuals, aged 7 to 32 years at the time of being trafficked, returning home HIV-positive.

Mental Health Issues

Post-traumatic stress disorder (PTSD) is an obvious effect of sexual exploitation, but perhaps even more insidious is the destruction of self-esteem. Women and children who have been trafficked view themselves as worthless and experience a kind of numbing of the soul. Some might call this clinical depression, and some of these women do try to kill themselves. Others find the strength to live on in the hope that their lives will change (de Chesnay, 2013a, 2013b).

LEGAL INTERVENTION

In March of 2013, President Obama signed the Trafficking Victims Protection Reauthorization Act (H.R. 972), after receiving unanimous congressional approval for the legislation (U.S. Department of State, 2014). This law reauthorizes and expands the original 2000 law, which focused on international human trafficking by targeting the purchasers of illegal sex acts—that is, the customers and traffickers who exploit domestic victims. That provision, known as the End Demand for Sex Trafficking Act, focuses on halting the trafficking of people, primarily women and children, in the United States for purposes of sexual slavery. The "End Demand" measure is designed to help police investigate and prosecute sex trafficking cases. It also will provide funds to assist trafficking victims, including the establishment of residential care centers for underage children. Under the legislation, studies and conferences to ascertain progress in this area will be conducted regularly (Strode, 2006).

While the United States' legislation centers around helping the victims, it is first necessary to identify and define them as victims. Similar to the treatment of rape and child molestation, it is useful to define them as "survivors" during treatment and when interacting with them, but make no mistake—these people are victims and if defining them as victims helps to obtain scarce resources for them, it is not only acceptable, but preferable to do so.

Child victims of traffickers are clandestine and may be hard to reach. Identifying victims becomes easier when one realizes that the behaviors of victims are similar to the behaviors linked with substance abusers (since they are sometimes drugged by their handlers in order to control them.) Other indicators are missing school (if they are even allowed to attend school) and worldly knowledge, gained by being shipped around or having contact with johns who move around and talk about their work.

The United States focuses on providing a safety net for victims through shelters, PTSD treatment, medical intervention for trauma and disease, psychological help, and medications. These interventions are obviously needed, but we need to go further in decriminalizing the victims of trafficking. What is wrong with the picture when a child like Luisa is locked in a juvenile detention center and the traffickers to whom she was sold go free?

POLICY IMPLICATIONS

At this writing, several measures are in place to protect trafficked victims. Some countries seem to be taking this more seriously than others and the U.S. Department of State (2014) rates many on their progress by publishing an annual report of the extent to which countries are creating and enforcing measures to address human trafficking within their borders. The Trafficking in Persons (TIP) report rates countries as Tier 1, 2, 3, or 4; with 1 being the best rating and 4 indicating little or no progress. Rankings are based on progress in victim services, criminal prosecution, partnering with nongovernmental organizations (NGOs), and reintegration of victims, among other criteria.

T-Visa

Despite the debates about immigration reform, it is possible to offer slaves who are trafficked into the United States a T-visa to avoid automatic deportation to their home countries where they may be captured by the original traffickers. Among the requirements are

- Are now or were a victim of trafficking, as defined by law
- Are in the United States, American Samoa, the Commonwealth of the Northern Mariana Islands, or at a port of entry due to trafficking
- Comply with any reasonable request from a law enforcement agency for assistance in the investigation or prosecution of human trafficking (or under the age of 18 or unable to cooperate due to physical or psychological trauma)
- Demonstrate that you would suffer extreme hardship involving unusual and severe harm if you were removed from the United States (U.S. Department of Homeland Security, 2013).

Domestic Minor Sex Trafficking

In the United States, we seem to be more comfortable emphasizing policies, laws, and services for children who find themselves in the sex trade. Certainly some advocate groups pay attention to migrant workers and news outlets that cover stories about foreign workers trafficked abroad, but nothing touches American hearts like the stories of children who are abused and enslaved. Thanks to Senator Renee Unterman, (R-45, GA) Georgia was the first state to develop a state-wide response to the commercial sex exploitation of children. A task force was created from the Governor's office and the honorary chair was Mrs. Sandra Deal, the First Lady of Georgia. As a member of the task force, my most significant contribution was to invite our student nurses to attend. The outcome was that not only are they members of the various working groups, but they also sponsored a resolution at both their state and national student nurses' conventions that schools of nursing should address human trafficking in the curricula (see the chapter by Collins, Chance, and Williams in this edition.)

Policies Needed: Reduce the Demand

Attention on the problem has been focused on decriminalizing the victim and prosecuting the traffickers, which is all well and good, but if there were no customers, there would be no profit and subsequently no trafficking. One of the leaders in reducing demand for sex trafficking is Shared Hope International, which issues its annual report card on the progress of states to address child sex trafficking (Shared Hope International, 2013). According to the most recent data, states that received an "A" meaning they are making substantial progress are: Washington, Louisiana, and Tennessee. States that received an "F" meaning little to no progress are: California, Michigan, South Dakota, Pennsylvania, Hawaii, and Maine.

A fairly new program to address the problem of American sex tourists going abroad for sex involves the passport as the essential document that enables citizens to travel. The Secretary of State can prohibit or withdraw passports for known sex offenders or tourists who are caught abroad (Legal Information Institute, n.d.)

CONCLUSION

When I worked in the early 1970s with my first patient who had been trafficked, I thought slavery had ended with the Emancipation Proclamation. Nothing is further from the truth. Human trafficking is fast-growing and profitable for those who prey on the vulnerable. Human trafficking is a global problem and the health effects are pandemic. Nurses need to educate themselves to recognize and treat survivors with compassion and not judge them for a choice they could not make for themselves.

ACKNOWLEDGMENTS

This chapter was derived from a paper presented to the Society for Applied Anthropology in Santa Fe, New Mexico, during their conference held April 5–10, 2005.

REFERENCES

Bales, K. (2009). *The slave next door: Human trafficking and slavery in America today*. Berkeley, CA: University of California Press.

Bauer, I. (2008). "They don't just come for Machu Picchu": Locals' views of tourist–local sexual relationships in Cuzco, Peru. *Culture, Health and Sexuality, 10*(6), 611–624.

Butcher, K. (2003). Confusion between prostitution and sex trafficking. *Lancet, 361*, 1983.

Cusick, L., Kinnell, H., Brooks-Gorden, B., & Campbell, R. (2009). Wild guesses and conflated meanings: Estimating the size of the sex worker population in Britain. *Critical Social Policy, 29*(4), 703–719.

de Chesnay, M. (1986a). Jamaican family structure and sex roles. *Journal of the Alabama Academy of Sciences, 57*(3), 153.

de Chesnay, M. (1986b). Jamaican family structure: The paradox of normalcy. *Family Process, 25*, 293–300.

de Chesnay, M. (2013a). Psychiatric-mental health nurses and the sex trafficking pandemic. *Issues in Mental Health Nursing, 34*(12), 901–907.

de Chesnay, M. (2013b). *Sex trafficking: A clinical guide for nurses*. New York: Springer Publishing.

Dharmadhikari, A., Gupta, J., Decker, M., Raj, A., & Silverman, J. G. (2009). Tuberculosis and HIV: A global menace exacerbated via sex trafficking. *International Journal of Infectious Diseases*, 13(5), 543–546.

Dickson, S. (2004). *Sex in the city: Mapping commercial sex across London*. London: The Poppy Project, Eaves Housing for Women. Retrieved from www.womeninlondon.org.uk

Jayasree, A. (2004). Searching for justice for body and self in a coercive environment: Sex work in Kerala, India. *Reproductive Health Matters*, 12(23), 58–67.

Kotrla, K. (2010). Domestic minor sex trafficking in the United States. *Social Work*, 55(2), 181–187.

Legal Information Institute. (n.d.). Retrieved from http://www.law.cornell.edu/uscode/text/22/212a

Miller, E., Decker, M., Silverman, J., & Raj, A. (2007). Migration, exploitation and women's health: A case report from a community health center. *Violence Against Women*, 13(5), 486–497.

Padilla, M. (2008). The embodiment of tourism among bisexually behaving Dominican male sex workers. *Archives of Sexual Behavior*, 37, 783–793.

Raymond, J. (2004). Prostitution on demand: Legalizing the buyers as sexual consumers. *Violence Against Women*, 10(10), 1156–1186.

Shared Hope International. (2013). *Protected innocence challenge: A legal framework of protection for the nation's children*. Retrieved from http://sharedhope.org/wp-content/uploads/2014/02/2013-Protected-Innocence-Challenge-Report.pdf

Strode, T. (2006). President Bush signs bill targeting sex trafficking, says U.S. has duty in fight. Retrieved from http://erlc.com/article/president-bush-signs-bill-targeting-sex-trafficking-says-us-has-duty-in-fig

Svrivankova, K. (2006). Combatting trafficking in human beings. *International Review of Law, Computers and Technology*, 20(1–2), 229–232.

U.S. Department of Homeland Security. (2013). Retrieved from http://www.uscis.gov/humanitarian/victims-human-trafficking-other-crimes/victims-human-trafficking-t-nonimmigrant-status

U.S. Department of State. (2014). U.S. laws on trafficking in persons. Retrieved from http://www.state.gov/j/tip/laws/

Vijeyarasa, R., & Stein R. (2010). HIV and human trafficking–related stigma: Health interventions for trafficked populations. *Journal of the American Medical Association*, 304(3), 344–345.

Williamson, C., & Prior, M. (2009). Domestic minor sex trafficking: A network of underground players in the Midwest. *Journal of Child and Adolescent Trauma*, 2, 46–61.

Xiao, Y., Kristensen, S., Sun, J., Lu, L., & Vermund, S. (2007). Expansion of HIV/AIDS in China: Lessons from Yunnan province. *Social Science and Medicine*, 64(3), 665–675.

Chapter 40

Impact of the Affordable Care Act on Health Policy and Advocacy for Vulnerable Populations

Kathryn Osborne

OBJECTIVES

At the end of this chapter, the reader will be able to

1. Describe federal health policies aimed at improving health outcomes for vulnerable populations.
2. Make the case for continued national healthcare reform.
3. Describe the implications for nursing of the passage of the bills described in the chapter.

INTRODUCTION

The creation of health policy as a mechanism to improve health outcomes for vulnerable populations has been a part of the national agenda in the United States for more than a century. Current efforts to improve health outcomes in the United States are occurring at the local, state, and national levels. This chapter focuses on federal health policy and healthcare reform. Readers are encouraged to investigate the impact of health policy on vulnerable populations in their individual states and local communities.

VULNERABLE POPULATIONS FROM A HEALTH POLICY PERSPECTIVE

In 1998, the President's Advisory Commission on Consumer Protection and Quality in the Health Care Industry identified that there were certain populations who were vulnerable to poor health outcomes. Moreover, the commission defined those vulnerable populations as "groups of people made vulnerable by their financial circumstances or place of residence; health, age, or functional or developmental status; or ability to communicate effectively … [and] personal characteristics, such as race, ethnicity, and sex" (Advisory Commission on Consumer Protection in the Health Care Industry, 1998, para. 1). Since that time, the Agency for Healthcare Research and Quality (AHRQ) has shifted the focus from vulnerable populations to "priority populations—groups with unique healthcare needs that require special focus" (AHRQ, 2013, p. 247). The definition of these groups was clarified with passage of the Healthcare Research and Quality Act of 1999 to include "racial and ethnic minority groups; low-income groups; women; children (age 0–17); older adults (age 65 and over); residents of rural areas; and individuals with special healthcare needs, including individuals with disabilities and individuals who need chronic care or end-of-life care" (AHRQ, 2013, p. 248). Since 1999, the list of priority populations has been expanded to include lesbian, gay, bisexual, and transgender (LGBT) individuals, men and women who are incarcerated, immigrants and refugees, pregnant women, veterans, and persons who used drugs (AHRQ, 2013; Centers for Disease Control and Prevention [CDC], 2014).

Healthy People 2020 provides over 1,200 national objectives relative to improving the health status of people in the United States. For over 20 years, one of the overarching goals of Healthy People has been to reduce disparate health outcomes. While the term *disparities* often implies racial and ethnic disparities, Healthy People recognizes the multidimensional nature of disparate health outcomes in the United States. In addition to race and ethnicity, an individual's ability to achieve optimal health status can be influenced by age, gender, sexual identity, disability, geographic location, living situation, and socioeconomic status (Healthy People 2020, 2014a). In an attempt to reduce disparities in health outcomes, Healthy People 2020 includes a new set of objectives aimed at addressing the social determinants of health. While the goals of Healthy People 2020 are aimed at improving the overall health of the U.S. population, it is clear that the health policy agenda of this government-sponsored program places a high priority on reducing disparities for vulnerable populations.

HISTORICAL BACKGROUND

The origins of health policy aimed at improving the health status of vulnerable populations in the United States can be traced as far back as the late 19th century. Early public policy attempts often focused on "upstream" interventions—meaning policy that dealt with root causes of poor health such as overcrowded housing, poor sanitation, waste management, poor working conditions, and other social and economic determinants of health (Lantz, Lichtenstein, & Pollack, 2007). The enactment of the Sheppard-Towner Act in 1921 was an early example of health policy aimed at altering the healthcare delivery system. This act was passed in response to research conducted by the Federal Children's Bureau, which revealed alarmingly high rates of maternal and infant mortality in the United States. The act allocated funds to individual states for the purpose of establishing maternal and child health services (Rooks, 1997).

Despite the efforts of several U.S. presidents during the first half of the 20th century, health policy, in the form of national healthcare reform, did not come about until the 1965 passage of Title XVIII and Title XIX of the Social Security Act, during the Lyndon Johnson administration (Morone, 2010). Title XVIII and Title XIX called for the establishment of Medicare and Medicaid. Medicare provided healthcare coverage for most Americans at or older than age 65, while the purpose of Medicaid was to expand the healthcare coverage available under existing federal–state welfare programs for low-income populations (Centers for Medicare and Medicaid Service [CMS], 2013). In 1972, passage of the federal Supplemental Security Income (SSI) program extended Medicare eligibility to persons younger than age 65 with long-term disabilities (and to persons of any age with end-stage renal disease), and allowed states to expand Medicaid eligibility to elderly, blind, and disabled individuals (CMS, 2013).

Over the next 3 decades, several modifications to Medicare and Medicaid were adopted. Perhaps most notable were the creation of the State Children's Health Insurance Program (SCHIP) in 1997, which expanded Medicaid coverage for children, and passage of the Medicare Prescription Drug, Improvement, and Modernization Act (MMA) in 2003, which was intended to improve drug benefits for senior citizens. Included in MMA was a provision to implement Medicare Part D, which further expanded drug benefits for senior citizens (CMS, 2013).

THE CASE FOR NATIONAL REFORM

Despite implementation of these programs, the overall health status of Americans continues to be relatively dismal. In 2012, total health expenditures in the United States rose to more than $2.8 trillion ($8,915 per capita), representing slightly more than 17% of the country's gross domestic product (CMS, 2014). Per capita spending on health care in the United States is higher than the equivalent rate in any other country (World Health Organization [WHO], 2012). Yet the United States has the lowest life expectancy at birth among industrialized nations and ranks 32nd in the world in terms of infant mortality rates (Organization for Economic Cooperation and Development [OECD], 2013). In 2007, the United Nations Children's Fund report card ranked the United States 26th, among 29 developed nations, for overall child well-being, and 25th on measures of child health and safety (United Nations Children's Fund, 2013). In 2010, Amnesty International referred to maternal health outcomes in the United States as a "human rights crisis," citing increased rates of maternal mortality (higher than those in 40 other countries), especially among African American women (Amnesty International, 2010).

Increased Access to Care: Is It Really the Answer?

Access to health care is defined by AHRQ as having "the timely use of personal health services to achieve the best health outcomes" (AHRQ, 2013, p. 234). Access to care is measured in three distinct ways: identification of resources that facilitate health care (such as insurance or a usual source of care); patient assessment of the ease with which access to care was gained; and identification of utilization measures (AHRQ, 2013). Given that the acquisition of health insurance facilitates entry into the U.S. healthcare system, the degree to which Americans are covered by health insurance is often used as a key indicator of access to care. Clearly, individuals without health insurance experience disparities in health outcomes and overall health status (AHRQ, 2013). It is with this understanding that current measures to improve disparities in health outcomes for vulnerable populations have focused on improving access to health insurance as a way to increase access to care.

Improved access to health care was clearly an outcome of the implementation of Medicare and Medicaid. However even many years after the introduction of these programs, Americans continue to have some of the poorest health outcomes in the world. For example, despite advances in perinatal care, racial and ethnic disparities persist with regard to death and disease related to pregnancy, preterm birth, and infant and fetal mortality in the United States. Reasons for these disparities remain largely unexplained (Healy et al., 2006; MacDorman & Kirmeyer, 2009), although limited access to quality health care has been cited as one of the contributing factors (MacDorman & Kirmeyer, 2009). During the past decade, expansion of statewide Medicaid programs has significantly improved access to care for pregnant women, but yielded little or no change in disparate perinatal outcome measures. Nonetheless, efforts to eliminate disparities in perinatal outcomes continue to focus on increasing access to early and adequate prenatal care.

According to the most recent statistics, 70.8% of women who delivered a live infant in the United States in 2007 received prenatal care in the first trimester although racial disparities persist in the utilization of early prenatal care (Healthy People 2020, 2014a, 2014b). Recognizing that early and adequate prenatal care is associated with an improvement in several perinatal outcome measures, the federal government, in an attempt to eliminate disparities, identified increased access to early and adequate prenatal care as one of the objectives of Healthy People 2010. However, the fact that access to early pre-natal care has vastly improved over the last decade without a corresponding reduction in racially disparate outcomes (Amnesty International, 2010; Healthy People 2020, 2014a; Paul, Lehman, Suliman, & Hillemeier, 2007) may suggest that simply improving access to care falls short when it comes to reducing racial disparities in health outcomes (Healy et al., 2006; Mainous, Hueston, Love, & Griffith, 1999; Schempf, Kroelinger, & Guyer, 2007). It is anticipated that the inclusion of new objectives aimed at addressing the social determinants of health in Healthy People 2020 will aid in the reduction of disparate health outcomes for vulnerable populations.

The passage of the Patient Protection and Affordable Care Act (ACA), described in the next section, has vastly increased access to affordable health insurance coverage for Americans. It established the groundwork for improvements in the healthcare delivery system so that issues such as the availability of appropriate healthcare providers and the delivery of culturally sensitive health care become priorities (Patient Protection and Affordable Care Act, 2010).

The Patient Protection and Affordable Care Act (H.R. 3590)

On March 23, 2010, President Barack Obama signed the Patient Protection and Afford-able Care Act (ACA) into law. Depending on how one defines vulnerability or vulnerable populations, it is possible to find provisions on any one of the 2,000-plus pages of the ACA that relate to one vulnerable population or another. This Act is so comprehen-sive that it focuses on vulnerable populations in a number of ways, many of which are embedded within larger provisions in which vulnerable populations are not explicitly mentioned. For example, one of the provisions in the ACA created state-based Health Benefit Exchanges (or Marketplaces when discussed later) through which individuals are able to purchase more affordable health insurance coverage. For example, farmers, who because of their geographic location, are considered a vulnerable population, and because of the dangerous nature of their work, have difficulty purchasing affordable health insurance policies, now have access to more affordable health insurance coverage through these exchanges (ACA, 2010). Another provision of the ACA increased Medicare reimbursement to certified nurse–midwives from 65% to 100% of the reimbursed rate for physicians. This provision increased access to primary care providers for women age 65 and older, as well as young, disabled women who qualify for Medicare. Under another provision of the act, dependent children up to age 26, many of whom are members of vulnerable populations, now qualify for coverage under their parent's private health insurance plans (ACA, 2010).

A complete review of the ACA is beyond the scope of this chapter. The Kaiser Family Foundation summarized the key provisions of the law (see **Table 40-1**) that directly affect

Table 40-1   Key Provisions of the Patient Protection and Affordable Care Act with Direct Implications for Vulnerable Populations

Individual mandate

All U.S. citizens are required to have qualifying health insurance coverage. Tax penalties for those without coverage will be phased in through 2016 with exemptions for certain populations.

Sources of coverage

Employers with more than 50 full-time employees are required to offer health insurance coverage.

Individuals and small businesses may purchase insurance coverage through state-based or federally established American Health Benefit Exchanges. Premium and cost-sharing credits, which substantially decrease the cost of coverage, are available for individuals and families with incomes between 100–400% FPL.

In its original form, the ACA required states to expand Medicaid coverage to include all individuals under age 65 with incomes up to 138% FPL. A Supreme Court ruling on the constitutionality of the act preserved the Medicaid expansion provisions but resulted in making Medicaid expansion optional for states. Despite the provision of enhanced federal funding to finance coverage for newly eligible Medicaid recipients, as of December, 2013, 25 states have not moved forward with Medicaid expansion.

Individuals age 65 and older will continue to qualify for coverage under Medicare. Included in the ACA are provisions to contain the costs of Medicare programs and limit expenditures for Medicare enrollees, including a provision that eliminates cost-sharing for preventive services that are recommended by the U.S. Preventive Services Task Force.

Benefit requirements

All qualified health benefits plans sold on exchanges, and plans purchased through individual and small group markets outside the exchanges, must offer an essential health benefits package with limited cost-sharing and no cost-sharing for preventive services recommended by the U.S. Preventive Services Task Force.

Dependent children up to age 26 must be covered under all individual and group policies.

Most plans are prohibited from using pre-existing condition exclusions.

All plans offered through exchanges and sold outside exchanges in individual and small group markets must create four levels of coverage, each with varying costs and subsequently cost-sharing (though all plans must provide the essential health benefits package). A separate catastrophic plan must be made available for individual purchase through and outside of exchanges.

Table 40-1 Key Provisions of the Patient Protection and Affordable Care Act with Direct Implications for Vulnerable Populations *(Continued)*

Changes in healthcare delivery

The Independence at Home demonstration program was established to provide high-need Medicare beneficiaries with the delivery of in-home primary care. This program offers incentives to healthcare providers who are able to demonstrate a reduction in preventable hospitalizations and readmission, improved health outcomes and patient satisfaction, and reductions in the cost of healthcare services.

The Community-Based Collaborative Care Network Program was established to provide support for coordinated healthcare services provided for low-income underinsured and uninsured populations.

Data regarding race, ethnicity, gender, primary language, disability status, and underserved rural and frontier populations must be collected and analyzed to monitor trends in disparate health outcomes.

Grant monies have been allocated to support evidence-based/community-based prevention and wellness services aimed at reducing chronic disease and addressing health disparities.

The Indian Health Care Improvement Act has been reauthorized and amended.

Provisions with implications for nurses serving vulnerable populations

Funds have been allocated to support the education and training of health professionals through scholarships and loans, and to increase the workforce in rural and underserved areas

Specific funding has been allocated to support the education and employment of nurse practitioners who provide primary care in FQHCs and nurse-managed clinics.

Funding has been allocated to support the establishment of school-based health centers and nurse-managed clinics.

Funding for National Health Service Corps was increased by $1.5 billion over 5 years.

Source: Data from the Kaiser Family Foundation, 2013a

vulnerable populations (Kaiser Family Foundation, 2013a). A full summary of the ACA can be found at http://www.kff.org/healthreform/8061.cfm

Although the ACA was signed into law in 2010, full implementation will not be complete until 2018. Moreover, the impact of the act on reducing disparities in health outcomes for vulnerable populations will not likely be realized for years to come. National estimates regarding changes in insurance coverage will not be available until late 2014. An early study examining these changes found an uninsured rate of 16.3% in April 2014, down from 21.0% in September 2013, just prior to open enrollment under the ACA (Sommers et al., 2014). This decline in uninsured rates suggests an estimated 10.3 million U.S. citizens gained health insurance coverage during the first open enrollment period in the Health Insurance Marketplace (Department of Health and Human Services [HHS], 2014). Although more adults during this same time period reported having a personal physician, further research is necessary to more clearly understand the impact of the ACA on declining uninsured rates and increased access to care (Sommers et al., 2014).

Expanding Medicaid coverage to adults with incomes at or below 138% Federal Poverty Level (FPL) was a key provision of the ACA, which aimed to increase access to health care for low-income individuals. However, the Supreme Court decision on the ACA had the effect of making Medicaid expansion optional for states; as of the date of this writing, 25 states have opted not to expand Medicaid. In many of these states, limited Medicaid coverage is available to parents below 100% FPL and there is no coverage for low-income childless adults. An estimated 5 million uninsured adults will fall into a "coverage gap" in these states (Kaiser Family Foundation, 2013b). Without Medicaid expansion, these individuals remain ineligible for Medicaid yet they do not have incomes high enough to qualify for premium tax credits to purchase coverage on the exchange (which begin at 100% FPL) and many will remain uninsured (Kaiser Family Foundation, 2013b). Moreover, significant racial and ethnic disparities exist in health coverage among adults, with people of color more likely to be uninsured than whites. Failure to expand Medicaid creates a coverage gap that disproportionately affects people of color and will likely widen racial and ethnic disparities in coverage and access to care (Kaiser Family Foundation, 2013b).

IMPLICATIONS FOR NURSING

For many years, the American Nurses Association (ANA) has been a leading advocate for healthcare reform, including the availability of universal health care. In 2008, this organization published The ANA's Health System Reform Agenda, which identified four critical issues that must be considered during the reformation of the healthcare delivery system:

- Access
- Cost
- Quality
- Workforce (ANA, 2008).

A comparative analysis of the ACA and The ANA's Health System Reform Agenda revealed that all four critical issues identified in the ANA agenda were addressed in the ACA. Further, most of the recommendations included in the Health System Reform Agenda will continue to be addressed with the implementation of the ACA through 2018 (ANA, 2010a).

Access

Provisions in the ACA ensure access to care in all geographic locations to all American citizens regardless of age, gender, ethnicity, and socioeconomic status. Other provisions call for health care to be delivered in a way that is acceptable to recipients, e.g., delivered with respect for patient autonomy, cultural sensitivity, and in a way that is patient centered.

Cost

The ACA also focuses on ensuring the affordability of health care for U.S. citizens, and inclusion of a standard package of essential health services (including mental health parity). While the ACA does not call for the public funding (including creation of a single-payer system) that was supported by the ANA, it does contain provisions that will control costs and protect the financial well-being of families with high medical expenses. The ACA also contains provisions for cost sharing between individuals and payers (based on income level) while recognizing the importance of personal responsibility on the part of the healthcare recipient. However, the act falls short with regard to the provision of health care for undocumented immigrants and fails to recognize health care as a basic human right (ANA, 2010a).

CASE STUDY

Trapped: Not Poor Enough—Not Rich Enough

Sue and Tom have been married for 30 years and both are 55 years old. Sue provides day-care services in her rural home for children with developmental disabilities. Tom works at a local hardware store. Neither Sue nor Tom work for employers that provide health insurance. As a result, they have been spending almost 30% of their monthly income to purchase high-deductible individual health insurance policies. They have one 24-year-old son who is newly unemployed and is no longer covered by employee-sponsored health insurance. Facing foreclosure on their home because they have been unable to afford their mortgage payment, Sue and Tom decided that the time had come to give up their health insurance. With a combined income of 250% FPL, neither of them qualify for the state Medicaid program.

On November 1, 2013, Sue paid a visit to the online Health Insurance Marketplace to investigate the possibility of purchasing coverage on the exchange. She discovered that for a cost that would not exceed 8.05% of their total income, they could purchase a policy that provided the essential benefits package with limited cost sharing of additional expenses. She also discovered that her son would be eligible for coverage under their policy. Sue purchased the policy on the exchange and now this family, who was soon to be uninsured or risk losing their home, has health insurance coverage, financial access to health services in their community, and peace of mind about their mortgage payment.

Quality

Recognizing the importance of improving both access to care and quality of care, the ANA identified six quality indicators to be addressed as the healthcare delivery system is reformed. The ACA include provisions to improve the quality of health care on all six of these measures: safety, effectiveness, patient-centeredness, timeliness, efficiency, and equitability. Consistent with the framework within which nursing research is often conducted, the ACA established the Patient-Centered Outcomes Research Institute. Also in keeping with the recommendations of the ANA, it includes provisions that support continuity of care and address chronic disease management. Moreover, the act includes provisions that promote health and that will, over time, lead to disease prevention. Finally, the ACA contains provisions that have established a national quality improvement strategy as well as the adoption of quality indicators for nursing (ANA, 2010a).

Workforce

Although the provisions related to workforce development may not be explicitly stated in terms of vulnerable populations, it is important to recognize that an estimated 32 million U.S. citizens, most of whom have lacked any form of health insurance, now have gained access to the healthcare system as a result of the ACA (Goodson, 2010). Further, only 30% of the physicians practicing in the United States are providing primary care services (Goodson, 2010).

In recognition of the shortage of primary care providers, the ACA supports expansion of the primary care workforce, including recognition of nurse practitioners and certified nurse–midwives as primary care providers. It also establishes grant programs for school-based health clinics and authorizes funds to support nurse-managed health centers operated by advanced practice nurses (ANA, 2010b). Finally, it includes measures to enhance the delivery of primary care and recognizes the economic value of nurses, including the recognition of advanced practice nurses as primary care providers (ANA, 2010a). These provisions will expand opportunities for nurses at all levels of practice. It is further anticipated that the mandate for expanded funding of nursing education will increase the size of the nursing workforce, both the number of practicing nurses and the faculty necessary to prepare new nurses.

CONCLUSION

The United States has a lengthy history of policy aimed at improving health outcomes for vulnerable populations. Passage of the ACA is anticipated to narrow the gap between health outcomes for affluent Americans and health outcomes for vulnerable populations. Nurses are poised to play a key role in implementation of the ACA, through their continued advocacy for the vulnerable populations whom they serve. In light of the fact that much of the implementation of the ACA is occurring at state and local levels, it is important for nurses to become involved in state and local government, including individual state legislative proceedings. This is especially true in states that have opted out of Medicaid expansion. The full effect of the ACA on health disparities for vulnerable populations will not be felt until well into the next decade. Even so, the future looks bright, both for the profession of nursing and for vulnerable populations served by nurses.

REFERENCES

Advisory Commission on Consumer Protection in the Health Care Industry. (1998). Quality first: Better health care for all Americans [Chapter 8]. Retrieved from http://archive.ahrq.gov/hcqual/final/chap08.html

Agency for Healthcare Research and Quality (AHRQ). (2013). 2013 National healthcare disparities report. Retrieved from http://www.ahrq.gov/research/findings/nhqrdr/nhdr13/2013nhdr.pdf

American Nurses Association (ANA). (2008). *Health system reform agenda*. Silver Spring, MD: American Nurses Association.

American Nurses Association (ANA). (2010a). ANA policy and provisions of health reform law. Retrieved from http://www.rnaction.org/site/DocServer/PPACAProvisions_April2010.pdf?docID=1261

American Nurses Association (ANA). (2010b). Health care reform: Key provisions related to nursing. Retrieved from http://www.rnaction.org/site/DocServer/KeyProvisions_Nursing-PublicLaw.pdf?docID=1241&verID=1

Amnesty International. (2010). Deadly delivery: The maternal health care crisis in the US. Retrieved from http://www.amnestyusa.org/dignity/pdf/DeadlyDelivery.pdf

Centers for Disease Control and Prevention (CDC). (2014). Minority health: Other at risk populations. Retrieved from http://www.cdc.gov/minorityhealth/populations/atrisk.html#Other

Centers for Medicare and Medicaid Services (CMS). (2013). History. Retrieved from https://www.cms.gov/About-CMS/Agency-Information/History/index.html?redirect=/History

Centers for Medicare and Medicaid Services (CMS). (2014). National health expenditure data: Historical. Retrieved from http://www.cms.gov/Research-Statistics-Data-and-Systems/Statistics-Trends-and-Reports/NationalHealthExpendData/NationalHealthAccountsHistorical.html

Department of Health and Human Services (HHS). (2014). New study: 10.3 million gained health coverage during the marketplace's first annual open enrollment period. Retrieved from http://www.hhs.gov/news/press/2014pres/07/20140723b.html

Goodson, J. (2010). Patient Protection and Affordable Care Act: Promise and peril for primary care. *American College of Physicians, 152*, 742–744.

Healthy People 2020. (2014a). Disparities. Retrieved from http://healthypeople.gov/2020/about/DisparitiesAbout.aspx

Healthy People 2020. (2014b). Objectives: Pregnancy health and behaviors. Retrieved from http://www.healthypeople.gov/2020/topicsobjectives2020/objectiveslist.aspx?topicId=26

Healy, A., Malone, F., Sullivan, L., Porter, F., Luthy, D., Comstock, C., ... D'Alton, M. E. (2006). Early access to prenatal care: Implications for racial disparity in perinatal mortality. *Obstetrics and Gynecology, 107*(3), 625–631.

Kaiser Family Foundation. (2013a). Summary of the Affordable Care Act. Retrieved from http://kff.org/health-reform/fact-sheet/summary-of-the-affordable-care-act/

Kaiser Family Foundation. (2013b). The impact of the coverage gap in states not expanding Medicaid by race and ethnicity. Retrieved from http://kff.org/disparities-policy/issue-brief/the-impact-of-the-coverage-gap-in-states-not-expanding-medicaid-by-race-and-ethnicity/

Lantz, P., Lichtenstein, R., & Pollack, H. (2007). Health policy approaches to population health: The limits of medicalization. *Health Affairs, 26*(5), 1253–1257.

MacDorman, M., & Kirmeyer, S. (2009). National vital statistics reports: Fetal and perinatal mortality, United States, 2005. Retrieved from http://www.cdc.gov/nchs/data/nvsr/nvsr57/nvsr57_08.pdf

Mainous, A., Hueston, W., Love, M., & Griffith, C. (1999). Access to care for the uninsured: Is access to a physician enough? *American Journal of Public Health*, *89*(6), 910–912.

Morone, J. (2010). Presidents and health reform: From Franklin D. Roosevelt to Barack Obama. *Health Affairs*, *29*(6), 1096–1100.

Organization for Economic Cooperation and Development (OECD). (2013). Health at a glance 2009. Retrieved from http://www.oecd-ilibrary.org/social-issues-migration-health/health-at-a-glance_19991312;jsessionid=3h1gf2q0r9hfn.x-oecd-live-01

Patient Protection and Affordable Care Act, H.R. 3590 (ACA). (2010). Retrieved from http://www.opencongress.org/bill/111-h3590/text

Paul, I., Lehman, E., Suliman, A., & Hillemeier, M. (2007). Perinatal disparities for black mothers and their newborns. *Maternal Child Health Journal*, *12*, 452–460.

Rooks, J. (1997). *Midwifery and childbirth in America*. Philadelphia: Temple University.

Schempf, A., Kroelinger, C., & Guyer, B. (2007). Rising infant mortality in Delaware: An examination of racial difference in secular trends. *Maternal Child Health Journal*, *11*, 475–483.

Sommers, B. D., Musco, T., Finegold, K., Gunja, M. Z., Burke, A., & McDowell, A. M. (2014). Health reform and changes in health insurance coverage in 2014. *The New England Journal of Medicine*, *371*(9), 867–874. Retrieved from http://www.nejm.org/doi/pdf/10.1056/NEJMsr1406753

United Nations Children's Fund. (2013). Child well-being in rich countries: A comparative overview. Retrieved from http://www.unicef-irc.org/publications/pdf/rc11_eng.pdf

World Health Organization (WHO). (2012). Spending on health: A global overview. Retrieved from http://www.who.int/mediacentre/factsheets/fs319/en/index.html

Chapter 41

Health Systems and Human Resources for Health: New Dimensions in Global Health Nursing

Patricia L. Riley and Maureen A. Kelley

OBJECTIVES

At the end of this chapter, the reader will be able to

1. Describe the Millennium Development Goals.
2. Identify the essential building blocks of a health system.
3. Identify three human resources for health (HRH) issues challenging health service delivery in low-income countries.
4. Define task shifting versus task sharing and explain the differences between the two.
5. Describe an approach for benchmarking and measuring an organization's competency and maturity.

INTRODUCTION

This chapter pertains to caring for vulnerable populations in global settings. It focuses on *health systems* and *human resources for health* (HRH). The global nurse needs skills that go beyond competency in the provision and management of health services. In addition to these abilities, current engagement in global health requires an understanding of the components of a health system and analytical capabilities for assessing, designing, and evaluating appropriate interventions at the system level. Because nearly every country, especially those designated as low-income countries, is experiencing a critical shortage of healthcare providers, competency in global nursing necessitates acquiring technical abilities that contribute to building the HRH base. Additionally, interdisciplinary collaboration and communication is essential for working with a diverse range of national stakeholders in a variety of settings (Institute of Medicine [IOM], 2010a; Joint Learning Initiative, 2004; Reich, Takeni, Roberts, & Hsiao, 2008).

Advancement in Global Health Policies and Initiatives

Over the past 30 years, there have been tremendous shifts and advancement in global health policies and initiatives. The past decade has introduced new paradigms that have revolutionized the way in which foreign assistance is provided. Governments are no longer the sole purveyors of health interventions. New players entering the arena include:

- Multilateral agencies (e.g., World Bank)
- Public–private partnerships (e.g., Global Fund to Fight AIDS, Tuberculosis and Malaria)
- Bilateral governmental initiatives (e.g., U.S. President's Emergency Plan for AIDS Relief [PEPFAR]; President's Malaria Initiative)
- The private sector (e.g., Bill and Melinda Gates Foundation)
- Philanthropic trusts (e.g., the Wellcome Trust)

Never before has such a wide array of donors supported so many global health initiatives with significant funding. For example, The PEPFAR Stewardship and Oversight Act (Public Law 113-56), enacted by the U.S. Congress into law in 2003 and reauthorized in 2013 through 2018, received $6.7 billion in 2014 (PEPFAR, Annex V—Health Systems Strengthening, n.d.). That same year, billionaire philanthropist Bill Gates, complemented the U.S. government's funding for the global HIV/AIDS program by committing up to $500 million, nearly doubling his foundation's previous contribution to the Geneva-based The Global Fund (TGF). When coupled with matching grants from other donors, this support could result in a $1.6 billion total contribution to TGF (*The Wall Street Journal*, 2013).

Another important factor influencing global health is the United Nations (UN) Millennium Declaration, with its eight time-bound goals, the Millennium Development Goals (MDGs). These goals have increased attention to the health needs of the world's most vulnerable populations (World Health Organization [WHO], 2005). The eight MDGs for global development (see **Table 41-1**) include poverty eradication; access to primary education; promoting gender equality and the empowerment of women; reduction of child mortality; improve maternal health; reduction of HIV/AIDS, malaria, and tuberculosis; and the promotion of environmental sustainability; and global partnerships (WHO, 2005).

Table 41-1   Health in the Millennium Development Goals

Health targets		Health indicators
Goal 1: Eradicate extreme poverty and hunger		
Target 1	Halve, between 1990 and 2015, the proportion of people whose income is less than $1 a day	
Target 2	Halve, between 1990 and 2015, the proportion of people who suffer from hunger	4. Prevalence of underweight children under 5 years of age 5. Proportion of population below minimum level of dietary energy consumption
Goal 2: Achieve universal primary education		
Target 3	Ensure that, by 2015, children everywhere, boys and girls alike, will be able to complete a full course of primary schooling	
Goal 3: Promote gender equality and empower women		
Target 4	Eliminate gender disparity in primary and secondary education, preferably by 2005, and at all levels of education no later than 2015	
Goal 4: Reduce child mortality		
Target 5	Reduce by two-thirds, between 1990 and 2015, the under 5 mortality rate	13. Under 5 mortality rate 14. Infant mortality rate 15. Proportion of 1-year-old children immunized against measles
Goal 5: Improve maternal health		
Target 6	Reduce by three-quarters, between 1990 and 2015, the maternal mortality ratio	16. Maternal mortality ratio 17. Proportion of births attended by skilled health personnel
Goal 6: Combat HIV/AIDS, malaria and other diseases		
Target 7	Have halted by 2015 and begun to reverse the spread of HIV/AIDS	18. HIV prevalence among pregnant women aged 15–24 years 19. Condom use rate of the contraceptive prevalence rate 20. Ratio of school attendance of orphans to school attendance of non-orphans aged 10–14 years

(Continues)

Table 41-1 Health in the Millennium Development Goals (*Continued*)

Health targets		Health indicators
Target 8	Have halted by 2015 and begun to reverse the incidence of malaria and other major diseases	21. Prevalence and death rates associated with malaria 22. Proportion of population in malaria-risk areas using effective malaria prevention and treatment measures 23. Prevalence and death rates associated with tuberculosis 24. Proportion of tuberculosis cases detected and cured under DOTS (Directly Observed Treatment Short-course)
Goal 7: Ensure environmental sustainability		
Target 9	Integrate the principles of sustainable development into country policies and programmes and reverse the loss of environmental resources	29. Proportion of population using solid fuels
Target 10	Halve by 2015 the proportion of people without sustainable access to safe drinking-water and sanitation	30. Proportion of population with sustainable access to an improved water source, urban and rural
Target 11	By 2020 to have achieved a significant improvement in the lives of at least 100 million slum dwellers	31. Proportion of population with access to improved sanitation, urban and rural
Goal 8: Develop a global partnership for development		
Target 12	Develop further an open, rule-based, predictable, non-discriminatory trading and financial system	
Target 13	Address the special needs of the least developed countries	
Target 14	Address the special needs of landlocked countries and small island developing states	
Target 15	Deal comprehensively with the debt problems of developing countries through national and international measures in order to make debt sustainable in the long term	
Target 16	In cooperation with developing countries, develop and implement strategies for decent and productive work for youth	

Table 41-1   Health in the Millennium Development Goals (*Continued*)

Health targets		Health indicators
Target 17	In cooperation with pharmaceutical companies, provide access to affordable essential drugs in developing countries	46. Proportion of population with access to affordable essential drugs on a sustainable basis
Target 18	In cooperation with the private sector, make available the benefits of new technologies, especially information and communications	

Sources: "Implementation of the United Nations Millennium Declaration," Report of the Secretary-General, A/57/270 (31 July 2002), first annual report based on the "Road map towards the implementation of the United Nations Millennium Declaration," Report of the Secretary-General, A/56/326 (6 September 2001); United Nations Statistics Division, Millennium Indicators Database, verified in July 2004; World Health Organization, Department of MDGs, Health and Development Policy (HDP). World Health Organization. (2005). Health and the Millennium Development Goals. Geneva: World Health Organization.

Each of these targets is matched with corresponding health indicators, which serve as guideposts for global organizations, donors, and stakeholders, and provide an overarching framework for measuring progress toward commonly agreed upon global priorities (WHO, 2005). Since the launch of this worldwide effort, the MDGs have garnered acceptance among rich and poor countries alike. The ambitious timeline, targeted for attainment by the year 2015, has created momentum within the field of global health (Travis et al., 2004; WHO, 2009). In 2013, the Millennium Development Report noted progress in several areas despite the global economic recession. Several MDG targets have been met or are within reach, specifically:

- The proportion of people living in extreme poverty has been halved at the global level. The world achieved this poverty reduction target 5 years ahead of schedule.
- Over 2 billion people gained access to improved sources of drinking water. The proportion of the global population using these sources improved to 89%—an increase of 13% from 1990.
- Mortality rates from malaria and tuberculosis have decreased by 25% and 50%, respectively.
- The proportion of urban slum dwellers with access to clean water, sanitation, and durable housing or sufficient space exceeded the MDG target.
- The combined ratio of debt burden to export revenue ratio for developing countries dropped 12% compared to 2000.
- The hunger reduction ratio was reduced by half and is now within reach of the 2015 target (*The Millennium Development Goals Report 2013*, 2013).

Targets in Need of Bolder Action

Bolder action and an accelerated action plan are needed to reach 2015 targets for other MDG goals, including:

- *Environment sustainability*: Decreasing global carbon emissions, deforestation, and over use of marine fish stocks
- *Childhood mortality*: Decreasing mortality for children less than 5 years of age
- *Maternal mortality*: Accelerated interventions to reduce the current ratio of 210 deaths per 100,000 live births by 2015
- *HIV/AIDS*: While new HIV infections are declining, universal access to antiretroviral therapy (ARV) is lagging; 2015 targets are realizable if current trends continue.
- *Primary education*: Progress is stalled and there is concern that this target will not be realized by 2015.
- *Sanitation*: 1.9 billion people lack access to a latrine, flush toilet, or an improved sanitation facility.
- *Reduced global assistance*: There has been a 4% drop in resources compared to 2011; in 2012, bilateral development assistance fell by 13% (*The Millennium Development Goals Report 2013*, 2013).

Inadequate infrastructure for providing service delivery, shortages of trained health workers, interruptions in the procurement and supply of health products, and poor governance are elements of a dysfunctional health system. These factors not only obstruct global health assistance, but become a systematic problem unto themselves (Hill, Mansoor, & Claudio, 2010; WHO, 2009). Difficulty in producing reliable morbidity and mortality data for benchmarking reflects weakened health systems. Although select, targeted initiatives have shown an overall trend of improved quality and equity in access to health care, low-income countries need to sustain steady progress in these areas to strengthen health systems (WHO, 2009). In the 2013 report, *Evaluation of PEPFAR*, the IOM underscored the importance of strengthening systems over time. It also advocated for health workforce capacity development to sustain management of HIV programs and to provide equitable access to services for populations most in need. (IOM, 2013). Because health systems and HRH are essential for realizing global advancement in all MDGs, each is discussed in further detail below.

HEALTH SYSTEMS

Overview

Due to weakened health infrastructure resulting from decades of neglect and insufficient investment, progress toward reaching the MDGs for health is compromised in most low-income countries (WHO, 2009). Reasons for inadequate health infrastructure include economic crises and political unrest that occurred in many developing countries during the 1980s. This was often followed by restricted budgets due to debt repayment and cuts in public health spending. These events, which negatively affected both health service delivery and health service providers, resulted in a dramatic rise in emigration of highly skilled, yet poorly paid healthcare providers. The exodus of the professional health workforce left the majority of developing countries unable to respond effectively to the HIV/AIDS epidemic by the time it was fully manifested. As noted by the WHO Maximizing Positive Synergies Collaborative Group, the impact of HIV/AIDS resulted in further crippling of damaged, overstretched health systems (WHO, 2009). The AIDS epidemic further exacerbated the inability of low-income countries to meet the general health needs of their populations.

The WHO defines health systems as including organizations, personnel and activities that promote health (WHO, 2007). This definition includes both the determinants of health and health-improving activities, such as public health and contributions to health protection seen with legislation and government policy (WHO, 2007). The overall goals of health systems are to improve health and health equity by making the best and most efficient use of available resources. Yet for many developing countries, this expectation is beyond their current reach (de Savigny & Adam, 2009). As noted in the 2000 World Health Report entitled *Health Systems: Improving Performance*, every country has a health system, however fragmented. Integration and oversight do not determine the system, but they may greatly influence how well it performs (WHO, 2000). An integrated health systems approach is essential. WHO's Framework for Action portrays the individual components of a health system, using discrete building blocks (see **Figure 41-1**). These building blocks represent a complete health system which, when functional, results in the overall goals of improved health, responsiveness to the health needs of the community, social and financial equity, and improved efficiency (WHO, 2007).

Individual building blocks do not constitute a health system; rather, the health system comprises multiple relationships and interactions between the components. The ease with which each component interacts with the others determines the function of the system. Most important, the interaction of the health system components can enable (or impede) health services to achieve the purpose for which they were created (de Savigny & Adam, 2009). Current approaches to furthering global healthcare builds on a systems concept that includes understanding the methods and processes of healthcare delivery, knowledge capacity of the health system, building and maintaining health information relationships, and encouraging a culture that values a functional health system (de Savigny & Adam, 2009).

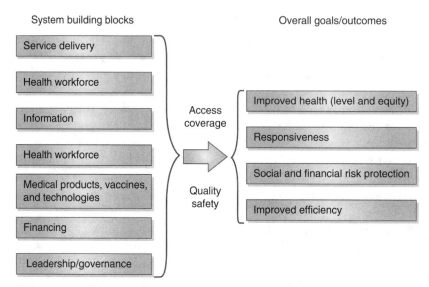

Figure 41-1 The WHO health system framework.

Reproduced from World Health Organization. (2007). *Everybody's Business: Strengthening Health Systems to Improve Health Outcomes—WHO's Framework for Action.* Geneva: WHO Press.

Policy and Research

Over the past decade, global health policy has embraced different strategies for advancing MDG attainment (see **Table 41-2**). One approach emphasizes disease-specific interventions, as illustrated by PEPFAR, the Global Fund to Fight AIDS, Tuberculosis and Malaria, and the Global Alliance for Vaccines and Immunizations (GAVI). Others promote a broad and integrated systematic approach to health improvement (de Savigny & Adam, 2009; WHO, 2000, 2007).

While disease-specific initiatives have been shown to improve health conditions in low-income countries (Reich et al., 2008), these targeted strategies have the potential to crowd out other health-promoting services within the health sector (Travis et al., 2004). For example, a WHO study of polio eradication reported that the majority of district level staff noted a disruption of routine health service delivery during the period leading up to national immunization days (Mogedal & Stenson, 2002). A disease-specific approach can fragment an already weakened health system and prevent the development of strategies to sustain focused initiatives (Chan et al., 2010). As a result, the prevailing opinion in global health has endorsed a more balanced approach between disease-specific mandates and systems-based interventions and methodology (Reich et al., 2008).

Table 41-2   Typical System Constraints and Possible Disease-Specific and Health-System Responses

Constraint	Disease-specific response	Health-system response
Financial inaccessibility: inability to pay, informal fees	Exemptions/reduced prices for focal diseases	Development of risk pooling strategies
Physical inaccessibility: distance to services	Outreach for focal diseases	Reconsideration of long-term plan facility for capital investment and siting of facilities
Inappropriately skilled staff	Continuous education and training workshops to develop skills in focal diseases	Review of basic medical and nursing training curricula to ensure that appropriate skills included in basic training
Poorly motivated staff	Financial incentives to delivery of particular priority services	Reward Institution of proper performance review systems, creating greater clarity of roles and expectations regarding performance of roles, review of salary structures and promotion procedures
Weak planning and management	Continuous education and training workshops to develop skills in planning and management	Restructuring ministries of health, recruitment and development of cadre of dedicated managers
Lack of intersectoral action and partnership	Creation of special disease-focused, cross-sectoral committees and task forces at national level	Building systems of local government that incorporate representatives from health, education, agriculture, and promote accountability of local governance structures to the people
Poor quality care amongst private sector providers	Training for private sector providers	Development of accreditation and regulation systems

Reprinted from *Lancet*, 364, Travis, P., Bennett, S., Haines, A., et al. Overcoming health-systems constraints to achieve the Millennium Development Goals, Pages 900–906, Copyright 2004, with permission from Elsevier.

The Obama Administration's investment in the Global Health Initiative (GHI), an intervention designed to facilitate coordination between disease-specific and issue-specific initiatives, provides a current example of this integrated construct. GHI focuses on formalizing partnership frameworks or agreements between the U.S. government and national ministries of health. This requires joint assessment of service delivery and workforce capacity, information, medical products and technologies, financing, leadership, and governance. This approach identifies the health system elements essential for redirecting U.S. global assistance to sustainable local ownership (PEPFAR, 2010).

While WHO's health systems definition, framework, and essential building blocks are accepted tenets for global engagement, relatively little is known about the best approaches for health systems improvement (Fryatt, Mills, & Nordstrom, 2010; Mgone et al., 2010; *Report from the Ministerial Summit on Health Research*, 2004; Sanders & Haines, 2006; *Strengthening Health Systems: The Country Perspective*, 2009; Task Force on Health Systems Research, 2004). This is due, in part, to the fact that until recently, support for health systems research was sparse, especially compared to the resources for drug and vaccine research (Mgone et al., 2010).

Health systems research is a complex science. Proven metrics for measuring impact are still evolving. As a consequence, health systems and health system interventions are infrequently evaluated. Despite the vast resources that have been allocated for a variety of disease-specific or targeted health interventions, to date there have been no robust prospective studies regarding the overall effects targeted interventions have had upon local health systems. There is insufficient data upon which conclusions can be drawn regarding the impact (either positive or negative) of disease-specific initiatives on local health systems (Hill et al., 2010; WHO, 2009).

Policy recommendations regarding health systems strengthening require a systematic and transparent approach capable of assessing the different types of evidence needed for complex decision making. The Grading of Recommendations Assessment, Development and Evaluation (GRADE) approach offers a format that is capable of discriminating the quality of scientific evidence and characterizing or grading the strength of recommendations for health systems interventions (Lewin et al., 2012). Priority questions confronting health systems decision makers and researchers working in low-income settings include:

- What are the best practices for integrating discrete health initiatives at the local level?
- What are optimal health management strategies, including the use of auxiliary (i.e., non-professionally educated) health workers?
- What are the costs and benefits analyses of different healthcare service models?

Investigating these questions requires improved data quality and availability, which in turn, necessitates strengthened country capacity in collecting, processing, analyzing, and using health data (Mgone et al., 2010). It is in tackling the health information gap that answers to these and many other health systems questions can be answered—and answers to these questions can improve the health and welfare of vulnerable populations, especially those at risk for morbidity, mortality, and the diseases of poverty.

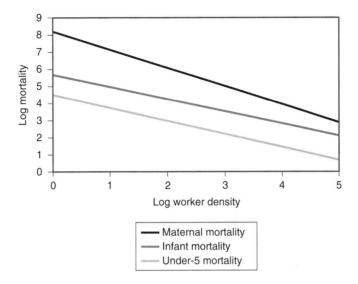

Figure 41-2 Association between worker density and mortality rates.

Reprinted from *Lancet, 364,* Chen, L., Evans, T., Anand, S., et al. Human resources for health: overcoming the crisis, Pages 1984–1990, Copyright 2004, with permission from Elsevier.

Human Resources

Overview

Workforce density makes a critical difference in mortality rates of mothers, infants, and children younger than 5 years of age (see **Figure 41-2**).

A similar association was noted with regard to workforce density, health services, and the impact of MDG interventions, such as achieving 80% coverage of childhood measles immunization and assuring that the majority of births are attended by skilled providers (Chen et al., 2004) (see **Figure 41-3**).

Global policies and resolutions in the early 2000s brought attention to the need for strengthened HRH capacity and information systems in developing countries (Pan American Organization and WHO, 2001; WHO, 2004). The first analysis of the impact of global workforce shortages on health services and health outcomes was reported by the Joint Learning Initiative, a consortium of more than 100 global health leaders. The Rockefeller Foundation launched this consortium with a supported secretariat at Harvard University's Global Equity Initiative (Chen et al., 2004; Joint Leaning Initiative, 2004).

Chen and colleagues postulate that the critical minimum HRH coverage threshold is 2.5 workers per 1,000 population. When the provider to population ratio falls below

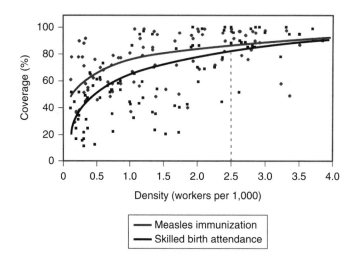

Figure 41-3 Association between worker density and service coverage.

Reprinted from *Lancet, 364,* Chen, L., Evans, T., Anand, S., et al. Human resources for health: overcoming the crisis, Pages 1984–1990, Copyright 2004, with permission from Elsevier.

this level, health outcomes and preventive health services are significantly compromised (Chen et al., 2004). While some pregnancy-related services and life-saving child health services, such as immunizations or the provision of HIV/AIDS care, can be adequately provided by auxiliary staff, effective health workforce planning consists of a balance of professional, paraprofessional, and community health workers (WHO, n.d.) Based on these criteria, WHO has identified 57 HRH crisis countries (36 of which are in Africa) that have an estimated combined deficit of 2.4 million doctors, nurses, and midwives (WHO, 2006). HRH issues include: HRH out-migration, retention, and maldistribution. Each of these topics is briefly discussed below.

Out-Migration

The majority of health worker migration occurs internally (i.e., when healthcare workers move within a country, usually from rural areas to urban centers). A more controversial migration occurs when highly skilled professionals from poorer countries move to richer and more developed countries. This out-migration crisis particularly impacts physicians and nurses, who are able to achieve equivalency credentialing in destination countries (Joint Learning Initiative, 2004). Additionally, recent HRH studies have found that professionals who out-migrate are among the most qualified providers. For example, findings from a Kenyan nursing workforce study document that the majority of nurses who out-migrate are RN or BSN prepared (Riley et al., 2007). Between the years 1999 and 2007, for every four nurses that Kenya added to its workforce through training, one existing nurse applied for out-migration (Gross et al., 2010). Similar impacts to the healthcare system occur with physician out-migration. While destination countries receiving physicians from low-income nations benefit from workforce additions, the reliance of the United States, United Kingdom, Canada, and Australia on international medical graduates is reducing the supply of physicians in many developing nations (Mullan, 2005).

Retention

In an attempt to offset the out-migration imbalance from HRH crisis countries, there is increased emphasis on identifying appropriate and effective workforce retention strategies. Current capacity-building approaches, such as PEPFAR's Medical and Nursing Education Partnership Initiatives, have focused on the production of health professionals as an immediate strategy to scale-up Africa's HRH workforce (Collins, Glass, Whitescarver, Wakefield, & Goosby, 2010). However, the emphasis on producing new providers may result in overlooking solutions for retaining currently employed health professionals (Haines & Sanders, 2005). Incentives for HRH retention in rural and underserved areas have not been addressed fully. A recent literature review of motivational and retention issues affecting healthcare providers cited limitations in promotion, career development, and living and working conditions as being of equal significance to low wages (Willis-Shattuck et al., 2008). Both the IOM report, *Preparing for the Future of HIV/AIDS in Africa*, and the Joint Learning Initiative report identify satisfactory remuneration, a positive work environment, and synchronization of support systems as core elements for sustaining an engaged and motivated workforce (IOM, 2010b; Joint Learning Initiative, 2004).

Maldistribution

Within developing countries, structural imbalances often result in provider maldistribution. Examples include the placement of providers without regard to local provider-to-population ratios, professional and specialty discrepancies (i.e., underinvestment in nurses and midwives at the expense of physician specialty training), and urban bias whereby political or economic forces within a country reinforce provision of services and health investments in urban areas (Fritzen, 2007). These may be the most critical barriers for achieving universal healthcare coverage, Chen describes maldistribution of healthcare workers as imbalances in skills and provider shortages. He attributes the shortages of healthcare coverage as being exacerbated by the pool of overly specialized professionals. This imbalance results in unnecessary tests and procedures, over-prescribing of drugs, and higher costs at the expense of the underserved (Chen, 2010).

In response to this problem, WHO convened an expert group to investigate access to health providers in remote and rural areas. After reviewing evidence-based retention strategies specific to rural and remote areas, this expert group developed global policy recommendations tailored to those ministries of health that face maldistribution of providers. These recommendations serve as an initial step for addressing HRH imbalances (WHO, 2010a).

Approaches to Strengthening Human Resources for Health Policy

Global awareness of the indiscriminate recruitment of professional healthcare providers from low-income to high-income countries has resulted in responsive global health policies. In a historic move in 2010, the 63rd World Health Assembly unanimously passed a resolution to adopt a voluntary global code of practice regarding the international recruitment of health personnel. By committing to this code, member states voluntarily agreed to adopt the principles and practices for the ethical recruitment of health personnel, taking into account the responsibilities and rights of both the source (low-income countries) and destination (high-income countries), other stakeholders, and those of the migrant health personnel themselves (WHO, 2010b). In passing this resolution, nations acknowledged the global dimension, complexities, and interconnected nature of the health workforce crisis.

Other recent policy developments affecting global HRH include the realignment of roles and responsibilities regarding healthcare delivery. Referred to as *task shifting*, this terminology refers to the process whereby specific provider tasks are transferred, as appropriate, to mid-level health cadres or to auxiliary health workforce with less professional training and fewer qualifications (WHO, 2008). The intent of this approach is to facilitate efficient use of existing human resources and to ease bottlenecks common to service delivery in low-income countries. In situations where additional providers are needed, task shifting may also involve the delegation of some clearly delineated tasks to newly created cadres, such as advanced nurse practitioners in low-resource nations. The IOM proposed a newer terminology, *task sharing*, in place of task shifting. Task sharing, they contend, more aptly describes the requirement for enhanced knowledge in the provision of delegated performance skills. Used in this way, task sharing decreases hierarchy and allows for role changes as needed (IOM, 2010b)

Research

Examples of current HRH research approaches include the "discrete choice methodology" and "the capability maturity model." Discrete choice methodology asks participants to state preferences in a hypothetical setting. Discrete choice experiments (DCEs) are interactions with choices described by various attributes to which participants respond.

Their responses determine how important the attributes are and how they influence preferences (Mangham, Hanson, & McPake, 2009). Using DCE, a recent multicountry study of nurses in Kenya, South Africa, and Thailand evaluated policy interventions designed to attract nurses in these countries to work in rural areas. The DCE involved asking individual nurses to state their work site preference using hypothetical alternative scenarios. Nurses in Kenya and South Africa identified better educational opportunities or rural allowances as being most effective in increasing their retention at rural health posts. In Thailand, health insurance coverage had the greatest impact in attracting nurses to rural posts (Blaauw et al., 2010). DCE provides policy makers with an efficient, evidence-based approach for identifying effective interventions for staff shortages and maldistribution.

The capability maturity model (CMM) is a research approach used to assess organizational improvement. Created by the Carnegie-Mellon University Software Engineering Institute, the CMM identifies critical functions of an organization (see **Figure 41-4**) and provides stepwise performance levels for each function, benchmarking capabilities and progression toward optimal performance (Humphrey, 1987).

The African Health Profession Regulatory Collaborative for Nurses and Midwives (ARC), a PEPFAR-supported, 17-country regional initiative in east, central, and southern Africa. is an example of CMM adaptation (McCarthy & Riley, 2012; McCarthy, Zuber, Kelley, Verani & Riley, 2014). ARC's modification of the CMM (entitled the Regulatory Function Framework) involved identifying essential nursing and midwifery regulatory functions and then staging performance levels for each respective function (McCarthy, Kelley, Verani, St. Louis, & Riley, 2014) (see **Table 41-3**).

This Regulatory Function Framework was used to align the region's nursing and midwifery regulatory functions to those of global bodies (i.e., International Council of Nurses, International Confederation of Midwives, World Health Organization, United

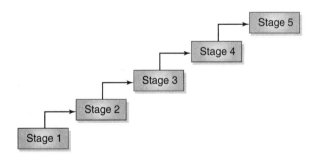

Figure 41-4 The Capability Maturity Model's stepwise progression through 5 discrete stages.

Reprinted from *Evaluation and Program Planning, 46,* McCarthy, C. F., Kelley, M. A., Verani, A. R., St. Louis, M. E., Riley, P. L. (2014). Development of a framework to measure health profession regulation strengthening, Pages 17–24, Copyright 2014, with permission from Elsevier.

Table 41-3 The ARC Regulatory Function Framework

	Stage 1	Stage 2	Stage 3	Stage 4	Stage 5
Nursing and midwifery legislation	Identification of key issues with participation of stakeholders Consensus around whether a new nursing and midwifery Act or amendments to existing legislation	Legislation drafted with stakeholders including MOH, nursing and midwifery council and/or professional associations, academia, and legislature or parliament	Approval, commencement, and publication of legislation	Implementation through dissemination and training of nurses and midwives in their rights and duties Issuance by Councils and/or ministry of health of rules or regulations	Monitoring and evaluation of compliance and impact
Registration system and use of registration data	Registration is not legally required for nurses and midwives to practice or Registration is lifelong (i.e., renewal not required) The register is primarily a paper-based system.	Renewal of registration (or license) is required. Both paper and electronic (e.g., Excel) system for registration is used. Registration system can answer basic queries (e.g., number of midwives in the country).	Registration system (including licensure and re-licensure) is primarily electronic (use of software). Database includes all public sector nurses and is regularly updated. Registration system can be queried to generate workforce reports.	Registration system is completely electronic and includes all public and private sector nurses. Database displays various registration statuses of nurses and midwives. Database can be programmed to automatically generate workforce reports.	Registration, licensure and re-licensure services are available online or are de-centralized. Registration database can exchange data with other health information systems. Registration data used by decision makers for policy and planning.

Licensure Process	Licenses not required to practice	Licenses are issued with initial registration (no separate licensure examination). Renewal of license is required at intervals specified by the regulatory authority.	An examination or assessment process is in place for initial registration and licensure. The examination or assessment is paper-based. National competency standards are being developed.	Examination or assessment content meets national competency standards. Various statuses of licenses issued (i.e., conditional, suspended). Licensure verification process facilitates entry of foreign educated nurses/midwives into workforce.	Registration and initial licensure examination content is updated regularly. Examination content aligns with global guidelines or regional competency standards. The licensure status is available to public via website or viewing in-person.
Scope of practice (SOP)	SOP is not defined by legal statute or regulation. SOP may be decided by the employer or based on health facility needs.	Council has the authority to formally define the SOP. SOP is under development. SOP has been reviewed or revised within 10 years.	Nationally standardized SOP for all nurse and midwife categories. SOP is based on nursing/midwifery job descriptions. SOP reviewed or revised within last 5 years.	SOP includes essential nursing/midwifery competencies. SOP is regularly and systematically reviewed and revised. SOPs allow for individuals to make decisions about task shifting or task sharing.	All SOPs align with global guidelines and standards for nursing and midwifery. SOP is reviewed and revised according to global standard. SOP is dynamic, flexible, and inclusive, not restrictive.

(Continues)

Table 41-3 The ARC Regulatory Function Framework (*Continued*)

	Stage 1	Stage 2	Stage 3	Stage 4	Stage 5
Continuing professional development (CPD)	CPD is voluntary. CPD framework for nursing and midwifery may be in planning stages.	Council has a mandate in legislation to require CPD. National CPD framework for nursing and midwifery is developed. Implementation of CPD requirement is in pilot or early stages.	CPD program for nurses and midwives is finalized and nationally disseminated. CPD is officially required for re-licensure. Strategy is in place to track compliance.	Electronic system is in place to monitor CPD compliance. Penalties for non-compliance with CPD exist. Available CPD includes content on national HIV service delivery guidelines for nurses and midwives.	Multiple types of CPD are available including web-based and mobile-based models. CPD content aligns with regional standards or global guidelines. Regular evaluations of CPD program carried out.
Accreditation of pre-service education	Council does not have legal authority to approve pre-service nursing/ midwifery schools or programs. Public schools/ programs may be "endorsed" by the council.	Council has legal authority to approve pre-service schools/ programs. Council issues standards for accreditation of nursing schools / programs. No time limit or expiration date on accreditation approval.	Initial assessment visits are carried out by the council or their designated authority. Standards for accreditation are regularly reviewed and revised. Requirement for accreditation renewal is enforced.	Assessment visits are regularly carried out by an independent body. Council has an electronic system to track accreditation status. Various levels of accreditation granted (i.e., probationary, conditional).	Group independent from council makes accreditation determination for both public and private schools/programs Accreditation standards align with global or regional guidelines. Accreditation status available to the public.

| Professional Misconduct and Disciplinary Powers | Council does not have authority to manage complaints and impose sanctions. Standards of professional conduct may not be defined. | Legislation authorizes council to define standards for professional conduct. Council has authority to investigate or initiate inquiries into professional misconduct. Basic types of complaints and sanctions exist. | Complaint investigation and misconduct hearings are separate processes. A range of disciplinary measures (penalties, sanctions, conditions) exist. Appeals processes are available and accessible. | The processes and documentation of complaints and sanctions is transparent. Processes and timelines are in place to review and remove penalties and sanctions. Processes are in place for member of the public to lodge a complaint. | Professional conduct standards align with regional standards or global guidelines. The complaint management process is regularly evaluated for transparency and timeliness. Information on complaints and sanctions is available to the public. |

Source: Data from McCarthy, C. F., Kelley, M. A., Verani, A. R., St. Louis, M. E., Riley, P. L. (2014). Development of a framework to measure health profession regulation strengthening. *Evaluation and Program Planning, 46* (2014), 17–24.

Table 41-4 Regulatory Function Framework: Assessing the Country's Performance in Revising Nursing and Midwifery Laws

Country X	Planning (Stage 1)	Developing (Stage 2)	Defining (Stage 3)	Managing (Stage 4)	Optimizing (Stage 5)
Revisions to nursing and midwifery law	There is consensus among key stakeholders on issue(s) to be reformed in legislation.	Draft of legislative change(s) has been approved by stakeholders. MoH supports and approvesproposed legislative change.	MoH fully engages, supports, advances, and represents updated draft of legislation.	Draft is referred to legislative body for induction and passage. Act is promulgated, published, and commenced.	Law is implemented in nursing and midwifery practice environments. Compliance and impact are monitored.
Documenting the country's progress in revising nursing and midwifery laws over time					
Revisions to nursing and midwifery law	There is consensus among key stakeholders on issue(s) to be reformed in legislation.	Draft of legislative change(s) has been approved by stakeholders. MoH supports and approvesproposed legislative change.	MoH fully engages, supports, advances, and represents updated draft of legislation.	Draft is referred to legislative body for induction and passage. Act is promulgated, published, and commenced.	Law is implemented in nursing and midwifery environments. Compliance and impact are monitored.

Source: Data from McCarthy, C. F., Kelley, M. A., Verani, A. R., St. Louis, M. E., Riley, P. L. (2014). Development of a framework to measure health profession regulation strengthening. *Evaluation and Program Planning, 46* (2014), 17–24.

Nations, and East, Central, and Southern Africa College of Nursing). This framework (see **Table 41-4**) was used to stage regulatory performance for each of the 17 ARC countries and to assess ARC's impact in improving the region's nursing and midwifery regulatory infrastructure (McCarthy et al., 2014).

Information Systems

Challenges associated with studying health workforce dynamics pertain to the absence of routine HRH data collection (Joint Learning Initiative, 2004). Workforce data in developing countries is sparse and often fragmented. A systematic review of 63 national HRH information systems identified that information was rarely used for HRH resource allocation and program planning. Those countries most in need of efficient utilization of scarce human and financial resources were largely lacking accurate and timely data on pre-service training capacity and production, workforce availability, qualification, deployment, and retention (Appiagyei et al., 2014; Riley et al., 2010). Current global health initiatives emphasize the need for human resources information systems (HRIS), which facilitate the collection and dissemination of workforce information.

When designed to operate within a health system, a national HRIS can provide information on health workforce size, composition, and deployment station (Riley et al., 2010). HRIS typically collect workforce "supply" data, such as professional registration, major qualifications, and continuing education maintained by professional regulatory boards. Well-designed HRIS have the capability to link supply data to workforce deployment data, maintained by an employer, such as the ministry of health. Functional HRIS provide current and accurate data that can be used for supporting HRH policy decisions. As an example, when Kenya's HRIS projected insufficient numbers of nurses available to replace those scheduled to retire within 5 to 10 years, the National Parliament voted to increase the mandatory retirement age of public health providers (all civil servants) from 55 years to 60 (Rakuom, Oywer, Arudo, Vidot, & Jones, 2010). *The Kenya Nursing Workforce Project: The Status of Nursing in Kenya 2012* (2012) offers a good example of how complete and accurate workforce information can assist with planning health services and scaling-up priority health interventions. The potential yield of information from HRIS has yet to be fully realized. Nevertheless, PEPFAR and other global initiatives have identified HRIS development as well as strengthening HRH data collection as priority areas for intervention (Dal Poz, Gupta, Quain, & Soucat, 2009; PEPFAR, 2009).

GLOBAL NURSING: REDUCING VULNERABILITY

Despite recognition that well-functioning health services and adequate numbers of well-prepared providers are essential in reaching global health goals, critical gaps remain in identifying best practices for addressing vulnerabilities in healthcare systems. The nursing profession, as the largest health professional cadre worldwide, has immense influence on expanding the knowledge base of best practices.

CASE STUDY

A Global Nursing Consultation

The country of Equatoria, which has been identified among those countries most impacted by the AIDS epidemic, recently received a large grant from a global organization to scale-up HIV services. Because nurses represent 80% of Equatoria's health workforce, this cadre of health professionals is expected to absorb additional duties in the care and treatment of HIV-infected clients. Your employer, a global nongovernmental organization (NGO) has received donor support to assist low-income countries in responding to the global AIDS epidemic. Specific funding in the organization's award has been earmarked for supporting nursing improvements in these countries.

In response to Equatoria's request for technical assistance, your organization has been asked to provide a 2-week nursing consultation to the Ministry of Health. You have been identified to provide the necessary technical assistance. In this capacity, you will be expected to:

- Conduct a needs assessment of the immediate HRH issues, and in particular, nursing issues, impacting Equatoria's ability to expand HIV services.
- Design an approach that targets HRH issues but also takes into account infrastructure of the country's health systems.
- Create a long-range strategy capable of being owned and sustained by both the Ministry of Health and Equatoria's nursing leadership.

Case Study Questions

1. In order to prepare for this assignment, what background information would be useful for you to know?
2. As part of this consultative process, what kinds of HRH issues will be important for you to assess immediately?
3. What sources of nursing data would be relevant for this assignment? Where might you begin your search for this data?
4. How might you go about benchmarking current nursing capacity and documenting progress?

REFERENCES

Appiagyei, A., Kirlinya, R., Gross, J., Wambua, D., Oywer, E., Kamenju, A., ... Rogers, M. (2014). Informing the scale-up of Kenya's nursing workforce: A mixed methods study of factors affecting pre-service training capacity and production. *Human Resources for Health*, *12*, 47.

Blaauw, D., Erasmus, E., Pagaiya, N., Tangcharoensathein, V., Mullei, K., Mudhune, S., ... Lagarde, M. (2010). Policy interventions that attract nurses to rural areas: A multicountry discrete choice experiment. *Bulletin of the World Health Organization*, *88*, 350–356.

Chan, M., Kazatchkine, M., Lob-Levyt, J., Obaid, T., Schweizer, J., Sidibe, M., ... Yamada, T. (2010). Meeting the demand for results and accountability: A call for action on data from eight global health agencies. *PLoS Medicine*, *7*, e1000223.

Chen, L. (2010). Striking the right balance: Health workforce retention in remote and rural areas. *Bulletin of the World Health Organization*, *88*, 323.

Chen, L., Evans, T., Anand, S., Boufford, J. L., Brown, H., Chowdhury, M., ... Wibulpolpraset, S. (2004). Human resources for health: overcoming the crises. *Lancet*, *364*, 1984–1990.

Collins, F., Glass, R., Whitescarver, J., Wakefield, M., & Goosby, E. P. (2010). Developing health workforce capacity in Africa. *Science, 330,* 1324–1325. Retrieved from http://www.fic.nih.gov/news/publications/Science-Article-Dec2010.pdf

Dal Poz, M. R., Gupta, N., Quain, E., & Soucat, A. (Eds.). (2009). *Handbook on monitoring and evaluation of human resources for health, with special applications for low- and middle-income countries.* Geneva, Switzerland: WHO Press.

de Savigny, D., & Adam, T. (Eds.). (2009). *Systems thinking for health systems strengthening. Alliance for Health Policy and Systems Research.* Geneva, Switzerland: WHO Press.

Fritzen, S. (2007). Strategic management of the health workforce in developing countries: What have we learned? *Human Resources for Health, 5,* 4. Retrieved from http://preview.human-resources-health.com/content/5/1/4

Fryatt, R., Mills, A., & Nordstrom, A. (2010). Financing of health systems to achieve the health millennium development goals in low-income countries. *Lancet, 375,* 419–426.

Gross, J. M., Rogers, M. F., Teplinskiy, I., Oywer, E., Wambua, D., Kamenju, A., … Waudo, A. (2010). *The impact of out-migration on the nursing workforce in Kenya.* Unpublished manuscript.

Haines, A., & Sanders, D. (2005). Building capacity to attain the millennium development goals. *Transactions of the Royal Society of Tropical Medicine and Hygiene, 99,* 721–726.

Hill, P., Mansoor, G. F., & Claudio, F. (2010). Conflict in least-developed countries: Challenging the millennium development goals. *Bulletin of the World Health Organization, 88,* 562–563.

Humphrey, W. S. (1987). Characterizing the software process: A maturity framework. In CMU-SEI (Ed.), *The software process feasibility project.* Pittsburgh, PA: Carnegie Mellon University Software Engineering Institute.

Institute of Medicine (IOM). (2010a). *Preparing for the future of HIV/AIDS in Africa: A shared responsibility.* Washington, DC: National Academies Press.

Institute of Medicine (IOM). (2010b). *Summary of the February 2010 Forum on the Future of Nursing.* Washington, DC: National Academies Press.

Institute of Medicine (IOM). (2013). *Evaluation of PEPFAR.* Washington, DC: National Academies Press. Retrieved from http://www.iom.edu/Reports/2013/Evaluation-of-PEPFAR.aspx

Joint Learning Initiative. (2004). *Human Resources for health: Overcoming the crisis.* Cambridge, MA: Harvard University Press.

The Kenya Nursing Workforce Project: The Status of Nursing in Kenya, 2012. (2012). Nursing Unit, Kenya Ministry of Health, Nairobi, Kenya.

Lewin, S., Bosch-Capblanch, X., Oliver, S., Akl, E. A., Vist, G. E., Lavis, J. N., … Haines, A. (2012). *Guidance for evidence-informed policies about health systems: Assessing how much confidence to place in the research evidence.* PLoS Medicine, 9, e1001187.

Mangham, L. J., Hanson, K., & McPake, B. (2009). How to do (or not to do): Designing a discrete choice experiment for application in a low-income country. *Health Policy and Planning, 24,* 151–158.

McCarthy, C. F., Kelley, M. A., Verani, A. R., St. Louis, M. E., & Riley, P. L. (2014). Development of a framework to measure health profession regulation strengthening. *Evaluation and Program*

Planning, 46(2014), 17–24. Retrieved from http://www.sciencedirect.com/science/article/pii/S0149718914000470

McCarthy, C. F., & Riley, P. L. (2012). The African health profession regulatory collaborative for nurses and midwives. *Human Resources for Health, 10,* 26. Retrieved from http://www.human-resources-health.com/content/10/1/26

McCarthy, C. F., Zuber, A., Kelley, M. A., Verani, A. R., & Riley, P. L. (2014). The African Health Profession Regulatory Collaborative (ARC) at two years. *African Journal of Midwifery and Women's Health, 8*(Suppl 2), 4–9.

Mgone, C., Volmink, J., Coles, D., Makanga, M., Jaffar, S., & Sewankambo, N. (2010). Linking research and development to strengthen health systems in Africa. *Tropical Medicine and International Health, 15,* 1401–1406.

The Millennium Development Goals Report 2013. (2013). Retrieved from http://www.un.org/millenniumgoals/pdf/report-2013/mdg-report-2013-english.pdf

Mogedal, S., & Stenson, B. (2002). *Disease eradication: Friend or foe to the health system? Synthesis report from field studies on the Polio Eradication Initiative in Tanzania, Nepal and the Lao People's Democratic Republic.* Geneva, Switzerland: WHO Press. Retrieved from http://www.who.int/vaccines-documents/DocsPDF00/www552.pdf

Motivation and retention of health workers in developing countries: A systematic review. *BMC Health Services Research, 8,* 247. Retrieved from http://www.biomedcentral.com/1472-6963/8/247

Mullan, F. (2005). The metrics of the physician brain drain. *The New England Journal of Medicine, 353,* 1810–1818.

Pan American Organization & World Health Organization. (2001). *35th Session of the Subcommittee of the Executive Committee on Planning and Programming: Development and strengthening of human resources management in the health services.* Washington, DC. Retrieved from http://www.paho.org/english/gov/ce/ce128index-e.htm

Rakuom, C. P., Oywer, E. O., Arudo, J., Vidot, P., & Jones, T. (2010). *Health workforce information system: Kenya's nursing experience.* Report prepared for the Commonwealth Secretariat.

Reich, M., Takeni, K., Roberts, M., & Hsiao, W. (2008). Global action on health systems: A proposal for the Tokyo G8 summit. *Lancet, 371,* 865–869.

Report from the Ministerial Summit on Health Research, Mexico City, 15–20 November 2004. (2004). Geneva, Switzerland: WHO Press.

Riley, P. L., Vindigni, S. M., Arudo, J., Waudo, A. N., Kamenju, A., Ngoya, K., ... Marum, L. H. (2007). Developing a nursing database system in Kenya. *Health Services Research, 42,* 1389–1405.

Riley, P. L., Zuber, A., Vindigni, S. M., Gupta, N., Verani, A., & Sunderland, N. (2010). *Information systems to monitor human resources for health (HRH): A systematic review.* Unpublished manuscript.

Sanders, D., & Haines, A. (2006). Implementation research is needed to achieve international health goals. *PloS Medicine, 3,* e186.

Strengthening health systems: The country perspective. (2009). A global initiative to strengthen country health systems surveillance (CHeSS): Summary report of a technical meeting and action plan. Retrieved from http://www.who.int/healthsystems/healthsystems_thecountryperspective_1_09.pdf

Task Force on Health Systems Research. (2004). Informed choices for attaining the millennium development goals: Towards an international cooperative agenda for health-systems research. *Lancet*, *364*, 997–1003.

Travis, P., Bennett, S., Haines, A., Pang, T., Bhutta, Z., & Hyder, A. (2004). Overcoming health-systems constraints to achieve the millennium development goals. *Lancet*, *364*, 900–906.

U.S. President's Emergency Plan for AIDS Relief (PEPFAR). (n.d.). Annex V—Health system strengthening priority-setting. Implementation of the Global Health Initiative Consultation Document, 2010. Retrieved from http://www.pepfar.gov/reports/guidance/framework/120741.htm

U.S. President's Emergency Plan for AIDS Relief (PEPFAR). (2009). *Technical guidance for human resources for health: State of the program area*. Unpublished document.

The Wall Street Journal. Gates Foundation to double donation to fight AIDS, (2013, December 2). Retrieved from http://blogs.wsj.com/washwire/2013/12/02/gates-foundation-to-double-donation-to-fight-aids/

Willis-Shattuck, M., Bidwell, P., Thomas, S., Wyness, L., Blaauw, D., & Ditlopo, P. (2008). World Health Organization (WHO). (n.d.). Health workforce: Achieving the health-related MDGs. It takes a workforce! Retrieved from http://www.who.int/hrh/workforce_mdgs/en/index.html

World Health Organization (WHO). (2000). *The world health report 2000. Health systems: Improving performance*. Geneva, Switzerland: WHO Press.

World Health Organization (WHO). (2004). World Health Assembly. International migration of health personnel: a challenge for health systems in developing countries. Retrieved from www.who.int/gb/ebwha/pdf_files/WHA57/A57_R19-en.pdf

World Health Organization (WHO). (2005). Health and the millennium development goals: World Health Organization. Retrieved from http://www.who.int/hdp/publications/mdg en.pdf

World Health Organization (WHO). (2006). *The world health report: Working together for health*. Geneva, Switzerland: WHO Press.

World Health Organization (WHO). (2007). *Everybody's business: Strengthening health systems to improve health outcomes: WHO's framework for action*. Geneva, Switzerland: WHO Press.

World Health Organization (WHO). (2008). *Task shifting: Rational redistribution of tasks among health workforce teams. Global recommendations and guidelines*. Geneva, Switzerland: WHO Press. Retrieved from http://www.who.int/healthsystems/TTR-TaskShifting.pdf

World Health Organization (WHO). (2009). Maximizing Positive Synergies Collaborative Group: An assessment of interactions between global health initiatives and country health systems. *Lancet*, *373*, 2137–2169.

World Health Organization (WHO). (2010a). *Increasing access to health workers in remote and rural areas through improved retention*. Geneva, Switzerland: WHO Press.

World Health Organization (WHO). (2010b). 63rd World Health Assembly. *International recruitment of health personnel: Global code of practice*. Geneva, Switzerland: WHO Press. Retrieved from http://www.who.int/workforcealliance/media/news/2010/codestatementwha/en/index.html

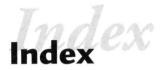

Index

Note: Page numbers followed by *f* or *t* indicate material in figures or tables respectively.

A

AARP, 543
ABA. *See* applied behavioral analysis
abortion methods, sex trafficking and, 503
abuse
    child, 483
    substance, 483, 485
    victims suffer psychological, 501
abusive families, 8
ACA. *See* Affordable Care Act
academic competencies, development of, 466
access to healthcare, 373
    barriers to, 363
    health insurance and, 5
    health outcomes and, 564–565
    health policy and advocacy and, 564–565
    PPACA provisions, 566t–567t
ACES. *See* Advancing Care Excellence for Seniors
ACHA. *See* American College Health Association
ACHRE. *See* Advisory Committee on Human Radiation
    Experiments
ACNM. *See* American College of Nurse-Midwifes
ACOG. *See* American Congress of Obstetricians and
    Gynecologists
acting on patient's behalf, 20
Action for Health committee (New York), 332
action theory research, 411–412
"activational effect," 313
activities of daily living, 527
acute coronary events, 165
acute myocardial infarction (AMI), 165–166
    CMS adapted for older adults diagnosed with,
        171–173
Ad Hoc Committee on Advocacy of NASW, 25
ADAAA. *See* Americans with Disabilities Act Amendments
    Act
ADAPT. *See* Association for Drug Abuse Prevention and
    Treatment

ADDM network. *See* Autism and Developmental Disabilities
    Monitoring network
ADHD and pet therapy, 313
adherence, 121–123
Administrative Procedures Act, 540
adolescent health promotion
    evidence-based template for, 398, 399t–400t
    resources for, 398, 401t–402t
adolescents
    autism in, 349–350
    with bipolar II disorder, 467–468
    case study, 402–405
    health indicators among, 396, 396t
    human capital, 393–394
    with mental health disorder, college-bound, 461–474
    pre-incarceration stage, 369
    programs to promote resilience, 397–398, 399t–402t
    promoting resilience among, 396–397
    risk and resilience among, 394–402
    risky behaviors among, 394, 394t–395t
    social capital, 393
    social status, 391–393
    strengths, 397
    in type 1 diabetes mellitus, 419–425
    vulnerabilities, 391–394, 397
adults, diet and mental health in, 463–464
advanced practice nurse, 514
Advancing Care Excellence for Seniors (ACES), 526
adversity, resilience to, 38
Advisory Committee on Human Radiation Experiments
    (ACHRE), 186
advocacy role of providers, 19–29
    activities of, 23
    attributes of, 20
    behaviors cited by nurses as, 22
    case study of Mr. Jackson, 27–29
    case study of Mrs. Smith, 26–27
    class advocacy, 23

advocacy role of providers (*Cont.*)
  communication typology of, 22
  compartmentalization, 26
  defined, 23–24
  implications for practice, 29
  institutional review boards (IRBs), 20
  interdisciplinary benefits and approach, 25–29
  nursing literature review, 20–23
  overview, 19–20
  paternalism in, 21
  patient advocacy concept, 20–21
  patient advocate's role, 21–23
  patients' perception of, 22
  political nature of health care, 19
  in public policy, 542
  relational ethics and, 23
  social justice in, 20, 25
  social work literature review, 23–25
  studying, 20, 22
Affordable Care Act (ACA), 374, 375
Afghanistan, 305
African Americans
  clinic services in poor neighborhoods, 433
  coping of ill elderly, 40
  cultural competence and, 34
  as high-risk mothers, 7
  maternal mortality of, 564
  racism's effect on, 34
  substance abuse in children, 12
African Health Profession Regulatory Collaborative for
  Nurses and Midwives (ARC), 587, 592
  Regulatory Function Framework, 587, 588*t*–592*t*
age, pre-incarceration stage, 367
Agency for Healthcare Research and Quality (AHRQ), 562
aggression issues, adolescents, 349–350
aging issues, incarceration, 373
AHRQ. *See* Agency for Healthcare Research and Quality
AIANGRC. *See* American Indian and Alaska Native Genetics
  Resource Center
AIDS Service Organization (ASO), 204
alcohol, 7
  awareness of, 473
  use of, 464–465
alleviation of social inequality by co-learning in CBPR, 248
ALS. *See* amyotrophic lateral sclerosis
Alzheimer's disease, 10, 525, 526
amelioration, social justice and, 58–59
America, factors to homelessness in, 481, 485
American Academy of Nursing (AAN), 429
American Academy of Pediatrics (AAP), 255
American Academy of Pediatrics' Council on Children with
  Disabilities, 342
American Anthropological Association, 545
American Association of Colleges of Nursing (AACN), 429
American College Health Association (ACHA), 13

American College of Nurse-Midwifes (ACNM), 255
American College of Obstetricians and Gynecologists, 152
American Congress of Obstetricians and Gynecologists
  (ACOG), 255
American Diabetes Association, 152
American Health Benefit Exchanges, 565, 566
American Heritage Online Dictionary, 37
American Indian and Alaska Native Genetics Resource
  Center (AIANGRC), 189
American Indians. *See* indigenous people
American Nurses Association (ANA)
  *Code of Ethics with Interpretive Statements, Nursing's
    Social Policy Statement and Nursing: Scope and
    Standards of Practice*, 51
  Health System Reform Agenda, 568
American Society for the Prevention of Cruelty to Animals
  (ASPCA), 312
Americans with Disabilities Act Amendments Act (ADAAA),
  469
Americans with Disabilities Act of 1990, 469
AMI. *See* acute myocardial infarction
Amnesty International, 564
amyotrophic lateral sclerosis (ALS), 129
ANA. *See* American Nurses Association
analysis of variance (ANOVA), 226
anger, caregiving and, 12
animal-assisted intervention (AAI), 313
animal-assisted therapy, websites for, 318–319
ANOVA. *See* analysis of variance
anthropology and life histories, 236
antidepressant use by college students, 13
antitrafficking organization, 457
anxiety, 172, 423
  disorder, 467
  in HIV-infected population, 12
Appalachian Patterns General Ethnographic Nursing
  Evaluation Studies in the State III, 360
applied behavioral analysis (ABA), 344
appraisal, 173
  concept of, 167, 171
ARC. *See* African Health Profession Regulatory
  Collaborative for Nurses and Midwives
Arizona Board of Regents, 189
Arizona State University (ASU), 189
ASD. *See* autism spectrum disorder
Ashkenazi Jews, breast cancer in, 218, 221
Asian and Pacific Islander American Health Forum, 385
ASO. *See* AIDS Service Organization
ASPCA. *See* American Society for the Prevention of Cruelty
  to Animals
Association for Drug Abuse Prevention and Treatment
  (ADAPT), 542
ASU. *See* Arizona State University
attention issues, adolescents, 349–350
attitudes, as variable in depression, 10

Australia, outmigration to, 584–585
Autism and Developmental Disabilities Monitoring (ADDM) network, 339
autism spectrum disorder (ASD), 339–353
    adolescents issues, 349–350
    applied behavioral analysis, 344
    comorbidity, 342
    cultural components of resilience, 345–347
    elements of resilience, 344–351
    environmental components of resilience, 344–345
    formal network of caregivers, 348
    key points for healthcare providers, 352
    nervous system, 341–342
    nursing intervention, 351–352, 353t
    nursing priorities and, 341
    parenting role stress and, 347
    physiological components of resilience, 350–351
    primary goals of treatment, 342
    protective factors, 340
    psychological components of resilience, 348–350
    resilience, 340–352
    resources available to nurses, 353t
    risk factors, 340
    rural poverty and, 344
    sleep disorders in, 347–348
    social components of resilience, 347–348
    social factors, 347–348
    social isolation, 340–341, 348
    social/psychological factors, 340, 340t
    symptoms of, 341–342
    treatment plan, 342, 344
    vulnerability, 342–344
autobiography, 236
autonomy, safeguarding, 20
awareness, 34, 510
    of available aid, 481
    social justice, 58–59

B

barriers to health care, 363
behavior-specific cognitions, 130
behavioral change process, 120
behavioral regression, 352
Belmont Report, 191
bias, ethnocentric, 430
biocultural ecology and workforce issues in cultural competence, 35
biological view of schizophrenia, 10–11
bipolar disorder, 463, 472
bipolar II disorder, adolescents with, 467–468
Blacks. *See* African Americans
blaming the victim, 5
body image dissatisfaction, 39
BRCA1/2 literature research, 220–224
BRCA1 Questionnaire, 225–227

breast cancer, 284t
    in Ashkenazi Jews, 218
    BRCA1/2 genetic mutations linked to, 216, 218
    factors associated with genetic mutation, 220
    genetic counseling and, 221
    genetic testing for, 216, 221
    Latinas and, 219–220
Breathe2Relax, 474
"bricherismo," 551
brigadista (community health worker), 331
BSN Essentials (AACN), 429
budget, business plans, 335
budget justification, 209, 209t
business plans, 334–336

C

C-section, 280t–281t
CAM. *See* complementary and alternative medicine
Camp Kudzu, 423–425
Campinha-Bacote, 35, 36
Campus Awareness, Resource and Empowerment (CARE) center, 489
Canada
    Canadian Nurses Association's (CNA) Revised Code of Ethics, 51
    outmigration to, 584–585
cancer
    in Native Americans, 513
    screening and management, 6
cancer susceptibility, genetic testing for, 221
Candido Godoi, 186
capability maturity model (CMM), 587, 587f
CAPS. *See* Coping and Promoting Strength Program
cardiopulmonary resuscitation (CPR) programs, 434
cardiovascular disease (CVD), 6, 165–166
CARE center. *See* Campus Awareness, Resource and Empowerment center
Caribbean, sex workers in, 551
CATT. *See* Coalition on Aging Think Tank
CATT-Rath Center model, 416–417
CBPR. *See* community-based participatory research
CCM. *See* chronic care model
CDC. *See* Centers for Disease Control
Center for International Nursing, 434–435
Centers for Disease Control (CDC), 185
cerebral palsy, pet therapy, 313–314
certified nurse midwives (CNMs), 257
Cesarean delivery rate, 291
Chance, Kaitlin, 453–459
Charity Organization Societies (COS), 24
CHC. *See* Community Health Clinic
child abuse, 483
children
    abuse of, 7, 337
    Afghan, 40

children (*Cont.*)
  resilience in, 38–39
  as sex trafficking victims, 550, 551
China, HIV/AIDS in, 555
chronic care model (CCM), 133–134
chronic illness issues, incarceration, 373
chronic obstructive pulmonary disease (COPD), 134
chronic pelvic pain, 502
chronically ill and disabled persons, as vulnerable
  population, 7
cigarette, 504
CINAHL. *See* Cumulative Index to Nursing and Allied
  Health Literature
"class advocacy," in social work, 23
client-nurse relationship, 144
clinical information systems, 133
clinical trials, 244
CMM. *See* capability maturity model
CNMs. *See* certified nurse midwives
co-learning, social inequality by, 248
co-payment for services, 371
Coalition on Aging Think Tank (CATT), 412
coenzyme Q10 (CoQ10), 327
cognitive coping processes, 170–171
cognitive illness representations, 170
  controllability, concepts of, 169–170
  identity and cause, concepts of, 168–169
  timeline and consequence, concepts of, 170
cognitive processing, 118
college-bound adolescent, with mental health disorder,
  461–474
Collins, Lady, 450–451, 453, 457–459
commercial pastoralism, 287
Commercial Sexual Exploitation of Children (CSEC), 459
common myth, 485
common sense model of illness behavior (CSM)
  adapted for older adults diagnosed with AMI, 171–173
  concepts of, 167–171
  evaluation of, 173
  overview, 166–167
  theoretical assumptions, 173
communication, 293–294
  schizophrenic families, difficulties in, 11
  techniques for public policy activism, 542
  therapeutic skills of, 539
  typology of roles in advocacy, 22
community and health systems, 133
community-based care, 431
community-based participatory research (CBPR), 243–251
  building on strengths in, 246–247
  clinical trials, 244
  collaboration, 247–248
  community as unit of study, 246
  implementing, 250–251
  integrating knowledge and action, 248
  iterative process, use of, 249

  overview, 244–245
  partnering in dissemination of findings, 249–250
  principles of, 246–250
  promoting alleviation of social inequality by
    co-learning, 248
  as qualitative method, 249
  saturation of data, 249
  vulnerable populations and, 250–251
  wellness and ecological perspective, 249
Community Health Clinic (CHC), 366
community health nurse, 130
community health nursing simulation, 525–526
  case study, 526–528
  for vulnerable populations, 523–530
community nurses, 325
community ownership, establishment of, 361
community programs, pre-incarceration, 370
compartmentalizing, 26
complementary and alternative medicine (CAM), 326
complementary medicine. *See* healers, traditional
conceptualization, advocacy, 24
conceptualize research ethics, 183
confidentiality of care, 392–393
congenital disorder, autism, 341–342
consent forms, 225
contemporary nursing care, 117
contracts
  as funding sources, 335
  population-based programs, 335
contractual justice, 54
controllability, concepts of, 169–170
COPD. *See* chronic obstructive pulmonary disease
Coping and Promoting Strength Program (CAPS), 39
coping mechanisms, 474
coping processes, 167, 170–171
cornerstone, 23
COS. *See* Charity Organization Societies
cost-effective care, 431
costs
  business plans, 335
  of healthcare, 5
couch surfing, 484
counseling and support, 22–23
counseling services, accessibility and quality of, 468
counterterrorism, 304
CPR programs. *See* cardiopulmonary resuscitation programs
cross-cultural communication, 36
cross-cultural training, 9
crowd funding, 336
CSEC. *See* Commercial Sexual Exploitation of Children
CSM. *See* common sense model of illness behavior
cues, 156
cultural competence, 33–37
  African Americans and, 33. *See also* African Americans
  biocultural ecology and workforce issues in, 35
  case study of Mr. Hernandez, 41–42

cultural blurring, 34
cultural proficiency, 35
cultural sensitivity comparison, 34–35
culture clues, 37
didactic materials to teach, 37
dimensions of, 34–35
holistic nursing and, 36
Hutterites, 37
immersion programs, 36–37, 432, 516–517
learning of, 36–37
Leininger on, 35, 37
models of, 34–36
native healing practices and, 36
overview, 33, 430–431
resilience and, 37–42
self-awareness in, 36
social justice and marginalization in, 34
Watson's theory of caring and, 35
cultural identity, 7
cultural values, 40
culture
    characteristics of, 142
    as context for societal problems, 536
    defined, 142
    homeless college students, 483–485
    of vulnerability, 4
culture care, theory of (Leininger), 141–146
Cumulative Index to Nursing and Allied Health Literature (CINAHL), 50, 535, 536
cure/control concept, 169
CVD. *See* cardiovascular disease

D
DCE methodology. *See* discrete choice experiment methodology
de Chesnay, Mary, 450–451, 456, 460
de salud faith-based programs, 224
death, 40
debriefing sessions, 530
decision-making ability, 125
decision-making process, 156, 159–160, 167, 169, 173
    advocacy and, 24
    of older adults, 171
Declaration of Helsinki, 191
delivery system design, goal of, 133
dementia, pet therapy, 315
demographic variables, 158
demographics of families, 8
deoxyribonucleic acid (DNA) testing for *BRCA1/2*, 216
Department of Health and Human Services, 6
depression, 10, 423
    antidepressant use by college students, 13
developmental regression, 352
diabetes
    in Americans, 513
    management of, 421

Diabetes Management Self-Efficacy Scale (DMSES), 121
Diabetes Prevention Program (DPP), 150, 151
Diabetes Project with the Havasupai Tribe, 189
diabulimia, 422
didactic approach, 37
diet
    and mental health, 463–464
    during pregnancy and postpartum, 299
disabled persons and chronically ill, 7
disaster relief, 306
discrete choice experiment (DCE) methodology, 586–587
discrimination, ethnocentric bias, 430
disparities in health
    access to care and, 564–565
    concept of, 536
disparities in Somali community, 291–293
distributive justice, 51, 59
diversity and universality, 142–144
DMSES. *See* Diabetes Management Self-Efficacy Scale
DNP. *See* doctor of nursing practice
DNP-prepared nurse
    development of, 442
    vulnerable populations, role of, 441–444, 445*t*–446*t*
DNP translational research, vulnerable populations, 444, 445*t*–446*t*
DNS. *See* doctor of nursing science
doctor of nursing practice (DNP)
    capstone project, 257
    degree, development of, 443–444
    programs, 326
doctor of nursing science (DNS), 443
doctoral nursing program, online, 435–436
dog-assisted interventions, 313
dogs, as co-therapist, 314
domestic violence, victims of, 483
domestication, 312
Dominican Republic, sex workers in, 551
DPP. *See* Diabetes Prevention Program
drug abuse, complexity of, 368
drugs, 502
    awareness of, 473
    use of, 464–465
Duquesne Model, 433–436
Dysfunctional Attitude Scale, 10

E
Earvolino-Ramirez, 38
Eastern Nursing Research Society (ENRS), 245
eating disorders, vulnerability to, 11
EBP. *See* evidence-based practice
ectopic pregnancy, 282*t*
Educating Children with Autism (National Research Council), 345
Education Department, 539
education, lack of, 493
educational intervention, development of, 159

educational programs, implementation of, 221
effective health education methods, 224
effective verbal communication, 293
elderly
    African Americans, 40
    in Appalachia, 359
    resilience in, 39–40
    vulnerability of, 5, 8
electronic event monitoring, 122
emic approaches to vulnerability, 6
emotion regulation instruction, 10
emotional arousal, 120
emotional illness representations, 170
empathetic communication, 120
employed adolescents, 394
employment opportunities, ex-prisoners, 377
empowerment
    in community-based participatory research, 246
    of vulnerable persons, 432, 542
enactive attainment, 119
Encyclopedia of Social Work, 23
End Demand for Sex Trafficking Act, 556
ENRS. *See* Eastern Nursing Research Society
entitlement, 52
epidural/spinal anesthesia, 254
Epsom salts, 326
equity in social justice, 52
"equivalence of care" principle, 371
Essential Early Education programs, 345
ethics
    context of relational, 23
    framework and orientations of, 50
    social justice and, 50
ethics foundations, 190
ethnicity, pre-incarceration stage, 367
ethnocentric bias, 430
ethonograph computer data management program, 206
etic approaches to vulnerability, 6
European Commission, 192
evidence-based practice (EBP), 443
evidence-based program, 256
evidenced-based projects, 256
ex-prisoners
    advocacy activities for, 377
    housing, 376, 377
    social network, 376
exercise, lack of, 464
experiential learning models, 433–437
external influencing sources, 168, 172, 173
eye contact, 497

F
FAFSA. *See* Free Application for Federal Student Aid
families
    Afghan, 40
    in Appalachia, 359

    Native American, 516
    vulnerable, 8
Family, Infant and Toddler (FIT) program, 345
family nurse practitioner (FNP), 134, 383, 384, 386
family nursing practice, 509–520
    community description, 512–515
    cultural immersion, 516–517
    domestic intercultural immersion project, 511–512
    evaluation, 517–520
    immersion design, 517
    immersion experience, 515–516
    Indian Child Welfare Program, 513
    Lake Superior Chippewa Indians (formerly Ojibwa), 512
    life expectancy of Native Americans, 513
    medical model in, 510
    noncompliance, 514
    overview, 509–511
    "relational practice," 518
    spiritual beliefs of, 515
family therapy, pre-incarceration, 369
FDA. *See* U.S. Food and Drug Administration
Federal Bureau of Prisons, 373
Federal Children's Bureau, 563
Federal Food, Drug, and Cosmetic Act, 190–191
federal medical privacy regulations, 393
Federal Register, 540
Federally Qualified Health Center (FQHC), 361
Federally Qualified Health Center Look-Alike (FQHC-LA), 361
Feed the Future Program, 488
feedback remediation, 22
female genital cutting (FGC), 294, 386–388
fetal-neonatal outcomes, 258
FGC. *See* female genital cutting
financial aid, 482
FIT program. *See* Family, Infant and Toddler program
Florida College System, 490
Florida Community College System, 490
FNP. *See* family nurse practitioner
focus group interviews, 330
focus groups, 248
folk practices, 143
food insecurity, 11
food travel course, 37
formal network of caregivers, 348
formative data, 541
"40-days rule," 296
FQHC. *See* Federally Qualified Health Center
FQHC-LA. *See* Federally Qualified Health Center Look-Alike
Framework for Action, WHO, 579
Free Application for Federal Student Aid (FAFSA), 481, 490
Frontier Nursing Service, 442
Functional Family Therapy, 369

functional health literacy, 122
functional support systems, 128
funding
  business plans, 335–336
  nurse practitioner-run center in rural
    Appalachia, 362

G

GANS. *See* Georgia Association of Nursing Students
garbage can model of organizations, 537
garden communities, 436
GAVI. *See* Global Alliance for Vaccines and Immunizations
GD. *See* gestational diabetes
gender differences, 10
genetic testing for breast cancer, 216, 221
genetics, 283*t*–284*t*
genogram, 237
Georgia Association of Nursing Students (GANS), 450, 451,
  453, 455
gestational diabetes (GD), 149–152
GHI. *See* Global Health Initiative
Global Alliance for Vaccines and Immunizations (GAVI),
  580
Global Fund to Fight AIDS, 580
Global Health Initiative (GHI), 574, 581
global health systems
  code of practice, 586
  coverage threshold, 583
  defined, 579
  developing countries and, 579
  discrete choice experiment (DCE) methodology,
    586–587
  disease specific interventions, 580, 581*t*
  Framework for Action, WHO, 579
  HIV/AIDS, 577, 579
  human resources information systems (HRIS), 593
  Joint Learning Initiative, 583–585
  maldistribution, 585–586
  Millennium Development Goals (MDGs), 574,
    575*t*–577*t*, 577–578
  nursing, case study, 593–594
  outmigration to, 584–585
  overview, 573–577, 583–584
  policy and research, 580–583, 586–592
  retention, 585
  task shifting/sharing, 586
  WHO on, 579
  workforce density, 583, 583*f*
glycemic control in type 1 diabetes mellitus, 419–425
Governor's Office of Children and Families Statewide
  Commercial Sexual Exploitation of Children
  (GOCF-CSEC) task force, 451, 452
grants as funding sources, 335
grants, population-based programs, 335
grass-roots fundraising, 335–336
Great Recession, 482

group facilitator role in advocacy, 22–23
Guidelines for Human Experimentation 1931, 190
gynecology, 277*t*–278*t*

H

habitual unhealthy behaviors, 153
Haiti, disaster aid to, 307
halal diet, 298
Harvard University's Global Equity Initiative, 583
Havasupai study, 189–190
Havasupai Tribe, 189
HAW. *See* Homelessness Awareness Week
Hawaiian natives. *See* indigenous people
HbA1C test, T1DM, 425
HBM. *See* health belief model
Head Start, 510
healers, traditional, 36
Health and Human Services (HHS) Department, 6, 539
health behavior, 153
health belief model (HBM), 11, 152–154, 217, 221–224
  concepts for adapted, 158
  evaluation of, 159–160
  to genetics, 217*t*
  to guide study, use of, 158–159
  major concepts and definitions of, 154–156
  theoretical assumptions, 157–158
  for women with gestational diabetes, 157
health care
  incarceration, provision of, 371
  price of, 482
health center providers, accessibility and expertise of,
  468–469
health disparities, 8, 243, 536
health insurance
  for farmers, 565
  immigrants and poor and, 5
  as indicator of access to care, 565
  Patient Protection and Affordable Care Act of 2010,
    565, 566*t*–567*t*, 567–568
Health Insurance Portability and Accountability Act
  (HIPAA) of 1996, 393
health issues, review of, 263–268
health literacy, 394
Health Plan Employer Data and Information Set (HEDIS),
  536
Health policy and advocacy for vulnerable populations,
  561–570
  access to care, 564–565, 568
  cost control, 569
  health policy perspective of vulnerability, 562
  historical background, 562–563
  implications for nursing, 568–570
  national reform, 563–568
  priority populations, 562
  quality indicators under PPACA, 569–570
  workforce development, 570

health promotion model (HPM), 130–131
    development of, 223
health promotion programs, 398
health protective behaviors, 222
    model's utility for, 222
health-related quality of life (HRQOL), 128–129
health screening, 373
health status in America, 441–442
health systems, 573–574
    consolidation of, 442
Health Systems: Improving Performance, WHO, 579
health threats, consequences of, 170
healthcare community, 366
healthcare costs, 366
healthcare delivery, 443
healthcare professionals, pet therapy, 316
healthcare providers, 253
healthcare reform, 6, 563–568
healthcare regimens, compliance of, 153
Healthcare Research and Quality Act of 1999, 562
healthy lifestyle behaviors, 151–152
    adoption of, 158, 159
healthy lifestyle for woman, benefits of, 155
Healthy People 2020, 562
    objectives, 562
Healthy People 2010, objectives, 7
HEDIS. *See* Health Plan Employer Data and Information Set
hepatitis C infection, 372
hermanamiento (sister school relationship), 435
HHS Department. *See* Health and Human Services
    Department
HIPAA of 1996. *See* Health Insurance Portability and
    Accountability Act of 1996
hippotherapy
    pet therapy, 313–314
    with sex trafficking survivors, 315
HIV/AIDS, 372
    needle exchange programs and, 542
    public policy and, 538
    sex trafficking and, 503, 555
    vulnerability to, 11–12
    WHO on, 577
HIV-infected mothers, 202
    diagnosis of, 198, 199, 201
    methods, 204–209
    rationale, 203
    significance, 199–202
    stigma, 201, 202
Homeland Security Department, 538
Homeless At-Risk Transitional Students Programs (HARTS),
    City College of San Francisco, 490
homeless college students, 479–491
    CARE Center, 489
    case study, 486–488
    contributing factors, 481–483
    culture, 483–485

FAFSA, 481
    health risk of, 486
    Homelessness Awareness Week (HAW), 489
    hypertension in, 486
    issue of, 480
    project requirements, 480
    risks, 485–486
    university-based programs, 490
    vulnerable populations and, 480–481
homeless persons
    social justice and, 58
    as vulnerable population, 8
Homelessness Awareness Week (HAW), 489
homicide, vulnerability to, 7
Honors Capstone Project, 494–506
    delivery, 495–506
    preparation, 494–495
Hospital Anxiety and Depression Scale, 129
hospital mission (vignette), navy nurses, 307–309
hotline sponsors, 500
Housing and Urban Development (HUD)
    Department, 433
housing, ex-prisoners, 376, 377
HPM. *See* Health Promotion Model
HRH. *See* human resources for health
HRIS. *See* human resources information systems
HRQOL. *See* health-related quality of life
HUD. *See* U.S. Department of Housing and Urban
    Development
human capital, adolescents, 393–394
human radiation experiments, 186
human resources for health (HRH), 574
    information systems, 592–593
    maldistribution, 585–586
    outmigration, 584–585
    overview, 583–584
    policy and research, 586–592
    retention, 585
human resources information systems (HRIS), 593
human trafficking, 449–460, 485
    Chance, Kaitlin, 453–459
    Collins, Lady, 450–451, 453, 457–459
    issue of, 493
    Meyers, Christine, 452–453, 459–460
    victims of, 496, 501
humanitarian mission (vignette), navy nurses, 306–307
Hurricane Katrina, 40
Hutterites, 37
hydrotherapy, 257
hyperglycemia, 422
hypertension, 486
hypoglycemia, 424

I

IBC. *See* inherited breast cancer
ICE office. *See* Immigration Customs Enforcement office

illness representation, cognitive element of, 167–168
IMF. *See* International Monetary Fund
immersion, 36–37, 432
    cultural, 516–517
    design, 517
    evaluation of, 517–520
    experience, 515–520
immersion planning, health implications for, 512–515
immigrant women, role transition for
    and intimate partner violence, 385–386
    mail-order bride, 383–384
    marriage and female genital cutting, 386–388
    overview, 381–382
    pregnant immigrant women, 384–385
    vulnerabilities and strengths, 381–388
immigrants/refugees, 382
    Asian survivors of sexual abuse, 39
    undocumented, 321–327
    as vulnerable population, 8
Immigration Customs Enforcement (ICE) office, 323
immunization, 6
imprisonment, complexity of, 368
in-prison program, 377
inadequate sleep, 462–463
incarceration
    aging and chronic illness issues, 373
    experience of, 370–371
    health care provision, 371
    infectious disease transmission risk, 372
    mental health disorders management, 372–373
    nursing interventions with prisoners, 373
    overview, 370
    post-incarceration, 374–377
    release from, 374–377
    social and ethical issues with, 371–373
income disparity, adolescents, 394
India, antitrafficking organization in, 457
Indian Child Welfare program, 513
indigenous people
    research and, 7
    working with cultural belief systems of, 36
individual-level middle-range theories, 118–121
inequality, health status and, 56
infants, mortality, 563, 564
infectious disease transmission incarceration, risk of, 372
informal network of caregivers, 348
information systems, HRH, 592–593
informed consent, 192
inherited breast cancer (IBC), 216
injury, treatment of, 497
innovative medical reperfusion therapies, 166
inpatients, pet therapy, 316
Institute of Medicine (IOM)
    landmark document, 442, 443
    policy document, 444
    Preparing for the Future of HIV/AIDS in Africa, 585

    public policy role, 545
    on racial and ethnic differences in health, 9
institutional review boards (IRBs), 20, 224, 494
insulin, 424
insulin sensitivity, 151
Integrated Library Information System, 208
integrative middle-range concepts and theories, 128–130
interdisciplinary benefits and approach, 25–29
internal cues, 156
internal influencing sources, 168, 172
international community, 184
International Consensus Conference on Breast Cancer Risk, Genetics, and Risk Management, 220
International Diabetes Federation, 151
International Monetary Fund (IMF), 287
international research with vulnerable populations, cross-cutting issues in, 192–193
Internet, patient use of, 22
intimate partner violence (IPV), immigration and, 385–386
intrapartum nurses
    in facilities, 257
    majority of, 257
intrauterine device (IUD), 385
introversion, schizophrenia and, 11
investigator role in advocacy, 22–23
IOM. *See* Institute of Medicine
IPV. *See* intimate partner violence
Iraq, 305
IRBs. *See* institutional review boards
Irmick, Dana, 509, 510, 513, 519
isolation, social, 340–341, 348
iterative processes in research, 249
IUD. *See* intrauterine device

J
Jewish Chronic Diseases study, 188
Joint Learning Initiative, 583–585
justice
    contractual, 54
    distributive and market, 51–53
    distributive justice, 59

K
Kaiser Family Foundation, 565
Katrina. *See* Hurricane Katrina
kava (Piper methysticum), 326–327
Kefauver-Harris Amendment, 190
Kennesaw State University (KSU) Model, 436–437, 488–490, 494
Kenya, nursing retention in, 585, 587, 593
Knowledge About Inherited Breast Cancer, 225–227
Knowledge About Inherited Breast Cancer and BRCA1 Questionnaire (National Center for Human Genome Research Cancer Studies Consortium), 225, 226
KSU. *See* Kennesaw State University

L

L-theanine, 327
La Clinica de Roberto Clemente, 435
labeling, 4, 14
Lac du Flambeau. *See* Family nursing practice
Lake Superior Chippewa Indians (formerly Ojibwa), 512
Lakeland Volunteers in Medicine (LVIM), 416
landmark document, IOM, 442, 443
Latinas, significance to, 219–220
Latinos
    diversity of, 8
    education methods for, 224
    genetic testing for breast cancer and, 219
Lavender-scented Epsom salts, 326
lead, level of, 350–351
learning cultural competence, modes of, 36–37
lecture content, Honors Capstone Project, 495–506
legislative process, 539
Leininger's culture care theory, 37, 141–146
    culturally congruent care in, 143
    culture, defined, 142
    diversity and universality, 142–144
    folk practices, 143
    generic and professional care, 143
    modes of action in, 143–144
    overview, 141–142
    research enablers, 144
    sunrise model, 142–145
    utility of, in nursing research and practice,
        144–146
liaison role in advocacy, 22
life expectancy
    of Native Americans, 513
    type 1 diabetes mellitus in, 420
life history methodology, 235–240
    autobiography, 236
    genogram, 237
    Jim (case study), 237–240
    methodology, 236–237
    oral history, 236
    overview, 235–236
    semi-structured interviews, 237
    support from loved ones, 239
    time lines, 237
    traditional ethnography, 236
lifestyle
    impact of self-management on, 421–422
    intervention strategies, 152
Likert-type scale, 121
LVIM. *See* Lakeland Volunteers in Medicine

M

"mail-order bride" industry, 383–384
majority groups, 56
maldistribution, 585–586
malnourishment, 485

malnutrition, risk for, 485
mammography adherence, 123
Marci Stidum, 480, 483, 484
marginalization
    distributive justice and, 59
    as factor in resource allocation, 6
    labeling and, 4
    as nursing research focus, 54
    of vulnerable populations, 5, 33, 35
marijuana use, 12
market justice, 51, 52
marriage and female genital cutting, 386–388
Martin, Jennifer, 484
"massage parlors," 454
maternal body mass index (BMI), 150
maternal mortality, 563, 564
maternal outcomes, 258
Matrix Method, 258
Maximizing Positive Synergies Collaborative Group, WHO,
    579
MDGs. *See* Millennium Development Goals
MealBux program, 490
Medicaid
    establishment of, 563
    as funding for Appalachian clinic, 362
    minimal services provided by, 53
    outcome of improved access to care, 564
    programs, 375, 393
Medical and Nursing Education Partnership
    Initiatives, 585
medical home model, 340*t*
Medical model, 510
Medicare
    drug benefit for, 5
    establishment of, 563
    as funding for Appalachian clinic, 362
    outcome of improved access to care, 564
    PPACA provisions, 565, 566*t*–567*t*
Medicare Current Beneficiary Survey, 537
Medicare Prescription Drug Improvement and
    Modernization Act of 2003 (MMA), 5, 543, 563
MEDRETE (planned medical readiness and training
    exercise), 306
mental health, 279*t*–280*t*
    of victims of sex traffickers, 555–556
    view of, in Appalachian communities, 362
mental health disorders
    background and significance, 461–462
    case study, 467–468
    environmental factors impacting vulnerability
        counseling services, 468
        health center providers, 468–469
        roommate compatibility, 470
        university housing, 469–470
        university policies related to accommodations
            for, 469

incarceration, management of, 372–373
mental health self-management, 471
nursing strategies to reduce risk, 471–474
personal factors impacting vulnerability
    academic competencies development, 466
    alcohol, tobacco, and drug use, 464–465
    lack of exercise, 464
    poor diet, 463–464
    self-management of, 465
    sleep disruption, 462–463
    social support structure alterations, 466–467
    stress management, 467
plan of action to promote optimum, 472–474
strategies to identify and stabilize, 471–472
mental health self-management, 471
mental health services, coordination of, 369
mental health treatment services, lack of, 367
mental illness, 486
    disabilities and, 482, 483
    and disabled persons, 7
    pre-incarceration stage, 367–368
Merriam-Webster Online Dictionary, 37
Mexico, 436–437
    by nurse practitioner students, 524
Meyers, Christine, 452–453, 459–460
middle-range concepts and theories, 117–118
    adherence, 121–123
    change, 123–126
    chronic care model (CCM), 133–134
    Health Promotion Model (HPM), 130–131
    individual-level middle-range theories, 118–121
    integrative, 128–130
    resilience, 131–133
    social middle-range theories, 126–128
Milgram Shock Experiment, 188
Milgram, Stanley, 187–188
Millennium Declaration, 574, 577
Millennium Development Goals (MDGs), 574, 575t–577t, 577–578
minimal health care, 53
minorities
    disparity of cultural groups, 6
    health disparity reduction and, 6
mission, navy nurses, 304
MMA of 2003. *See* Medicare Prescription Drug Improvement and Modernization Act of 2003
Model for Evidence-Based Practice Change, 256
modern nursing, evolution of, 509
modifiable life behaviors, 151
morbidity in adolescent vulnerability, 396, 396t
mortality in adolescent vulnerability, 396, 396t
mothers, as vulnerable population, 7
motivational approaches to substance abuse, 12
MTFs. *See* U.S. Military Treatment Facilities
multifinality, 431
myocardial tissue, 166

N
NAACP. *See* National Association for the Advancement of Colored People
NAEH. *See* National Alliance to End Homelessness
NASW. *See* National Association of Social Workers
national agenda, 538
National Alliance on Mental Illness, 462
National Alliance to End Homelessness (NAEH), 481
National Association for the Advancement of Colored People (NAACP), 367
National Association of Social Workers (NASW)
    Ad Hoc Committee on Advocacy, 25
    Code of Ethics, 25
    Task Force on Urban Crisis and Public Welfare Problems, 25
National Association of Student Financial Aid Administrators, 484
National Center for Health Statistics, 8
National Center for Human Genome Research Cancer Studies Consortium, 225
National College Health Assessment (NCHA), 462
National Commission for the Protection of Human Subjects of Biomedical and Behavior Research, 191
National Committee for Quality Assurance, 536–537
National Governors Association (NGA), 443
National Health Service, 13
National Human Trafficking Resource Center sponsored by Polaris Project, 500
National Institutes of Health (NIH), 6, 185, 244, 250, 545
National League for Nursing (NLN), 525, 526
National Research Act, 191
National Student Nurses Association (NSNA), 454
Native American Network for Health, 336
navy nurses, 303–309
    clinical competence, 304
    deployed to war (vignette), 305–306
    hospital mission (vignette), 307–309
    humanitarian mission (vignette), 306–307
    mission, 304
    overview, 303–304
    planned medical readiness and training exercise (MEDRETE), 306
    Reserve nurses, 304–305
Nazi human experiments, 185–186
NCHA. *See* National College Health Assessment
needle exchange programs, 542
negative/unsupportive parental behavior, 421
neoliberal policy, 288
neonatal mortality rates, 254
NGA. *See* National Governors Association
Nicaragua, nursing immersion programs in, 434–435
NIH. *See* National Institutes of Health
NLN. *See* National League for Nursing
noncompliance with medical instructions, 514
nonpharmacological pain management, 254–255
Not For Sale campaign awareness program, 450

NSNA. *See* National Student Nurses Association
Nuremberg Code, The, 190
nurse-client relationship, Leininger on, 144
nurse educator graduate student, role of, 523
nurse-managed wellness centers, 433–434
nurse-patient relationship, 325
nurse practitioner-run center in rural Appalachia, 357–364
    acceptance, 359
    access to services, 363
    barriers to care, 363
    being hardy, 358
    case study, 360
    center development, 360–364
    core values, 358–360
    demographic characteristics, 358
    family, 359
    Federally Qualified Health Center Look-Alike, 361
    funding, 362
    health promotion, 362–363
    mobile unit of, 363
    neighboring, 360
    obesity, 363
    operational plan, 361–362
    opportunities, 363–364
    outcomes, 362–363
    population characteristics, 358–360
    problem statement, 358
    social services incorporation, 362
    spirituality, 359
nurses
    intention for, 495
    resilience in, 40–41
    social justice and, 56
nursing
    global, 573
    holistic, 36
    navy nursing, 304–305
    opportunity, undocumented immigrants, 325–327
    pet therapy in, 311–319
nursing course, vulnerable populations, 480
nursing education articles, views of justice in, 53–54
nursing educator, 510
nursing interventions, 120
    with prisoners, incarceration, 373
nursing literature, definitional limitations in, 56–57
nursing practice articles, views of justice in, 55–56
nursing practice, family, 515
nursing research articles, views of justice in, 54–55
Nursing Research journal, 536, 544
nursing theories applied to vulnerable populations, 141–142
nursing workforce, underutilization of, 442–443

O
obesity
    in Appalachia, 363
    of Native Americans, 513

Office of Information Technology Services, 208
Office of Management and Budget (OMB), 545
Ojibwa, 511–512
Oman, women of. *See* women of Oman
Omani census data (2010), 263
OMB. *See* Office of Management and Budget
operating room (OR), 308
oral history, 236
Oregon State University's, 490
outmigration, 584–585

P
pain control, 295–296
pain management options in childbirth, 254–255
Pan American Sanitary Bureau, 185
pancreatic beta cell function, 151
PAR. *See* participatory action research
parenting, autistic children, 342, 352
parenting education, pre-incarceration, 369
participant observation and interviewing, 433
participatory action research (PAR), 245, 411
Passion Conference in Atlanta, 454
paternalism, advocacy and, 21
patient advocacy, 509
patient education, 259
Patient Protection and Affordable Care Act (ACA) of 2010,
    394, 442, 565, 566t–567t, 567–568
peer-reviewed literature, integrative analysis of, 255
pelvic inflammatory disease (PID), 502
Pennsylvania Department of Health, 363
PEPFAR, 578, 580, 585, 593
perceived barriers, 155–156
perceived benefits, 155
perceived severity, 155
perceived susceptibility, 154–155
Perception of Risk for BRCA1 and BRCA2 (National
    Center for Human Genome Research Cancer Studies
    Consortium), 225
perinatal health care of Somali women, transcultural aspects
    of, 287–289
    communication, 293–294
    death, pregnancy termination, and miscarriage,
        297–298
    disparities, 291–293
    frequently eaten food choices, 298–299
    health and illness, 290–291
    labor and delivery, 295
    pain control, 295–296
    postpartum care needs, 296–297
    prenatal care, 294–295
    Somalis in the United States, 289–290
personal mastery experiences, opportunities for, 120
personality, schizophrenia and, 11
Peru
    clean water project in, 435
    sex tourism in, 551

pet-human bond, historical accounts of, 312–313
pet therapy, in nursing, 311–319
    ADHD and, 313
    case scenarios, 314–316
    cerebral palsy and hippotherapy, 313–314
    implications for, 316–317
    uses of, 313–314
Peter Christensen Health Center Clinic (Wisconsin), 509, 511
Pets Evacuation and Transportation Standards Act, 312
Pew Charitable Trusts, 544
PHS. *See* U.S. Public Health Services
physical abuse, signs of, 496
physiological feedback, 120
PI. *See* Principal Investigator
PID. *See* pelvic inflammatory disease
Piper methysticum (kava), 326–327
planned medical readiness and training exercise
    (MEDRETE), 306
Polaris Project, 499
policy entrepreneurs, 542
policy process, 537–538
population-based programs, 329–338
    balancing efficiency with need and effectiveness,
        329–330
    brigadista (community health worker), 331
    business plans, 334–336
    capturing data, 333–334
    costs and budget, 335
    crowd funding, 336
    definition and role in seeking funding, 334
    design process, 332–334
    evaluation, 336
    feasibility study, 332–333
    focus of program, 330–332
    formal dinners, 335–336
    funding sources, 335–336
    gatekeepers, 331
    grants and contracts, 335
    grass-roots fundraising, 335–336
    mission, 332
    overview, 329
    participant observation, 333, 433
    problem statement, 330
    public campaigns, 335
    raffles, 335–336
    recruitment of team, 332
    stakeholders, 330–331
    values, 331
post-abortion sepsis, 503
post-incarceration
    adjustment, 374–377
    nursing interventions to reduce vulnerability, 377
post-traumatic stress disorder (PTSD), 505, 555
postdatism, 292
postpartum care needs, 296–297
postpartum, diet during, 299

postpartum practices, 299
potential victim, 498
poverty, 5, 344, 352
pranic healing, 327
pre- and post-tests, 494–495, 506
pre-incarceration
    community and school-based programs, 370
    ethnicity and age, 367
    family therapy, 369
    intervention at, 369–370
    mental health services coordination, 369
    mental illness, 367–368
    overview, 366–367
    parenting education, 369
    risk factors at, 367–369
    socioeconomic factors, 368–369
    substance abuse, 368
predisposition, genetic, 4
pregnancy
    co-morbidities, 271*t*–272*t*
    complications, 273*t*–276*t*, 503
    diet during, 299
pregnant immigrant women, 384–385
prenatal care, 7, 294–295, 564–565
Preparing for the Future of HIV/AIDS in Africa, 585
Prescott House, 337
Presidential Commission for the Study of Bioethical Issues,
    185
prevention, levels of, 223
primary care center, development of
    barriers to care, 363–364
    goals of, 361
    operational plan, 361–362
    outcomes, 362–363
    overview, 360–361
primary prevention, Health Belief Model (HBM), 223
Principal Investigator (PI), 237
priority populations, 562
prison health services, 371
prison population, vulnerability of, 365–366
prison system, nurses role in, 373
prisoners, pet therapy, 316
privilege, 57, 58
professional communication skills, 120
prostitution, legalizing, 550
protective factors and resilience, 37, 39
protocol variables, 258
psychiatric-mental health nursing simulation, 524–525
    case study, 528–530
    for vulnerable populations, 523–530
PTSD. *See* post-traumatic stress disorder
public campaigns, population-based programs, 335
public health concept of vulnerability, 4
public policy, 535–546
    advocacy in, 542
    agenda setting, 538, 541–542

public policy (*Cont.*)
    definitions, 535–537
    evaluation, 541, 544–545
    garbage can model of organizations, 537
    government response, 538–540, 542–543
    health disparities, 536
    implementation, 540–541, 544
    linking policy process and vulnerable populations,
        541–545
    policy communities, 538
    policy entrepreneurs, 542
    policy process, 537–538
    regulatory process, 540
    role of research in, 545
    special *vs.* vulnerable populations, 535–536
    therapeutic communications skills, 539
    uninsured, 537

Q

Quality and Safety Education for Nurses (QSEN), 526
quality of health care, 6, 569
quantitative sample research proposal (breast cancer),
    197–209
    abstract, 197–198
    Ashkenazi Jews, breast cancer in, 218, 221
    assumptions, 217–218
    background, 216–217
    BRCA1/2 genetic mutations, 216, 218
    budget, 227
    data analysis, 226
    definitions, 218–219
    demographic data, 226
    design, 224
    education methods for Latinas, 224
    ethnic group differences, 224
    feasibility and application, 220
    genetic counseling, 221
    genetic testing for BRCA1/2, 216
    health behavioral action, 222
    Health Belief Model (HBM), 217, 221–224
    health protection, 223
    instrumentation, 225
    limitations, 219
    literature review, 220–224
    methodology, 224–227
    methods, 204–209
    null hypothesis, 216
    procedures, 226–227
    rationale, 203
    research questions, 216
    sample, 224–225
    setting, 225
    significance, 199–202
    significance to Latinas, 219–220
    study overview, 198–199, 216–220
    theoretical framework, 217
    timeline, 227
    validity and reliability, 226
Quit Line (New York), 333

R

racism, effect of on African Americans, 34
raffles, population-based programs, 335–336
Rahab's Rope, 457
Rath Senior ConNEXTions and Education Center
    development strategy, 414
    journey through aging, 415
    model development, 416–417
    partnerships for sustainability, 415–416
    research activity, 412–414
    transitions and technology, 414–415
RCM. *See* Royal College of Midwives
RCOG. *See* Royal College of Obstetricians and
    Gynaecologists
red flag, 498
regulatory process, 540
rehabilitation for drug offenses, 376
rehabilitation programs, 377
reiki, 327
reintegration, in society, 375–376
"relational practice," 518
rescuing victims of human trafficking, 501, 502
research enablers (Leininger), 144
research with vulnerable populations, 183–193
    codes and principles, 190–191
    cross-cutting issues in international, 192–193
    historical background for, 184–190
    overview, 183–184
    public policy role in, 545
    range of conditions addressed, 9–10
resilience, 37–42
    adolescents, promotion of, 396–398, 399*t*–402*t*
    antecedents to, 38
    autistic children and, 342–352
    body image dissatisfaction and, 39
    case study of Mr. Hernandez, 41–42
    in children, 38–39
    cultural competence and, 33–42
    defined, 37
    in families, 39
    importance of, 432
    in nurses, 40–41
    in older adults, 39–40
    overview, 37–38
    spiritual needs and, 40
    in survivors of disasters, 40
    vulnerability and, 342–344
    in women, 39
resource availability, 6, 12
right to healthcare, 53
Robert Wood Johnson Foundation, 544
round table programs, 416

Royal College of Midwives (RCM), 256
Royal College of Obstetricians and Gynaecologists (RCOG), 256
rural communities
    cultural risk in, 345
    lack of healthcare services in, 537
    poverty in, 344, 352

S

San Antonio Contraceptive study, 188–189
Saranac trail initiative, 332
saturation of data, 249
schedules, for optimum mental health, 472–473
SCHIP. *See* State Children's Health Insurance Program
schizophrenia, biological view of, 10–11
school-based programs, pre-incarceration, 370
schools, support children with ASD, 345
Seattle University College of Nursing (SUCN), 436
Seattle University Model, 436
secondary prevention, Health Belief Model (HBM), 223
sedentary lifestyles, 150
seizure disorder, 350–351
self-advocacy, 542
self-awareness, 36, 431, 437, 438
self-care behavior, 121
self-efficacy theory, 118–120, 125, 126, 154, 156
    of diabetes management, 121
    immigrants, 382
    sources, 119–120
self-esteem, 501
Self-hypnosis for Complete Relaxation, 474
self-identity, immigrants, 382
self-management of mental health disorder, 465, 471
settlement house movement, 24
sex offenders, 550–551
sex slavery, 551
sex tourism and trafficking, 485, 493–508, 549–559
    attitudes of, 497
    "bricherismo," 551
    clinical reports, 552–555
    defined, 550
    HIV/AIDS and STDs, 555
    Honors Capstone Project, 494–506
    intervention, 556
    legalizing prostitution, 550
    mental health issues, 555–556
    original fieldwork, 552
    overview, 549–550
    policy implications, 556–558
    post-traumatic stress disorder (PTSD), 555
    samfie man, 550
    sex offenders, 550–551
    sex tourism, 551
    sex trafficking, 551–552
    "staged authenticity," 551
    victims of, 495, 497–506

Sex Trafficking: A Clinical Guide for Nurses (de Chesnay), 451
sexual abuse, 8
Sexual Transmissible Diseases Inoculation Studies in Guatemala, The (1946–1948), 185
sexually transmitted infections (STIs), 366, 502
shared decision-making, 382
Sheppard-Towner Act of 1921, 563
simulations, 524–526
    community health nursing simulation, 525–526
    psychiatric-mental health nursing simulation, 524–525
situational factors, in depression, 10
Six Sigma concepts, 330
sleep deprivation, 463
sleep disorders in autism, 347–348
sleep disruption, 462–463
smart phone applications, for mental health disorder, 472
smoke-free policies, implementation of, 330
smoking, schizophrenia and, 10
social capital, adolescents, 393
social cognitive theory, 119
"social health survey," 189
social impairment, 343
social injustice, 56
social justice in nursing, 49–60
    advocacy and, 20, 25
    alternative views of, 57–58
    awareness, amelioration, and transformation, 58–59
    championing, 20
    contractual justice, 54
    costs and, 6
    critique, 57
    cultural competence and, 34
    defining justice in nursing, 50–51
    definitional limitations in literature, 56–57
    distribution of wealth and, 56
    distributive justice, 51–53, 59
    education articles, views, 53–54
    ethics and, 50
    literature search methodology, 50–51
    majority groups and, 56
    market justice, 51–53
    overview, 49–50
    points of intervention for, 58
    practice articles' views, 55–56
    research articles' views, 54–55
    social justice, 51–53
    view of vulnerable persons, 6, 57
social middle-range theories, 126–128
social network, ex-prisoners, 376
social-psychological work of Lewin, 222
Social Security Act
    Title XVIII, 563
    Title XIX, 563
social services, incorporation of, 362
social status, adolescents, 391–393

social support systems, 126–127
    structure alterations in, 466–467
social work advocacy, 24–25
Social Work Dictionary, 23
Somali community, 296
Somali culture, 292
Somali immigrants, 287, 289, 295
Somali refugees, 289
Somalis in United States, 289–290
South Africa, nurse retention in, 587
spiritual grounding, 39
spirituality
    in Appalachia, 359
    in elderly, 40
    of Native Americans, 513
spree killings, 13, 14
SPs. *See* standardized patients
SPSS software. *See* Statistical Package for the Social Sciences
    software
staff education, 259
"staged authenticity," 551
stakeholders
    policy makers as, 251
    population-based programs, 330–331
standard educational approaches, 221
standardized patients (SPs), 525
State Children's Health Insurance Program (SCHIP), 563
State University of New York (SUNY), 336
Statistical Package for the Social Sciences (SPSS) software,
    412
stereotyping, 4, 35
Stewart B. McKinney Act of 1987, 544
stigma, 201, 202
STIs. *See* sexually transmitted infections
strengths, building on in CBPR, 246–247
stress, 484
stress management, 467
stress reduction mobile apps, 474
stress reduction techniques, 474
structural variables, 158
structured brainstorming and teamwork, 256
students
    depression and, 10
    familial types and alcoholism, 13
    violence and alcohol use in college, 13
    as vulnerable population, 13–14
Study of Untreated Syphilis in Negro Males in Tuskegee,
    Alabama (1932-1972), 184–185
substance abuse, 483, 485
    in African American children, 12
    motivational approaches to, 12
    pre-incarceration, 368
    violence and alcohol abuse in college students,
        13–14
    vulnerability to, 12–13
SUCN. *See* Seattle University College of Nursing

suicide
    by college students, 13
    vulnerability to, 7
summative data, 541
sunrise model (Leininger), 142–145
SUNY. *See* State University of New York
Supplemental Security Income (SSI) program, 563
survivors of disasters, resilience in, 40
susceptibility to health problems, 4
sustainability, Rath Senior ConNEXTions and Education
    Centerm partnerships for, 415–416
symptom management strategies, 170
system context view of vulnerability, 6
system monitoring, 23

T
Task Force on Health Systems Research, 582
teaching nurses about vulnerable populations, 429–438
    chart audit system, 434
    cost-effective care, 431
    CPR programs, 434
    cultural competence overview, 430–431
    Duquesne Model, 433–436
    ethnocentric bias, 430
    garden communities, 436
    hermanamiento (sister school relationship), 435
    Kennesaw State University Model, 436–437
    key components of educational experience, 437–438
    models of experiential learning, 433–437
    multifinality, 431
    nurse-managed wellness centers, 433–434
    online doctoral program, 435–436
    participant observation and interviewing, 433
    Seattle University Model, 436
    self-awareness, 431, 437, 438
Tearoom Trade Study, 189
terrorism
    in schools, 13
    September 11 attacks, 538
tertiary prevention, Health Belief Model (HBM), 223
Thailand, 587
Thalidomide tragedy, 187
The Kenya Nursing Workforce Project: The Status of
    Nursing in Kenya 2012, 593
Theory of Reasoned Action, 398
Theory of Self-Regulation (SRT), 166
time lines, 237
time management, 466
TIP. *See* Trafficking in Persons
Title X Family Planning Programs, 393
tobacco-free worksite policies, development of, 330
tobacco, use of, 464–465
traditional nomadic pastoralism, 288
trafficked children, community action by undergraduate
    students, 449–460
Trafficking in Persons (TIP), 556

Trafficking Victims Protection Reauthorization Act, 556
transformation, social justice and, 58–59
translational research, 248
translators, 307
Transtheoretical Model of Change (TTM), 123, 124
    central constructs of, 124–125
Treasury Department, 540
treatment-seeking behavior, 173
treatment seeking delay (TSD), 166
troubleshooting, 22–23
TSD. *See* treatment seeking delay
TTM. *See* Transtheoretical Model of Change
Tuberculosis and Malaria (Global Fund), 580
Tuskegee Institute, 184
"Tuskegee Study of Untreated Syphilis in the Negro Male," 184
type 1 diabetes mellitus (T1DM)
    complications, 420
    developmental stage of adolescence, 421
    disease management, 420–421
    internalized problems, 423
    overview, 419–420
    patient adherence to treatment protocols, 420
    psychological problems, 423
    treatment complexities, 424
type 2 diabetes mellitus (T2DM), 485
    risk of, 149–152

U

undocumented immigrants, 321–327
    Grace, 324–325
    Lester, 324
    Maria/Hector, 324
    nursing opportunity, 325–327
    overview, 321–322
    Roberto, 323
    Talia, 322
    treatments, 326–327
unethical clinical medical studies, 184
UNICEF, 297
United Kingdom, outmigration to, 585
United Nation Population Fund, 385
United Nations Children's Fund report card, 563
United Nations (UN) intervention in Somalia, 288
United States
    health status in, 441–442
    obstetrical culture in, 256
    outmigration to, 585
    political climate in, 255
    prisoner population, 365–366
    Somalis in, 289–290
    trafficking victims in, 496
    type 1 diabetes mellitus in, 419–420
    unaffordable health care in, 482
    women in, 254
Universidad Politecnica de Nicaragua (UPOLI), 434, 435

university housing, 469–470
University of Washington, 37
UPOLI. *See* Universidad Politecnica de Nicaragua
U.S. adolescents
    health indicators among, 396, 396*t*
    risky behaviors among, 394, 394*t*–395*t*
U.S. army, waterbirth protocol in, 257–259
U.S. Department of Housing and Urban Development (HUD), 481, 483
U.S. Food and Drug Administration (FDA), 187
U.S. Military Treatment Facilities (MTFs), 256, 259
"US/PHS STD Inoculations Studies in Guatemala," 185
U.S. Public Health Services (PHS), 184
"US/Tuskegee/Alabama Study," 185
U.S. Venereal Disease Research Laboratory (VDRL), 185
USNS Comfort, 304, 306
USSR, 288

V

VDRL. *See* U.S. Venereal Disease Research Laboratory
verbal persuasion, 120
vicarious experience, 119–120
victims
    of domestic violence, 483
    potential, 498
    of sex trafficking, 495, 497–506
    treatment of, 494
video-based educational intervention on knowledge, 220
video education program, 224
violence, 5, 13, 14
Violence Risk Assessment tool, 13
Visiting Nurse Association, 433
vulnerability, 3–14
    Aday's framework of, 6
    aggregate *vs.* individual, 3
    blaming the victim, 5
    caregiver, 10
    in childbirth, 253–254
        evidence-based approach to practice change, 256–257
        pain management options in childbirth, 254–255
        positions of professional organizations on waterbirth, 255–256
        waterbirth protocol in U.S. army, 257–259
    in community-based participatory research, 250–251
    concepts and theories, 6
    contextual, 4
    cost issues in, 6
    defined, 4, 144, 536, 537
    to depression, 10
    disparities in health, 6–9
    to eating disorders, 11
    ecological approach to, 6
    emic *vs.* etic approaches, 6
    of ethnic minorities, 5
    in families, 8

vulnerability (*Cont.*)
    health insurance and, 5
    to HIV/AIDS, 11–12
    of impoverished to health problems, 5
    infants and, 6
    Institute of Medicine study, 9–14
    labeling process and, 4, 14
    linking policy process to, 541–545
    marginalization and, 5, 6, 33, 35, 54, 59
    as nursing research focus, 54–55
    of populations, 5
    public health concept of, 4, 14
    resilience and, 342–344
    resource availability and, 6
    to schizophrenia, 10–11
    social justice view of, 5, 57
    to specific conditions or diseases, 9–10
    stereotyping, 4, 35
    of students, 13–14
    to substance abuse, 12–13
    "susceptibility" and, 4
    WHO's dimensions of health, 6
vulnerable populations
    adherence, 122
    caring for, 441–444, 445*t*–446*t*
    change, 125
    chronic care model (CCM), 133
    DNP translational research, 444, 445*t*–446*t*
    health promotion, 130
    individual-level middle-range theories, 120
    integrative middle-range concepts and theories, 129
    resilience, 132
    social middle-range theories, 127
    teaching nurses about, 429–438. See also teaching
        nurses about vulnerable populations

W

Wachniak, Lana, 489
water labor, 254
waterbirth, 254, 255
    positions of professional organizations on, 255–256
    protocol in U.S. army, 257–259
Watson's theory of human caring, 35

wealth, theory of inequality of distribution of, 5, 56
websites for animal-assisted therapy, 318–319
wellness and ecological perspective in CBPR, 249
wellness centers, 433–434
WellStar School of Nursing, 436
White Americans, inappropriately used for comparison, 56
WHO. *See* World Health Organization
WIC program. *See* Women, Infants, and Children program
Willowbrook hepatitis study, 188
Wisconsin Department of Health and Family Services, 513
WMA. *See* World Medical Association
women
    Asian survivors of sexual abuse, 39
    domestic violence and, 7
    to eating disorders, 11
    exclusion from clinical trials, 244
    health and social issues of, 9
    maternal mortality, U.S., 563, 564
    mothers as vulnerable population, 7
    resilience in, 39
    specific vulnerability issues of, 9
Women, Infants, and Children (WIC) program, 126, 516
women of Oman, 263–264
    methodology, 264–265
    purpose, 264
    results, 265–266
workforce density, 583, 583*f*
workforce development, 570
World Bank, 288
World Health Assembly (63rd), 586
World Health Organization (WHO), 6, 149–150, 580*f*
    definition of health systems, 579
    dimensions of health and, 6
    Framework for Action, 579
    on health research, 582
    Health Systems: Improving Performance, 579
    on HRH maldistribution, 586
    Maximizing Positive Synergies Collaborative Group,
        579
World Medical Association (WMA), 191

Y

YouTube, 474